Modern System of Ophthalmology (MSO) Series

Neuro-Ophthalmology

Modern System of Ophthalmology (MSO) Series

Neuro-Ophthalmology

Editor-in-Chief

AK Khurana MS, CTO (London), FAICO
Fellow, Moorfields Eye Hospital, London
Senior Professor and Head
Regional Institute of Ophthalmology
Pt BD Sharma Postgraduate Institute of Medical Sciences
Rohtak, Haryana

Editors

Rashmin A Gandhi DNB, FRCS
Managing Director, Beyond Eye Care and
Visiting Consultant
Center for Sight
Hyderabad

Aruj K Khurana DNB
Consultant Ophthalmologist
Cataract and Medical Retina Services
Nirmal Eye Institute
Rishikesh (UK)

Associate Editors

Devendra Venkatramani DNB, FRCS, FICO
Fellow, LVPEI, Hyderabad
Consultant Vitreo-retinal Surgeon
Laxmi Eye Institute
Panvel

Bhawna Khurana MS, DNB, FICO
Department of Ophthalmology
All India Institute of Medical Sciences (AIIMS)
Rishikesh (UK)

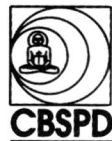

CBSPD

CBS Publishers & Distributors Pvt Ltd

New Delhi • Bengaluru • Chennai • Kochi • Kolkata • Lucknow • Mumbai
Gujarat • Hyderabad • Jharkhand • Nagpur • Patna • Pune • Uttarakhand

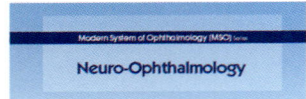

ISBN: 978-81-239-2446-5

Copyright © AK Khurana

First Edition 2014
Reprint: 2019, **2026**

Published by Satish Kumar Jain and produced by Varun Jain for

CBS Publishers & Distributors Pvt Ltd

4819/XI Prahlad Street, 24 Ansari Road, Daryaganj, New Delhi 110 002, India
Ph: 011-23289259, 23266838   Website: www.cbspd.com   e-mail: delhi@cbspd.com

Corporate Office: 204 FIE, Industrial Area, Patparganj, Delhi 110 092, India
Ph: 011-49344934   Fax: 011-49344935
e-mail: publishing@cbspd.com; publicity@cbspd.com

Branches

- Bengaluru: Seema House 2975, 17th Cross, KR Road, Banasankari 2nd Stage, Bengaluru 560 070, Karnataka, India
  Ph: +91-80-26771678/79   Fax: +91-80-26771680   e-mail: bangalore@cbspd.com
- Chennai: No.18/8B, Subbarayan Street, Shenoy Nagar, Chennai 600 030, Tamil Nadu, India
  Ph: +91-44-42032115, 26681266   e-mail: chennai@cbspd.com
- Kochi: 42/1325, 1326, Power House Road, Opposite KSEB, Power House, Ernakulam 682018, Kochi, Kerala, India
  Ph: +91-484-4059061–67   Fax: +91-484-4059065   e-mail: kochi@cbspd.com
- Kolkata: 147, Hind Ceramics Compound, 1st Floor, Nilgunj Road, Belghoria, Kolkata 700056, West Bengal, India
  Ph: +91-33-25330055/56   e-mail: kolkata@cbspd.com
- Lucknow: Basement, Khushuma Complex, 7 Meerabai Marg (behind Jawahar Bhawan), Lucknow 226001, UP, India
  Ph: +91-522-4000032   e-mail: tiwari.lucknow@cbspd.com
- Mumbai: PWD Shed, Gala No. 25/26, Ramchandra Bhatt Marg, Next JJ Hospital Gate No. 2, Opp. Union Bank of India, Noorbaug, Mumbai 400009, Maharashtra, India
  Ph: +91-22-66661880/89   e-mail: mumbai@cbspd.com

Representatives

• Gujarat	0-9879558667	• Hyderabad	0-9885175004	• Jharkhand	0-9811541605
• Nagpur	0-8692091830	• Patna	0-9334159340	• Pune	0-9664372571
• Uttarakhand	0-9716462459				

Printed at Nutech Print Services, Faridabad, Haryana, India

to
the Teachers and Residents in Ophthalmology for
their endeavor to dissipate and acquire knowledge
to our Parents and Teachers for their blessings
to our Families for their understanding and encouragement
to our Patients for letting us learn

Foreword

Neuro-Ophthalmology has gained importance in the last two decades as most of the neurological disorders are reflected in the eye. It is a complex specialty wherein specially trained ophthalmologists with the help of integrated findings of gadgets like ultrasound, UBM, and mainly neuro-imaging techniques like MRI and CT scans come to a diagnosis and management.

It is indeed a pleasure for me to write the foreword to *Neuro-Ophthalmology* one of the eleven books in the series *Modern System of Ophthalmology* by Dr AK Khurana (Editor-in-Chief). A concise and comprehensive series like this was much needed for the residents in ophthalmology.

This book on neuro-ophthalmology gives a total picture of the complex neuro-ophthalmic disorders which will be useful for the practitioners as well as residents in ophthalmology.

The volume has good chapters with updated references and the reader will find a greater clarity in the subject. I appreciate the efforts of the editorial team in this regard for presenting a complete and up-to-date text in a very systematic manner with the help of abundant high quality photographs, line diagrams, visual field charts, and neuro-imaging scans.

I am sure this book will be a boon to all students, teachers and practitioners. I wish and congratulate the author for all success in publishing this wonderful book.

TS Surendran
Vice Chairman and Director of
Pediatric Ophthalmology
Sankara Nethralaya, Chennai
President, Strabismus and Pediatric
Ophthalmological Society of India

Preface

*M*odern System of Ophthalmology (MSO) series comprises separate volumes on different subspecialities of ophthalmology. Each volume is planned with a very specific aim to cater to the needs of postgraduate students in ophthalmology.

Salient Features of MSO Series

- Each volume is edited by different editors, yet the layout and organization has been kept similar for all the volumes.
- Editors of different volumes are masters in their subspeciality with an uncanny knack of picking up the right perspectives.
- Text matter is designed to meet the needs of residents in ophthalmology with a comprehensive coverage in a concise manner. Text is complete and up-to-date with recent advances incorporated.
- Text is organized in such a way that the students can easily understand, retain and reproduce it. Various levels of headings, subheadings, bold face and italics given in the text will be helpful for a quick revision of the subject.

Neuro-Ophthalmology, though an interesting and fascinating subject, has always been an untouchable entity for most of the residents and practising ophthalmologists because of intricate neurological pathway and neuro-ophthalmic lesions with their complex pathophysiology. An effort has been made in this book to present the text as a readable compendium in a more easily understood form. In a bid to simplify the text, at places the description looks more dogmatic than is warranted by the facts. To keep the book a basic text, advanced description of many lesions has not been included.

The text has been arranged in eight sections. *Section I* on Clinico-investigative Neuro-ophthalmology includes chapters on examination and essential investigations required for a neuro-ophthalmic case. *Sections II to IV* are devoted to Anatomy, Physiology and various Disorders of Pupil, Visual Pathway and Optic Nerve, respectively. *Section V* includes various Symptomatic Disturbances of Vision. *Sections VI to VIII* cover comprehensively the Ocular Manifestations of Diseases of Central Nervous System, Ocular Motor System, and Neurological Disorders of Eyelids, Face, Orbital Syndromes and Headache, respectively.

Editor of this volume Dr Rashmin A Gandhi, Visiting Consultant, Centre for Sight, Hyderabad, is an internationally renowned faculty on neuro-ophthalmology. Second Editor, Dr Aruj K Khurana, Consultant at Nirmal Eye Institute, Rishikesh and the Associate Editor, Dr Devendra Venkatramani are dedicated disciples of Dr Rashmin A Gandhi from Sankara Nethralaya, Chennai. Second Associate Editor, Dr Bhawna Khurana, trained at Guru Nanak Eye Centre, New Delhi, is presently at AIIMS, Rishikesh. This volume is an outcome of dedicated team work.

Compilation of this volume has been made possible due to the chapters received from many selfless contributors. My sincere thanks are due to all of them. I want to express my gratitude to Prof CS Dhull, Director, PGIMS, and Prof SS Sangwan, Vice-Chancellor, UHS, Rohtak, for providing an atmosphere conducive to such academic activities. I shall also like to thank Dr MPS Sachdev, Chairman, Center for Sight Centers, for providing an excellent academic atmosphere and encouraging Dr Rashmin A Gandhi. My gratitude is also due to Dr DP Kar, Medical Director, Nirmal Eye Institute, Rishikesh, for encouraging Dr Aruj K Khurana from his center for academic activities.

The affection and moral support, in addition to editorial help, rendered by my daughter Dr Arushi, MD, University of Connecticut, USA, and my wife Dr Indu Khurana, Senior Professor, Department of Physiology, PGIMS, Rohtak made my task untiring. My special thanks are due to dear friends, Prof RV Azad, Prof PS Sandhu, Prof Amod Gupta, Prof Sunandan Sood, Prof GS Bajwa, Prof Atul Kumar, Prof VP Gupta, Prof BP Guliani, Prof MR Dogra, Prof Jagat Ram, Prof SM Bhati, Prof KP Chaudhri, Prof TS Surendran, Prof Kamlesh and Prof Subhash Dadeya for their guidance and encouragement. I acknowledge with humble thanks, the respect, affection and cooperation received from faculty members of RIO, PGIMS, Rohtak, namely Dr SV Singh, Dr JP Chugh, Dr VK Dhull, Dr RS Chauhan, Dr Manisha Rathi, Dr Neebha Passi, Dr Manisha Nada, Dr Urmil Chawla, Dr Ashok Rathi, Dr Sumit Sachdeva, Dr Jitender Phogat and Dr Reena Gupta. I also acknowledge the help received from Jr. Residents, RIO, especially Dr Vipul Gupta and Dr Sujay Chauhan.

The enthusiastic cooperation received from Mr SK Jain, Managing Director, Mr YN Arjuna, Senior Director—Publishing, Editorial and Publicity, and Mrs Ritu Chawla, Manager—Production, CBS Publishers & Distributors, New Delhi, needs special acknowledgement. Mr Sanju, graphic artist, and Mr Tarun, DTP operator, need special mention because of their efforts to provide considerable beauty to this volume.

In spite of the best efforts, a venture like this is unlikely to be error-free. Constructive criticism and suggestions from the readers are invited for further improvements in this volume.

AK Khurana
Editor-in-Chief

Editorial Board and Contributors

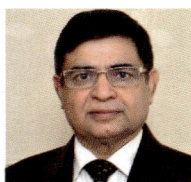
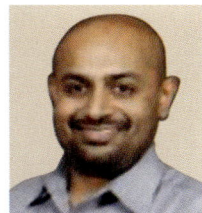
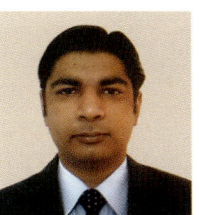
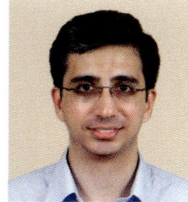
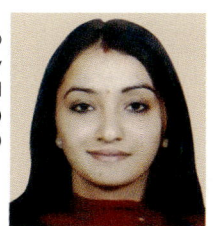

List of Contributors

Akshay Gopinathan Nair
LV Prasad Eye Institute, Road No. 2
Banjara Hills, Hyderabad 500 034
akshaygn@gmail.com

Amit Gupta
LV Prasad Eye Institute, Road No. 2
Banjara Hills, Hyderabad 500 034
amitg.dr@gmail.com

Ankita Phogat
Senior Resident, RIO
PGIMS, Rohtak

Ashwin Mohan
Sankara Nethralaya (Medical Research
Foundation), College Road
Nungambakkam
Chennai 600 006
drashwinm@gmail.com

Chekitan Singh DNB
Consultant, Ishwar Eye Institute, Rohtak

Indu Khurana MD
Senior Professor
Physiology, PGIMS, Rohtak

Mahesh Kumar
Aravind Eye Hospital, 1, Anna Nagar
Madurai 625 020, Tamil Nadu
neuro@aravind.org

Mayav J Movdawalla
mayavjm@gmail.com
Sankara Nethralaya (Medical Research
Foundation), College Road
Nungambakkam, Chennai 600 006

Neebha Passi MS
Professor
RIO, PGIMS, Rohtak

Neha D Shrirao
Sankara Nethralaya (Medical Research
Foundation), College Road
Nungambakkam, Chennai 600 006

Nikhil Choudhari
LV Prasad Eye Institute, Road No. 2
Banjara Hills, Hyderabad 500 034
nkl164@gmail.com

Ramesh Kekunnaya
LV Prasad Eye Institute, Road No. 2
Banjara Hills, Hyderabad 500 034
rameshak@lvpei.org

Reena Gupta MS
Asst Professor
RIO, PGIMS, Rohtak

Rohit Saxena
All India Institute of Medical Sciences
Ansari Nagar, New Delhi 110 029
rohitsaxena80@yahoo.com

Shikha Bassi
Sankara Nethralaya
(Medical Research Foundation), College
Road, Nungambakkam, Chennai 600 006
drsrb@snmail.org

Swati Phuljhele
All India Institute of Medical Sciences
Ansari Nagar, New Delhi 110 029

Urmil Chawla MS, DNB
Professor
RIO, PGIMS, Rohtak

Vijay Ananth
Sankara Nethralaya (Medical Research
Foundation), College Road
Nungambakkam, Chennai 600 006
vijaymedic@gmail.com

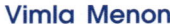

Vimla Menon
All India Institute of Medical Sciences
Ansari Nagar
New Delhi 110 029
vimalamenonj@yahoo.com

Virendra Sachdeva
LV Prasad Eye Institute, GMR Varalakshmi
Campus, 11-113/1, Hanumanthawaka
Junction Visakhapatnam 530 040
Andhra Pradesh
vsachdeva@lvpei.org

Contents

SECTION I: CLINICO-INVESTIGATIVE NEURO-OPHTHALMOLOGY

SECTION II: PUPIL AND ITS DISORDERS

SECTION III: VISUAL PATHWAYS

SECTION IV: OPTIC NERVE

SECTION V: SYMPTOMATIC DISTURBANCES OF VISION

SECTION VI: OCULAR MANIFESTATIONS OF DISEASES OF CENTRAL NERVOUS SYSTEM

SECTION VII: OCULAR MOTOR SYSTEM

SECTION VIII: NEUROLOGICAL DISORDERS OF EYELIDS, FACE, ORBITAL SYNDROMES, AND HEADACHE

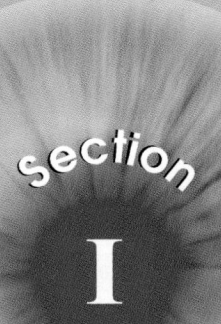

Section

I

Clinico-investigative Neuro-ophthalmology

1 EXAMINATION OF A NEURO-OPHTHALMIC CASE

Neha D Shrirao, Rashmin A Gandhi,
Reena Gupta, Chekitan, AK Khurana

INTRODUCTION

Examination of a neuro-ophthalmic case basically includes a thorough ocular, neurological and systemic clinical work-up and investigations including neuro-imaging to reach up at the proper diagnosis.

- *Visual loss,* i.e. either transient visual loss or visual impairment due to lesions of visual pathway and or cortical centers and psychosomatic condition.
- *Diplopia,* primarily because of palsies of cranial nerves supplying various extraocular muscles.
- *Visual field defects* due to various lesions of visual pathway.
- *Deranged higher visual functions* in the form of visual-hallucinations, illusions and agnosia.
- *Papilledema* is an important neuro-ophthalmic manifestation.
- *Anomalous pupillary reflexes* make up essential clues in a neuro-ophthalmic case.

In this text examination of a neuro-ophthalmic case is discussed as:
- Clinical investigative approach to a patient with visual loss, and
- Clinico-investigative approach for a patient with diplopia.

CLINICO-INVESTIGATIVE APPROACH TO A PATIENT WITH VISAUL LOSS

Visual loss can be broadly classified into
- Transient visual loss, and
- Visual impairment.

TRANSIENT VISUAL LOSS

Transient loss or blurring of vision in one or both eyes is not an uncommon visual complaint. The approach to such a patient is complicated by challenging differential diagnosis and overlapping disease profiles. It is an important sign of cerebrovascular diseases in some patients and thus warrants a systematic approach in examining, investigating and treating such patients.

TERMINOLOGY

Transient visual obscuration (TVO), i.e. fleeting loss of vision lasting just a few seconds

Monocular transient visual loss includes:
- *Amaurosis Fugax,* i.e. partial or total (rare) monocular blindness lasting a few seconds to minutes.
- *Transient monocular blindness* refers to more prolonged (30 minutes to hours to days) episodes of partial or total loss of monocular vision.

Binocular transient visual loss includes episodes of bilateral loss of vision lasting from 5–30 minutes and occasionally longer, involving either homonymous field, inferior or superior altitudinal fields or the central fields.

CAUSES OF TRANSIENT VISUAL LOSS (TVL)

1. Non-ischemic causes of TVL

- *Ocular surface disorders* such as dry eye, blepharitis (anterior or posterior) and recurrent corneal erosions.
- *Corneal endothelial disorders* such as dystrophies and decompensation
- *Intermittent angle closure*
- *Uveitis*
- *Vitreous floaters*
- *Optic disc disorders* such as papilledema, papillitis, drusen and colobomas.

2. Ischemic causes of TVL

i. *Embolic diseases*
- Carotid embolic diseases, e.g. atheromas and obstruction.
- Cardiac embolic diseases, e.g. valvular—rheumatic, prosthetic valves, fibrillation and myxomas.
- Great vessels embolic diseases, e.g. aortic arch embolus

ii. *Vasculitis*
- Giant cell arteritis

iii. *Hypoperfusion* as seen in:
- Carotid obstruction
- Vertebrobasilar insufficiency
- Ocular ischemic syndrome

iv. *Vasospasm,* e.g. migraine

v. *Hyperviscosity,* e.g. polycythemia
vi. *Hypercoagulability*

APPROACH TO A PATIENT WITH TRANSIENT VISUAL LOSS

1. History

A meticulous history is very important. It should include:

i. *Age:* In less than 50 years of age vasospasm and migraine are the commonest causes of TVL and in more than 50 years of age carotid embolic disease is a common cause.

ii. *Associated medical conditions:* To be enquired include hypertension, diabetes, coronary artery diseases and Raynaud's phenomenon.

Features of TVL:
- Monocular or Binocular TVL
- Duration of visual loss
- Number of episodes of visual loss
- Pattern of visual loss and recovery should be noted:
  – Shade or curtain coming down and then lifting is typical of amaurosis fugax due to carotid disease.
  – Positive visual phenomenon, e.g. scintillating scotomas in migraine.
  – Transient blurring of vision with exercise and increased body temperature is typical of *Uhthoff* phenomenon seen in optic neuritis associated with multiple sclerosis.
  – Abrupt change in vision may be associated with posterior circulation ischemia.

iii. *Associated symptoms:* To be noted include headaches, weight loss, fever, scalp tenderness, loss of consciousness, diplopia, dizziness, dysarthria and focal weakness.

2. Examination and investigations in a patient with transient visual loss

In a patient with monocular visual loss
Examination tests include:
- Visual acuity
- Ocular motility in cardinal positions of gaze
- Orbital examination for proptosis. Gaze evoked blurring of vision is reported in intraconal mass lesions.
- Pupillary evaluation for RAPD, and anisocoria
- Slit lamp biomicroscopy for lids, lashes, cornea, anterior chamber (cells, flare), cataract and anterior chamber angle depth

- Applanation tonometry
- Gonioscopy to note open, closed or occludable angles
- *Fundus examination* for evalution of optic disc, retinal vessel calibre, emboli, and signs of ischemia (hemorrhages, cotton wool spots)
- *Auscultation* of carotids for bruit and cardiac murmurs
- Palpation of temporal artery
- *Pulse rate* and *blood pressure* recording

Investigations should include:
- Complete hemogram
- Erythrocyte sedimentation rate (ESR)
- C-reactive protein (CRP)
- Coagulation profile
- Lipidogram
- Serum glucose levels
- Carotid Doppler
- Magnetic resonance imaging (MRI)
- Magnetic resonance angiography (MRA)
- Carotid angiography—Gold standard for the assessment of carotid stenosis
- Echocardiography
- ECG, Holter monitoring

CLINICAL ENTITIES ASSOCIATED WITH TVL
Non-ischemic transient visual loss

- *Ocular surface diseases and corneal abnormalities* are one of the commonest causes of non-ischemic TVL. Patients usually complain of transient visual obscurations of vision at specific times of the day, many times a week and more so in certain seasons. Slit lamp exam reveals abnormal tear break up time, anterior or posterior blepharitis. Patients usually respond well to warm compresses, anti-inflammatory and antibiotic therapy of short duration supplemented with tear substitutes.
- Patients with *corneal endothelial diseases and dystrophies* report episodes of blurring of vision lasting many hours usually more pronounced in the mornings. Slit lamp exam, pachymetry and specular count are diagnostic. Hyperosmotic drops, ointments and IOP lowering drugs help in symptomatic relief. Lamellar or full thickness corneal transplants can completely cure symptoms.
- *Intermittent angle closure* is an important cause of episodes of TVL. Patients usually complain of episodes of transient blurring of vision accompanied by ocular discomfort, seeing colored haloes and mild headaches. Slit lamp exam to grade AC depth along with gonioscopy show occludable angles and help clinch the diagnosis. Symptoms are completely relieved by YAG peripheral iridotomy.
- *Papilledema and optic disc drusen* can be associated with episodes of transient visual obscurations or episodes of gray, black or white vision. The episodes are usually associated with changes in posture. The likely etiology for TVL in these cases is axonal compression/stasis at the elevated optic nerve head.
- *Papillitis/optic neuritis* is associated with TVS similar to cases of papilledema. The likely etiology is demyelination and inflammation of the optic nerve.

Ischemic transient visual loss

Characteristic of transient visual loss are:
- Ischemic transient visual loss occurs due to temporary interruption of the blood supply to the retina, optic nerve or retrochiasmal visual pathways in the brain.
- Patients tend to be more specific, descriptive and discrete about the pattern of visual loss and recovery—onset, duration, number of episodes, central or peripheral field involvement.

Carotid artery stenosis or occlusion is the commonest cause of ischemic TVL. Atherosclerosis is the commonest cause but other causes like Takayasu arteritis, trauma, radiation arteritis and carotid dissection should be kept in mind. Carotid related amaurosis fugax results either from emboli originating from the diseased proximal internal carotid segment to the retinal arterial circulation or from decreased blood flow to the retina. The typical features of embolic monocular TVL are sudden onset, painless, described as a shade or a curatin coming down on the field of vision which lifts and vision clears in 1–5 minutes (sometimes up to 30 minutes).

Emboli that cause TVL can often be visualized with an ophthalmoscope or slit lamp fundus biomicroscopy (78 D, 90 D lens) and often appear distinctive, their probable site of origin can be inferred which becomes crucial directing appropriate patient evaluation.

- *Cholesterol emboli (Hollenhorst plaques)* appear as yellow-orange refractile deposits at bifurcations of vessels and are typically a sign of carotid disease.
- *Platelet fibrin emboli* are dull grey or white in color, concave meniscus at each end, lodge along the course of vessel and are likely a result of carotid thrombosis, thrombosis associated with recent myocardial infarction or heart valves.
- *Calcium* emboli are chalky white in color, large round or ovoid, lodge in the first or second vessel bifurcations or may overlie the optic disc. They can arise from the heart (rheumatic heart disease, calcification of mitral valve) or great vessels (calcific aortic stenosis).

Stroke and transient visual loss

- The risk of stroke from *amaurosis fugax* per annum is approximately 2% and a 1% risk of permanent visual loss.
- In patients *with carotid stenosis*, ipsilateral eye symptoms may be accompanied by those *of ipsilateral cerebral ischemia* like contralateral hemiparesis, sensory loss, language deficits and hemianopia.

Clinical work-up

- *General examination* should include pulse rate (irregular in arrhythmias, fibrillation), cardiac auscultation (murmurs) and carotid auscultation (bruit). However, presence or absence of a carotid bruit is generally not help-ful for diagnosing significant carotid stenosis or predicting a carotid source of emboli.
- *Carotid ultrasound and Doppler* are effective screening tools for identification and estimation of the degree of internal carotid artery stenosis.
- *Magnetic resonance imaging–angiography* (MRA) is another non-invasive test for carotid stenosis, however, it tends to overestimate the degree of stenosis.
- *Computed tomographic angiography* (CT angio) is another screening test and can be used to confirm MRA or ultrasound findings.
- *Conventional angiography* is the gold stan-dard test for evaluation and quantification of carotid stenosis as its specificity and sensitivity exceed those of any non-invasive tests.

- In a elderly patient if the all the general workup including carotid tests are unrevealing then an atheroma arising from the more proximal vessels like the aorta or an acephalgic migraine should be considered as possible etiologies for TVL.
- In a young patient with an unrevealing work-up, vasospasm and hypercoagulable states, due to antiphospolipid antibodies, protein C, protein S and antithrombin III levels should be considered possible causes for TVL.

Treatment

If not contraindicated, antiplatelet therapy with aspirin should be immediately started in patients with amaurosis fugax to reduce the risk of stroke. Addition of clopidogrel or anti-coagulants can also be considered in consulta-tion with an interventional cardiologist. Multiple clinical trials have established the benefit of carotid surgery for symptomatic (retinal or hemispheric TIA) carotid stenosis greater than 70%. The management of asymptomatic carotid stenosis is however extremely controversial.

VISUAL IMPAIRMENT

A patient presenting with diminution of vision without any evidence of structural abnormali-ties in the eye is a puzzle for an ophthalmologist. It is important to have a logical and meticulous approach to evaluate such patients so as to come to a conclusion regarding the cause of visual loss. This includes detailed history, thorough clinical examination and appropriate investigations.

COMMON CAUSES

Visual impairment can be broadly classified to belong to the following pathologies:
1. Refractive errors and media opacities
2. Lesions of visual pathway
   - Optic nerve lesions
   - Chiasmal lesions
   - Retrochiasmal lesions
3. Macular lesions
4. Amblyopia
5. Psychogenic/malingering

We will further see how to rule out each of them and come to a problem oriented working diagnosis. Figure 1.1 is the flow chart for assess-ment of visual impairment and segregating patients with refractive errors, media opacities.

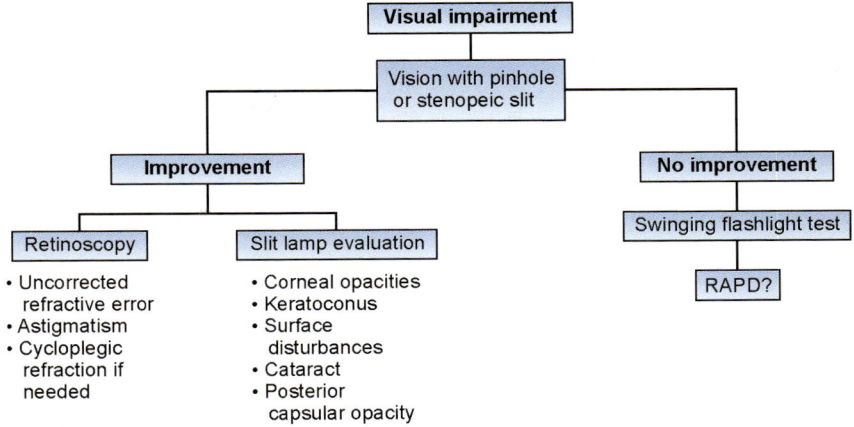

Fig. 1.1 *Flow chart for a patient with visual impairment.*

CLINICAL WORK-UP AND TESTS

TESTS FOR REFRACTIVE ERRORS, MEDIA OPACITIES AND VISUAL PATHWAY LESIONS

PINHOLE TEST AND STENOPEIC SLIT TEST

As refractive errors are one of the leading causes of decreased vision they should be the first ones to be ruled out. Use of pinhole and stenopeic slit determines whether or not vision will improve with refractive correction. Improvement by two lines on Snellen's chart or more on looking through the pinhole or stenopeic slit makes it clear that the visual impairment is due to optical problems.

As the pinhole eliminates paraxial rays of light, minimizing blurring of the image falling on the retina, all optical defects can be neutralized to some extent with this method, not only the refractive ametropias. However, many patients, especially children and old people find it difficult to peek through the pinhole and do not give reliable responses. The method is uncertain, and improvement of less than two lines should certainly be interpreted with caution. Repeated subjective and cycloplegic *refraction* will usually uncover an undetected and irregular corneal astigmatism or hypermetropic error.

- Limitations of pinhole are that vision may apparently worsen in patients with central media opacities (such as posterior subcapsular cataract) and macular pathologies. Vision does not improve to 6/6 if refractive error exceeds ±4 DS.
- Detailed slit lamp examination will reveal any obvious corneal opacities, surface irregularities, keratoconus and not to mention presence of cataract or posterior capsular opacity.
- If the vision does not improve with the pinhole, the next step will be checking the pupils for relative afferent pupillary defect.

SWINGING FLASHLIGHT TEST

This is performed to detect the presence of relative afferent pupillary defect (RAPD).

Remember: Relative = compared to the other eye, and Afferent = problem in the afferent pathway.

The main use of RAPD is in evaluating a patient who has decreased vision in one eye and normal vision in the other. If it is present, there is lesion in one of the eyes, or asymmetric optic nerve or retinal lesion. If it is not present, retina or optic nerve of both eyes are normal or symmetrically involved. But brisk pupillary reaction to light definitely rules out optic nerve pathology.

Technique of swinging flashlight test

The swinging flashlight test is performed as follows:

- *Patient is seated* in a dimly lit room and asked to fixate at a distant target. This provides maximum relaxation of the iris sphincter muscle.

- *Torchlight is shone* into one eye. The light should be directed from below so that it does not act like a near target and induce miosis associated with accommodation. It should be shone into the eye for about 2–3 seconds.
- *Pupillary reaction is observed* and the light is quickly moved across the bridge of the nose and directed into the opposite eye. If the light is moved too slowly; the pupil is seen to constrict when finally the light falls on it and thus gives a false impression of a normal reaction.
- *Pupillary reaction of the other eye is observed* and compared in amplitude and speed to the first eye.
- *The light should be moved across one eye to the other* briskly and rhythmically at least 5 times. This is important to be sure that any papillary dilatation on one side is not just the sphincter movement due to physiological pupillary unrest. The light should be bright, but not so bright that it makes the patient photophobic.
- *RAPD can be identified even in cases where the reaction of both pupils cannot be studied,* for example single eyed individuals, patients in whom one pupil is distorted, non-dilating and fixed or constricted due to neurological disease, iris trauma or synechiae.

Observations

While performing the swinging flashlight test, we observe the pupil that is being illuminated. But the opposite pupil also reacts in an identical manner. Thus in these cases the examiner must observe only the reactive pupil. If the abnormal eye is the eye with the fixed pupil, then the normal eye will react briskly when the light is shone into it and will dilate when the light is shone into the opposite eye. On the other hand, if the eye with the apparently normal pupil is the affected eye, then its pupil will dilate when the light is shone onto it and constrict when the light is directed on the other eye (with the fixed pupil).

Normal response (RAPD absent)

When light is shone into one eye, the pupil constricts. When it is transferred to the other eye, its pupil is either already constricted (due to consensual reflex) or constricts further. When it is shone back into the first eye, the same response takes place.

Abnormal response (RAPD present)

When light is shone into the normal eye, its pupil constricts. When light is transferred to the other abnormal eye, it will either consistently constrict more weakly compared to the normal eye; or does not react; or actually dilates on light stimulation (phenomenon called as pupillary escape); RAPD is said to be present. At this point the other eye's pupil will also be dilated.

Presence of RAPD means that cause of visual loss is unilateral or asymmetric bilateral retinopathy or neuropathy.
- Interpretation of presence of RAPD is shown in Fig. 1.2.
- On dilated fundus examination, a retinopathy severe enough to cause RAPD will be easily appreciated.
- However, optic neuropathy may be present in the absence of any fundus abnormalities.

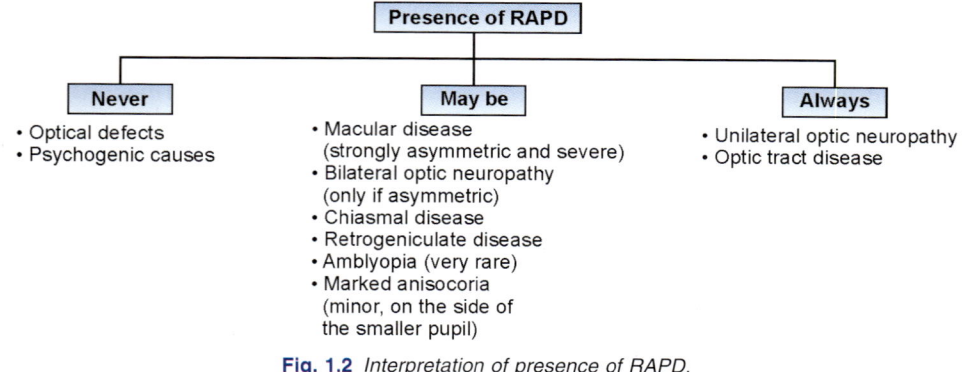

Fig. 1.2 *Interpretation of presence of RAPD.*

Retinal pathologies capable of causing RAPD are:
- Central retinal artery occlusion
- Central retinal vein occlusion
- Total retinal detachment

These will have substantial changes in the fundus and a careful dilated fundus examination can help differentiated them from neuro-ophthalmological disease.

If RAPD is absent, visual loss in these cases may be due to:
- Macular pathologies
- Amblyopia
- Psychogenic causes/malingering

Use of neutral density filters

The neutral density filters are available ranging from 0.3 log units to 2 log units; in steps of 0.3 log units. Neutral density filters can be used for:
- *Quantifying the RAPD.* The neutral density filters are placed in front of the normal eye. The density of the filter that neutralizes the RAPD is the measure of the defect.
- *Unequivocal findings.* The neutral density filters are successively placed in front of either eye. If RAPD is present in an eye it becomes more obvious when the filter is placed in front of that eye. If it is absent, when the filter is placed in front of one eye the pupil will dilate on shining light onto it; and this will repeat when the filter is shifted to the other eye, i.e. there will be an 'Artificially created RAPD'.

Grading of RAPD

- *Grade I.* A weak initial constriction and greater re-dilatation
- *Grade II.* Initial stall and greater re-dilatation
- *Grade III.* Immediate pupillary dilatation
- *Grade IV.* Immediate pupillary dilatation following prolonged illumination of the good eye for 6 seconds
- *Grade V.* Immediate pupillary dilatation with no secondary constriction.

Note

As mentioned before, the presence of a relative afferent papillary defect almost always confirms a neuro-ophthalmological cause, but the absence of it does not rule out the same. So either ways, we must go ahead with further optic nerve function tests which complement our findings and which assume special importance in case of unequivocal results or if pupil cannot be examined.

OPTIC NERVE HEAD EXAMINATION

A meticulous optic nerve head examination using slit lamp biomicroscope and high power lenses like 78 D or 90 D gives valuable information about the acuteness of the condition and to some extent the etiology.

COLOR VISION TESTING

Testing the color vision helps to differentiate optic nerve pathology from other pathologies. Usually in day-to-day clinical practice, Ishihara pseudo-isochromatic tests plates are used. Inability of indentifying a number at all is considered as defective color vision. The D 15 color vision test is based on a set of colored plates or disks which have to be arranged in the correct order. Tests like Farnsworth-Munsell 100 hue test and Hardy-Rand-Ritter (HRR) charts are more detailed tests which include various colors which have a very subtle difference of hue which the patient has to compare and obtain the nearest match. Though these tests can identify very early or fine changes, they are very time consuming and very difficult to carry out in day-to-day busy clinics.

To determine whether the color vision deficit is due to optic nerve involvement we need to note if:
- There is relevant history (acquired loss of color vision)
- Color vision worse in dim light
- Preferential inability to discriminate between red and green colors (in macular abnormalities there will be preferential loss of ability to differentiate blue and yellow colors).

Color saturation

To patients with optic nerve disease colors appear less bright, faded (desaturated) or darker in the affected eye than the normal eye. To check for this, a red stimulus (brightly colored stimulus preferred) is presented to each eye in succession and patient is asked if to one eye the color appears 'brighter' or 'richer' than the other. If the patient clearly says yes it is taken as a positive response. To the eye with defective optic nerve function the red color may appear as a faded color such as orange, pink or faded red (indicating decreased saturation) or brown, gray (indicating decreased brightness).

BRIGHTNESS COMPARISON TEST

This test detects decreased brightness sensitivity in the affected eye if any. Bright torchlight is shone into each of the eyes and patient is asked which appears brighter. Taking the brighter one as 100% patient is asked to compare it with the other eye and determine how much is the decrease in the brightness perception in the other eye. This test is slightly more sensitive than the RAPD and may help detect an early defect.

CONTRAST SENSITIVITY TESTS

Visual acuity determines the smallest spatial detail that can be resolved for a high contrast stimulus, whereas measurement of contrast sensitivity checks the responses of visual system to different sizes and contrasts. These tests are thus useful adjuncts to reveal the deficit in patients with normal visual acuity but who may have a visual pathway lesion.

• It is usually determined by measuring the contrast thresholds for sinusoidal gratings, an alternating pattern of light and dark bars, the luminance of which varies sinusoidally in a direction perpendicular to the orientation of the grating. The size of the grating is specified according to the spatial frequency which is the number of cycles of the grating pattern (i.e. the pair of dark and light bars) per degree of visual angle. The contrast sensitivity function measures between 3 and 10 spatial frequencies from 0.5 to 30 cycles per degree.

• Other tests available to measure the contrast sensitivity are Pelli-Robson contrast sensitivity chart, Vistech contrast sensitivity chart and a low contrast version of the Bailey-Lovie visual acuity chart. These charts make use of contrast letters to measure contrast sensitivity. However, whether these tests are superior to the ones using sinusoidal gratings to measure contrast sensitivity is controversial.

Note. One must note that sensitivity losses have little specificity for differential diagnosis purposes. Similar patterns of loss can be obtained by a wide variety of conditions and at the same time many types of disorders can produce similar amounts of visual acuity loss.

VISUAL FIELD TESTING

Confrontation test

The next step is to determine any defect or decreased sensitivity in the visual fields. This can be done in the OPD performing the confrontation test which is done as follows:

1. *Patient should be comfortably seated.* The clinician is seated about 1 meter in front of and at the level of the patient, who is asked to fixate on the bridge of the examiner's nose. While testing patient's right eye, his left eye should be occluded and the clinician's right eye should be closed.

2. *Firstly ask the patient* if he can see the examiner's full face clearly. If not, then ask him to elaborate which parts are missing or not clearly visible to him. This will tell us about any gross defects in the field of vision.

3. *Testing of single quadrants.* One or two stationary fingers are presented randomly in each quadrant of the right eye taking care that the stimulus remains well within 30 degrees of the visual field; and the patient is asked to count the fingers. Children can be asked to simulate the number of fingers seen and at the same time the examiner looks for the eye movements brought forth by the stimulus.

4. *Delineating the scotoma.* If the patient is not able to see the fingers—move the finger from the defective quadrant slowly towards the vertical meridian. Patient is asked to identify as soon as he sees the stimulus. This way we can recognize if the border of the defect is aligned to the vertical meridian. Same procedure should be repeated to if there is presence of a defect respecting the horizontal meridian.

Steps 2, 3, 4 are repeated in the left eye.

5. *Testing double quadrants.* This is performed if the patient correctly identifies stimuli in single quadrant testing but the clinician suspects presence of defect in a certain quadrant. One or two fingers of both the hands are simultaneously presented in two different quadrants and the patient is asked to count the total number of fingers seen.

6. *Brightness comparison.* If the patient responds correctly to the above tests he may be asked to compare the clarity or brightness of two fingers simultaneously presented in two different quadrants and if there is any reduction in brightness of one of them.

7. **Red desaturation test.** Two identical bright colored objects (preferably red) are presented to the patient in two different quadrants and asked if there is any difference in the brightness of the color in any of the quadrant. If yes, the object is moved slowly from the defective quadrant towards the vertical meridian and the patient is asked if the object becomes brighter or duller in the course. If there is marked difference, a hemianopic defect exists. Same maneuver is repeated with the horizontal meridian.

The confrontation test gives a rough idea about presence of any gross visual field defects. It has very less specificity and sensitivity as it depends largely on the patient's ability to understand how to perform the test and maintain fixation. Though it should never replace formal visual field testing, it assumes importance in certain scenarios like examination of a bed ridden patient where technical investigations may not be possible.

Automated visual field examination

One of the most important investigations in neuro-ophthalmology is the automated visual fields examination. Central 30 degrees of field testing in standard automated perimetric programmes is preferred.

Visual field analysis must be considered

1. If RAPD is present
2. If any of the adjunctive clinical tests (color vision, color saturation, brightness sensitivity, contrast sensitivity) are abnormal
3. Optic nerve head examination shows pallor/ edema/optic atrophy/glaucomatous changes

Visual field examination helps greatly to quantify the defect and localise the lesion along the afferent visual pathway and thereby can be called an important part of visual testing.

While trying to localize the lesion we must try to differentiate between a non-hemianopic and hemianopic defect. The loss of entire hemifield is not necessary for the diagnosis of hemianopic defect, it is enough that the border of the defect is aligned to the vertical fixation meridian. If the field defect is hemianopic, it points towards the cause of an optic neuropathy or retinopathy, whereas a hemianopic defect would point to a chiasmal lesion.

TESTS FOR MACULAR PATHOLOGIES

Tests that can be used to rule out macular pathologies are as follows.

Amsler's grid test

In the standard Amsler's grid chart the patient is presented a grid of black lines on a white background and a central black dot for fixation at a reading distance. The patient must wear his refractive correction. First the patient is asked if he can see the central dot. He is then asked to mark on the chart if any of the squares seem bent or distorted or of unequal sizes; or if he is unable to see any parts of the grid. The presence of meta-morphopsia is diagnostic of macular disease, as it is caused by the separation, distortion or crowding of foveal cones by edema, fluid or scarring.

There are other types of Amsler's grids:
- White squares on black background and central white dot
- White squares on a black background with a central white dot and diagonal white limits of his scotoma
- Red squares on a black background with a central red dot. This chart helps to diagnose optic nerve, chiasmal, or toxic amblyopia related problems.

Photostress test

Baseline visual acuity of the patient is deter-mined. Bright light is directed into one of the eyes for ten seconds. This bleaches the photo-receptors. After ten seconds the patient's Snellen's visual acuity is recorded again. The time between bleaching and recovery to within one Snellen line of the original visual acuity is measured. If the time taken to recover is substantially greater in one eye than the other, it indicates impaired regeneration of photoreceptor pigment in the retinal pigment epithelium. However, this is a highly subjective test and can hardly be relied upon for the diagnosis.

Electroretinogram (ERG)

In the standard full field (Ganzfield) ERG the potentials are excited by short flashes of light and detected by recording electrodes contacting the anterior surface of the eye. The stimulus covers the entire retina, and the recorded responses are a summation of the electrical potentials generated by the entire retina. It thus is a mass response and will detect generalized outer retinal disease and fails to detect isolated macular or other localized pathologies. Multifocal ERG (Mf ERG) is the new specialized type of ERG which is capable of highlighting such localized pathologies.

This is useful in determining the cause of visual disabilities when there are no visible findings on ophthalmoscopy.

Fundus fluorescein angiography

This is done to identify subtle macular lesions and vascular pathologies and is capable of detecting defects in the RPE and choroid too. It occasionally spots lesions not visible even on high magnification ophthalmoscopy.

TESTS FOR AMBLYOPIA

If there is absence of retinal lesion, the visual loss can be attributed to amblyopia. Amblyopia refers to poor vision caused by abnormal visual development secondary to abnormal visual stimulation.

History of squinting or cataract in childhood or congenital ptosis which occludes the visual axis may give a clue towards the presence of amblyopia. Binocular amblyopia may be considered in the cases of children with high hypermetropia. There are no confirmatory investigations for this entity and the diagnosis of amblyopia is made when all other causes are ruled out. A few simple clinical tests may aid in the diagnosis:

Testing for 'crowding phenomenon'

An amblyopic patient when asked to read single letters, is said to have a higher visual acuity then when he is asked to read an entire line. This is called *crowding phenomenon*.

Neutral density filter test

A 2 log unit neutral density filter is used in this setting. It is placed in front of the normal eye and the visual acuity is checked. It causes a drop in the visual acuity. When the same procedure is repeated in front of the other suspected amblyopic eye, it degrades the visual acuity less.

Base out prism test

This test detects the presence of a central fixation scotoma <5 degrees and is not specific for amblyopia. A 4 PD prism is placed in front of the normal eye in the base out position. The image is thus shifted temporally in that eye. There is bilateral vergence movement away from the eye behind the prism to take up fixation and similar movement of the other eye. However, since the image falls within the small scotoma the eye does not show any refixation movement. Similarly, when the prism is placed in front of this eye, there is no movement of either eye.

NEUROIMAGING

Neuroimaging is essential in certain scenarios to come to the correct diagnosis. It should be considered in cases of:

1. *Acute loss of vision*; unilateral (suspicion of hemorrhagic, ischemic, embolic phenomenon) or bilateral (suspecting a lesion above the level of chiasma)
2. *Hemianopic field defects* on visual field analysis indicating chiasmal lesion
3. *Trauma*; to rule out hemorrhage, fractures, optic nerve injury or compression
4. *Suspicion of compressive pathology*.

The choice of imaging modality depends upon the clinical diagnosis, available facilities and the cost factor. Magnetic resonance imaging (MRI) and computed tomography (CT) are the most commonly ordered investigations by a neuro-ophthalmologist.

Magnetic resonance imaging (MRI)

MRI is the investigation of choice in neuro-ophthalmology; especially for a patient with acute vision loss. It is more useful in:
• Identifying small lesions
• Identifying vascular lesions
• Characterization of lesion
• Extent and invasion of surrounding lesion
• Surgical planning if necessary

MRI offers better delineation of soft tissues and thus an improved differentiation between retrobulbar soft tissues (fat, muscle and optic nerve), between normal components of the brain (gray and white substances) and between differing forms of pathological change (infarction, hemorrhage, inflammation, and neoplasms).

MRI with gadolinium contrast enhances the blood vessels, extraocular muscles and active lesions and is preferred in this setting.

The most important advantage of MRI scanning lies in the fact that the signal strength in the image determined by tissue-specific parameters, the T1 and T2 relaxation times. This produces a high-resolution image with excellent tissue identification. Normal anatomy is best demonstrated in **T1-weighted** images, whereas **T2-weighted** images are better for demonstrating intracranial or other pathology.

Magnetic resonance angiography (MRA) and Magnetic resonance venography (MRV) are performed when the MRI does not yield any results but there is a strong suspicion of vessel pathology.

Absolute contraindications to MRI:
- Cardiac pacemakers
- Incorporated ferromagnetic foreign bodies/implants
- Shrapnel wounds
- Aneurysm clips of uncertain origin.

Computed tomography (CT)

CT is the imaging method of choice for patients with skull/brain injuries. The presence and course of fractures in the orbit can be studied, using the windows that allow the best definition of bones' anatomy (**Bone window**). The effects of direct ocular trauma, or retrobulbar hemorrhages, are best studied when using the window settings for soft tissues (**Soft tissue window**). Thus, ophthalmic vein distension may be detected because of a traumatic carotid cavernous fistula.

In soft tissue tumors where we expect calcification or hyperostosis (like meningioma) or an orbital tumor CT scan is a better choice of investigation. Also for detection of foreign bodies CT scan is preferred as such cases are a potential contraindication for MRI.

CT with contrast is done for better visualization of blood vessels.

Contraindication of contrast: It is important to remember the contraindications for the use of contrast materials:
- Allergy to iodinated compounds
- Hyperthyroidism
- Poor renal function
- Paraproteinemia

SUMMARY

If all the above mentioned causes of visual loss are eliminated with the aid of clinical tests, visual field examination, neuroimaging and other diagnostic investigations; and still no cause is found; the visual loss can then be attributed to psychogenic causes.

It is often tempting enough to refer such a patient with unexplained visual loss to the neuro-ophthalmologist but what is essential is a systematic and rational approach to come to a working diagnosis and thus save the patient of anxiety, dissatisfaction and expenses.

Clinico-investigative approach to a patient with visual loss is summarized in Fig. 1.3.

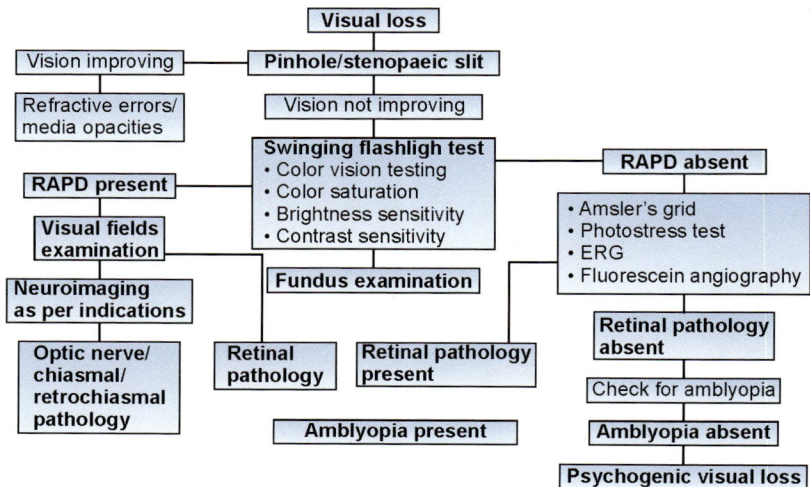

Fig. 1.3 *Summary of clinico-investigative approach to a patient with visual loss.*

CLINICO-INVESTIGATIVE APPROACH FOR A PATIENT WITH DIPLOPIA

INTRODUCTION

Diplopia essentially means "double vision". Causes of diplopia range from benign and common entities such as a decompensated phoria to ominous entities such as aneurysmal third nerve palsy or sixth nerve palsy due to increased intracranial pressure. Dysfunction of the extraocular muscles may be the result of an abnormality of the muscle itself or an abnormality of the motor nerve to the muscle. The major symptom associated with this dysfunction is diplopia. Diplopia is a common presenting symptom to ophthalmologists and emergency room physicians with many potential causes that can involve many different structures. Given that the etiology of diplopia spans such a broad spectrum, it is important to have a systematic approach in evaluating patients presenting with this symptom.

CAUSES OF DIPLOPIA

MONOCULAR DIPLOPIA

Monocular diplopia is defined as double vision that is present in the affected eye while the other eye is occluded. Monocular diplopia in nearly all circumstances is the result of local ocular aberration (defects of the cornea, iris, lens or retina). Neurologic misalignment causes binocular diplopia, whereas ocular causes such as refractive error, lead to monocular diplopia. Patients with optical causes of monocular diplopia like media opacity such as subtle changes in the optical density of anterior and posterior layers of lens in the case of incipient cataract generally describe blurring and glare and the patient may see a ghost image that is much lighter and less defined. Other causes include defects of cornea like irregular astigmatism, corneal scars (Fig. 1.4A), scars due to laser eye surgery (LASIK), iris defects (Fig. 1.4B) or in appropriately placed peripheral iridectomy, subluxated crystalline lens or IOLs

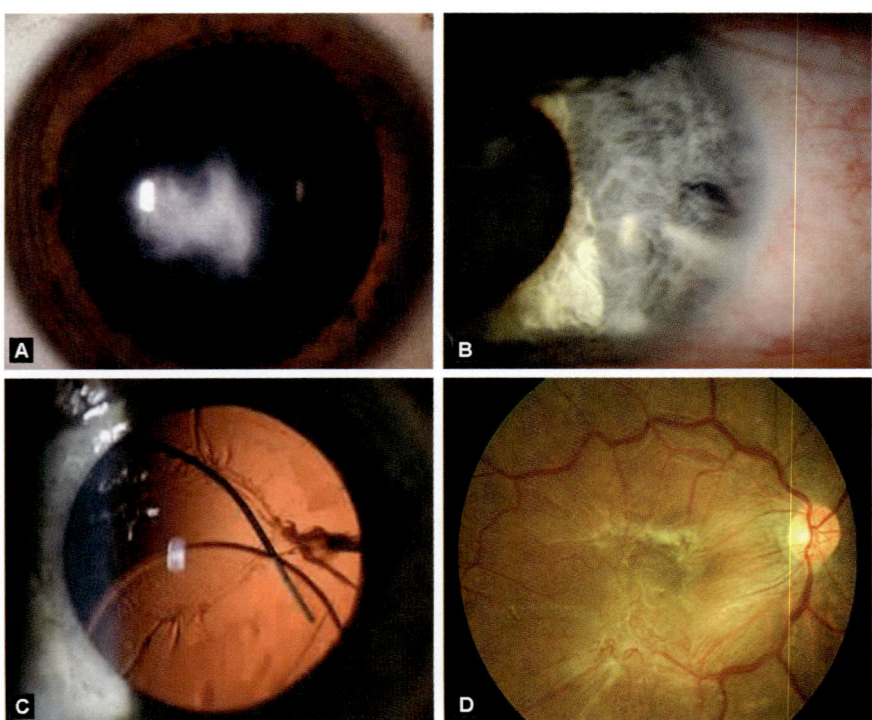

Fig. 1.4 *Common causes of monocular diplopic: (A) Corneal scar; (B) Iridotomy; (C) Subluxated IOL; (D) Macular pucker.*

(Fig. 1.4C). In all these conditions monocular diplopia resolves with pin hole. Patients with macular disorders generally describe a break, bend or distortion of the viewed edge leading to a distorted image. This type of monocular double vision generally does not improve when the object is viewed through a pinhole, in fact, vision is often worse in these cases. Common disorders of macula include choroidal neovascular membrane or an epiretinal membrane (Fig. 1.4D). The other cause of monocular diplopia which does not resolve with pinhole is central diplopia which is caused by lesion involving visual cortex and is associated with visual field defects. In this setting the patient may also complain of triple or quadruple vision.

BINOCULAR DIPLOPIA

Binocular diplopia, on the other hand, resolves with closure of either eye. From the eye to the brain, the following seven mechanisms and their associated locations should be kept in mind while gathering historical information regarding binocular diplopia:
- Orbital/ocular displacement
- Extraocular muscles restriction
- Extraocular muscles weakness
- Neuromuscular junction dysfunction
- 3rd, 4th and 6th cranial nerve dysfunction
- Cranial nerve nuclear dysfunction in brainstem
- Supranuclear dysfunctions (pathways to and between nuclei of 3rd, 4th and 6th cranial nerves)

Common causes of binocular diplopia are summarized in Table 1.1.

Table 1.1 *Common causes of binocular diplopia*

Types of lesion	Causes
Orbital disorders	• Trauma • Tumor/mass • Infection
Extraocular muscle restriction	• Thyroid associated ophthalmopathy • Mass/tumor • Extra-ocular muscle entrapment • Injury/hematoma due to ocular surgery
Extraocular muscle weakness	• Congenital myopathies • Muscular dystrophy
Neuromuscular junction dysfunction	• Myasthenia gravis • Botulism
3rd, 4th and 6th cranial nerve dysfunction	• Ischemia • Hemorrhage • Tumor/mass • Vascular malformations • Aneurysm • Trauma • Multiple sclerosis • Meningitis
Cranial nerve nuclear dysfunction in brainstem	• Stroke • Hemorrhage • Tumor/mass • Vascular malformations
Supranuclear dysfunction	• Internuclear ophthalmoplegia • Convergence spasm • Convergence and divergence insufficiency • Pseudoabducens palsy • Skew deviation • Monocular elevator palsy

SUPRANUCLEAR PATHWAY LESIONS

GAZE PALSIES

1. *Conjugate gaze palsy.* If both eyes are equally paretic in the same direction of gaze and causes no diplopia. These are of two types:

- *Horizontal—conjugate* gaze palsies localize to pons or frontal cortex.
- *Vertical—*conjugate gaze palsies localize to midbrain.

2. *Disconjugate gaze palsy* results in diplopia. It is of two types:

- *Horizontal,* e.g. internuclear ophthalmoplegia.
- *Vertical—*skew deviation.

INTERNUCLEAR OPHTHALMOPLEGIA

Disruption of the MLF in the pons or midbrain results in an internuclear ophthalmoplegia (INO). There is adduction deficit in the eye on the same side of lesion and simultaneous nystagmus of the abducting eye in lateral gaze. The side of the adduction deficit determines the side of the INO. It is most commonly associated with multiple sclerosis and stroke.

Clinical features

The patients with INO may complain of horizontal diplopia, particularly when there is profound adduction weakness. Those patients with subtle paresis may have no symptoms or complain of blurred vision with eccentric gaze only. Since a skew deviation is frequently associated with lesions of the MLF, vertical diplopia may be another complaint. Oscillopsia may be the other symptom which may result from either the abduction nystagmus or an impaired vertical vestibular ocular reflex.

- The hallmark finding of INO is impaired adduction of the eye. Subtle cases may be evident only upon fast eye movements from midline to eccentric gaze which is known as medial rectus float. The demonstration of intact convergence in INO establishes the supranuclear localization of the medial rectus weakness and usually signifies a lesion of the MLF within the pons. In contrast patients with MLF lesions close to the third nerve nucleus may have impaired convergence. However, some patients with INO have poor conver-

gence because of the vertical misalignment produced by the associated skew deviation. Therefore, the absence of convergence may not be a totally reliable sign to localize the lesion in a discrete part of the MLF pathway.

- The eye that is contralateral to the MLF lesion typically exhibits an abducting nystagmus in end gaze. Evidence suggests that this abducting nystagmus is an adaptive phenomenon to increase the innervation to the weak adducting eye.
- Since the otolith pathways project through the MLF, a skew deviation is commonly observed with an INO. Typically, the hypertropic eye is on the same side as the adduction weakness. There is downbeating nystagmus in the eye ipsilateral to the MLF lesion and torsional nystagmus in the contralateral eye.
- Bilateral lesions of the MLF usually produce additional eye findings, including impaired vertical pursuit and vertical gaze holding defects. Severe bilateral INOs may also result in a large angle exotropia in primary gaze in so called WEBINO (wall eyed bilateral INO).

Diagnosis

The diagnosis of INO is usually straightforward, especially when there is impaired medial rectus dysfunction in lateral gaze with normal convergence. A unilateral INO in an older patient usually results from a brainstem infarction, while bilateral INO in a young patient typically signifies a demyelinating process such as multiple sclerosis. However, a variety of lesions may be associated with INOs including vascular malformations, tumors; head trauma, infections, vasculitides such as systemic lupus erythematosus, Behçet's disease and giant cell arteritis; nutritional disorders such as Wernicke's disease; metabolic disorders such as hepatic encephalopathy; Arnold-Chiari malformation; and degenerative conditions, progressive supranuclear palsy.

- The combination of an INO with an ipsiversive conjugate palsy is a pontine "one-and-half" syndrome due to simultaneous ipsilateral involvement of the PPRF and the MLF. Damage to the MLF in addition to the corticospinal tracts results in the Raymond.

Cestan syndrome, characterized by an INO and contralateral hemiparesis.

SKEW DEVIATION

Skew deviation is an acquired vertical misalignment of the eyes that commonly occurs from acute brain stem dysfunction. It may also result from peripheral vestibular or cerebellar lesions. Patients may complain of binocular vertical diplopia, sometimes with a torsional component. The associated neurologic symptoms and signs often helps in differentiating skew deviation from other causes of vertical misalignment such as third and fourth nerve palsies.

Ocular tilt reaction. The combination of skew deviation with ocular torsion and a head tilt is known as the *ocular tilt reaction (OTR)*. This syndrome typically develops because of loss of otolithic input to the INC from a central lesion, which may be in the medulla, pons, or midbrain. With an ocular tilt reaction, if the head is tilted to the left, the right eye becomes hypertropic, and both eyes rotate toward the lower ear. The opposite response of the eyes occurs if the head is tilted to the right. A fourth nerve palsy is the motility disorder that may be the most difficult to distinguish from a skew deviation since both conditions may be associated with a positive head tilt or three step test. With a fourth nerve palsy, the compensatory head tilt is opposite the side of the higher eye (similar to ocular tilt reaction), but the hypertropic eye is extorted which is opposite of the skew deviation.

Thalamic esodeviation is an acquired horizontal deviation that occurs with lesions near the junction of the diencephalon and midbrain. This disorder may be seen in younger patients with pineal tumors or craniopharyngioma or in older patients with cerebral hemorrhage.

CONVERGENCE SPASM

This condition, characterized by convergence, accommodation, bilateral papillary miosis, and pseudomyopia, may mimic bilateral sixth nerve palsies. The distinction is important because convergence spasm is almost always indicative of a functional disorder. Patients usually complain of double vision, and they often have obvious personality disorders or other hysterical symptoms. The hallmarks are pupillary constriction on attempted abduction and a variable esotropia. Other features include normal abducting saccades, intact abduction during the oculocephalic maneuver or testing of monocular ductions, and resolution of the myopia following cycloplegia. The miosis may resolve upon occlusion of the fellow eye by disrupting the binocular input necessary for convergence. Convergence spasm should be distinguished from convergence retraction nystagmus or pseudoabducens palsy from pretectal lesions.

CONVERGENCE INSUFFICIENCY

Patients with convergence insufficiency describe horizontal diplopia at near, typically after a period of reading. Medial rectus function is normal when ocular ductions are tested, but patients typically have an exodeviation worse at near. A common sequela of head trauma, the condition may also be seen in association with dorsal midbrain syndrome, may be a decompensation of long standing exophoria or may be idiopathic.

DIVERGENCE INSUFFICIENCY

This ocular motility deficit is characterized by acquired horizontal diplopia at distance but not near, a comitant esophoria or esotropia at distance, motor fusion at near, and full ocular ductions without evidence of a sixth nerve palsy. Divergence insufficiency is typically benign, and affected patients are usually neurologically normal otherwise. However since small bilateral sixth nerve palsies may mimic divergence insufficiency, elevated intracranial pressure, masses, and pontine lesions must be excluded with neuroimaging. Small vessel ischemic disease is a relatively common finding on magnetic resonance imaging studies of older patients with this condition.

- Prenuclear vertical misalignment seen in brainstem and cerebellar lesions may be comitant or incomitant with full motility but vertical misalignment decreases when patient lays supine.

CLINICAL EVALUATION OF DIPLOPIA

Diplopia may be the initial presentation of the potentially life-threatening disorder or it may be secondary to a harmless process. So, a detailed history as well as physical examination of a patient with diplopia is must to review the most common associated features that help localise the cause of diplopia.

HISTORY

The examiner should first determine whether the patient rarely sees double or has blurred vision of one eye, an overlay of the image or sees a halo surrounding the image. This information is obtained by a careful history and also we can ask the patient to draw a picture of what he sees. Once it has been confirmed that the images are truly separated, placing a cover over either eye will determine whether the diplopia is monocular or binocular.

The following questions should be kept in mind while approaching a patient with diplopia:
- Is the diplopia monocular or binocular?
- Is the onset acute or gradual?
- Is it constant or intermittent?
- Is there any variability/remission?
- Are there any associated signs and symptoms?
- History of ocular surgery/trauma?
- Any systemic diseases—Diabetes, hypertension, hyperlipidemia, hyperthyroidism, parkinsonism?

Features of diplopia

- *On set.* Diplopia is almost always sudden in onset. The only exceptions are thyroid ophthalmopathy, divergence insufficiency and myasthenia gravis where gradual progression is seen.
- *Constant or intermittent.* We should always enquire from the patient whether the diplopia is constant or intermittent in nature. Most common causes of intermittent diplopia by far are decompensating phorias, vergence problems, accommodative spasm, headache (temporal arteritis) and myasthenia gravis. Myasthenia gravis is one condition which should be investigated in detail in a patient complaining of intermittent diplopia.

- *Separation of images.* Normally we do diplopia charting to look for separation of images. But we can always narrow down group of muscles which are affected by asking about the separation of images.
- *Horizontal separation* of two images indicates 6th nerve palsy.
- *Vertical separation* if pure can be due to 4th nerve palsy.
- *Oblique separation* of images Occurs in 3rd nerve palsy.
- *Orbital processes* can cause horizontal, vertical or oblique diplopia.
- *Horizontal diplopia* worse at distance is associated with esotropia and implies lateral rectus palsy.
- If mainly at near, medial recti are implicated and is diagnosed as convergence insufficiency.
- Internuclear ophthalmoplegia and myasthenia gravis are other causes of horizontal diplopia.
- *Thyroid associated ophthalmopathy*, skew deviation and myasthenia gravis present as vertical diplopia.

Associated symptoms

Associated signs and symptoms are vital to localize the site of injury.
- Elderly patient with severe headache and isolated 3rd nerve palsy with dilated non-reacting pupil implicates a compressive injury of 3rd nerve in subarachnoid space. Most likely cause would be intracranial aneurysm of posterior communicating artery.
- Symptoms of jaw claudication, headache, scalp tenderness and arthralgias should be enquired in older patients with diplopia to rule out temporal arteritis.
- Patient should be asked about associated neurological symptoms like facial numbness or weakness, hearing loss, dysphagia, dysarthria, vertigo, incoordination or numbness or weakness of extremities to rule out brainstem injury and supranuclear pathway injuries.
- If a patient reports with eye pain and diplopia, then common causes like cellulitis, any mass lesion, inflammatory disorders like pseudo-tumor should be ruled out.

Diurnal variation of diplopia

Diplopia that progressively worsens throughout the day or worsens with reading is common with neuromuscular junction disorders that affect extraocular muscles like myasthenia gravis. More than 50% patients of myasthenia gravis present with ptosis and diplopia alone.

Palinopsia refers to seeing multiple images of an object immediately after turning away from the object or after the object is removed from the sight. This is known as after image or strobe effect. This condition is seen in discrete lesions with occipitoparietal or occipitotemporal cortex and homonymous visual field defects are also associated with these cortical visual illusions.

EXAMINATION

Examination of all basic visual sensory and ocular motor functions is necessary in the evaluation of diplopia.

GENERAL EXAMINATION

- In general examination of a patient note should be made of gait, physical appearance, stature, head posture, facial symmetry, moist hands or tremors on a hand shake.
- Blood pressure, random blood sugar and resting pulse rate should be recorded.
- *Unaided and best corrected visual acuity followed by visual fields* to confrontation, pupillary appearance and reaction to light and pupil response to viewing a near target should be recorded. An invaluable tool for measuring visual acuity is a hand held pin hole device (Fig. 1.5) that allows a patient to have monocular view of an eye chart through small holes. Pin hole can eliminate refractive errors, ocular aberrations and correct monocular diplopia caused by the same. On the other hand macular disorders of the retina do not improve with pin hole.
- *An Amsler grid* can be used to identify macular diseases which can be confirmed on indirect ophthalmoscopy and fundus biomicroscopy.

GLOBE, ORBIT AND EYELID EXAMINATION

- The examiner should note periorbital swelling (Fig. 1.6), forward displacement proptosis (Fig. 1.7), backward displacement enophthalmos (Fig. 1.8) or sideways displacement (dystopia) of the globe.

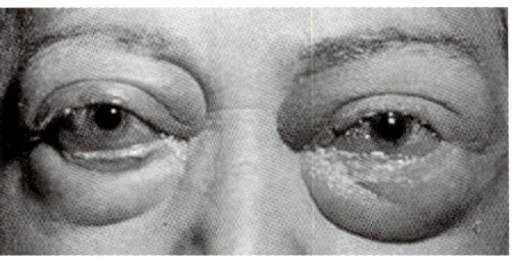

Fig. 1.6 *Periorbital swelling.*

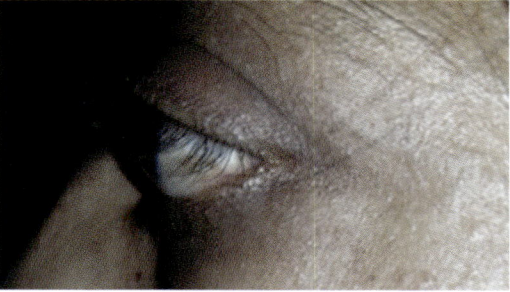

Fig. 1.7 *Proptosis.*

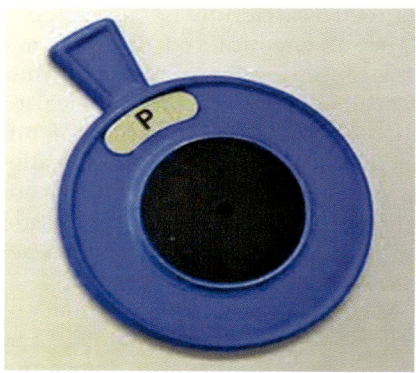

Fig. 1.5 *Pinhole.*

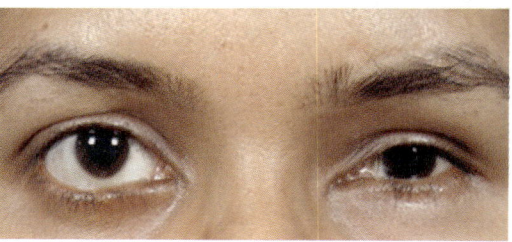

Fig. 1.8 *Enophthalmos.*

- An exophthalmometer is used to detect and measure proptosis. Reading greater than 21 mm for either eye or a differences of more than 2 mm between each eye indicates proptosis/enophthalmos.
- *Eyelid position and function* should be examined. When the upper eyelid is above the upperborder of iris and sclera is showing, lid retraction is diagnosed and if the eyelid "lags" behind the eye on downward eye pursuits lid lag is present (Fig. 1.9). These two signs are commonly present in thyroid associated ophthalmopathy, whereas eyelid retraction without lid lag is seen in dorsal midbrain disease. Ptosis is present if there is less than 4 mm between corneal light reflex and the upper eyelid with the patient fixating in primary gaze. Neurologic causes of ptosis result from dysfunction of the levator palpebrae muscle, controlled by the third cranial nerve or from dysfunction of the Müller's muscle, controlled by sympathetic innervations.

EXTRAOCULAR MUSCLE EXAMINATION

Ocular movement

The cardinal positions of gaze are examined by asking the patient to follow a target or the examiners finger held approximately 12 to 14 inches away from the patient's eyes. Ocular motility of each eye should be tested separately called ductions. Normal ductions rule out mechanical restriction of extraocular muscles but do not exclude possibility of paresis of extra ocular muscles as paretic eye may move normally into the paretic field due to maximal innervation. Paresis is diagnosed by testing the versions (binocular eye movements). We should note that whether both eyes move fully and

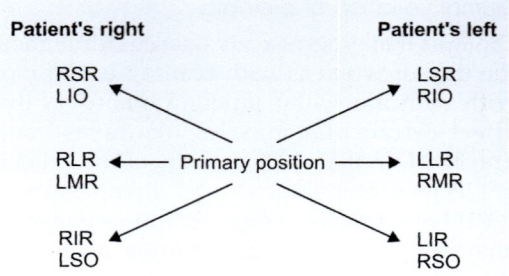

Fig. 1.10 *Eye movements in cardinal positions of gaze and corresponding muscles responsible for different directions of gaze.*

simultaneously or whether there is limitation or excessive movement of non-fixating eye. If duction/versions are limited, then one has to determine whether the limitation is caused by restrictive process, muscle weakness, neuro-muscular junction dysfunction, cranial nerve palsy or supranuclear injury. Figure 1.10 shows eye movements in cardinal positions of gaze and corresponding muscles responsible for different directions of gaze.

Forced duction test

Forced duction testing is done to detect mechanical restriction. When there is an actual restriction of movement, it becomes essential to determine, whether the restriction of movement is due to the primary underaction of paretic muscle or is it because of presence of contractures in the antagonist muscle. Under topical anesthesia the eye is moved with two toothed forceps, applied to the conjunctiva near the limbus in the direction opposite that in which mechanical restriction is suspected. If no resistance is encountered then the motility defect is caused by the paralysis of muscle. If resistance is encountered mechanical restrictions do exist and contracture of muscle, conjunctiva, tenon's capsule or myositis must be considered. Restrictive diplopia, due to orbital processes such as thyroid-associated ophthalmopathy, is associated with positive forced duction testing.

Active force generation test

Active force generation test determines the active force generated by a contracting muscle

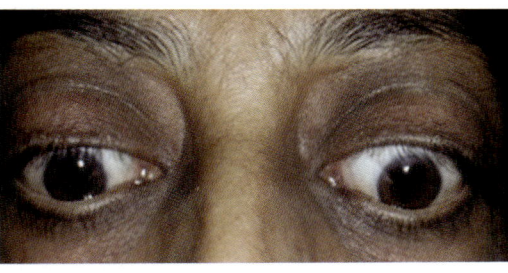

Fig. 1.9 *Lid lag.*

and is useful in assessing the function of apparently paretic muscles. The examiner stabilizes the eye with forceps while the patient tries to move the eye in the direction of paretic muscle against this obstacle. The presence of tug on the forceps indicates that residual innervation is present and there is incomplete or partial paralysis whereas absence of tug is due to complete paralysis of muscle.

The examination of a patient with ocular misalignment involves more than the evaluation of movement of eyes. The examiner should measure ocular alignment in various directions of gaze and with a right or left head tilt.

Measurement of deviation

Methods to measure diviation include:
1. Objective method
   - Prism bar cover test
2. Subjective methods
   - Red-green glasses
   - Maddox rod test
   - Maddox wing test
   - Hess and diplopia charting
   - Lees screen test

The motility disturbance will be obvious after inspection and testing of vergences. However, more subtle problems will require quantification of the misalignment using prism alternative cover or Maddox rod techniques.

Maddox rod test

Maddox rod can be used to determine the presence and degree of ocular misalignment. The red line is held over either the right or left eye while the patient focuses on a distant, pinpoint light source. The ridges are placed in the horizontal direction to evaluate for horizontal misalignment and in the vertical direction to evaluate for vertical misalignment. The relationship of the line to the light that the patient sees determine the type of misalignment (Fig. 1.11). The red line seen by the patient is oriented vertically, when the ridges are placed horizontally over the right/left eye and vice versa. The Maddox rod test is also useful in quantitating the degree of torsional misalignment.

BRAINSTEM EXAMINATION

The brainstem examination includes examination of all the cranial nerves (Fig. 1.12).

- 2nd, 3rd, 4th and 6th cranial nerve exam— visual acuity, eye movements in cardinal positions of gaze
- Facial strength and sensation
- Corneal sensations
- Masseter strength
- Hearing

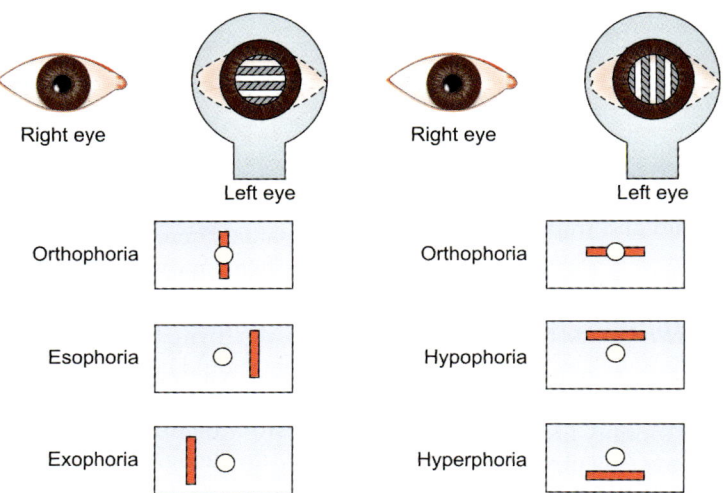

Fig. 1.11 *(A) Horizontally placed Maddox rod over left eye to detect horizontal misalignment; (B) Vertically placed Maddox rod over left eye to detect vertical misalignment.*

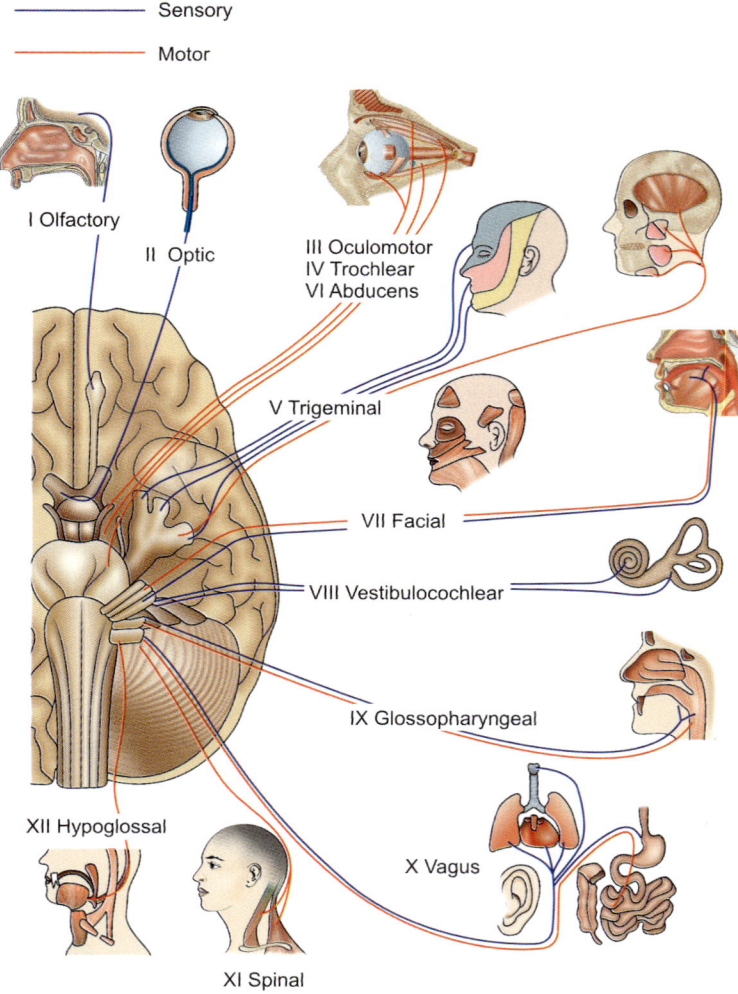

— Sensory

— Motor

I Olfactory

II Optic

III Oculomotor
IV Trochlear
VI Abducens

V Trigeminal

VII Facial

VIII Vestibulocochlear

IX Glossopharyngeal

XII Hypoglossal

X Vagus

XI Spinal

Fig. 1.12 *Cranial nerves: Origin and organs supplied.*

- Elevation of palate and uvula
- Sternocleidomastoid and trapezius strength
- Gag reflex
- Position and strength of tongue

SUPRANUCLEAR PATHWAY EXAMINATION

The most important examination feature of a supranuclear motility deficit is the ability to overcome the ocular motility limitation with an oculocephalic maneuver (oculocephalic reflex) depicted in Fig. 1.13.

In cases of supranuclear injury, the nuclei of 3rd, 4th and 6th cranial nerves are still intact and the cranial nerve fascicles are functioning normally. Therefore, stimulation of the nuclei with head movements should result in full ocular ductions.

To perform the oculocephalic reflex the patient should be instructed to fixate at a object/ target 14 to 16 inches away. Then, while the patient is fixating the patient's head is tilted slowly to the right/left and up/down. This head movement during fixation should overcome any limitations of ductions or versions due to supranuclear pathway dysfunction.

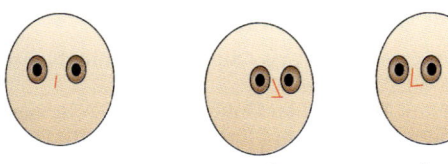

Head turns to side, but eyes are still facing forward, or move back to midline–infact brainstem

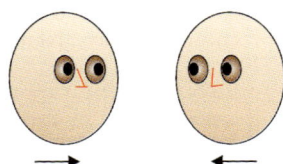

Head turns to side, eyes turns with the head, i.e. do not correct–brainstem affected

Fig 1.13 *Demonstration of oculocephalic reflex.*

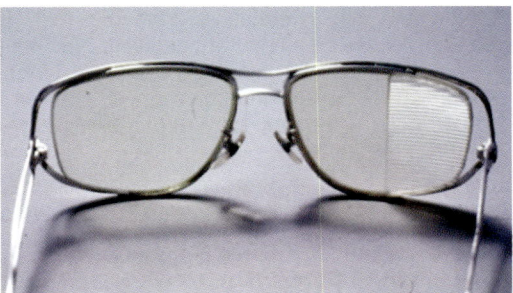

Fig. 1.14 *Stick on Fresnel prisms.*

INVESTIGATIONS

Investigations required depend on the suspected etiology of diplopia as follows:
- **Monocular diplopia**—refraction, pinhole vision
- **Orbital disorders**—USG/CT/MRI orbit
- **Neurological causes**—CT/MRI/MRA
- **Suspected Myasthenia**—Edrophonium test

TREATMENT

The ophthalmoparesis in some of the disorders described, such as ischemic and traumatic oculomotor palsies, will often resolve spontaneously. Other cases, such as those due to myasthenia gravis or bacterial meningitis, will improve as the underlying cause is treated.

Treatment modalities for diplopia are as under:
- *Glasses*
- *Stick-on occlusive lenses*
- *Fresnel prisms* (Fig. 1.14). Temporary Fresnel paste on prisms can be used initially followed by ground-in-prisms in chronic cases.
- *Patching.* Children patched for symptomatic relief should have the patch alternated daily between eyes to prevent occlusion amblyopia.
- *Chemo-denervation.* Botox therapy (Fig. 1.15)— Botulinum toxin injections into the antagonist muscle of a paretic one, even in supranuclear disorders.

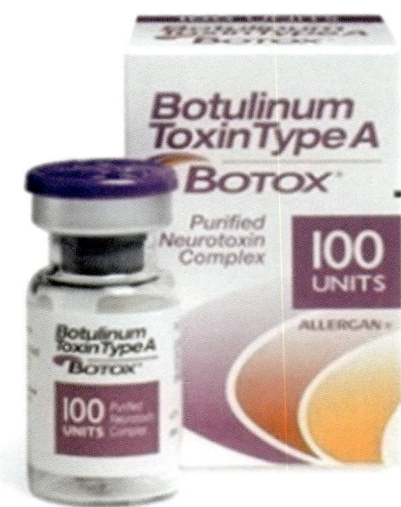

Fig. 1.15 *Botulinum toxin vial.*

- *Immunomodulation*—steroids, immunosuppressives
- *Surgical correction of strabismus*—individuals with paresis who do not improve spontaneously, and whose condition remains stable for 6 months, are candidates for corrective eye muscle surgery.
- *Speciality consultations*—neurology, endocrinology.

BIBLIOGRAPHY

CLINICO-INVESTIGATIVE APPROACH TO A PATIENT WITH VISUAL LOSS

1. Burde RM. "Amaurosisfugax. An overview". J Clin Neuro-ophthalmol 1989;9(3):185–9.

2. Newman NJ. "Cerebrovascular disease". In Hoyt, William Graves; Miller, Neil; Newman, Nancy J.; Walsh, Frank. Walsh and Hoyt's Clinical Neuro-ophthalmology. 3 (5th ed.). Baltimore: Williams & Wilkins 1998;3420–6. ISBN 0-683-30232-9.

3. Ravits J, Seybold ME. "Transient monocular visual loss from narrow-angle glaucoma". Arch. Neurol. 1984;41(9):991–3.

4. Sadun AA, Currie JN, Lessell S. "Transient visual obscurations with elevated optic discs". Ann. Neurol 1984;16(4):489–94.

5. Smit RL, Baarsma GS, Koudstaal PJ. "The source of embolism in amaurosisfugax and retinal, 1994.

CLINICAL WORK-UP FOR DIPLOPIA

1. Friedman DI. Pearls: diplopia. Semin Neurol Feb 2010;30(1):54–65.

2. Lutwak N. Binocular Double Vision—A Review. American Journal of Clinical Medicine 2011;8(3): 166–9.

3. Pelak VS. Evaluation of diplopia: an anatomic and systematic approach. Clinical review article. Hospital Physician March 2004;6–25.

4. Rucker JC, Tomsak RL. Binocular diplopia. A practical approach. Neurologist 2005;11(2):98–110.

5. Torun N. A practical approach to a patient with diplopia. Journal of Experimental and Clinical Medicine 2012;28:S55–57.

2 | IMAGING IN NEURO-OPHTHALMOLOGY

Urmil Chawla, AK Khurana, Neebha Passi

GENERAL CONSIDERATIONS
- Introduction
- Indication
- Neuroimaging modalities

COMPUTED TOMOGRAPHY (CT)
- Conventional CT
- Multislice helical CT
- Indication
- Disadvantages

MAGNETIC RESONANCE IMAGING (MRI)
- Basics of MRI
- Relaxation time
- Images
- Enhancement
- Limitations
- Comparison of CT and MRI capabilities

IMAGING IN SPECIFIC NEURO-OPHTHALMIC CONDITIONS
- Optic nerve disorders
- Chiasmal compressive lesions
- Cranial nerve palsies and ocular motality disorders
- Carotid cavernous fistula

NEUROVASCULAR IMAGING
- CT and MRI angiography
- MR venography
- Proton MR spectroscopy
- Catheter angiography

CONCLUSION
- Guidelines
- Common errors
- Suggestions for improving the results

GENERAL CONSIDERATIONS

INTRODUCTION

Neuro-ophthalmology is the speciality that deals with ophthalmic diseases with neurological problems and various optic nerve disorders. Eye being a superficial organ is easily accessible to the ophthalmologist for assessment using clinical tests. Although initial clinical assessment plays a vital role in assessment of the visual neural pathway, diagnostic imaging is required subsequently to assess the anatomy and pathology of the visual neural pathways.

Neuroradiological evaluation of visual disorders using computed tomography and magnetic resonance imaging has advanced dramatically during the past two decades. Plain radiographs, arteriograms, and pneumoencephalograms have been replaced by modern computed imaging using better signal characteristics, resulting in sound clinicopathological and biochemical correlations. Even more exciting is the advent of functional imaging techniques such as positron emission tomography (PET), single photon emission computed tomography (SPECT), and functional magnetic resonance imaging (fMRI) that reveal both pathophysiology and pathology of the visual apparatus. Other techniques such as computed tomographic and magnetic resonance angiography (CTA and MRA), super-selective catheter angiography, use of newer embolization materials, magnetic resonance spectroscopy, carotid and transcranial Doppler, and color-flow imaging provide valuable information to the modern neuro-ophthalmologist and neuro-diagnostician. A word of caution: although modern neuroimaging techniques have improved considerably our diagnostic speed and accuracy, they should not be used as a substitute for an excellent and thorough clinical evaluation.

INDICATIONS

Common indications for which radiological imaging is requested in neuro-ophthalmology cases are as follows:

- Visual loss, unilateral or bilateral
- Field defects and scotomas
- Anisocoria or ptosis
- Proptosis
- Diplopia or ophthalmoplegia
- Oscillopsia (for example, nystagmus)
- Ophthalmoscopic abnormalities (papilledema, drusen)
- Pupillary defects

NEUROIMAGING MODALITIES

Neuroimaging modalities available include:
- Computed tomography (CT)
- Magnetic resonance imaging (MRI)
- CT and MR angiographic techniques
- Catheter DSA
- fMRI
- PET and
- SPECT

Note. MRI is the imaging modality of choice in most of the conditions pertaining to neurophthalmology. CT would be preferred in patients where MRI is contraindicated, viz. metallic foreign bodies, pacemakers and cochlear implants.

COMPUTED TOMOGRAPHY (CT)

First results and descriptions of clinical CT were published in British Journal of Radiology in December 1973, by Hounsfield. CT rapidly became an excellent modality for investigation of CNS, because of relatively static CNS structures and ability to immobilize the head. It depends on relative attenuation of the radiation beam by tissues with different density and atomic number. With rapid advances in computational technology and radiological hardware, it is now possible to image large volumes in very short time, effectively removing the deleterious effects of even physiological movements such as respiration and cardiac motion.

Conventional CT was limited to scanning in one plane, i.e. the axial plane and other planes had to be reconstructed using computer manipulation leading to loss of resolution in the Z axis.

Multi slice helical CT allows acquisition of isometric volumes leading to spatial resolution in the sub mm range in all three planes, removing one of the big disadvantages of conventional CT.

CLINICAL INDICATIONS

In general, CT is easier and faster to perform than MRI but exposes the patient to ionizing radiation.
- The main advantage over MRI lies in detecting bony lesions such as fractures and erosions, and demonstrating skull anatomy. CT is therefore very useful for evaluating patients with orbital trauma and can display fractures and foreign bodies as well as blood, herniation of extraocular muscles and emphysema.
- CT can also detect intraocular calcification (optic disc drusen and retinoblastoma).
- CT is preferable for acute cerebral or subarachnoid hemorrhage because the lesions may not appear on MRI for hours.
- CT is as good or superior to MRI with fat suppression in demonstrating enlarged extraocular muscles in thyroid eye disease.
- CT can be used when MRI is contraindicated (i.e. patients with ferrous foreign bodies).

Disadvantages of CT include exposure to radiation, no direct sagittal imaging, possibility of contrast reactions, and dental or bony artifacts. The X-ray dose for a standard scan is 3–5 rads and 10 rads for a high-resolution scan. This is a very small dose as compared with 750–2000 rads needed to induce changes in the crystalline lens. The adjunctive intravenous injection of iodinated contrast provides enhancement in cranial CT to areas of increased vascularity and to areas of blood–brain barrier breakdown, through which seepage of iodinated contrast occurs. Contrast enhancement is used to detect intracranial extension of orbital tumors and evaluation of chiasmal and parachiasmal lesions. The use of intravenous iodinated contrast must be weighed against its risks, which include allergic reactions, nephrotoxicity, and anaphylactic shock that can be life-threatening. CT has the advantage over MRI of being a procedure that takes shorter time, is less expensive, and is useful in patients with contraindications or inability to perform MRI.

MAGNETIC RESONANCE IMAGING (MRI)

In current practice, MRI is the imaging modality of choice in all neuro-radiological imaging. With dense bone surrounding the optic nerve at the apex of orbit, MRI provides unique possibilities of assessing the intrinsic lesions of the optic nerves and tracts. The study depends on interaction of protons (hydrogen nuclei) with a strong magnetic field in which they are placed. The CT was an extension of conventional imaging where it studied attenuation differences in tissues. The use of detectors and computers to enhance the difference in attenuation, changed the amount of information available, but did not change the kind of information available. The MRI has proven to be a paradigm shift in imaging as it involves fundamentally different principles and physics for assessment of anatomy and pathology. MRI offers the possibility of varying many factors thus opening up a large vista of different protocols and sequences and thus can have a long learning curve.

BASICS OF MRI

MRI is based on the principle of nuclear magnetic resonance (NMR).

MRI depends on the rearrangement of hydrogen nuclei (protons—positively charged) when a tissue is exposed to a short electromagnetic pulse (the "Nuclear" bit).

The subject is placed inside a giant superconducting magnet that causes randomly aligned protons to align with the axis (north-south) of the magnet (the "Magnetic" bit).

When these protons are stimulated by a radiofrequency (RF) pulse they absorb energy and spin in the direction of the pulse (the "Resonance" bit).

When the RF pulse is turned off, the protons relax back to their original alignment—and give off the energy absorbed during the RF pulse. These energy signals are detected and converted into MRI image (the " Imaging" bit).

RELAXATION TIMES

T1 and T2 weighing refers to two methods of measuring the relaxation times of the excited protons after the magnetic field has been switched off. Various body tissues have different relaxation times so that a given tissue may be T1- or T2-weighted (that is best visualized on that particular type of image). In practice both types of scans are performed.

IMAGES

1. **T1-weighted images**
   - Best for normal anatomy
   - Water (vitreous/CSF) appears dark (hypo-intense)
   - Fat (orbit) appears bright (hyperintense)

2. **T2-weighted images**
   - Preferred for viewing pathological changes
   - Water (vitreous/CSF) appears very bright (hyperintense)
   - Fat (orbit) appears dark (hypointense)

Enhancement

1. Contrast MRI (gadolinium) image

Gadolinium is a substance which acquires a magnetic moment when placed in an electromagnetic field. It is administered intravenously.
- Looks like T1 image but blood vessels/extraocular muscles appear bright.
- Active lesions enhance (infections/MS plaques)
- Contraindicated in pregnancy/allergy to gadolinium.

Hence, contrast MRI is very helpful in the detection of tumors and inflammatory lesions. It is safer than iodine; adverse effects are uncommon and usually relatively innocuous (nausea, hives and headache).

FLAIR image
- Fluid attenuation inversion recovery sequence
- Water is suppressed and appears dark.
- Used in brain studies.
- Looks like a T2 image in that pathology appears bright but water (CSF) appears dark.
- Useful in studying deep white matter plaques adjacent to ventricles (the bright plaques are easily seen contrasted against the adjacent dark ventricles)

2. Fat suppression

The bright signal of orbital fat on conventional T1-weighted imaging frequently obscures other orbital contents. Fat suppression helps in eliminating this bright signal and better delineates both normal structures (optic nerve and extraocular muscles) as well as tumors, inflammatory lesions and vascular malformations.

SPIR/STIR images

- STIR (Short tau inversion recovery).
- SPIR (Spatial presaturation inversion recovery).

However, fat suppression may be associated with various artefacts and should be used in conjunction with, rather than instead of, conventional imaging.

Diffusion Weighted Image (DWI)

Usually an axial brain image looks like a T1 image (water dark) but pathology may appear either as dark or bright patches).

Limitations of MRI

- Imaging of bone not possible (which appears black), although this is not necessarily a disadvantage.
- It does not detect recent hemorrhage and is therefore inappropriate in patients with acute intracranial bleeding.

- Its use is contraindicated in patients with magnetic foreign objects (e.g. cardiac pacemakers, intraocular foreign bodies).
- It requires the patient to cooperate and remain motionless.
- It is difficult to perform in claustrophobic patients.

Brief comparison of CT and MRI capabilities as shown in Table 2.1.

IMAGING IN SPECIFIC NEURO-OPHTHALMIC CONDITIONS

Optic nerve disorders

MRI with contrast is the imaging modality of choice in patients suspected to have
- Optic neuritis
- Optic neuropathy
- Optic nerve tumors

Optic neuritis

- Coronal and axial T2 fat saturation images are most sensitive in identifying signal in the optic nerves.
- Post contrast study should include axial, coronal and sagittal T1 fat saturation images parallel to the optic nerves (Fig. 2.1).

Table 2.1 *Comparison of CT and MRI capabilities*

CT	MRI
Ionizing radiation	Magnetic field
Limited planes (axial and coronal images)	Multiplanar imaging (axial, coronal, sagittal, and angled images)
Excellent visualization of acute hemorrhage	Difficult visualization of acute hemorrhage
Useful in assessing retro-orbital mass in proptosis	Fat suppression with contrast essential for assessment
Excellent for bone and bony lesions, sinuses and calcification	Excellent for soft tissue delineation
Posterior fossa degraded by artifact	Well visualized
Limited visualization near dense bone	Dense bone does not impose any limitation
Poor resolution of demyelinating lesions	Demyelinating lesions well seen at all stages
Iodinated contrast agent	Paramagnetic contrast agent
Metal artifacts (skull plates, clips)	Ferromagnetic artifacts
Quick to attain, easily available, inexpensive	Limited availability, time consuming, expensive
Indications: orbital inflammation, trauma, tumor, thyroid ophthalmopathy, disc drusen, foreign body	Orbital tumor, optic nerve glioma, orbital apex and parasellar lesions

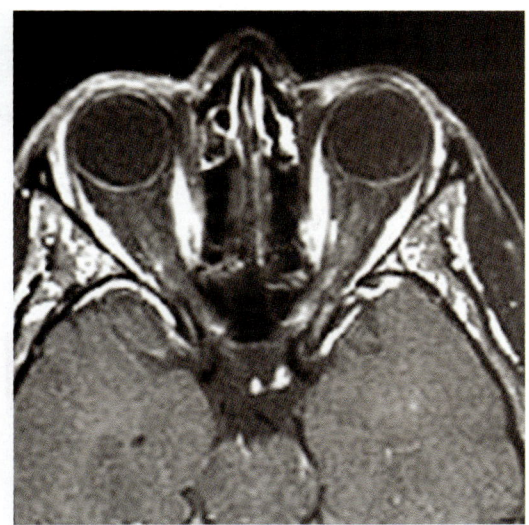

Fig. 2.1 *Axial, fat-suppressed, postcontrast, T1-weighted image demonstrates enhancement in the intracanalicular portion of the left optic nerve.*

- In patients suspected to have demyelination—brain and spine screening should always be performed.
- Brain contrast in patients with demyelinating plaques should be performed using magnetization transfer techniques.
- MR spectroscopy can be performed in patients with diagnostic dilemma.

Optic nerve tumors

The two most commonly encountered tumors of the optic nerve are meningioma and glioma which need to be differentiated (Table 2.2).

Traumatic optic neuropathy

- CT scan of the brain and orbit should be done to look for fracture of the optic canal.
- 1–2 mm thick sections should be obtained in both axial and coronal planes if patient's general condition permits coronal imaging. The axial sections should be parrelel to the optic nerves. Coronal sections are perpendicular to the axial sections.
- If CT scan does not show fracture, it should be followed by MRI to look for optic nerve contusion, avulsion or hematoma.
- MRI using surface coil is preferred in patients suspected to have optic nerve avulsion clinically.

Chiasmal compressive lesions

MRI should be done in patients suspected to have chiasmal lesions (Fig. 2.5). CT would be a cost effective modality in patients who cannot afford MRI.

MRI is superior to CT in:

- Identifying small lesions especially vascular
- Characterization of the lesion

	Table 2.2 *Differences between optic nerve glioma and optic nerve meningioma*	
	Optic nerve glioma	*Optic nerve meningioma*
Age	Young	Relatively older
Clinical History	Visual loss is earlier proptosis +	Visual loss is later proptosis +/–
Imaging CT	• Intraconal heterogenous fusiform mass inseparable from the optic nerve • Optic canal widening • Calcification absent • Cystic changes +	• Intraconal homogenous mass inseparable from the optic nerve • Optic canal normal • Calcification +/– • No cystic changes (Fig. 2.2)
Imaging MRI	• Fusiform heterogenous intraconal mass inseparable from the optic nerve • A mixed signal in T2-weighted images • Intracranial extension better visualized (Fig. 2.3)	• Fusiform homogenous perioptic mass, encased optic nerve seen separately • Homogenous signal in T2-weighted images—mostly hypointense • Intracranial extension is better visualized (Fig. 2.4)

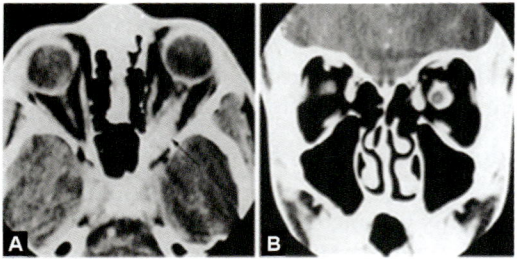

Fig. 2.2 *Axial and coronal images of CT scan orbit showing high density mass around optic nerve, favoring left optic nerve meningioma.*

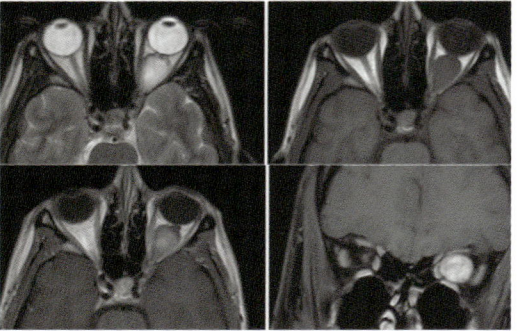

Fig. 2.3 *MRI of orbit (T2, T1 axial and coronal fat sat sequences) showing left optic nerve glioma.*

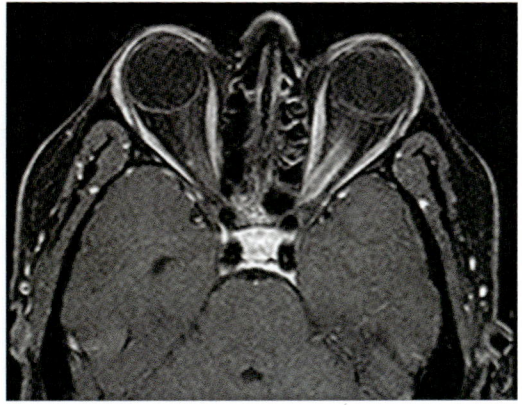

Fig. 2.4 *MRI of a patient with optic nerve sheath meningioma.*

- Extent and invasion of the surrounding structures
- Helps in surgical planning

CT is superior in identifying calcification and bony erosion.

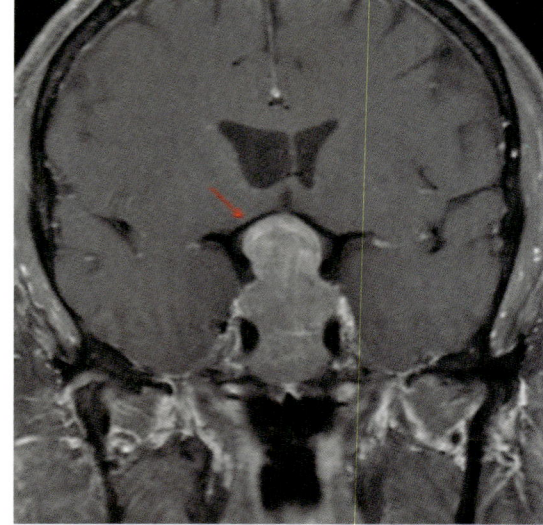

Fig. 2.5 *MRI of the sella in coronal image of post contrast T1 sequence shows pituitary macroadenoma compressing chiasma from below (arrow).*

Cranial nerve palsies and ocular motility disorders

- MRI is the modality of choice.
- MRI with contrast is preferable in patients suspected to have cranial nerve palsies.
- MR angiogram should be done in patients with pupil involving third nerve, followed by DSA if MRI is negative.
- Thin axial and coronal sections should be obtained to include the orbit, cavernous sinus and brainstem.

Carotid cavernous fistula (CCF)

- Dynamic contrast enhanced MRI should be done in patients suspected to have CCF to confirm the diagnosis as it is noninvasive and helps to exclude other lesions (Fig. 2.6). A negative MRI does not exclude CCF.
- MRI cannot completely delineate the type of fistula.
- DSA is the confirmatory imaging modality.

Note. The choice of the imaging modality should depend on the patient's clinical diagnosis, availability of the facility and cost factor.

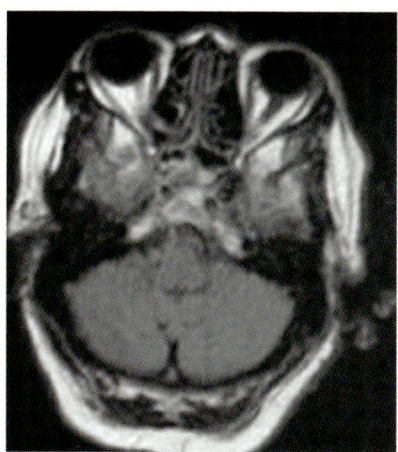

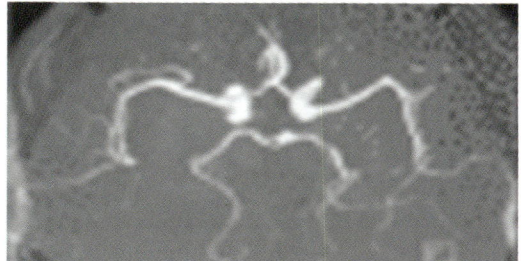

Fig. 2.8 *MR angiography showing normal vasculature at the skull base.*

Fig. 2.6 *MRI showing abnormal flow void in the left cavernous sinus region in a patient with an underlying carotid-cavernous fistula.*

- Images are not of the actual blood vessel itself as in a conventional arteriogram but blood flow characteristics within the vessel (Fig. 2.8).

Uses. Clinical diagnosis/MR study suggests aneurysm or AV malformation.

NEUROVASCULAR IMAGING

CT and MR angiography

The patients with suspected vascular abnormalities may undergo assessment using MR or CT angiographic techniques.

CT angiography entails assessment of arteries after intravenous injection of iodinated contrast; it provides anatomical information (Fig. 2.7). On the contrary, MR depends on flowing blood to provide contrast, and MRA can be done with or without intravenous contrast.

MR angiography (MRA)

- MRA is of two types: 2D or 3D Time of Flight MRA (common), and Phase Contrast MRA (less common).

MR venography (MRV)

Similar to MRA except it is commonly used to image dural venous sinuses.

Uses. Cavernous sinus thrombosis, idiopathic intracranial hypertension (hypoplasia or thrombosis of venous sinuses).

Proton MR spectroscopy (MRS)

Profiles biochemical alterations within brain lesions.

Common metabolites studied—choline, creatine, N-acetyl aspartate, lactate, lipids.

Image. Appears as a spectroscopic graph with various metabolite peaks, and a corresponding brain image with a box marking the area studied.

Uses. Brain tumor, stroke, focal cerebral lesions, MS, and intracranial hemorrhage. Not used for orbit lesions owing to smaller lesion size.

Catheter angiography and treatment

Prior to advent of the CT and MR angiography, catheter angiography formed the basis of all vascular assessment in the CNS. Besides being an invasive procedure, it has the potential to precipitate potentially devastating neurological sequelae. As a result, the CT and the MR angiographic techniques are supplanting catheter

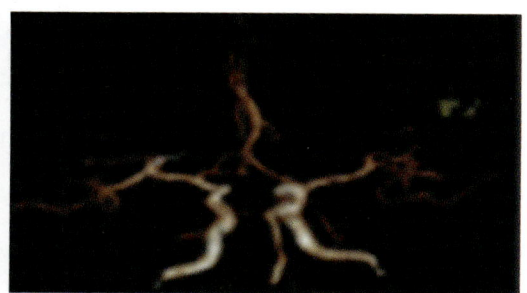

Fig. 2.7 *CT angiography showing a right middle cerebral artery aneurysm.*

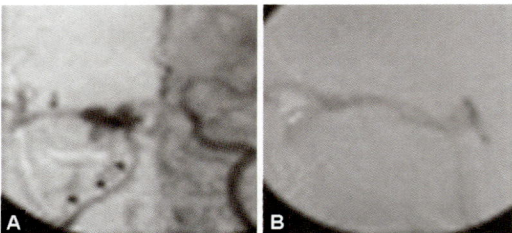

Fig. 2.9 *Catheter DSA in a patient with caroticocavernous fistula: The black arrows and arrowheads in (A) show orbital veins, and in (B) show catheterization of fistula prior to endovascular treatment.*

angiography for diagnostic purposes. However, with advances in catheter techniques and materials, catheter angiography has come to play a central role in endovascular management of many CNS vascular lesions with excellent results (Fig. 2.9).

CONCLUSION

GUIDELINES

In general, MRI is the investigation of choice for most neuro-ophthalmological assessments. CT is better for evaluation of bony orbit in patients of trauma or suspected destructive osseous lesions. It is also superior for detection of presence of calcification such as in optic nerve drusen. The fact that MRI entails so many different variables leading to many sequences such as T1, T2-weighted, FLAIR, GRE, diffusion weighted imaging, spectroscopy, etc. means that the studies need to be tailored to the patients' needs and clinical requirement. As in CT, IV contrast improves visualization of the lesions. Typically, the clinician need not worry about different sequences, as the imaging radiologist will decide which sequences will provide maximum information, depending on the patients' clinical picture in the shortest time. This in turn places extra responsibility on the shoulder of the referring physician to provide complete and accurate information regarding the patients' clinical profile, as it will determine what imaging the patient should undergo. Typically, the clinical information must include the site of suspected lesion and if possible the nature of suspected lesion. The information on site is important to allow detailed study of the

relevant area. As detailed study of multiple areas in one examination ends up adding the time required for each examination individually; which leads to a very long and time consuming examination which in turn reduces the patient cooperation. Another potential down side in trying to cover a large area is reduced resolution in an attempt to reduce time of examination. The information regarding the nature of the suspected pathology is important in deciding the protocol of examination and if intravenous contrast is required. In case of any doubt or confusion regarding which examination would best serve the interests of the patient, the best course of action would be to contact the radiologist. Direct interaction with the radiologist will reduce the potential for miscommunication and allow the radiologist to ask for supplementary information and give his suggestions regarding the best course of action.

COMMON ERRORS

Wolintz et al. in 2004 reviewed their case material for assessing the errors in use of MRI for neuro-ophthalmic disorders. According to them the errors could be divided into prescriptive and interpretive errors. Each of these categories could further be divided into four types.

Prescriptive errors

The four prescriptive errors are:
• Failure to apply a dedicated study.
• Inappropriate application of a dedicated study.
• Omission of intravenous contrast.
• Omission of specialized sequences.

Interpretive errors

The interpretive errors are:
• Failure to detect a lesion because of misleading clinical information.
• Rejection of a clinical diagnosis because an expected imaging abnormality was absent.
• Assumption that a striking abnormality accounted for the clinical abnormality.
• Failure to consider lack of clinical specificity of the imaging abnormalities.

After reviewing the above points it is clear that most of the errors resulted directly from inadequate communication between the referring clinician and the performing and interpreting radiologist.

SUGGESTIONS FOR IMPROVING THE RESULTS

The most common point of dispute is when either the imaging is normal in face of definite clinical signs or the imaging finding is not able to explain the clinical profile of the patient. In these cases the solution is to call the radiologist and discuss the case. Preferably, the neuro-ophthalmologist and the radiologist should together see the images and ensure the adequacy of the study. In such cases, the clinician brings his clinical acumen and possibly additional clinical data to the table and then the radiologist can make sure that the clinically relevant areas are imaged adequately without any artifacts. In case, the clinical symptomatology is progressive, it is also appropriate during this discussion to see if additional imaging with different imaging parameters such as different magnification or slice thickness will improve or add to the quality of imaging. Finally the referring clinician must realize that the images are representation of different processes in the patient and could be normal in face of definite clinical findings.

BIBLIOGRAPHY

1. Johnson LN, et al. Magnetic Resonance Imaging of Craniopharyngioma. Am J Ophthalmol 1986; 102:242–4.
2. Kanski JJ. Orbit. In: Clinical Ophthalmology: a systematic approach, 6th edn. Elsevier Butterworth Heinemann; 2007; p 170.
3. Kanski JJ. Neuro-ophthalmology. In: Clinical Ophthalmology: a systematic approach, 6th edn. Elsevier Butterworth Heinemann 2007; p 811.
4. Lindblow B, Truwit C, Hoyt WF. Optic nerve sheath meningioma: definition of intraorbital, intracanalicular and intracranial components with Magnetic Resonance Imaging. Ophthalmology 1992;99:560–6.
5. Lee AG, Johnson MC, Policeni BA, Smoker WR. Imaging for neuro-ophthalmic and orbital disease—a review. Clin Experiment Ophthalmol 2009;37(1):30–53.
6. Mandell N, Abrahams JJ. The Orbit. In: Computed Tomography and Magnetic Resonance Imaging of the whole body, 3rd edn. Mosby Year Book 1994;1:423.
7. Pusey E, et al. Magnetic Resonance imaging of Craniopharyngioma: tumour delineation and characterization. AJ NR 1987;8:439–44.
8. Zonneveld FW: Normal direct Multiplanar CT anatomy of the orbit with correlative anatomic cryosections. Radiol Clin North Am 1987; 25:381–407.

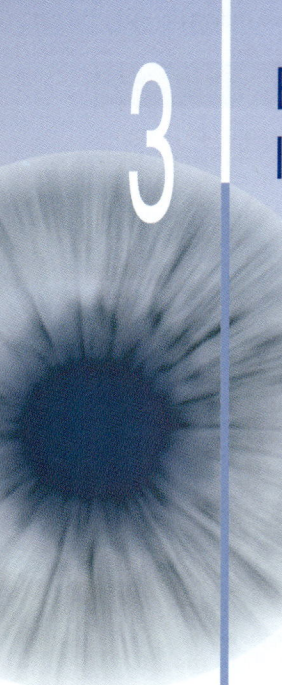

3

ELECTRODIAGNOSTIC TECHNIQUES IN NEURO-OPHTHALMOLOGY

Devendra V Venkatramani, Rashmin A Gandhi

VISUAL-EVOKED POTENTIAL (VEP)
- Types of VEP recording
- Aanlysis of VEP record
- Clinical uses of the VEP
- Multifocal VEP

ELECTRORETINOGRAPHY
- Origin of ERG waves
- Recording of ERG
- Analysis of ERG waveforms
- Pattern ERG
- Photopic negative response (PNR)
- Multifocal ERG

ELECTRO-OCULOGRAM (EOG)
- Recording of EOG
- Clinical uses

ELECTROMYOGRAPHY (EMG)
CLINICAL SCENARIOS
- Discriminating between a suspected optic neuropathy or maculopathy
- Evaluation of suspected functional visual loss
- Determining potential visual function in an eye with media opacity

VISUAL-EVOKED POTENTIAL (VEP)

The visual-evoked potential (VEP) is, as the name suggests, a record of electric activity obtained after providing a visual stimulus. In this regard, it is similar to other evoked potentials, like brain-evoked response audiometry (BERA) and somatosensory evoked potentials. The VEP recording can be considered to be part of an electroencephalographic (EEG) recording, in which the electrodes are placed over the occipital cortex. Signal averaging techniques help to amplify the VEP signal.

Retinal topographic representation of the VEP. The VEP is known to grossly over represent the macular region (the central visual field) for two reasons. Anatomically, it is the macular fibers which project to the occipital lobe cortex; those from the peripheral retina project deeper within the calcarine fissure. Hence, signal activity closest to the surface recording electrodes originates from the macular area. Additionally, as the visual impulse progresses from the retina

to the occipital cortex, the macular field gets 'amplified'.

TYPES OF VEP RECORDING

The VEP is an evoked potential. Hence, it is logical to suppose that the electric activity produced should vary with the nature of the stimulus provided. For testing purposes, two types of stimuli are used—either a flash of light (flash VEP—fVEP) or a pattern (pattern VEP—pVEP).

Flash VEP

To record a flash VEP, flashes of light are produced by a xenon-arc photostimulator. The flash has an intensity of 3 cd.s/m² against a background intensity of 15–30 cd/m². The flash should subtend a visual field of at least 20 degrees. This test is performed in a dimly illuminated room.

Pattern stimuli are in the form of a checkerboard pattern, which is a grid of alternate black and white squares. This pattern can be presented in either an 'onset-offset' manner,

34

wherein the pattern is displayed for a brief period and then replaced with a blank screen of the same intensity, or in a 'pattern reversal' manner in which the black and white checks reverse their orientation. In either case, it is important to note that the potential evoked by the stimulus should be due solely to a change in the pattern, and not due to a change in the light intensity (brightness). Any change in brightness during the test would result in luminance contamination.

As the fovea picks up finer stimuli compared to the parafoveal area, these areas can be differentially tested by varying the pattern check size from 10–15 to 50 minutes.

The VEP is recorded monocularly with undilated pupils. The patient should wear his/her refractive correction and sit in a relaxed position at a recording distance of one meter from the monitor.

ANALYSIS OF VEP RECORD

Like any electric potential tracing, the VEP is recorded and analysed as a waveform, with potential (microvolts) on the y-axis and time (milliseconds) on the x-axis. Properties which lend themselves to analysis are the amplitude, latency, and waveform (Figs 3.1 and 3.2).

1. *Amplitude* is the vertical height of the wave measured in microvolts from the preceding trough. In general, if the absolute amplitude of the P100 (the positive deflection at or around 100 milliseconds after stimulus presentation) is less than 5 microvolts, it is considered abnormal. However, it is difficult to standardize absolute values of amplitude because of the large variation between normal persons and variations in sensitivities of recording equipment. Relative amplitude (difference between the two eyes) is more commonly used when looking for unilateral or asymmetric disease.

2. *Latency* (milliseconds) is the delay between stimulus presentation and the peak of the wave in question. Latency shows less variation between subjects, but it can be affected by a number of factors such as pupil size, refractive error, age and stimulus factors (pattern size, luminance and contrast). The latency of the P100 wave should not exceed 110 ms in patients under the age of 60 years.

3. *Waveform* is the overall appearance of the wave.

There are two other methods of presenting a stimulus depending on whether the brain is allowed to adapt in between repetitive stimuli. If the visual stimulus is presented intermittently, allowing the brain to recover its resting state in between, the VEP obtained is called a transient VEP. If however the stimulus is projected at a faster rate that the brain does not regain its resting state, a sinusoidal waveform called the steady-state VEP is obtained. The transient VEP is used for all practical purposes—the steady-state VEP, though easy to describe quantitatively does not allow analysis of specific amplitude or latency components.

CLINICAL USES OF THE VEP

The VEP tests the integrity of the visual pathway, right from the retina up to the occipital cortex.

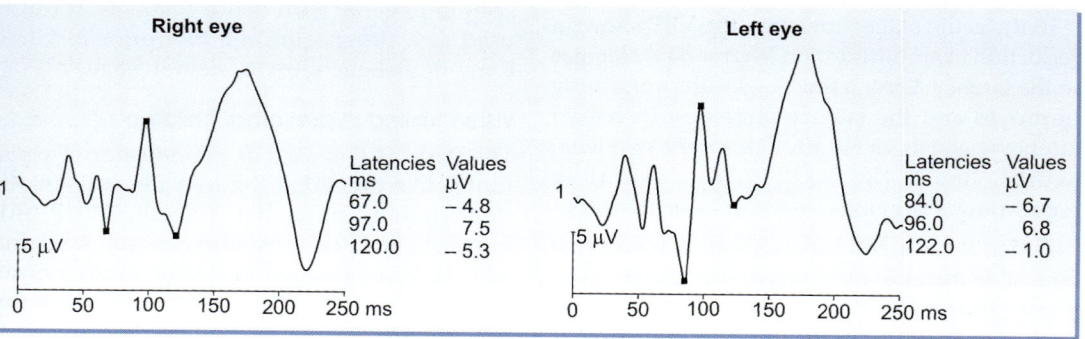

Fig. 3.1 *Flash VEP in a normal subject.*

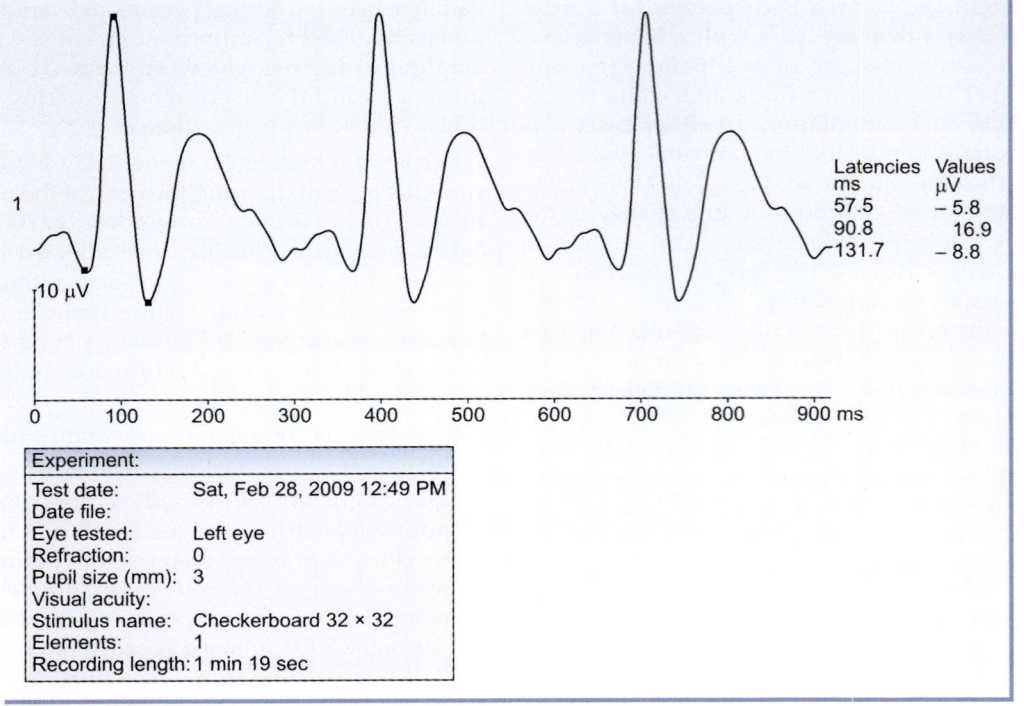

Latencies ms	Values µV
57.5	− 5.8
90.8	16.9
131.7	− 8.8

Experiment:

Test date:	Sat, Feb 28, 2009 12:49 PM
Date file:	
Eye tested:	Left eye
Refraction:	0
Pupil size (mm):	3
Visual acuity:	
Stimulus name:	Checkerboard 32 × 32
Elements:	1
Recording length:	1 min 19 sec

Fig. 3.2 *Pattern VEP in a normal subject.*

Optic neuritis and multiple sclerosis (MS)

The myelin sheath provides insulation to the neuron as well as greatly increases the speed of conduction. The electric impulse jumps from one node of Ranvier to the next, a process called salutatory conduction. Therefore the hallmark of demyelinating disease is slowing of conduction velocity. This is detected by the pattern VEP as a delayed P100 latency (Fig. 3.3).

In the acute stage, however, the VEP shows a reduction in amplitude and less marked changes in the latency. Over a few weeks, the amplitude improves and the latency increases. Increased latency persists even after recovery of visual acuity, hence the VEP can be useful in confirming a previous attack of optic neuritis.

Patients with MS but without a history or clinical features of optic nerve involvement can show abnormal VEP responses to pattern stimulation, suggesting subclinical visual pathway involvement.

In eyes with media opacity

The flash VEP is the test of choice in this situation. It can be performed in eyes with very poor vision, as the test does not need active patient participation.

The flash VEP can test the visual pathway in adults and children with dense media opacity.

A good correlation between VEP prediction and actual postoperative visual acuity has been seen in patients with dense cataracts. It can be used as a prognosticating tool prior to vitrectomy in diabetic vitreous hemorrhage.

Vision testing in preverbal children

The flash VEP is used as an indicator of visual function in preverbal children. Once again, it is important to note that a normal VEP only indicates an intact visual pathway. A normal VEP may be obtained in a structurally normal but behaviourally blind child, suggesting that the problem lies in visual association areas and not in the primary visual cortex . Flash VEP ha

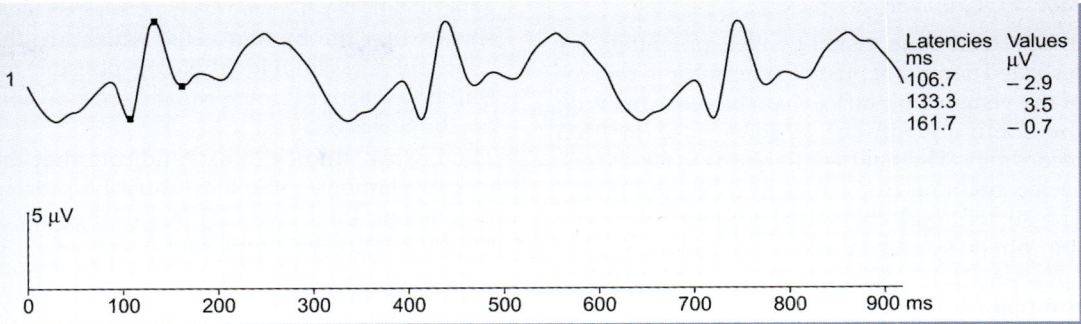

Latencies ms	Values μV
106.7	− 2.9
133.3	3.5
161.7	− 0.7

Fig. 3.3 *VEP in optic neuritis showing increased latency of the P100 wave.*

been noted to be abnormal in most studies in infants with delayed visual maturation.

The flash VEP has also been used to evaluate the central nervous system in neonates born prematurely, with intraventricular hemorrhage, or hydrocephalus. Controlled studies have shown a significantly higher proportion of abnormal flash VEP in high-risk infants as compared to normal full-term neonates.

Sweep VEP, originally described in 1985, is a specialized testing method. The stimulus is in the form of a grating, that is, a pattern of alternating dark and light bands. The width of the band (spatial frequency) can be altered. The VEP amplitude obtained is recorded over a range of spatial frequencies. A graph is then plotted of amplitude (microvolts) versus spatial frequency (cycles per degree). Grating acuity can be derived from this graph by extrapolating the spatial frequency to zero microvolts. This technique provides an objective assessment of visual acuity (grating acuity) in preverbal children.

Children with motor disorders may appear behaviorally blind, because the eyes may be unable to track a moving object. In such children preferential looking tests can falsely underestimate visual acuity. Additionally, seizure activity, wandering eye movements, and depressed cortical activity due to anti-epileptic drugs confound examination. In this situation, the VEP provides objective data.

In eyes with nystagmus, using a stimulus in the form of parallel stripes oriented along the plane of nystagmus reduces blur, and can

provide a more accurate measure of visual acuity. Pattern onset rather than pattern reversal stimulus may provide more accurate information.

In non-organic visual loss

In patients with normal or innocuous ocular findings and uncertain history, one may require to depend upon more objective tests to distinguish between organic and non-organic (functional) visual loss. In such patients, a normal pattern VEP to small checks (which tests the foveal region) establishes the presence of an intact visual pathway.

However, voluntary suppression of the VEP has been shown to be possible by using techniques such as concentrating beyond the plane of the checks, transcendental meditation, or by convergence. Some of these techniques involve defocusing the pattern, which correlates with the finding that optimum refractive correction is needed for recording the VEP. These can be overcome by special testing methods (described later).

In compressive lesions

The VEP shows a prolonged latency at an early stage, though not as much as in optic neuritis. There is a much higher incidence of waveform abnormalities than in patients with demyelinating disease.

In AION

Both flash and pattern VEPs show reduced amplitudes but normal latencies.

MULTIFOCAL VEP

In this technique visual-evoked potentials are recorded simultaneously from multiple regions of the visual field. mfVEP can be recorded with the same equipment available for mfERG recordings. The field is divided into 60 sectors, each containing 16 checks—8 black and 8 white. The sectors and checks are scaled differently (peripheral sectors larger) so that they are all of approximately equal effectiveness for cortical stimulation.

Pseudo-random sequences and a software algorithm allow the on-board computer to rapidly extract information simultaneously from each of the stimulated sectors.

Data is presented in topographic form, as well as the averaged signal waveforms for each quadrant. A probability plot is also provided.

The mfVEP has the ability to detect small abnormalities in visual signal transmission from centric and eccentric field. The mfVEP can be used to rule out non-organic visual loss, diagnose and follow-up patients of optic neuritis and multiple sclerosis, and confirm unreliable or questionable visual field examinations.

ELECTRORETINOGRAPHY

The electroretinography (ERG) is a method of recording the electrical activity of the retina, where the summative waveform is produced by individual retinal layers.

ORIGIN OF ERG WAVES

- The a-wave of the human ERG is generated by the photoreceptors, namely the rods and cones, and relates well with the phototransduction reaction. It is electronegative because the photoreceptor impulse occurs by hyperpolarization (i.e. becoming more negative) rather than by depolarization.
- The b-wave origin is less clear. In eyes following central retinal artery occlusion the b-wave is abolished whereas the a-wave is largely preserved, showing that the b-wave is derived from the inner retinal layers supplied by the central retinal artery. Subsequent studies suggested that the Müller cells

generate the b-wave; more recent reports have shown that the bipolar cells, which are the source of potassium ion fluxes responsible for Müller cell activity, are ultimately responsible for the b-wave.

- The c-wave studies in cats indicate that the retinal pigment epithelium must be present to generate the c-wave, although the photoreceptors also contribute to it.

RECORDING OF ERG

The ERG is recorded using a silver electrode mounted in a contact lens (active electrode). The lid speculum can be converted into an inactive electrode, the combination forming a bipolar electrode.

It is possible to differentiate rod and cone responses on the basis of either their spectral sensitivities, or using their optimal temporal rates of stimulation.

- *The scotopic ERG* (rod-dominant) is performed in the dark-adapted state. Blue light is used as a stimulus against a dim background illumination.
- *The photopic ERG* represents the cone response. Temporal summation occurs in rods at lower stimulation rates; flickering stimuli presented at 30 Hz, therefore, elicit a cone response. A combined rod and cone response can be obtained using relatively intense white stimuli.
- *Oscillatory potentials* are small wavelets superimposed on the ascending limb of the b-wave in normal subjects. Special recording techniques allow these to be isolated. They represent the activity of the inner retinal layers and often absent in patients with inner retinal ischemia such as in diabetic retinopathy.

ANALYSIS OF ERG WAVEFORMS

The ERG waveform can be described in terms of:

1. *Latency.* The time interval between the stimulus onset and the response onset.
2. *Implicit time.* Time required for the response to reach maximum amplitude.
3. *Amplitude.* Wave height measured from the baseline.
4. *b : a ratio.* Can be used as an index of inner to outer retinal function.

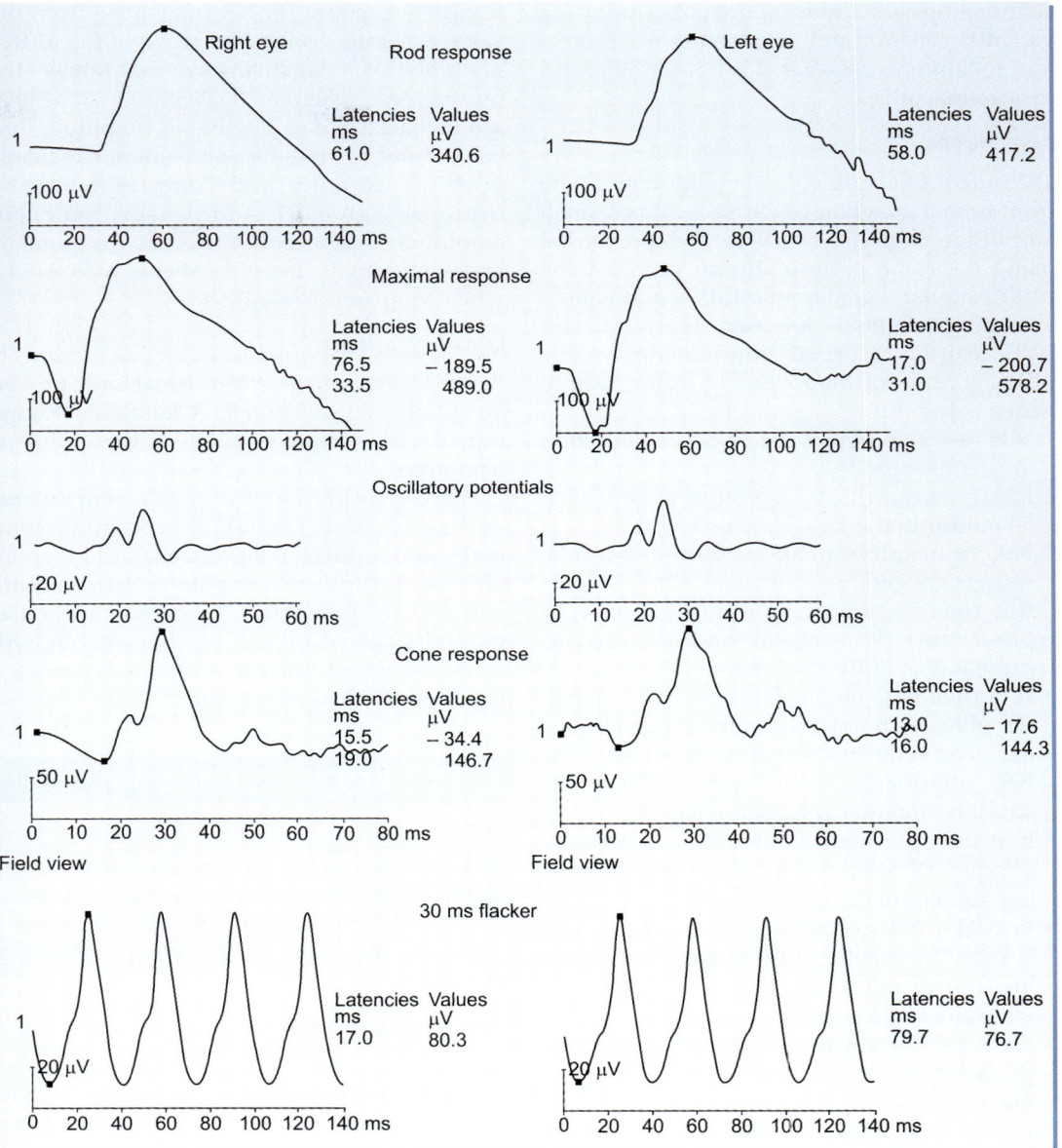

Fig. 3.4 *Flash ERG in a normal subject.*

Just like the VEP, the ERG can also be elicited using flash or pattern stimuli. The flash ERG represents the sum of responses obtained from over the entire retina ('mass response') (Fig. 3.4). Hence, it is not sensitive to focal abnormalities in the retina. On the other hand, it is quite useful to detect rod and cone dystrophies that diffusely affect the entire retina. The flash ERG is also sensitive to retinal ischemia, and can be used to monitor patients with dense vitreous hemorrhage due to diabetic retinopathy.

The ERG can help differentiate retinal disorders from neuro-ophthalmic disease. It is abnormal in congenital stationary night blindness, congenital achromatopsia, retinitis pigmentosa (including variants), cone-rod and cone dystrophies, cancer- and melanoma-associated retinopathies, and toxic retinopathies.

PATTERN ERG

The pattern ERG (pERG) is thought to originate from retinal ganglion cell activity. It is a small amplitude response (1 µV to 4 µV) recorded using the same pattern stimuli used for the pVEP; similar signal-amplification and signal-averaging techniques are used. The pERG and pVEP can be recorded simultaneously. The pERG consists of the following major components:

1. N35 (a-wave) which is a negative deflection at 30 milliseconds.
2. P50 (b-wave) which is a positive peak at 45 to 50 milliseconds.
3. N95, a negative peak at 95 milliseconds, reflects ganglion cell function.

It is convenient to think of the P50 wave as representative of the macula and N95 wave as representative of the optic nerve.

- A normal ERG but an abnormal P50 wave in the pERG thus suggests pathology relatively localized to the macular area. Affection of the N95 component with a normal P50 wave strongly suggests optic nerve pathology.
- In acute optic neuritis the pERG is severely affected. With time, the P50 wave is restored but absence of the N95 persists.
- In AION, N95 reduction may occur, but P50 is more frequently affected than in demyelinating disease, probably reflecting more widespread vascular dysfunction.
- The N95 : P50 ratio is another useful parameter to differentiate between optic nerve and macular disease. The ratio is decreased in nerve pathology but remains constant in macular disorders.

PHOTOPIC NEGATIVE RESPONSE (PNR)

Until recently, it was believed that measurable contributions from retinal ganglion cells were absent in the full-field flash ERG (unlike the pattern ERG). Hence, the flash ERG was thought to be of little use in diagnosis of optic nerve diseases. Evidence now suggests that a component of the photopic ERG called the photopic

negative response (PhNR) may arise from the same generator as the N95 wave of the pERG. The PhNR is a negative wave that follows the b-wave, seen when red flashes are used against a blue background. The PhNR amplitude has been found to be reduced in anterior ischemic optic neuropathy and compressive optic neuropathy (tumor). Additionally, the PhNR amplitude was lower in both the asymptomatic and symptomatic eyes of patients with AION, when compared to controls.

MULTIFOCAL ERG

In this technique, up to 256 retinal locations can be simultaneously tested. A false color-coded topographical representation of waveforms is displayed.

The test is of great utility in evaluating patients with poor vision, central or cecocentral scotomata, and reduced color vision, and in whom clinical findings are unable to differentiate between an optic nerve disease and a macular pathology. A pVEP will be abnormal in both these conditions, but an mfERG will pick up a localized macular pathology.

ELECTRO-OCULOGRAM (EOG)

There is a potential difference between the front and the back of the normal eye even in the resting state. Thus it behaves like an electric dipole with a potential difference of about 6 millivolts, the cornea being more positive than the retina.

RECORDING OF EOG

For purposes of recording the EOG electrodes are placed near the inner and outer canthi. The EOG is measured in light and dark conditions. Recording in the dark state is performed for about 20 minutes, and for about 15 minutes in the light state. The patient is asked to make saccades every second between two stimuli placed about 30 degrees apart.

A change in the potential difference between the two electrodes in these different positions of the eye is measured. The potential consists of two components—the light-sensitive and the light-insensitive components. The light-

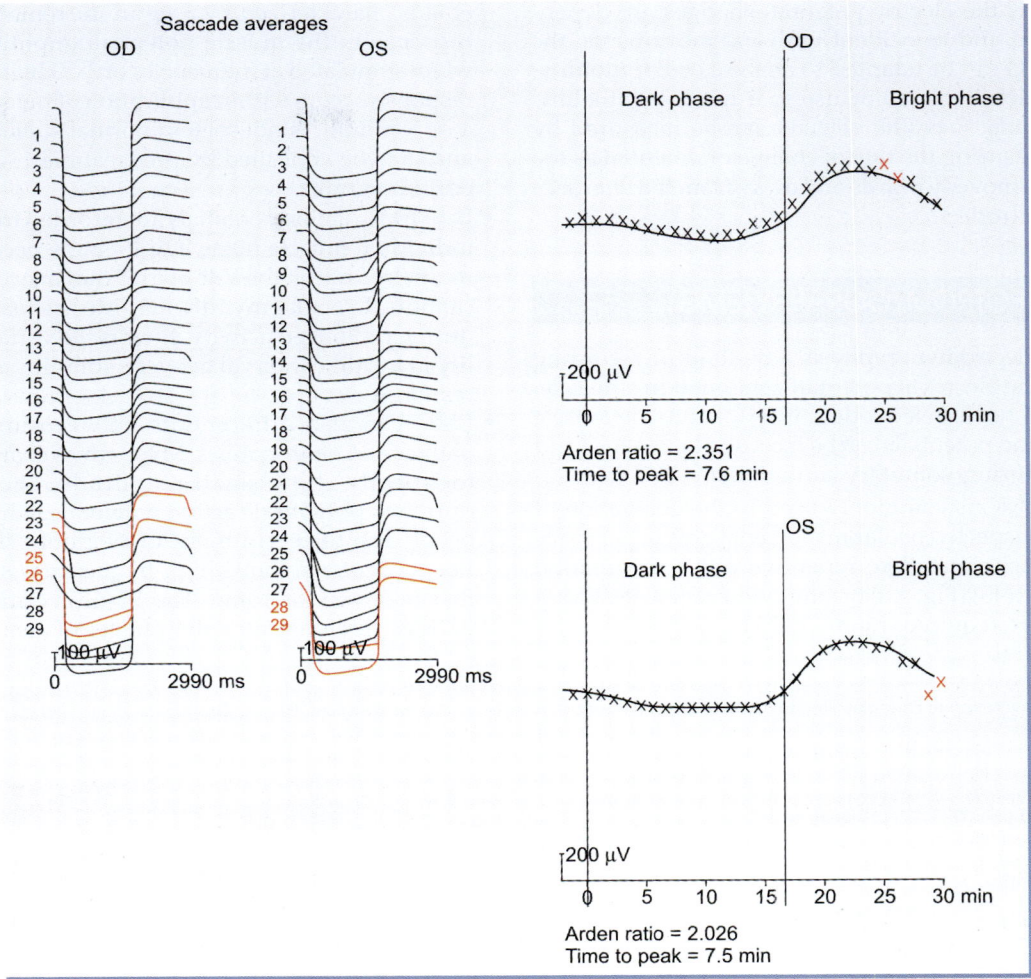

Fig. 3.5 *Electro-oculogram in a normal subject.*

insensitive potential (standing potential) decreases over a period of time in the dark-adapted state to reach a steady state called the dark trough. Following re-exposure to light the potential gradually increases to reach a peak (the light peak). The EOG is represented as a ratio of the light peak to the dark trough—the Arden ratio. This ratio is greater than 1.8 in normal subjects (Fig. 3.5).

Clinical studies show that the retinal pigment epithelium (RPE) is responsible for the EOG. The light-sensitive component appears to be produced by the photoreceptors.

CLINICAL USES

The EOG usually goes hand-in-hand with ERG, in that the EOG is usually abnormal if the ERG is so. However there are four conditions where the ERG may be normal but the EOG abnormal, namely Stargardt disease (fundus flavimaculatus), Best disease or Vitelliform dystrophy, advanced drusen, and butterfly-shaped pigment dystrophy of the fovea. An abnormal EOG may be found in asymptomatic 'carriers' of Best disease in whom the fundus appears normal. The EOG can also distinguish between dominant and recessive stationary night blindness.

As the electric potential changes are dependent and coincident with eye movements, the EOG can be adapted to analyse ocular motility, which is its major use in a neuro-ophthalmic setting. Saccadic velocity can be measured by measuring the rate of change of potential as the eye moves towards and away from the reference electrode.

ELECTROMYOGRAPHY (EMG)

- Electromyography is a method of recording the electrical potential generated in a muscle. A needle electrode is inserted into the muscle and potentials can be recorded both at rest and during voluntary contraction.
- EMG is commonly used in the evaluation of suspected ocular myasthenia gravis. Sensitive techniques like repetitive nerve stimulation (RNS) (Fig. 3.6) or single-fiber EMG (SFEMG) are required. By the RNS technique, myasth-

enia is characterized by a rapid decremental response in the muscle potential amplitude when stimulated at frequencies of 2–3 Hz. This response occurs within application of the first 4 or 5 stimuli, is not seen in normal subjects, and may be abolished by pre-treatment with edrophonium.
- In SFEMG, action potentials are recorded from individual muscle fibers employing a needle multielectrode in the side of a 0.5 mm injection cannula. In ocular myasthenia, jitter increases during prolonged activity. Jitter is the variability in the time interval between stimulus and response.
- EMG can also differentiate between myopathies and neuropathies. Myopathies characteristically show small amplitude, short-duration, polyphasic action potentials, which occur due to recruitment of neighbouring fibers. Myotonia shows high-frequency waves that may wax or wane. The EMG in neuropathies demonstrates the effects of dener-

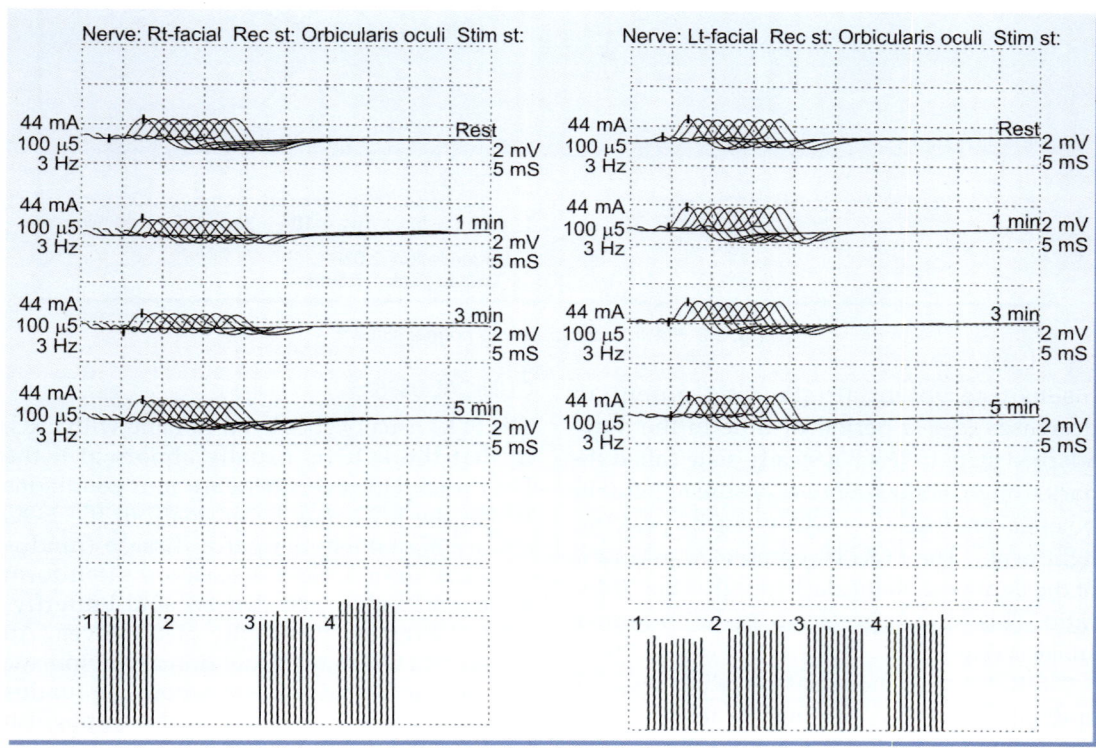

Fig. 3.6 *Repetitive nerve fiber stimulation.*

vation, namely a decrease in the number of activated motor units, with an increase in their rate of firing. Fibrillations and fasciculations also favor a diagnosis of neuropathy.

• Botulinum toxin has also been administered with EMG assistance.

CLINICAL SCENARIOS

DISCRIMINATING BETWEEN A SUSPECTED OPTIC NEUROPATHY OR MACULOPATHY

Some patients with inconclusive history and clinical findings may require electrophysiological testing, especially those with centro-caecal scotomata, reduced visual acuity, and subnormal color vision. This clinical picture may be seen in optic neuropathies as well as maculopathies.

A normal pVEP essentially excludes a diagnosis of optic neuropathy or maculopathy. However, an abnormal pVEP must be followed by further testing. An abnormal pVEP with an abnormal pERG, namely the P50 component, points strongly towards a maculopathy. In a neuropathy, the pERG may be normal or may show an abnormal N95 wave.

Multifocal ERG is another useful technique to evaluate a patient with suspected maculopathy (Fig. 3.7).

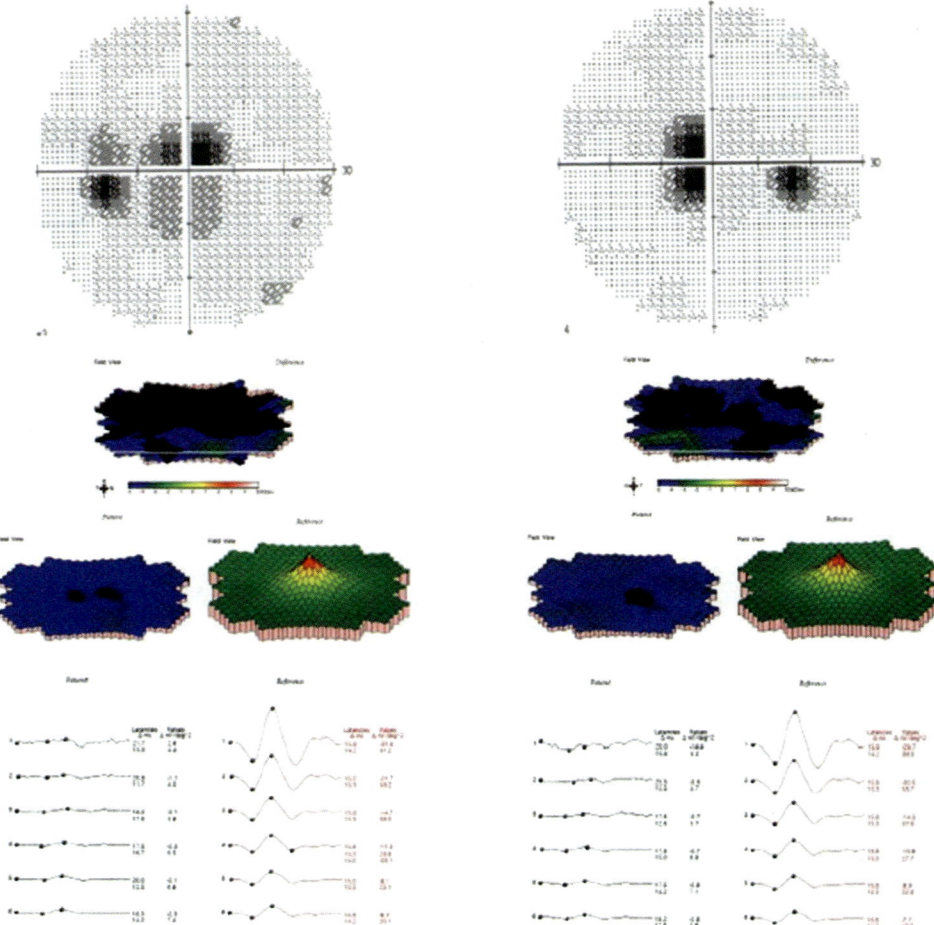

Fig. 3.7 *Multifocal ERG in a patient with bilateral chloroquine toxicity. Visual fields (top panel) show bilateral central scotomata.*

EVALUATION OF SUSPECTED FUNCTIONAL VISUAL LOSS

Functional visual loss includes malingering (deliberate exaggeration or misrepresentation of disability) and conversion disorder (also known as hysterical visual loss, usually for secondary gain). Many organic disorders also have a functional overlay.

A normal pVEP in a cooperative patient is good evidence of a lack of dysfunction in the primary visual pathway. An uncooperative patient may be tested with a flash VEP.

As described earlier, subjects may voluntarily suppress the VEP. However, the P300 response (positive wave at 300 milliseconds) is not directly produced by the sensory stimulus and persists even if the subject is able to suppress the P100 response.

Using larger check sizes, or testing with both eyes open, can mitigate artificial suppression of the VEP. However, these strategies are contrary to ideal test conditions.

DETERMINING POTENTIAL VISUAL FUNCTION IN AN EYE WITH MEDIA OPACITY

In eyes with dense cataract or vitreous hemorrhage examination of the posterior segment may not be possible. Imaging modalities such as ultrasound provide only a structural analysis. In this scenario, flash electrodiagnostic techniques are appropriate to evaluate visual potential, because opacities generally scatter or diffuse the incoming light rather than reflecting or absorbing it. Flash testing can be performed in eyes with very poor visual acuity, unlike pattern tests.

One may begin with a flash VEP. If normal, a significant maculopathy or optic neuropathy may be ruled out. In patients with unilateral pathology, comparing the amplitude with that of the other eye is useful. A reduction in fVEP amplitude by greater than 50 percent or delay of more than 30 milliseconds is suggestive of central visual field disturbance. A normal fVEP, however, is definitely not synonymous with normal postoperative visual acuity; this may need to be explained to the anxious patient.

An abnormal flash ERG suggests a diffuse rod and/or cone disease.

BIBLIOGRAPHY

1. Brigell M, Celesia GG. Electrophysiological Evaluation of the Neuro-ophthalmology Patient: An Algorithm for Clinical Use. Semin Ophthalmol 1992;7(1):65–78.
2. Glaser JS, Laamme P. The visual-evoked response: methodology and application in optic nerve disease. In: Thompson HS (Ed). Topics in Neuro-ophthalmology. Williams & Wilkins: Baltimore, MD 1979:199–218.
3. Halliday AM, McDonald WI, Mushin J. Delayed visual evoked response in optic neuritis. Lancet 1972; i: 982–5.
4. Halliday AM, McDonald WI, Mushin J. Visual evoked response in diagnosis of multiple sclerosis. British Medical Journal 1973;4(5893): 661–4.
5. Hoffmann MB, Seufert PS, Bach M. Simulated nystagmus suppresses pattern-reversal but not pattern-onset visual evoked potentials. Clin Neurophysiol 2004;115(11):2659–65.
6. Holder GE, Gale RP, Acheson JF, Robson AG. Electrodiagnostic Assessment in Optic Nerve Disease. Curr Opin Neurol 2009;22:3–10.
7. Holder GE. Electrophysiological assessment of optic nerve disease. Eye 2004;18:1133–43.
8. Holder GE. Ischaemic optic neuropathy. In: Heckenlively JR, Arden GB (Eds). Principles and Practice of Clinical Electrophysiology of Vision. Mosby Year Book: St Louis, MO 1991; 636–9.
9. Holder GE. Pattern Electroretinography (PERG) and an Integrated Approach to Visual Pathway Diagnosis. Prog Retin Eye Res 2001;20(4): 531–61.
10. Hood DC, Odel JG, Winn BJ. The Multifocal Visual-evoked Potential. J Neuro-ophthalmol 2003;23:279–89.
11. Kraemer M, Abrahamsson M, Sjöström A. The neonatal development of the light flash visual-evoked potential. Doc Ophthalmol 1999;99: 21–39.
12. Kurtzberg D. Event related potentials in the evaluation of high risk infants. Ann N Y Acad Sci 1982;388:557–71.
13. Lambert SR, Kriss A, Taylor D. A longitudinal clinical and electrophysiological assessment. Ophthalmol 1989;96(4): 524–7.
14. McBain VA, Robson AG, Hogg CR, Holder GE. Assessment of Patients with Suspected Nonorganic Visual Loss using Pattern Appearance Visual Evoked Potentials. Graefes Arch Clin Exp Ophthalmol 2007;245:502–10.
15. Miller N, Newman Nancy J, Biousse V, Kerrison J (Eds). Walsh & Hoyt's Clinical Neuro-ophthalmology. 6th edn. Baltimore. Lippincott Williams & Wilkins 2004;133–45.

16. Norcia AM, Tyler CW. Spatial frequency sweep VEP: visual acuity during the first year of life. Vision Res 1985;25(10):1399–408.

17. Odom JV, Bach M, Barber C, et al. Visual-evoked Potentials Standard. Doc Ophthalmol 2004;108: 115–23.

18. Placzek M, Mushin J, Dubowitz LMS. Maturation of the visual evoked response and its correlation with visual acuity in preterm infants. Dev Med Child Neurol 1985;27:448–54.

19. Rangaswamy NV, Frishman LJ, Dorotheo EU, Schiffman JS, Bahrani HM, Tang RA. Photopic ERGs in patients with optic neuropathies: comparison with primate ERGs after pharmacologic blockade of inner retina. Invest Ophthalmol Vis Sci 2004;45(10):3827–37.

20. Scherfig E, Edmund J, Tinning S, Trojaborg W. Flash visual-evoked potential as a prognostic factor for vitreous operations in diabetic eyes. Ophthalmology 1984;91(12):1475–9.

21. Sokol S. The Visually Evoked Cortical Potential in Optic Nerve and Visual Pathway Disorders. In: Fishman GA, Sokol S (Eds). Electrophysiologic Testing in disorders of the Retina, Optic Nerve and Visual Pathway. American Academy of Ophthalomology 1990;105–42.

22. Stalberg E, Ekstedt J, Broman A. Neuromuscular Transmission in Myasthenia Gravis studied with Single Fiber Electromyography. Journal of Neurology, Neurosurgey, and Psychiatry 1974; 37:540–7.

23. Towle VL, Sutcliffe E, Sokol S. Diagnosing functional visual deficits with the P300 component of the visual-evoked potential. Arch Ophthalmol 1985;103(1):47–50.

24. Viswanathan S, Frishman LJ, Robson JG. The uniform field and pattern ERG in macaques with experimental glaucoma: removal of spiking activity. Invest Ophthalmol Vis Sci 2000;41: 2797–810.

4 HAEMATOLOGICAL INVESTIGATIONS IN NEURO-OPHTHALMOLOGY

Ashwin Mohan, Rashmin A Gandhi

INTRODUCTION

BLOOD TESTS AS NON-INFECTIOUS SYSTEMIC PARAMETERS
- Erythrocyte sedimentation rate
- C-reactive protein
- Anti-nuclear antibody
- Antibodies in neuromyelitis optica (NMO)

- Non-arteritic anterior ischaemic optic neuropathy
- Sarcoidosis
- Nutritional optic neuropathy

BLOOD TESTS FOR INFECTIOUS AGENTS
- Tests for syphilis
- Tests for lyme disease
- Tests for HIV, CMV and VZV

INTRODUCTION

An ophthalmologist often faeces a diagnostic dilemma when a patient with visual loss as his sole complaint with inconclusive or almost normal findings comes to him for treatment.

Blood investigations have always been the cornerstone of medical diagnostic tests for systemic diseases. They help to us not only to identify the cause of the pathology but also to uncover underlying systemic conditions (which may be life-threatening) and effect appropriate referral.

In the following text we will discuss the blood tests requested in a neuro-ophthalmology setting and elucidate the disorders related to them.

BLOOD TESTS: AS NON-INFECTIOUS SYSTEMIC PARAMETERS

ERYTHROCYTE SEDIMENTATION RATE

The erythrocyte sedimentation rate (ESR), also called Biernacki reaction, is the rate at which red blood cells sediment in a period of 1 hour. It is a common hematology test that is a non-specific measure of inflammation. To perform the test, anticoagulated blood is placed in an upright Westergren tube, and the rate at which the red blood cells fall is measured and reported in millimeters at the end of 1 hour (mm at 1 hr).

An elevated ESR strongly supports a clinical suspicion of giant cell arteritis (GCA)—an important cause of arteritic anterior ischemic optic neuropathy—but a normal ESR does not rule out a diagnosis of GCA. According to the American College of Rheumatology, an ESR by Westergren method is elevated if it is >50 mm at 1 hr. Approximately 85% of patients with GCA have an ESR >50 mm at 1 hr.

C-REACTIVE PROTEIN

C-reactive protein (CRP) is a protein found in the blood, the levels of which rise in response to inflammation (i.e. C-reactive protein is an acute-phase protein). Its physiological role is to bind to phosphocholine expressed on the surface of dead or dying cells (and some types of bacteria) in order to activate the complement system via the C1Q complex.

CRP levels greater than 2.45 mg/dl and elevated platelet count show a positive correlation with the temporal artery biopsy in patients with GCA. Its advantages over the ESR are faster responsiveness to inflammation (within 4–6 hr), insensitivity to age, gender and hematological factors, and notably higher sensitivity and specificity for GCA in the appropriate clinical setting. The disadvantages of CRP include the higher cost of testing compared to ESR and perhaps a relative unfamiliarity with the test amongst clinicians.

ANTI-NUCLEAR ANTIBODY

These are antibodies directed against the cell nucleus and are elevated in autoimmune disease. All ANAs are elevated in systemic lupus erythematosus (SLE) which can manifest as a non-infectious cause of optic neuropathy. Serum ANA levels can be used as a screening test with 95% sensitivity. ESR and CRP may also be elevated in SLE.

ANTIBODIES IN NEUROMYELITIS OPTICA (NMO)

Neuromyelitis optica, also known as Devic's disease, is an inflammatory disease of the central nervous system (CNS) characterized by severe attacks of optic neuritis and myelitis, and which, unlike multiple sclerosis (MS), commonly spares the brain in the early stages. NMO used to be considered as a special form of MS. During the past 10 years, however, the two diseases have been shown to be clearly different. NMO is a B-cell-mediated disease associated with anti-aquaporin-4 (AQP4) antibodies in many cases and its pathophysiology seems to be near the acute lesion of necrotizing vasculitis.

The available data clearly point to the high specificity of anti-aquaporin-4 antibodies for Devic's disease.

The detection of antibodies against AQP4 has improved the diagnosis of neuromyelitis optica (NMO). Researchers recently evaluated an established cell-based anti-AQP4 assay in 273 patients with inflammatory CNS demyelination. The assay had a specificity of 99% and a sensitivity of 56% to detect all NMO patients and of 74% to detect recurrent NMO patients.

BLOOD TESTS FOR NON-ARTERITIC ANTERIOR ISCHEMIC OPTIC NEUROPATHY

NAION is caused by a non-arteritic occlusion of the arteries resulting in disruption blood flow and subsequent ischemia.

Blood sugar, fasting lipid profile and coagulation studies, serum homocysteine levels and serum test for antiphospholipid antibody will be helpful in investigating a case of suspected NAION.

Diabetes has been documented in up to 24% of patients with NAION. Repka et al. indicated that the prevalences of both hypertension and diabetes are increased over those of the control population in NAION patients in the age range 45–64 years, but that in patients over 64 years of age, no significant difference exists from those of the general population.

Deficiency of the enzymes involved in methionine metabolism result in abnormal accumulation of homocysteine producing an increased risk for strokes and carotid stenosis. The findings in the study by Pianka et al. suggest that hyperhomocystinemia is a risk factor for NAION and CRAO. Serum B_{12} levels are found to be low.

Anti-phospholipid syndrome is characterized by hypercoagulability of blood and an increased risk of thrombosis and vascular occlusion leading to ischemia.

BLOOD TESTS FOR SARCOIDOSIS

Sarcoidosis can be a cause of non-infectious optic neuritis, sometimes presenting with an optic nerve head granuloma. Chest X-ray and HRCT are used commonly to diagnose sarcoidosis, but raised ACE levels in the blood along with hypercalcemia can support the diagnosis of sarcoidosis. Angiotensin converting enzyme (ACE) is secreted by the non-caseating granuloma cells and can be an indicator of total body granuloma load. It is elevated in 60% of patients with sarcoidosis.

BLOOD TESTS IN NUTRITIONAL OPTIC NEUROPATHY

Temporal pallor associated with a centrocaecal scotoma should raise the suspicion of nutritional or toxic optic neuropathy. Tobacco-associated optic neuropathy and malnutrition in chronic alcoholics have been implicated in the pathogenesis of this neuropathy. Serum vitamin levels for B_1, B_2, B_{12} and pyruvate levels provide supportive evidence for nutritional optic neuropathy.

BLOOD TESTS FOR INFECTIOUS AGENTS

Syphilis, lyme disease, HIV, cytomegalovirus (CMV) and varicella-zoster virus (VZV) can all present with infectious optic neuritis or neuroretinitis.

TESTS FOR SYPHILIS

Veneral Disease Research Laboratory (VDRL), Rapid Plasma Reagin (RPR) and Fluorescent Treponemal Antibody (FTA-ABS) tests are used in syphilis serology. VDRL and RPR are screening tests employing a non-treponemal antigen, while FTA-ABS is more specific.

TESTS FOR LYME DISEASE

ELISA and immunofluorescence assay for IgM against *Borrelia burgdorferi* antigens are used as diagnostic serological tests for lyme disease.

TESTS FOR HIV, CMV AND VZV

Tests for HIV, CMV and VZV viruses should be ordered in suspected cash. Hence, a number of serological tests can be used to diagnose diseases in neuro-ophthalmological disorders which should be guided by appropriate clinical suspicion of the disease based on history and clinical findings. A few tests like ESR, CRP, blood sugar and ACE levels are supportive whereas parameters like NMO antibody levels and aquaporin-4 are diagnostic tests.

BIBLIOGRAPHY

1. Collongues N, de Seze J. Current and future treatment approaches for neuromyelitis optica 2011;4(2):111–21.

2. Dellevance A, et al. Anti-aquaporin-4 antibodies in the context of assorted immune-mediated diseases. Eur J Neurol 2011.

3. Hunder GG, Bloch DA, Michel BA, et al. The American College of Rheumatology 1990 criteria for the classification of giant cell arteritis. Arthritis Rheum 1990;33:1122–8.

4. Ischemic Optic Neuropathy Decompression Trial Research Group: Characteristics of patients with nonarteritic anterior ischemic optic neuropathy eligible for the Ischemic Optic Neuropathy Decompression Trial. Arch Ophthalmol 1996; 114:1366–74.

5. Kawasaki A, Purvin V. Giant cell arteritis: an updated review. Acta Ophthalmologica 2009; 87(1):13–32.

6. Ketelslegers IA, et al. Antibodies against aquaporin-4 in neuromyelitis optica: distinction between recurrent and monophasic patients. Mult Scler 2011.

7. Pianka P, Almog Y, Man O, et al. Hyperhomocysteinemia in patients with nonarteritic anterior ischemic optic neuropathy, central retinal artery occlusion, and central retinal vein occlusion. Ophthalmology 2000;107:1588–92.

8. Repka MX, Savino PJ, Schatz NJ, Sergott RC. Clinical profile and long-term implications of anterior ischemic optic neuropathy. Am J Ophthalmol 1983;96:478–83.

9. Thompson D, Pepys MB, Wood SP. "The physiological structure of human C-reactive protein and its complex with phosphocholine". Structure Feb. 1999;7(2):169–77.

5 OPTICAL COHERENCE TOMOGRAPHY IN NEURO-OPHTHALMOLOGY

Ashwin Mohan, Rashmin A Gandhi

INTRODUCTION

RNFL MEASUREMENTS

RNFL IN SPECIFIC DISEASE ENTITIES
- Multiple sclerosis
- Neurodegenerative disease
- Toxic optic neuropathies
- Ischemic optic neuropathy
- Papilledema

- Traumatic optic neuropathy
- Optic disc anomalies
- Hereditary optic neuropathy
- Amblyopia

CONCLUSIONS
- OCT—non-invasive
- Reproducibility of OCT in neuro-ophthalmology

INTRODUCTION

The retinal nerve fiber layer (RNFL) is populated by the axons of retinal ganglion cells, as they proceed in an organized fashion towards the optic nerve head. The fibers are non-myelinated and have a specific topographic course—the papillomacular bundle runs between the macula and the optic disc, arcuate fibers originate from the temporal retina, and straight fibers from the nasal retina. The horizontal raphe separates the superior and inferior retinal hemispheres.

Optical coherence tomography (OCT) is a non-invasive and quick imaging modality in widespread use today. It uses the principle of Michelson's interferometry; the interference pattern obtained between rays of light incident upon and reflected from a particular structure can be used to determine that structure's optical density. This property can be used to differentiate it from neighbouring structures, thus providing imaging data in the form of a 'slice' of tissues, just like an *in vivo* histology section.

This information is color-coded, hot colors (red and white) representing areas of high reflectance and cool colors (black and blue) representing areas of low reflectance, with green for an intermediate value. Layers of a tissue can be visually identified, and thicknesses can be measured.

RNFL measurements have been widely studied in the early diagnosis of glaucoma ('pre-perimetric glaucoma'). Interest in the RNFL has been kindled among neurologists and neuro-ophthalmologists, especially in patients with chronic and progressive neurological disease. The rationale behind this is that the RNFL is an easily examined neural tissue, and changes in this layer may act as an indicator of ongoing damage in the central nervous system. Retrograde, as opposed to anterograde degenertion, may be caused by diseases of the central nervous system such as multiple sclerosis. The common end-result is a reduction in thickness of the nerve fiber layer. Thus, OCT measurements provide a non-invasive and objective means of following up these patients in the hope of detecting disease progression. Occasionally in other diseases, disease-specific patterns of RNFL loss may also be seen.

RETINAL NERVE FIBER LAYER MEASUREMENTS BY DIFFERENT DEVICES

While the resolution of OCT has been improving by leaps and bounds, the reproducibility of OCT measurements has become a matter of great concern. In order to determine progression based on RNFL thickness measurements, it is obvious that exactly the same area must be scanned in subsequent tests. The RNFL thickness varies in different peripapillary sectors, and also increases with increasing proximity to the optic disc.

Time domain optical coherence tomography (TD-OCT) has been used commonly in clinical practice, but is difficult to perform in patients with fixation problems. Decentration also produces significantly differing results. Spectral domain (SD)-OCT produces three-dimensional (3-D) data volumes. The Heidelberg Spectralis (Heidelberg Engineering, Heidelberg, Germany) SD-OCT also incorporates an eye-tracking mode, which overcomes fixation problems. A circular target can be positioned over the optic disc margin in an infrared image, and the scan is then run along a second outer ring. These measures greatly improve inter-test reproducibility.

Direct comparisons of RNFL thickness measurements among OCT instruments may be misleading as there are considerable differences among devices. Physicians should consider this fact before judging a change of RNFL thicknesses if they were measured by different devices. OCT scan location matching may provide follow-up comparability between TD-OCT circular scan data and 3-D SD-OCT scan data.

RETINAL NERVE FIBER LAYER MEASUREMENTS IN DIFFERENT DISEASE ENTITIES

MULTIPLE SCLEROSIS

RNFL measurements in patients with multiple sclerosis (MS) were found to be heterogeneous and varied from normal to showing marked thinning. Thinning of the RNFL correlates with the number of episodes of prior optic neuritis, disease duration, and MS subtype (the most significant reductions occurring in primary and secondary progressive subtypes).

RNFL thinning in MS can occur due in two settings. Focal, gross areas of thinning are seen after optic neuritis. More subtle, global and progressive thinning seems to be related to the disease process itself. This progressive rarefaction may be beyond the resolution limits of even advanced SD-OCT techniques.

RNFL measurements were thought to be a possible method of monitoring disease progression in MS. However, there are drawbacks to this approach. Firstly, it is unknown whether diffuse RNFL loss occurs in all patients with MS (or only certain subtypes). Doubts also exist as to why and whether a diffuse CNS disease like MS would actually produce a retrograde trans-synaptic degeneration of the RNFL.

Additionally, the range of 'normal' RNFL thickness values is large, ranging from 75 μm to 125 μm with a mean of 97.2 ± 9.7 μm. Hence, it is difficult to draw any conclusions from a single RNFL reading. Serial RNFL measure-ments will be needed to detect progressive thinning, with a minimum observation period of at least 2 years being suggested in MS patients without optic neuritis. A global RNFL reduction about 2 μm to 4 μm per year was suggested in MS patients without optic neuritis. Progressive thinning must be differentiated from 'physiological' RNFL thinning due to age.

Lastly, RNFL measurements need to be performed under essentially the same conditions and need special testing algorithms to ensure comparability across machines and technologies (time domain vs. spectral domain).

The study with the longest follow-up (two years) in a well-defined cohort of relapsing-remitting (RRMS) and secondary-progressive (SPMS) forms without optic neuritis in the preceding 12 months did not find significant RNFL reduction. They suggested that OCT as yet cannot replace MRI, or even serve as new surrogate marker in MS.

A recent study in patients with longitudinally-extensive transverse myelitis found localized RNFL loss even in the absence of previous episodes of optic neuritis, suggesting subclinical optic nerve damage in these patients.

NEURODEGENERATIVE DISEASE

Alzheimer's disease is the prototypical neurodegenerative disorder. Mild cognitive impairment (MCI) may represent an early stage of this disease. OCT measurements of the RNFL were performed in subjects with MCI, patients with Alzheimer's disease, and in age-matched normal controls. There was a significant decrease in RNFL thickness in patients with both MCI and Alzheimer's disease, compared to controls. However, the difference between the MCI group and Alzheimer's group was not significant, and there was no relation between RNFL thinning and the severity of dementia.

TOXIC OPTIC NEUROPATHIES

In tobacco-alcohol induced toxic optic neuropathy temporal quadrant thinning has been demonstrated. Thickening of the RNFL may be due to edema. These findings correlated with bilateral central or centrocecal scotomata on perimetric testing.

OCT has also been performed in patients on ethambutol (Fig. 5.1). Findings vary with the duration of exposure, with thickening of the papillomacular bundle seen in the early stage and thinning in the chronic stage. RNFL measurements may also be a useful objective

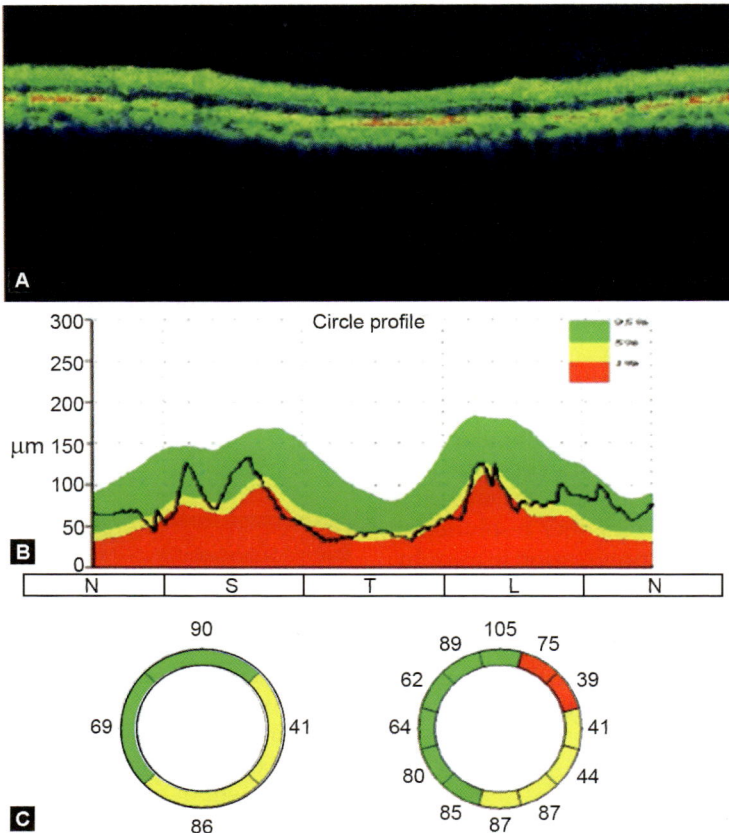

Fig. 5.1 *RNFL OCT of the left eye of a patient with ethambutol toxic optic neuropathy: (A) The false color OCT scan; (B) The 'unravelled' circular scan data, showing the RNFL thickness graph against color-coded probability zones; (C) The quadrantic and clock-hour thickness displays, showing thinning in the inferior and temporal sectors.*

surrogate marker in patients who are unable to perform visual field examination.

ISCHEMIC OPTIC NEUROPATHY

A clinical clue in favor of a diagnosis of non-arteritic anterior ischaemic optic neuropathy (NA-AION) is the presence of a small disc with a small cup in the fellow eye. This has been confirmed with OCT measurements of the optic nerve head. An excellent correlation between the peripapillary RNFL thickness and the visual field has also been found, suggesting that RNFL OCT may be used in place of perimetry in the follow-up of such patients.

A novel new technique utilizes the Doppler shift that occurs when two segments of the same blood vessel are scanned with a Fourier-domain OCT. This provides information about the blood flow rate and velocity within that vessel. Cross-sectional measurements also provide data regarding the vessel caliber. Patients with NA-AION had significantly lower blood velocity, vessel caliber and arterial corss-sectional area in comparison to normal controls, but there was no significant reduction in venous velocity. This exciting approach thus combines the classic 'structural' yield of OCT with information about vascular function.

PAPILLEDEMA

OCT can be used to objectively measure RNFL swelling, and serial examinations over time can show resolution or progression to optic atrophy.

Scanning of the RNFL in the peripapillary area can help to distinguish between true and pseudo-papilledema. In the former situation, serial scanning will reveal either resolution of the RNFL thickening or progression to atrophy. Nerve fiber layer measurements will remain stable in pseudo-papilledema due to con-genitally crowded or anomalous discs, unless associated optic nerve heard drusen exist, which may be produce RNFL thinning over time.

TRAUMATIC OPTIC NEUROPATHY

The RNFL undergoes progressive thinning after trauma to the optic nerve. Thinning has been noted to continue up to 70 days post-injury. When compared to macular thickness, RNFL thickness shows greater and faster reductions in traumatic neuropathy.

OPTIC DISC ANOMALIES

OCT can be used in the evaluation of eyes with optic disc drusen. Features seen are shadowing and RNFL thinning which corresponds to visual field defects. A characteristic lacy pattern of cavitation in the anterior portion of the optic nerve head can be seen in morning glory anomaly.

HEREDITARY OPTIC NEUROPATHY

Dominant optic atrophy has been linked to mutations in the OPA1 gene. A study of the RNFL thickness in 40 patients with DOA found a significant reduction in average RNFL thickness in the OPA1 group compared with normal controls. There was a severe involvement of the temporal papillomacular bundle, with relative sparing of the nasal fibers. The rarefaction of the RNFL was greater in patients with the more severe disease phenotype (DOA+), which has additional neuromuscular features.

AMBLYOPIA

SD-OCT performed in eyes with strabismic and anisometropic amblyopia, as well as a third control group of anisometropia without amblyopia, found that the mean RNFL thickness was similar in the amblyopic and the fellow eye. Central macular thickness was however significantly higher in those eyes with anisometropic amblyopia when compared with the fellow eye.

CONCLUSIONS

OCT—NON-INVASIVE

Due to the non-invasive nature of optical coherence tomography, it is a widely used imaging modality. Excellent image resolution and post-acquisition processing add to its popularity. After establishing its utility in the diagnosis and management of glaucoma and retinal diseases, it has now found use in neuro-ophthalmology, where measurements of the retinal nerve fiber layer thickness provide a useful and objective method of detecting disease progression.

REPRODUCIBILITY OF OCT IN NEURO-OPHTHALMOLOGY

Reproducibility of scanned areas has been a major concern. Newer devices, such as the spectral domain OCT, attempt to overcome this issue by the use of eye-tracking mechanisms and operator-dependent and-independent scan area selection. These ensure that the same area is scanned in subsequent tests, and minimize motion and fixation artifacts.

BIBLIOGRAPHY

1. Alasil T, Tan O, Lu AT, et al. Correlation of Fourier domain optical coherence tomography retinal nerve fiber layer maps with visual fields in non-arteritic ischaemic optic neuropathy. Ophthalmic Surg Lasers Imaging 2008;39(4): S71–9.

2. Al-Haddad CE, El Mollayess GM, Cherfan CG, et al. Retinal nerve fiber layer and macular thickness in amblyopia as measured by spectral-domain optical coherence tomography. Br J Ophthalmol 2011 Mar 11. [Epub ahead of print].

3. Bellusci C, Savini G, Carbonelli M, et al. Retinal nerve fiber layer thickness in nonarteritic anterior ischaemic optic neuropathy: OCT characterization of the acute and resolving phases. Graefes Arch Clin Exp Ophthalmol 2008;246(5):641–7.

4. Chan CK, Cheng AC, Leung CK, et al. Quantitative assessment of optic nerve head morphology and retinal nerve fiber layer in non-arteritic anterior ischaemic optic neuropathy with optical coherence tomography and confocal scanning laser ophthalmoscopy. Br J Ophthalmol 2009;93(6):731–5.

5. Clayton LM, Dévilé M, Punte T, et al. Retinal nerve fiber layer thickness in Vigabatrin-exposed patients. Ann Neurol 2011;69(5):845–54. doi: 10.1002/ana.22266. Epub 2011 Jan 19.

6. Cunha LP, Costa-Cunha LV, Malta RF, et al. Comparison between retinal nerve fiber layer and macular thickness measured with OCT detecting progressive axonal loss following traumatic optic neuropathy. Arq Bras Oftalmol. 2009;72(5):622–5.

7. Garcia-Martin E, Pueyo V, Ara J, et al. Effect of optic neuritis on progressive axonal damage in multiple sclerosis patients. Mult Scler 2011 Feb 7. [Epub ahead of print].

8. Hedges TR III. Optical coherence tomography in neuro-ophthalmology. In: Schuman JS, Puliafito CA, Fujimoto JG, editors. Optical coherence tomography of ocular diseases. Thorofare, NJ: Slack; 2004.

9. Henderson AP, Trip SA, Schlottmann PG, et al. An investigation of the retinal nerve fiber layer in progressive multiple sclerosis using optical coherence tomography. Brain 2008;131:277–87.

10. Henderson AP, Trip SA, Schlottmann PG, et al. A preliminary longitudinal study of the retinal nerve fiber layer in progressive multiple sclerosis. J Neurol 2010;257:1083–91.

11. Hong S, Kim Y, Shim J, Kim CY, Seong GJ. Inter-device Agreement of Retinal Nerve Fiber Layer Thickness Measurements Using Spectral Domain Cirrus HD OCT. Korean J Ophthalmol 2011;25(2):105–09.

12. Karam EZ, Hedges TR. Optical coherence tomography of the retinal nerve fiber layer in mild papilledema and pseudopapilloedema. Br J Ophthalmol 2005;89:294–8.

13. Kee C, Hwang JM. Optical coherence tomography in a patient with tobacco-alcohol amblyopia. Eye (2008) 22, 469–70; doi:10.1038/sj.eye.6702821; published online 13 April 2007.

14. Kesler A, Vakhapova V, Korczyn AD, et al. Retinal thickness in patients with mild cognitive impairment and Alzheimer's disease. Clin Neurol Neurosurg 2011 Mar 29. [Epub ahead of print].

15. Khanifar AA, Parlitsis GJ, Ehrlich JR, et al. Retinal nerve fiber layer evaluation in multiple sclerosis with spectral domain optical coherence tomography. Clin Ophthalmol 2010;4:1007–13.

16. Kim JS, Ishikawa H, Gabriele ML, et al. Retinal Nerve Fiber Layer Thickness Measurement Comparability between Time Domain Optical Coherence Tomography (OCT) and Spectral Domain OCT. Invest. Ophthalmol. Vis. Sci 2010(1);2:896–902.

17. Kim U, Hwang JM. Early stage ethambutol optic neuropathy: retinal nerve fiber layer and optical coherence tomography. Eur J Ophthalmol 2009;19(3):466–9.

18. Lee ES, Kang SY, Choi EH, et al. Comparisons of Nerve Fiber Layer Thickness Measurements between Stratus, Cirrus, and RTVue OCTs in Healthy and Glaucomatous Eyes. Optom Vis Sci 2011; 88(6):751–8.

19. Medeiros FA, Moura FC, Vessani RM, et al. Axonal loss after traumatic optic neuropathy documented by optical coherence tomography. Am J Ophthalmol 2003;135(3):406–8.

20. Moura FC, Fernandes DB, Apóstolos-Pereira SL, et al. Optical coherence tomography evaluation of retinal nerve fiber layer in longitudinally extensive transverse myelitis. Arq Neuro-psiquiatr 2011;69(1):69–73.

21. Petzold A, de Boer JF, Schippling S, et al. Optical coherence tomography in multiple sclerosis: a systematic review and meta-analysis. Lancet Neurol 2010;9:921–32.

22. Roh S, Noecker RJ, Schuman JS, et al. Effect of optic nerve head drusen on nerve fiber layer thickness. Ophthalmology 1998;105:878–85.

23. Serbecic N, Aboul-Enein F, Beutelspacher SC, et al. Heterogeneous pattern of retinal nerve fiber layer in multiple sclerosis. High resolution optical coherence tomography: potential and limitations. PLoS One 2010;5:e13877.

24. Serbecic N, Aboul-Enein F, Beutelspacher SC, et al. High Resolution Spectral Domain Optical Coherence Tomography (SD-OCT) in Multiple Sclerosis: The First Follow-up Study over Two Years. PLoS ONE 2011;6(5): e19843. doi:10.1371/journal. pone. 0019843.

25. Serbecic N, Beutelspacher SC, Aboul-Enein FC, et al. Reproducibility of high-resolution optical coherence tomography measurements of the nerve fiber layer with the new Heidelberg Spectralis optical coherence tomography. Br J Ophthalmol 2011;95:804–10.

26. Serbecic N, Beutelspacher SC, Aboul-Enein FC, et al. Reproducibility of high-resolution optical coherence tomography measurements of the nerve fiber layer with the new Heidelberg Spectralis optical coherence tomography. Br J Ophthalmol 2010: doi:10.1136/bjo.2010.186221.

27. Serbecic N, Beutelspacher SC, Kircher K, et al. (2010). Interpretation of RNFLT values in multiple sclerosis-associated acute optic neuritis using high-resolution SD-OCT device. Acta Ophthalmol 2010; doi: 10.1111/j.1755–3768.2010.02013.x.

28. Talman LS, Bisker ER, Sackel DJ, et al. Longitudinal study of vision and retinal nerve fiber layer thickness in multiple sclerosis. Ann Neurol 2010; 67:749–60.

29. Wang Y, Fawzi AA, Varma R, et al. Pilot study of optical coherence tomography measurement of retinal blood flow in retinal and optic nerve diseases. Invest Ophthalmol Vis Sci 2011; 52(2):840–5.

30. Yu-Wai-Man P, Bailie M, Atawan A, Chinnery PF, et al. Pattern of retinal ganglion cell loss in dominant optic atrophy due to OPA1 mutations. Eye (Lond) 2011;25(5):596–602. Epub 2011 Mar 4.

31. Zoumalan CI, Agarwal M, Sadun AA. Optical coherence tomography can measure axonal loss in patients with ethambutol-induced optic neuropathy. Graefes Arch Clin Exp Ophthalmol. 2005;243(5):410–6. Epub 2004 Nov 23.

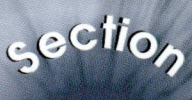

Pupil and its Disorders

6

ANATOMY, PHYSIOLOGY AND PHARMACOLOGY OF PUPIL

AK Khurana, Indu Khurana,
Aruj K Khurana, Bhawna Khurana

ANATOMY OF NORMAL PUPIL

GENERAL CONSIDERATIONS

The pupil is an aperture present in the center of the iris. It limits the amount of light reaching the retina and also, to some extent, controls the amount of chromatic and spherical aberration in the retinal image.

Number

Normally, there is one pupil in each eye. Rarely, there may be more than one pupil. This congenital anomaly is called *polycoria.*

Location

Normal pupil is placed almost in the center (slightly nasal) of the iris. Rarely, it may be congenitally eccentric (*corectopia).*

Size

Normal pupil size varies from 3 to 4 mm depending upon the illumination. The size of the pupil at any given time is the end result of a very complex interplay of hormonal, vascular and neural factors acting on the iridial muscles. There is probably no significant difference in pupillary size between blue irises and brown irises, nor between males and females.

Variation with age: Pupils are relatively small at birth, largest during adolescence, and tend to slowly grow smaller with increasing age.

Physiological changes in size: Pupil tends to dilate during emotional stress and constrict during sleep.

Isocoria: Normally, the two pupils are equal in size (isocoria). A slight (one tenth of a millimeter) anisocoria is present in a significant percentage of normal pupil.

Pupillary unrest: It refers to constant fluctuation in pupillary diameter under normal environmental conditions. It is detected on inspection of a magnified image of the pupil. Both pupils fluctuate identically and simultaneously. Pupillary unrest is influenced by emotional states, illumination and other factors.

Hippus: It refers to exaggeration of the pupillary unrest, i.e. it is fluctuation in pupillary diameter which can be easily detected on visual inspection without magnification. It has been seen in a number of pathological conditions, but is also seen in normal individuals and thus of no diagnostic significance.

Shape

Normal pupil is almost circular in shape. Irregularities in pupil shape are noticed in many pathological conditions.

Color

Of course, the pupil is a hole in the iris, but the pupillary area does exhibit a color, depending upon the condition of the structures located behind it. Normally, it is greyish black. It becomes jet black in aphakia. Leukocoria (white-colored pupil) is seen in a number of ocular conditions.

MUSCLES CONTROLLING THE PUPIL

Sphincter pupillae muscle

It forms one millimetre broad circular band in the pupillary part of iris. It consists of flat bar of plain muscle fibers which are derived from the ectoderm. It is supplied by the parasympathetic fibers through the third nerve. It constricts the pupil.

Dilator pupillae muscle

It lies in the posterior part of the stroma of ciliary zone of the iris. Its myofilaments are located in the outer part of the cells of anterior pigment epithelial layer. It is supplied by the cervical sympathetics and dilates the pupil.

PHYSIOLOGY OF THE PUPIL

LIGHT REFLEX

When light is shone in one eye, both the pupils constrict. Constriction of the pupil to which light is shone is called *'direct light reflex'* and that of the other pupil is called *'consensual (indirect) light reflex'*. In normal subjects, the direct and consensual reactions are almost, always identical in time, course and magnitude. If both

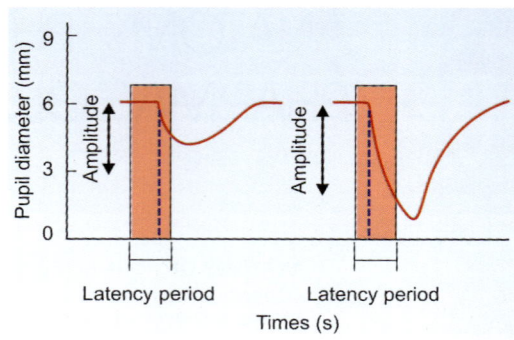

Fig. 6.1 *Pupillary response to a flash of light (intensity of flash 37 A) in a dark adapted subject.*

pupils are illuminated simultaneously, the response summates, i.e. the constriction of each pupil is greater than the constriction noted when only one pupil is illuminated. Of course, the amount of constriction depends upon the state of adaptation of the retina, the individual's emotional state, alertness and other factors.

Light reflex is initiated by rods and cones. With light intensity up to 9 log units above threshold strength and duration of pupillary contraction increases and the latency period decreases. At intensities above 9 log units, the pupillary response plateaus off (Fig. 6.1). The latent period is 0.2–0.5s; less than that for constriction induced by accommodation. The pupil is not capable of responding to stimuli with a frequency greater than 5 Hz.

Pathway of light reflex (Fig. 6.2)

The afferent fibers extend from the retina to the pretectal nucleus in the midbrain. Information from the rods and cones reaches the ganglion cells and travels centrally along the optic nerve to the chiasma, where fibers from the nasal retinae decussate and travel along the opposite optic tract to terminate in the contralateral pretectal nucleus, while the fibers from the temporal retina remain uncrossed and travel along the optic tract of the same side to terminate in the ipsilateral pretectal nucleus.

Internuncial fibers connect each pretectal nucleus with Edinger-Westphal nucleus of both sides as follows: Half of the postsynaptic fibers from the pretectal area curve around the

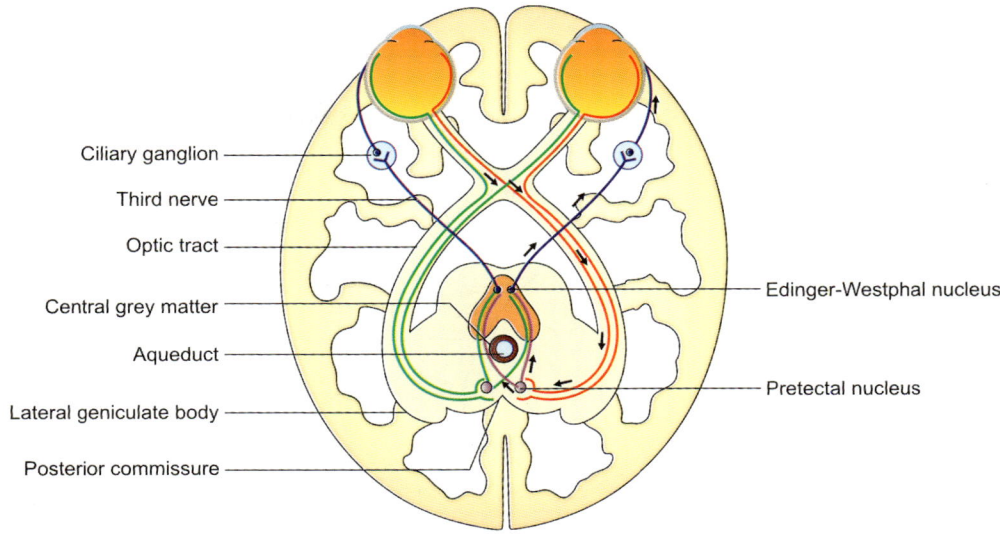

Fig. 6.2 *Pathway of light reflex.*

Ciliary ganglion

Third nerve

Optic tract

Central grey matter

Aqueduct

Lateral geniculate body

Posterior commissure

Edinger-Westphal nucleus

Pretectal nucleus

periaqueductal grey matter to terminate in the ipsilateral Edinger-Westphal nucleus, while the other half cross, mainly via the posterior commissure, to the contralateral Edinger-Westphal nucleus. This connection forms the basis of consensual light reflex. It is assumed that any given pretectal neuron behaves functionally as though it receives similar inputs from each eye and projects equally in each Edinger-Westphal nucleus.

Efferent pathway consists of the parasympathetic fibers which arise from the Edinger-Westphal nucleus in the midbrain and travel along the third cranial (oculomotor) nerve. The pupilloconstrictor fibers are situated on the surface of the third nerve, but their location on the surface changes along its intracranial course. For this reason and because of the long intracranial course of the nerve, unilateral deficits in pupilloconstriction can sometimes be of significant localizing value in cases of unilateral pathology, such as tumors and aneurysms. The preganglionic fibers enter the inferior division of the third nerve and via the nerve to the inferior oblique reach the *ciliary ganglion* to relay. Post-ganglionic fibers travel along the short ciliary nerves to innervate the sphincter pupillae.

Normally, there is a tonic inhibitory input from the cerebral cortex to the Edinger-Westphal nucleus, and it is a diminution of this input that results in pupillary constriction during sleep.

Functions of light reflex

1. Pupillary constriction associated with light reflex protects against excessive bleaching of the visual pigments by reducing the amount of light entering the eye.

2. Light reflex helps in light and dark adaptations; thus it plays a role in maximizing visual acuity at different light levels. A large pupil will admit more light and so can allow greater acuity in dim illumination. On the other hand, a smaller pupil will limit the aberrations produced by the eye's refractive system and so allows greater acuity. It has been found that at any given moderate light level, the size of the pupil strikes an optimum balance between these two factors.

NEAR REFLEX

Near reflex occurs on looking at near objects. It consists of two components:

a. *Convergence reflex* which comprises convergence of the visual axes of the eyes and associated constriction of the pupil.

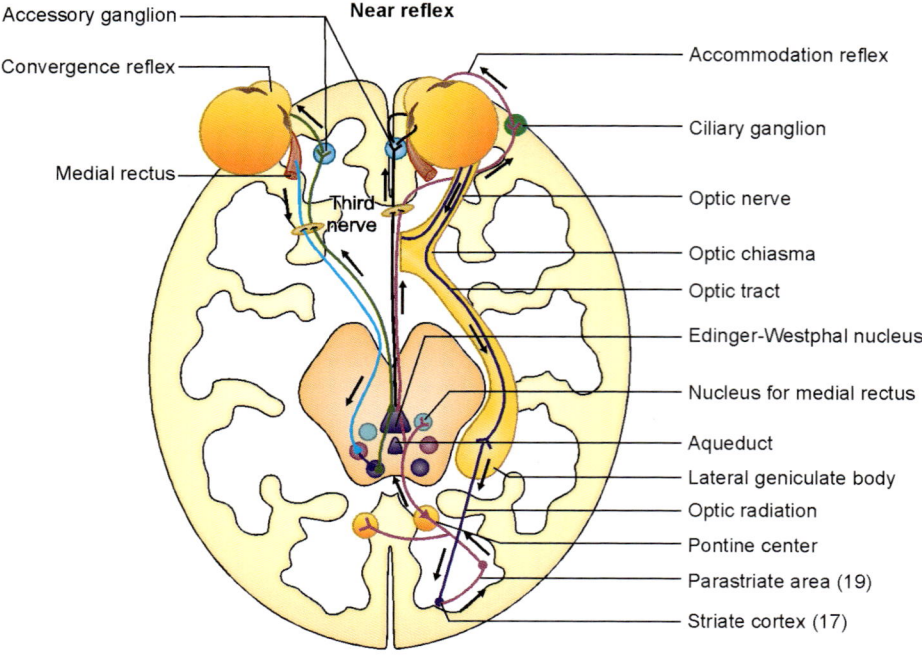

Fig. 6.3 *Pathway of near reflex.*

b. *Accommodation reflex* which includes increased accommodation and associated constriction of the pupil. In other words, the near reflex triad consists of:

1. Increased accommodation
2. Convergence of visual axes
3. Constriction of the pupils.

Pathway of convergence reflex (Fig. 6.3)

Afferent pathway of convergence reflex is still not elucidated. It is assumed that the afferents from the medial recti travel centrally via the third nerve to the mesencephalic nucleus of the fifth nerve, to a presumptive *convergence center* in the tectal or pretectal region.

Internuncial fibers from the so-called convergence center perhaps go to the Edinger-Westphal nucleus.

Efferent pathway of the convergence reflex is along the third nerve (similar to that of light reflex). From the third nerve, efferent fibers of convergence reflex relay in the *accessory ganglion*, before reaching the sphincter pupillae.

Pathway of accommodation reflex (Fig. 6.3)

Afferent impulses extend from the retina to the parastriate cortex (via the optic nerve, chiasma, optic tract, lateral geniculate body, optic radiations and striate cortex).

Internuncial fibers relay the impulses from the parastriate cortex to Edinger-Westphal nucleus of both sides via the occipitomesencephalic tract and the pontine center.

Efferent fibers. From the Edinger-Westphal nucleus the efferent impulses travel along the 3rd nerve and reach the sphincter pupillae and ciliary muscle after relay in the accessory and ciliary ganglia.

DARKNESS REFLEX

When a person goes from a lighted environment to darkness, the pupils dilate. It has been found that dilatation has two causes. The first is simply abolition of light reflex with consequent relaxation of the sphincter pupillae. The second is contraction of dilator pupillae supplied by sympathetic nervous system. The pathways involved in dark reflex are presumably the same as those of light reflex, since the redilatation at the end of long light stimulation also involves both relaxation of the sphincter pupillae and contraction of dilator pupillae.

PSYCHOSENSORY REFLEXES

Psychosensory reflexes refer to dilatation of pupil in response to sensory and psychic stimuli. A large number of differently described reflexes fall into this category. The psychosensory reflexes are not seen in a newborn, but appear in the first few days of life, developing fully by the age of six months. Their mechanism is very complex and their pathways have still not been elucidated. In general, it is believed that the mechanism of psychosensory reflexes is a cortical one and apparently the pupillary dilatation in these results from two components—a sympathetic discharge to the dilator pupillae and an inhibition of the parasympathetic discharge to the sphincter pupillae.

Pathway of sympathetic discharge

It is believed that some how sensations are conveyed to the hypothalamus, from where the impulses descend to the intermediolateral cell column of the cervical and thoracic parts of the spinal cord. However, the *ciliospinal reflex* (dilatation of pupil in response to painful stimuli in the neck region) has been reported to be elicited from patients with damaged sympathetic pathways in brainstem and even from patients with cervical cord transections; indicating thereby that at least "sympathetic discharge related to some of the psychosensory reflexes is mediated at the level of spinal cord.

LID-CLOSURE REFLEX

The lid-closure reflex is a non-specific term, (since the lid-closure may be accompanied by either pupillary contraction or pupillary dilatation), and hence should be used sparingly. In the literature the term lid-closure reflex has been used by different workers for the following entities:

1.Constriction of pupil associated with blinking

Following a blink, either voluntary or spontaneous, both pupils constrict transiently. It has been observed that such a reflex does not occur in darkness, so it has been assumed that perhaps this lid-closure reflex is nothing but simply a type of darkness reflex.

2. Homolateral pupillary constriction associated with closure of the lid

Which is evoked if the lid is held open whilst the effort of closure is made, is another entity which has also been referred to as lid-closure reflex. The effect is not large, however, if the subject is instructed to keep his gaze fixed on a distant object, while trying to close the eyes, this reaction does not occur. From this, it has been concluded that perhaps the pupillary contraction reported with this reflex is the result of an unconscious attempt at near gaze during the lid-closure effort.

3.Pupillary dilatation associated with lid-closure on touching the cornea (oculopupillary reflex)

It has also been considered by some a lid-closure reflex. However, it has also been reported that it is simply a type of psychosensory reflex.

PHARMACOLOGY OF THE PUPIL

MIOTICS

The drugs which constrict the pupil are known as miotics. These include two groups: the parasympathomimetic (sphincter stimulators) and sympatholytics (dilator inhibitors).

Parasympathomimetic drugs

Parasympathomimetics also called as cholinergic drugs either imitate or potentiate the effects of acetylcholine. Depending upon the mode of action, these can be classified as follows:

1. *Direct acting or agonists,* e.g. pilocarpine. These drugs are structurally similar to acetylcholine and act directly on the muscarinic receptors on the muscle membrane (Fig. 6.4A).

2. *Indirect acting parasympathomimetics or cholinesterase inhibitors.* As the name indicates, these drugs act indirectly by destroying the enzyme cholinesterase, thereby sparing the naturally acting acetylcholine for its actions

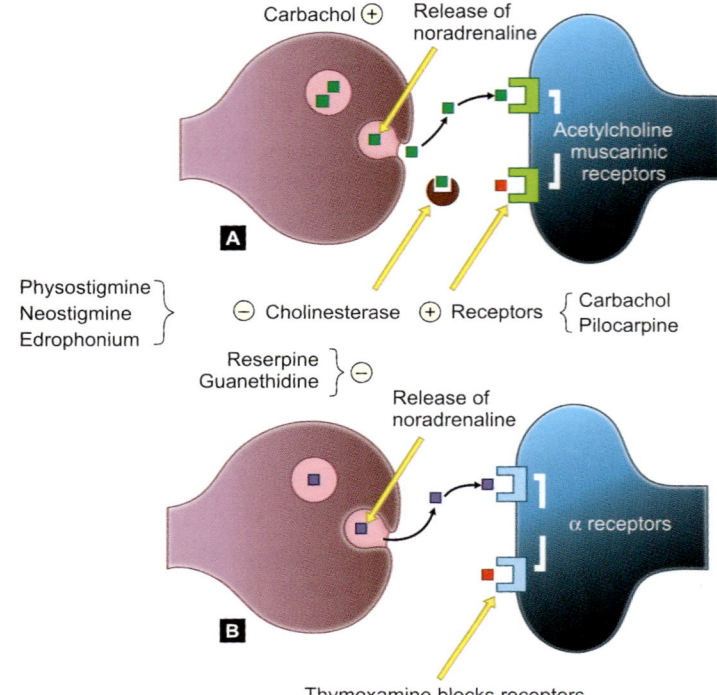

Fig. 6.4 *Mode of action of miotics: (A) Parasympathomimetic drugs; (B) Sympatholytic drugs.*

(Fig. 6.4A). These drugs have been divided into two subgroups: *reversible cholinesterase inhibitors* (e.g. physostigmine) and *irreversible cholinesterase inhibitors* (e.g. echothiophate iodide, demecarium and diisopropyl fluorophosphate, i.e. DFP or DFP3).

Normally, acetylcholine is liberated at the cholinergic nerve endings by the neural action potential. As soon as the acetylcholine is released, it is hydrolyzed by cholinesterases, which are probably present in the presynaptic axonal membrane. The anticholinesterase drugs either block the action of cholinesterase or deplete the stores of the enzyme in the tissue. These are thus able to potentiate the action of the chemical mediator by preventing its destruction by the enzyme cholinesterase. Thus, it follows from their mode of action that these drugs will lose their cholinergic activity after the nerve supply has been completely blocked.

3. *Dual action parasympathomimetics*, i.e. which act as both.

Sympatholytic drugs

Dilator pupillae can be inhibited either by preventing transmitter release at the neuro-muscular junction or by preventing the transmitter from affecting the dilator fibers.

Alpha-adrenergic blocker drugs such as thymoxamine, phenoxybenzamine, dibenamine and tolazoline produce miosis by preventing dilator contraction (Fig. 6.4B). These drugs occupy alpha-receptor sites on the iris dilator muscle. However, these drugs are seldom used in ophthalmology. *Guanethidine* is the commonly used sympatholytic drug. It disrupts norepinephrine release from the nerve ending and depletes norepinephrine stores. Continued topical administration of this drug to the eye causes Homer's syndrome characterized by ptosis, miosis and supersensitivity to adrenergic drugs.

Other miotics

Histamine acts as a protoplasmic irritant and affects the sphincter fibers directly. It even

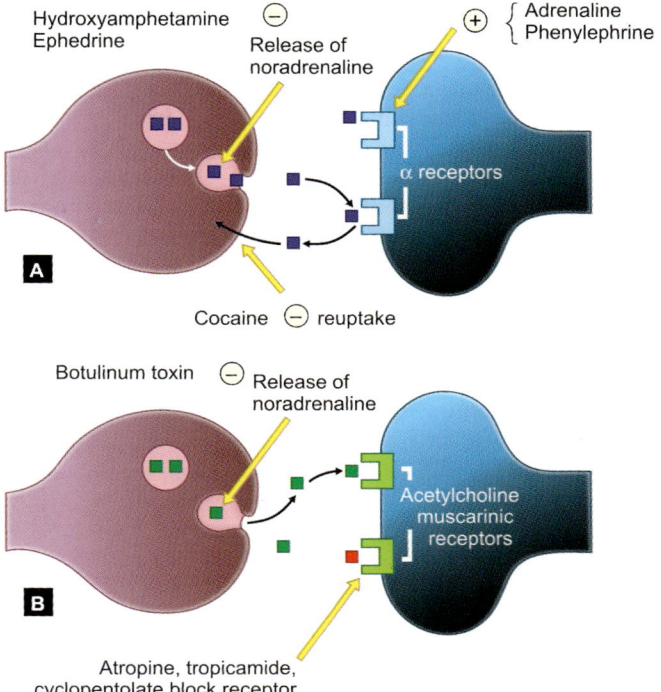

Fig. 6.5 *Mode of action of mydriatic drugs: (A) Sympathomimetic drugs; (B) Parasympatholytic drugs.*

constricts the pupil of a thoroughly atropinized eye. *Morphine* causes miosis by cutting off cortical inhibition of the Edinger-Westphal nucleus. It may also have a direct stimulating action on the Edinger-Westphal nucleus.

MYDRIATICS

Sympathomimetic mydriatics (dilator stimulators)

At the neuroeffector junction of the dilator pupillae norepinephrine is stored in vesicles at the presynaptic terminal and is constantly released. After the release, some of the norepinephrine is taken up into the presynaptic vesicle, some is metabolized and destroyed by monoamine oxidase, a small portion is washed away and the last portion may be degraded by the enzyme catechol-O-methyl transferase.

Sympathomimetics increase the dilator activity by any of the three ways:

1. Increasing norepinephrine release

2. Preventing its reuptake by presynaptic vesicle

3. Directly stimulating the dilator fibers.

Adrenaline (epinephrine), which acts directly on the α-receptors on the dilator pupillae, produces dilation after instillation of four drops of 1 in 1000 solution (Fig. 6.5A). Instillation is repeated every 5 min. However, topically applied epinephrine is not very effective in normal eyes, because it is readily taken up or inactivated. This makes it useful in testing for certain denervation syndromes in which dilator becomes hypersensitive.

Phenylephrine is a synthetic analog of epinephrine. It stimulates the normal dilator, when used in fairly high concentration (5 to 10%) (Fig. 6.5A). It may also cause local release of norepinephrine.

Hydroxyamphetamine and ephedrine cause norepinephrine to be rapidly released from peripheral nerve terminals, resulting in a mydriasis of short duration (Fig. 6.5A). Perhaps, they may also stimulate the dilator directly.

Cocaine, in addition to acting as a local anesthetic, prevents the reuptake of norepinephrine at the presynaptic terminal (Fig. 6.5A). Thus norepinephrine released from the nerve remains in the synaptic cleft and activates the dilator fibers. Cocaine and hydroxyamphetamine, are therefore, ineffective and adrenaline remains effective when the sympathetic nerve is paralyzed.

Parasympatholytic mydriatics

These drugs compete with acetylcholine at the myoneural junction and thus cause mydriasis by blocking sphincter activity (Fig. 6.5B). Some of the clinically used drugs are as follows:

Atropine is the strongest mydriatic which completely paralyses the sphincter pupillae and ciliary muscle (cycloplegia). It is used as 1% drops or ointment. It causes complete dilation in 30–40 minutes and cycloplegia in about 2 hours. Its effect persists for a week or more.

Homatropine (2% drops) acts more quickly than atropine. It causes cycloplegia and mydriasis in about 45 minutes to one hour. Its effect passes completely in about 48 hours.

Cyclopentolate (1.0% drops) is a short-acting cycloplegic. It causes mydriasis and cycloplegia in about 1 hour and the effect lasts for 6–12 hours.

Tropicamide (1%) is also a quick and short-acting drug.

BIBLIOGRAPHY

1. Adie WV: Complete and incomplete forms of the benign disorder characterized by tonic pupils and absent tendon reflexes. Br. J. Ophthalmol 1932;16:449–61.

2. Argyll Robertson D: Four cases of spinal myosis: with remarks on the action of light on the pupil Edinburgh Med. J 1869;15:487–93.

3. Arieff AJ, Pyzik SW. The ciliospinal reflex in injuries of the cervical spinal cord in man. Arch Neurol Psychiatry 1953;70:621–29.

4. Bonnet P. L' historique du syndrome de Claude Bernard. Le syndrome paralytique du sympathique cervical, Arch. Ophthal 1957;17:121.

5. Borgmann H. Grundlage fur eine klinische Pupillographic. IV. Abhangigkeit der Pupillenweite und der Lichtreaktion von Geschlecht, Irisfarbe und Refraktion. Albrecht v Graefes Arch. Ophthalmol 1972;185:11–21.

6. Gunn M. Discussion of retro-ocular neuritis, Lancet 1904;2:412–13.

7. Jones IS. Anisocoria: attempted induction by unilateral illumination. Arch Ophthalmol 1949;42: 249–253.

8. Kerr FWL, Brown JA. Pupillomotor pathways in the spinal cord. Arch. Neurol 1964;10:262–270.

9. Loewenfeld IE. The Argyll Robertson Pupil, 1869–1969. A critical survey of the literature. In Schwartz, B., editor: Syphilis of eye, Baltimore, 1970, The Williams and Wilkins Co. (represented from Surv. Ophthalmol 1669;14:199).

10. Lowerstein O, Loewenfeld IE. The pupil, In Davson H (ed): The Eye, Vol 3. New York, Academic Press, 1969.

11. Pilley SJF, and Thompson HS. Edge-light pupil cycle time, Br. J. Ophthalmol 1975;50:731.

12. Reeves AG, Posner JB. The ciliospinal response in man, Neurology 1969;19:1145–52.

13. Scheie HG. Site of disturbance in Adie's syndrome. Arch Ophthalmol 1940;24:225–37.

14. Thompson HS. Franceschetti AT, Thompson PM. Hippus, Am. J. Ophthalmol 1971;71:1116.

15. Thompson HS. Diagnostic pupillary drug tests. In Blodi FC, editor: Current concepts in ophthalmology, St. Louis, 1972, The CV Mosby Co., Vol. 3, Chapter 6.

16. Thompson LC. Binocular summation within the nervous pathways of the pupillary light reflex. J Physiol (Lond.) 1947;106:59–65.

17. Woodhouse JM, Campbell FW. The role of the pupil light reflex in aiding adaptation to the dark. Vision Res 1975;15:649–53.

7

DISORDERS OF PUPIL

AK Khurana, Rashmin A Gandhi, Indu Khurana
Aruj K Khurana, Bhawna Khurana

MORPHOLOGICAL ABNORMALITIES OF PUPIL
- Corectopia
- Polycoria
- Anisocoria

ABNORMALITIES OF PUPILLARY REFLEX

Afferent pathway defects
- Total afferent pathway defect
- Relative afferent pathway defect
- Wernicke's hemianopic pupil

Efferent pupillary defects
- Common causes
- Tonic pupil

Pupillary light-near dissociation
- Causes
- Argyll Robertson pupil

Sympathetic paresis
- Sympathetic supply of the eye
- Horner's syndrome

CLINICAL EXAMINATION OF PUPIL

Size, shape and color of pupil
- Measurement of pupil size
- Shape of pupil
- Color of pupil

Tests for pupillary reflexes
- Direct light reflex
- Consensual light reflex
- Kestenbaum pseudo-anisocoria test
- Swinging's flash light test
- Edge light pupil cycle time
- Near reflex
- Dark reflex
- Ciliospinal reflex

MORPHOLOGICAL ABNORMALITIES OF PUPIL

CORECTOPIA

Corectopia refers to congenital abnormal placement of pupil normally pupil is placed slightly nasal to the center.

POLYCORIA

In this rare congenital anomaly, there are more than one pupil.

ANISOCORIA

Normal size of pupil varies from 3 to 4 mm depending upon the illumination. Difference between the size of two pupils is called anisocoria.

Clinical types of anisocoria

1. Physiologic anisocoria

Also named, simple, central, or essential anisocoria, is characterized by following clinical features:
- Minimal anisocoria (mostly <0.4 mm)
- Both pupils react well to light

- Normal dilatation in dark (no dilatation lag)
- Equal dilatation of both pupils with topical cocaine.
- *Isolated condition.* No associated symptoms like ptosis, dilatation lag, normal iris on slit lamp examination, no exposure of pharmacologic agents.

2. *Miosis of one pupil*
- Effect of local miotic drugs (parasympatho-mimetic drugs).
- Effect of systemic morphine.
- Iridocyclitis (narrow, irregular, non-reacting pupil).
- Horner's syndrome.
- Head injury (pontine hemorrhage).
- Senile rigid miotic pupil.
- Due to effect of strong light.
- During sleep pupil is pinpoint.

3. *Mydriasis of one pupil*
- Effect of topical sympathomimetic drugs (e.g. adrenaline and phenylephrine)

- Effect of topical parasympatholytic drugs (e.g. atropine, homatropine, tropicamide and cyclopentolate).
- Sphincter damage, e.g. acute congestive glaucoma (vertically oval large immobile pupil).
- Internal ophthalmoplegia
- 3rd nerve paralysis
- Belladonna poisoning.

Evaluation

- A difference of pupil size greater than 2 mm is considered pathological and warrants further evaluation.
- Anisocoria is *not* caused by optic nerve or afferent pupil pathway dysfunction.
- Assuming the sphincter is structurally normal on slit lamp examination, anisocoria is a sign of autonomic (parasympathetic or sympathetic) dysfunction.
- The onset of anisocoria (especially if isolated and discovered as an incidental finding) can be determined by examination of pupil size in old photographs of the patient using good magnification (20D lens of the indirect ophthalmoscope).
- Evaluate pupil size in bright and dim illumination as mentioned under "Pupil Size" (page 74).
- A pupil with a **brisk sustained light reflex** is a **normal pupil** whether or not it appears larger or smaller than its fellow (Fig. 7.1A).
- *Anisocoria same in bright or dim illumination:* Physiological anisocoria
- *Anisocoria increases in bright illumination:* The larger pupil is the abnormal pupil with a parasympathetic palsy (Fig. 7.1B).
- *Anisocoria increases in dim illumination:*
  - The smaller pupil is the abnormal pupil with a sympathetic palsy (Fig. 7.1C).
  - Physiological anisocoria sometimes behaves in this manner.

ABNORMALITIES OF PUPILLARY REFLEXES

AFFERENT PATHWAY DEFECTS

Total afferent pathway defect (TAPD) or amaurotic pupil

It is caused by a complete optic nerve or retinal lesion leading to total blindness on the affected side. It is characterized by the following:

- Absence of direct light reflex on the affected side (say right) and absence of consensual light reflex on the normal side (i.e. left).
- When the normal eye is stimulated, both pupils react normally.
- In diffuse illumination, both pupils are equal in size.
- The near reflex is normal in both eyes.

Relative afferent pathway defect (RAPD) or Marcus Gunn pupil

It is the paradoxical response of a pupil to light in the presence of a relative afferent pathway defect (RAPD). It is caused by an incomplete optic nerve lesion or a severe retinal disease. It is best tested by 'swinging flashlight test'. For details see page 77.

Wernicke's hemianopic pupil

It indicates lesion of the optic tract. In this condition, light reflex (ipsilateral direct and contralateral consensual) is absent when light is thrown on the temporal half of the retina of the affected side and nasal half of the retina of

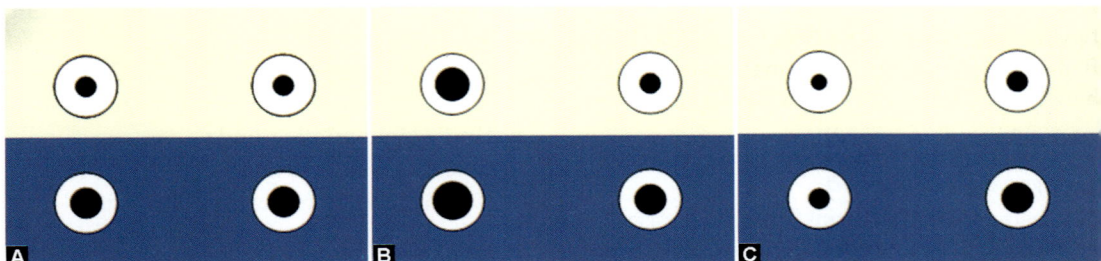

Fig. 7.1 *(A) Normal response—no difference in pupil size between the eyes either in light or dark; (B) RE parasympathetic palsy—anisocoria worse in light; (C) Sympathetic palsy—anisocoria worse in dark.*

the opposite side; while it is present when the light is thrown on the nasal half of the affected side and temporal half of the opposite side.

EFFERENT PUPILLARY DEFECTS

Efferent pupillary defects are characterized by absence of both direct and consensual light reflex on the affected side (say right eye) and presence of both direct and consensual light reflex on the normal side (i.e. left eye). On the affected side, near reflex is also absent and pupil remains fixed and dilated.

Common causes of efferent pupillary defects

1. **Brainstem lesions** at the level of the superior colliculus and red nucleus. Lesions here are often accompanied by long tract signs.
2. **Fascicular third nerve lesions.** Compressive third nerve lesions classically have pupillary involvement, although an efferent defect is not pathognomonic of a compressive lesion, as 20% of microvascular palsies will affect the pupillary fibers. An efferent pupillary defect may be a false localizing sign when raised intracranial pressure causes uncal herniation and compression of third nerve.
3. **Lesions of the ciliary ganglion** or short ciliary nerves.
4. **Iris damage** secondary to previous surgery or grossly elevated intraocular pressure.
5. **Drugs:** Inadvertent exposure to a mydriatic agent such as atropine is a common cause of fixed dilated pupil. Pilocarpine 1% will constrict a dilated pupil secondary to a neurological lesion; it will have no effect on a dilated pupil caused by a mydriatic agent.

Tonic pupil

Damage to the ciliary ganglion or short ciliary nerves produces tonic pupil which is characterized by following:
- The affected pupil is larger (moderately dilated pupil).
- *Reaction to light* is absent
- *Near reflex* is very slow and tonic.
- *Accommodative paresis.*
- *Cholinergic supersensitivity* of the denervated muscle (i.e. constricts with 0.125% pilocarpine, while normal pupil does not).

Causes of tonic pupil

A. *Local tonic pupil*
- Viral ciliary ganglionitis (e.g. herpes zoster).
- Orbital or choroidal trauma or tumors.
- Blunt trauma to the globe may injure branches of short ciliary nerves at the iris root.

B *Neuropathic tonic pupil*
Part of picture of peripheral neuropathy of:
- Diabetes
- Alcoholism.

C. *Idiopathic tonic pupil with benign areflexia (Adie's tonic pupil)*

Adie's tonic pupil

As discussed above, Adie's tonic pupil is caused by denervation of the postganglionic supply of the sphincter pupillae and ciliary muscle of unknown etiology. Its characteristic features are as below:
- It is usually unilateral (in 80%).
- It typically affects healthy young women more often than men.
- It may be associated with absent knee jerk.
- The affected pupil is large and irregular (anisocoria).
- The light reflex is absent or slow.
- Near reflex is slow and tonic.
- Accommodative paresis
- There may be associated mild regional impairment of corneal sensations.

Oculomotor nerve palsy

- Pupil mid-dilated
- Light, consensual, and near reflexes affected.
- Pilocarpine test:
  - No constriction (or occasionally a mild constriction) with 0.125% pilocarpine
  - Will constrict with 1% pilocarpine
- Look for other signs of TNP including pupil gaze dyskinesis (indicating aberrant regeneration).

Pharmacologic mydriasis

- Usually a widely dilated pupil (10–12 mm). (Tonic pupil and TNP pupil are mid-dilated)
- Dilatation with adrenergics (e.g. phenylephrine)
  - Blanched conjunctival vessels
  - Residual light reaction

– Upper lid retraction (Müller's muscle stimulation)
- *Pilocarpine test.* No constriction with either 0.125% or 1% pilocarpine.

Evaluation of parasympathetic palsy

Slit lamp examination

i. Examine pupil sphincter
   - Sphincter tears—trauma/surgery
   - Sphincter paresis due to ischemia in acute angle closure glaucoma
   - Sphincter atrophy—post acute angle closure glaucoma
   - Congenital aplasia of sphincter
ii. Look for segmental pupil contraction (vermiform movement) by increasing/decreasing illumination
   - Causes: Tonic pupils, TNP
iii. Contraction induced by ocular motility—elevation, adduction, or depression
   Cause: III nerve palsy with aberrant regeneration (Czarnecki sign—segmental contraction during adduction in TNP).
iv. Iris and anterior chamber
   Any other structural abnormality?

Pilocarpine test

Contraindication

Documented hypersensitivity, acute anterior uveitis pupillary block glaucoma, pregnancy (?).

Precaution

Acute cardiac failure, peptic ulcer, hyperthyroidism, GI spasm, bronchial asthma, Parkinson disease, recent myocardial infarction, urinary tract obstruction, and hypertension or hypotension.

Miosis may cause difficulty with dark adaptation and night driving.

Preparation 0.125% pilocarpine eye drops

- Withdraw 0.25 ml of commercially available 1% pilocarpine eye drops into a 2 ml syringe.
- Dilute by withdrawing normal saline up to the 2 ml mark (x 8 dilution)
- Fit a cannula to the syringe for topical instillation.
   Note. If 2% pilocarpine is available, it can be made into a 1% solution first as follows:

- Withdraw 0.25 ml of commercially available 2% pilocarpine eye drops into a 2 ml syringe.
- Dilute by withdrawing 0.25 ml (an equal amount) of normal saline (1:1 dilution). The syringe now contains 0.5 ml solution of 1% pilocarpine.
- Mix thoroughly and then discard 0.25 ml. What is left is 0.25 ml of 1% pilocarpine.
- Now follow steps (c) and (d) described above to prepare 0.125% solution of pilocarpine.

Method

- Measure pupil size in both eyes (in ambient or bright illumination)
- Instill 0.125% pilocarpine in both eyes every 10 minutes for half an hour.

Note. Make sure enough medication has been instilled equally in both eyes, making allowance for squeezing of the patients eye while applying medication in the second eye.
- Measure pupil size every 10 minutes

Result

- *Tonic pupil* dramatic constriction of the tonic pupil with no change in the size of the smaller pupil (known as denervation supersensitivity).
   Reversal of anisocoria in some cases, as the larger pupil becomes more miotic than its fellow.
- *TNP pupil and pharmacologic pupil.* No change in anisocoria (the larger pupil remains approximately the same size).

Note. Cholinergic supersensitivity may occasionally occur in TNP. Two ways to clinically judge a tonic pupil from TNP by this test are:

- Be suspicious of "moderate" constriction of the pupil with weak pilocarpine. It could be TNP.
- Look for a larger pupil that becomes smaller in darkness after instillation of weak pilocarpine. It is more likely to be a tonic pupil.

PUPILLARY LIGHT-NEAR DISSOCIATION

The term pupillary light-near dissociation refers to any situation in which the pupillary near reaction is present and the light reaction is absent.

Causes of light-near dissociation

Of course Argyll Robertson pupil is one of the important causes of light-near dissociation; but it is not synonymous with the condition. Argyll Robertson pupil has certain other peculiar features and is described separately. In general, the causes of light-near dissociation are shown in Fig. 7.2 and depicted below:

1. *Bilateral complete afferent pathway defect,* e.g. in bilateral old total retinal detachment (Fig. 7.2A) or bilateral optic atrophy (Fig. 7.2B), the light reflex is absent but near reflex is present.

2. *Lesions in the midbrain.* The light reflex path can be interrupted here in the pretectal area (Fig. 7.2C), without damaging the more ventrally located input for the near reflex. Causes include tumors (e.g. pinealomas manifesting as Parinaud's syndrome or 'Sylvian aqueduct syndrome'), vascular lesions, encephalitis and demyelinization. Neuro-syphilis causing Argyll Robertson pupil also causes a damage in the area of pretectum to the intercalated neuron (Fig. 7.2D).

3. *Third nerve palsy with aberrant regeneration of medial rectus innervation into the sphincter innervation pathway* (Fig. 7.2E) leads to presence of near reflex but absence of light reflex. This condition is termed 'pseudo-Argyll Robertson pupil'.

4. *Ciliary ganglion or short ciliary nerve lesions with aberrant regeneration of accommodation* impulse fibers into the sphincter pupillae (tonic pupil) has also been reported to result in light-near dissociation (Fig. 7.2F).

5. *Pupillary light-near dissociation* associated with peripheral neuropathies in diabetes, alcoholism, amyloidosis, etc. can also be explained on the basis of aberrant regeneration.

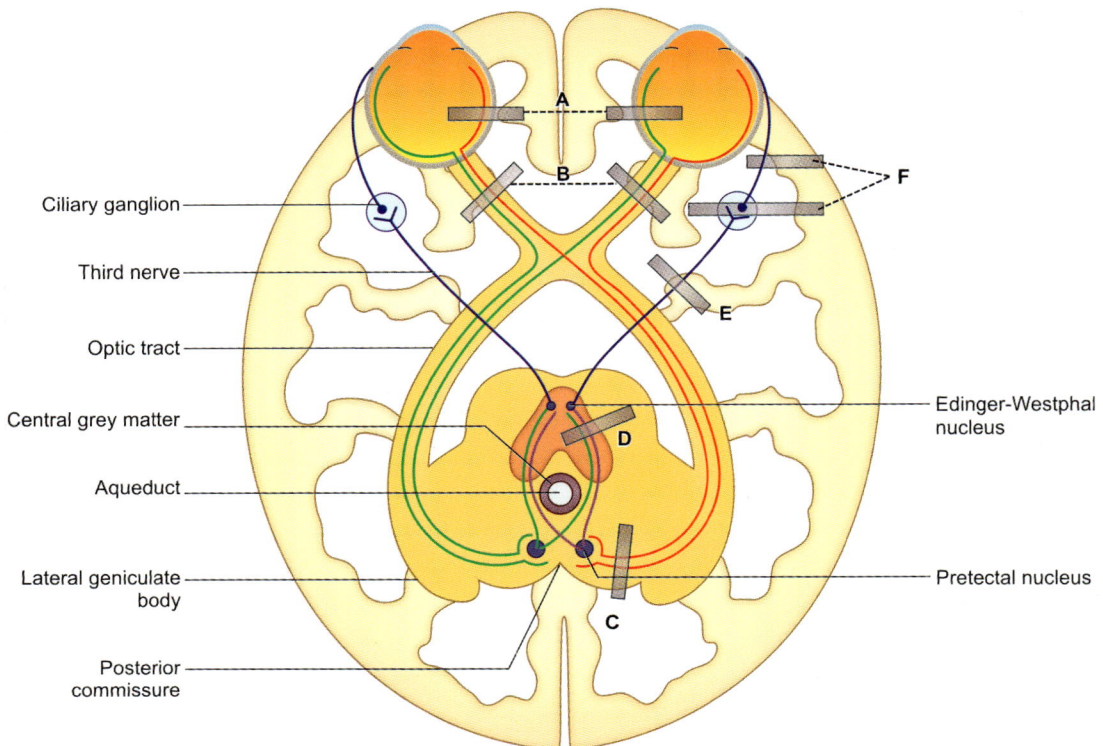

Fig. 7.2 *Site of lesions producing light-near dissociation: A. Retinal lesions; B. Optic nerve lesions; C. Lesions in pretectal region; D. Lesions in the intercalated neurons (e.g. Argyll Robertson pupil; E. Third nerve lesions with aberrant regeneration of sphincter innervation; F. Ciliary ganglion or short ciliary nerve lesions with aberrant regeneration of sphincter innervation.*

Argyll Robertson Pupil

The Argyll Robertson pupil (ARP) was originally described in 1869 in a series of patients with tabes dorsalis. It is thought to be caused by a lesion (neurosyphilis) in the region of tectum (rostral midbrain near the Sylvian aqueduct interfering with the light reflex fibers and the supranuclear inhibitory fibers as they approach the Edinger-Westphal nucleus) (Fig. 7.2D). Characteristic features of Argyll Robertson pupil are as follows:

- Involvement is usually bilateral but asymmetrical.
- The retinae are sensitive to light (usually good vision is present).
- The pupils are small in size and irregular in shape.

- The light reflex is absent, but near reflex is present (light-near dissociation) (just to remember the acronym ARP may be thought for accommodation reflex present).
- The pupils dilate very poorly with mydriatics like atropine.
- Physostigmine causes further constriction.

SYMPATHETIC PARESIS

Sympathetic supply of the eye

It consists of three neurons (Fig. 7.3).
Central neuron (first) starts in the posterior hypothalamus. It descends, uncrossed, traverses the brainstem and terminates in the *'cilio-spinal center of Budge'* located in the intermediolateral cell column of C8, T1 and T2.

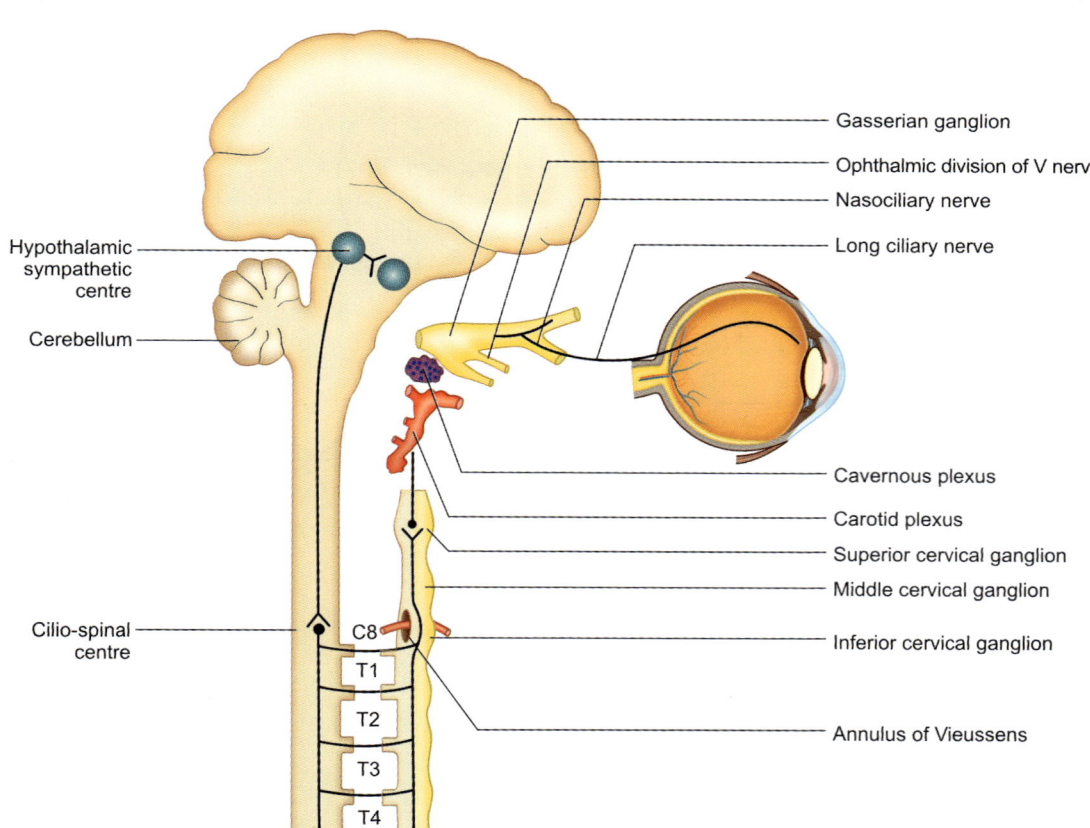

Hypothalamic sympathetic centre

Cerebellum

Cilio-spinal centre

C8
T1
T2
T3
T4

Gasserian ganglion

Ophthalmic division of V nerve

Nasociliary nerve

Long ciliary nerve

Cavernous plexus

Carotid plexus

Superior cervical ganglion

Middle cervical ganglion

Inferior cervical ganglion

Annulus of Vieussens

Fig. 7.3: *Sympathetic supply of the eye.*

Second neuron passes from the ciliospinal center of Budge (*preganglionic neuron*) to terminate in the *superior cervical ganglion* in the neck. During this long course, the preganglionic fibers are closely related to the apical pleura where these may be damaged by bronchial carcinoma (Pancoast's tumor) or during surgery on the neck.

Postganglionic neuron (third) arises from the superior cervical ganglion and ascends along with the internal carotid artery to enter the skull, where the postganglionic fibers join the ophthalmic division of the trigeminal nerve. Ultimately, the postganglionic sympathetic fibers reach the ciliary body and the dilator pupillae via the nasociliary and long ciliary nerves.

Horner's syndrome

Types of Horner's syndrome

Presently, the term *Horner's syndrome* is used to describe any oculosympathetic paresis, wherever the lesion may be (though Horner's own case was presumably of a neck lesion). Consequently, Horner's syndrome has been divided into three types:

1. Central Horner's syndrome

It occurs due to lesions located from hypothalamus to the cilio-spinal center of Budge at C8–T2.

Causes. Brainstem vascular lesions, demyelination and tumors; syringomyelia and spinal cord lesions at C8–T2.

2. *Preganglionic Horner's syndrome*

It occurs due to lesions located from C8 to T2 of spinal cord to the course of preganglionic fibers (in chest and neck) to the superior cervical ganglion.

Causes. Pancoast's tumor of the lung (very important cause), carotid and aortic aneurysms, lesions in the neck (e.g. malignant cervical lymph nodes, trauma or surgery), congenital (birth trauma).

3. *Postganglionic Horner's syndrome*

It is labelled when the lesion is in the course of postganglionic fibers in the head.

Causes. Benign vascular headache syndrome affecting the internal carotid artery, head trauma, intra-aural or retroparotid trauma and cavernous sinus lesions.

Clinical features of Horner's syndrome

Horner's syndrome usually occurs due to ipsilateral interruption of the sympathetic outflow to the head and neck. Its characteristic features are as follows:

1. *Ptosis.* Mild to moderate ptosis results from paralysis of Müller's muscle of the upper eyelid.
2. *Upside down ptosis* (elevation of inferior eyelid). It results from weakness of inferior tarsal muscle.
3. *Miosis.* There is moderate miosis due to unopposed action of the sphincter pupillae following paralysis of dilator pupillae. In bright light both pupils are nearly equal. The anisocoria is much more evident in dim illumination.
4. *Pupillary reactions* are normal to light and near.
5. *Dilation lag.* When lights are turned off the Horner's pupil dilates more slowly than the normal pupil does because it lags the pull of dilator pupillae and thus anisocoria is increased in dim light.
6. *Facial anhydrosis.* Reduced sweating on the ipsilateral face and neck is characteristic of preganglionic Horner's syndrome, i.e. when the lesion is below the superior cervical ganglion. Thus, not present in lesions beyond bifurcation of common carotid artery.
7. *Heterochromia irides.* When the sympathetic ocular innervation is interrupted early in life (congenital Horner's syndrome) the pigment of the iris stroma fails to develop producing heterochromia irides.
8. *Other signs* include ocular hypotony in the acute phase and increased amplitude of accommodation.

Localizing the lesion in Horner's syndrome

A patient with Horner's syndrome can be assigned to the category of central, preganglionic or postganglionic Horner's syndrome depending upon the associated signs and symptoms and certain pharmacological tests as below:

Associated signs and symptoms

1. *Central Horner's syndrome*

It may be associated with any of the following signs and symptoms:

- *Hypothalamic signs.* Diabetes insipidus, disturbed temperature regulation, altered sleep patterns.
- *Brainstem signs.* Contralateral IV/VI N palsy, vertigo, sensory deficits, anhidrosis of the body
- *Meningeal signs*
- *Signs of cervical cord disease*, or signs of syringomyelia.

2. *Preganglionic Horner's syndrome*

It may have any of the following associations:

- Lung or breast malignancy that has spread to thoracic outlet.
- History of injury or surgery in the region of neck, chest or cervical spine.
- Anhydrosis involves the face and neck.
- Brachial plexus palsy may be associated.
- Vocal cord paralysis due to phrenic nerve (3, 4, 5) palsy.

3. *Postganglionic Horner's syndrome*

Common causes of postganglionic Horner's syndrome are:

- Ipsilateral vascular headache.
- Head injury, intra-aural or retroparotid trauma (causing damage to carotid sympathetic plexus).
- A tumor of middle cranial fossa or cavernous sinus may involve parasellar cranial nerves and effect the sympathetic fibers of the eye. It is important to note that facial anhidrosis is absent in postganglionic Horner's syndrome since the postganglionic sympathetic fibers that control facial sweating travel on the external (not the internal) carotid artery and are, therefore, not affected by a postganglionic Horner's syndrome.

Associated features with post-ganglionic Horner's syndrome thus include:

- *Ipsilateral cluster/migraine headache* characterized by face pain, tearing, facial flushing, and rhinorrhea

- *Cavernous sinus signs*
  - Associated III, IV, VI, V1 palsy
  - Pseudo-pupil sparing
  - Simultaneous TNP and sympathetic palsy results in a normal sized but poorly reactive pupil (poor light reflex and position dilatation lag)
- No facial anhidrosis (but anhidrosis of forehead may be present)
  - Reason: sweat glands of forehead innervated by terminal branches of internal carotid nerve which may be involved
- *Internal carotid artery dissection signs*
  - Orbital/face/neck pain
  - Amaurosis fugax or retinal artery occlusion
  - Neck bruit or swelling
- Other neurologic signs
  - Dysgeusia, tinnitus, syncope, cranial neuropathy (VI, IX, X, XI, XII)

Pharmacological tests employed to localized Horner's syndrome

1. *Cocaine test*

Cocaine prevents the reuptake of noradrenaline at the adrenergic synapse and thus when 4% cocaine is instilled in both eyes, the normal pupil will dilate but the Horner's pupil will not. All Horner's pupils, no matter where the defect in the pathway is located, will dilate poorly to cocaine. Thus cocaine helps in establishing the diagnosis of sympathetic denervation and not in localizing the site of lesion.

Method

- Measure pupil size in both eyes and determine pre-test anisocoria
- Instill the drops in the conjunctival sac in both eyes, applying in the miotic (Horner's syndrome) eye first. Wipe both eyes with a tissue
- After 20–40 seconds instill a second drop of the drug to each eye (to balance the dosage)
- Measure post-test anisocoria 30 minutes after second instillation.

Note

a. Cocaine stings the eye and the patient may squeeze the lids during instillation of the drop in the second eye. This may result in less drug availability in that eye. Therefore it is important to apply the drug in the apparently affected (miotic) eye first.

b. Cocaine must be applied in eyes with intact corneal epithelium. This means that the test cannot be performed on the same day if the patient has undergone applanation tonometry, corneal sensitivity testing, or any procedure that could affect the integrity of the epithelium.

c. Dark irides dilate poorly with cocaine and the test result must be interpreted with more caution.

2. Hydroxyamphetamine test

When 10% drops of this drug are instilled into both eyes, in a patient with preganglionic lesion both pupils will dilate whereas in postganglionic lesion, the Horner's pupil will not. It is because, since the hydroxyamphetamine acts by releasing norepinephrine from the nerve endings at the myoneural junction, so in postganglionic lesions the drug will have no effect.

Note. A 48 hour interval between the cocaine test and the hydroxyamphetamine test is recommended. Both tests cannot be performed on the same day because cocaine inhibits the uptake of hydroxyamphetamine into the presynaptic vesicle, reducing accuracy of the hydroxyamphetamine test.

Comparison of the cocaine versus hydroxyamphetamine test is given in Table 7.1.

3. Adrenaline test or phenylephrine test

When either adrenaline 1 in 1000 or phenylephrine 10% is instilled in both eyes, the Horner's pupil due to postganglionic lesion dilates more than the normal pupil does (because of denervation supersensitivity).

Phenylephrine 1% correlates well with the results of hydroxyamphetamine 1% in localizing the lesion to the post-ganglionic neuron and is a reliable alternative to hydroxyamphetamine 1% should pharmacological testing be desired and hydroxyamphetamine 1% not be available.

Table 7.1 *Cocaine versus hydroxyamphetamine*

Drug	Cocaine	Hydroxyamphetamine
Action	Inhibits reuptake of norepinephrine at neuromuscular junction	Releases stored norepinephrine from postganglionic adrenergic nerve endings at the dilator pupillae.
Effect	Dilatation of the normal pupil (by about 1 mm only)	Preganglionic lesion—pupil dilatation
	No effect on Horner's syndrome pupil regardless of location of lesion (minimal dilatation may occur in partial palsy or central Horner's syndrome)	Postganglionic lesion—no pupil dilation
Interactions	Increases toxicity of MAO inhibitors	Beta-blockers may cause systemic adverse effects; exaggerated adrenergic effects may result as long as 21 d after MAO inhibitors
Contraindications	Documented hypersensitivity, pregnancy (?)	Documented hypersensitivity; narrow-angle glaucoma; anatomically narrow (occludable) angle without glaucoma, pregnancy (?)
Precautions	Hypertension, severe cardiovascular disease, thyrotoxicosis	Hypertension, diabetes, hyperthyroidism, cardiovascular abnormalities, arteriosclerosis
	The concaine test results in positive urine drug screens for cocaine for at least 48 hours	Rebound congestion may occur with frequent or extended use; rebound miosis may occur in older persons 1 day after phenylephrine treatment; re-instillation may produce reduction in mydriasis

CLINICAL EXAMINATION OF PUPIL

SIZE, SHAPE, AND COLOUR OF PUPIL

MEASUREMENT OF PUPIL SIZE

Measure and record pupil size (in mm) in both eyes in:
- Bright illumination
- Dim illumination.

Method

Use a scale or preferably a pupil gauge (with 0.5 mm steps) to determine pupil size.
- The illumination should be equal in both eyes.
- It is difficult to see the pupils in dim illumination especially in dark irides. For practical purposes a "dim" torch or any minimal illumination is useful to visualize the pupil, for evaluation of pupil size in dim illumination in dark irides. Allow the illumination to fall evenly on both eyes at the same time, during measurement (Fig. 7.4).

Result

Physiological anisocoria is considered if the difference in pupil size is less than 2 mm. Sometimes, there may be a physiological slight increase in anisocoria is dim illumination.
Pathological anisocoria is defined as any difference in pupil size greater than 2 mm. This has to be evaluated in detail (see Anisocoria, page 65).

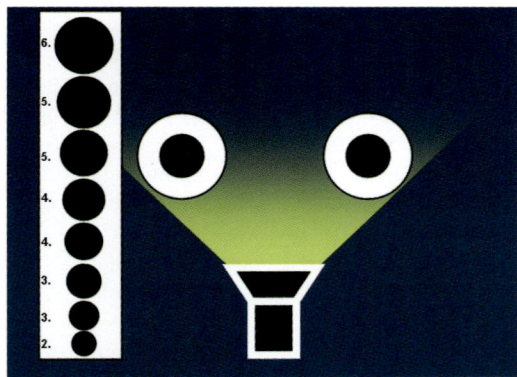

Fig. 7.4 *Dim but even illumination on both pupils to assess pupil size in dark. A pupil gauge (next to RE) is used to measure pupil size in mm.*

Table 7.2 *Distribution of afferent inputs*

Pathway	RE (50% APD)	LE
Ambient light	100	100
Optic nerve	50	100
Pretectal nucleus	50	100
WE nucleus	75	75
	(25 + 50)	(25 + 50)
III Nerve	75	75
Sphincter pupillae	75	75
Pupil size		

Anisocoria always indicates a lesion involving the efferent pupillary pathway (either parasympathetic or sympathetic).
Anisocoria is not a sign of afferent pupil pathway (optic nerve) disease. Even if one eye is completely blind due to optic nerve disease, the pupils of both eyes will be equal in size. This is because afferent inputs from both eyes are distributed equally to both Edinger-Westphal nuclei by each pretectal nucleus (Table 7.2).

Table 7.2 depicts explanation of why no anisocoria can occur in optic nerve disease. The numbers indicates hypothetical "units" of impulses. For example, 100 units of light result in 100 units of impulses in the L optic nerve but only 50 units of impulses are transmitted along the R optic nerve since there is a "50% weakness" of the R optic nerve. Working through the pupil pathways we can see that equal sharing of impulses by each pretectal nucleus to both Edinger-Westphal nuclei, results in final inputs into both pupil sphincters being equal (75 units). As a result the pupil size in both eyes are equal.

PUPIL SHAPE

Record any difference from the normal circular shape. Normal pupil is circular in shape.

Abnormalities of shape

- *Irregular narrow pupil* is seen in iridocyclitis.
- *Festooned pupil* is the name given to irregular pupil obtained after patchy dilatation (effect of mydriatics in the presence of segmental posterior synechiae).
- Vertically oval pupil (pear shaped pupil or updrawn pupil) may occur post-operatively due to incarceration of iris or vitreous in the wound at 12 o'clock position.

PUPIL COLOR

Of course, pupil is a hole in the iris, but the pupillary area does exhibit color depending upon the condition of the structures located behind it. Pupil looks:

- *Greyish black* normally;
- *Jet black* in aphakia;
- *Greyish white* in immature senile cortical cataract;
- *Pearly white* in mature cortical cataract;
- *Milky white* in hypermature cataract;
- *Brown* in cataracta brunescence, and
- *Brownish black* in cataracta nigra.
- *Leucocoria* (white reflex in pupil) in children is seen in congenital cataract, retinoblastoma, retrolental fibroplasia (retinopathy of prematurity), persistent primary hyperplastic vitreous and toxocara endophthalmitis. The yellowish white, semidilated, non-reacting pupil seen in retinoblastoma and pseudogliomas is also called as *ammaurotic cat's reflex.*

TESTS FOR PUPIL REFLEXES

DIRECT LIGHT REFLEX

Equipment

- A good bright uniform light source-usually a pen torch is required.
- The light stimulus should be adequately bright (Fig. 7.5A).
- A very bright light (indirect ophthalmoscope) causes discomfort. Blinking and tearing make pupil evaluation difficult.

- A weak light source produces a correspondingly weak pupil constriction that can be misinterpreted as being sluggish.
- Some torches have patchy uneven illumination. Do not use such torches with "scotomas" (Fig. 7.5B) as they may cause variable constriction of the pupils that can be misinterpreted.

Method

a. Keep room as dim as possible
b. Ask patient to look at a distant target (e.g. fixation target in mirror)
c. Swing bright light source in a quick motion onto the eye.
- The direction of illumination should be from below and slightly temporal.
  i. This keeps the corneal images of the light source (1st and 2nd Purkinje images) outside the pupillary area allowing a good visualization of the entire pupil (Fig. 7.6).
  ii. Keeping a light source directly in front of the eye will stimulate the near reflex that will produce a pupil constriction
- Record the following two aspects of the reaction of the pupil:
  i. Speed of reaction: Brisk or sluggish?
  ii. Sustaining of pupil constriction on continued illumination: Well-sustained or ill-sustained?
- To observe the sustaining of pupil constriction, keep the illumination directed at least 3–4 seconds on the eye being examined.
- Hippus—any exaggeration or difference between the two eyes may be significant.

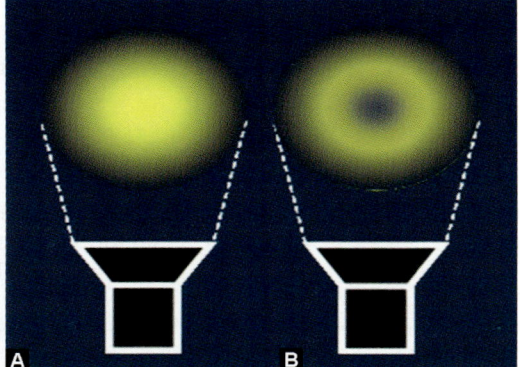

Fig. 7.5 *(A) Torch with evenly bright illumination; (B) Torch with uneven illumination with a "central scotoma".*

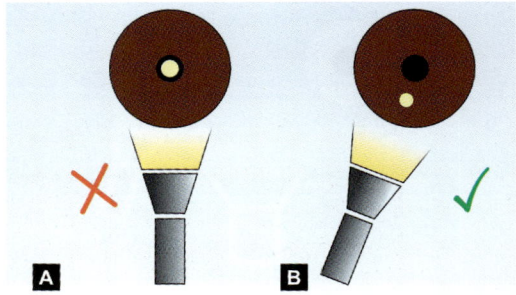

Fig. 7.6 *(A) Torch held directly in front of right eye—corneal image of torch falls on pupil making visualization difficult and also stimulates near reflex constriction; (B) Torch held below and slightly temporal to right eye—pupil clearly visible.*

- Observing pupil constriction by slit lamp biomicroscopy is not the correct method of evaluating the direct reflex.

CONSENSUAL LIGHT REFLEX

Method

a. Keep room as dim as possible.
b. Ask patient to look at a distant target (e.g. fixation target in mirror)
c. Swing bright light source in a quick motion onto the opposite eye.
d. Record the following two aspects of the reaction of the pupil:
  i. Speed of reaction: Brisk or sluggish?
  ii. Sustaining of pupil constriction on continued illumination: Well-sustained or ill-sustained?

To observe the consensual reflex in dark irides in a dim illumination is difficult as the bright light source is on the opposite eye. This may be overcome by using a dim light source on the eye whose pupil reflex is being evaluated. This light should be dim enough not to elicit a significant direct pupil reflex (Fig. 7.7).

Result

In the statement "Right eye: Direct sluggish; consensual normal" the laterality (right or left) should refer to the pupil and not the optic nerve. This statement should be taken to mean that the right optic nerve is affected resulting in a sluggish direct reflex, but the right pupil constricts normally by the consensual reflex when the left eye (optic nerve) is stimulated.

KESTENBAUM'S PSEUDO-ANISOCORIA TEST

- This test is not commonly preformed nowadays being superseded by its refinement— the swinging-flashlight test.
- Useful if a torch is unavailable.

Method (Fig. 7.8)

a. Patient in bright ambient illumination
b. Measure pupil size of one eye, keeping opposite eye occluded.
c. Repeat (b) for fellow eye

Result

The more dilated pupil has optic nerve disease (afferent pupillary defect).

The pupil size is a gross indicator of optic nerve disease (provided the III nerve and the

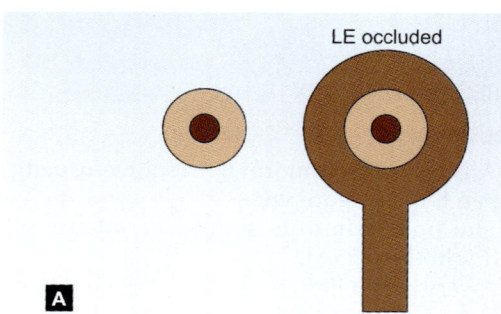

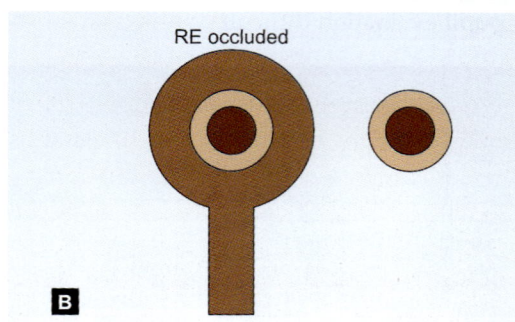

Fig. 7.8 *Measure each pupil in bright ambient illumination keeping the opposite eye occluded: (A) R pupil measures smaller than L pupil; (B) indicating left afferent pupillary defect (note that this is a pseudo-anisocoria since the occluded pupil is actually of the same size as the unoccluded pupil).*

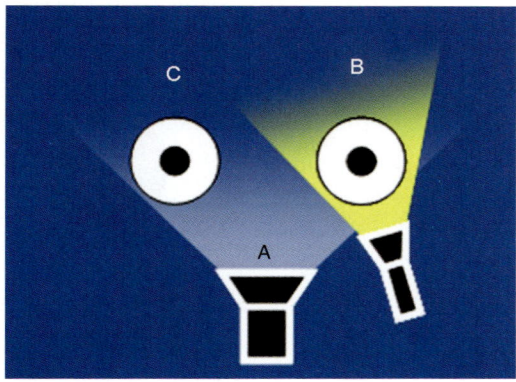

Fig. 7.7 *(A) Dim illumination over both eyes serves to visualize pupils in the dark; (B) bright illumination on LE allows easily visible direct pupil reflex; (C) Consensual reflex R pupil also visible because of the dim "background" illumination.*

pupil sphincter in both sides are normal). Inequality of pupil size indicates optic nerve dysfunction—the eye with the larger pupil being the affected one.

The test will be positive in unilateral or grossly asymmetric bilateral optic nerve disease.

It will not be positive in normals, and cannot be detected in patients with bilateral symmetric or subtle unilateral optic nerve disease.

SWINGING FLASHLIGHT TEST

- The test is named after Levatin
- The pupil with the relative afferent pupillary defect (RAPD) is described as a Marcus Gunn pupil.
- The test compares optic nerve function between the two eyes.
- The test requires a normal efferent pathway (III nerves) and pupillary sphincter, on at least one side.

Method

a. Keep room as dim as possible

b. Ask patient to look at a distant target (e.g. fixation target in mirror). Both pupils are equally dilated in dim light (Fig. 7.9A).

c. Swing bright light source in a quick motion onto the eye and observe the reaction of the pupil (Fig. 7.9B).

d. After about 3 seconds, rapidly swing the light source to the opposite pupil and observe its reaction (Fig. 7.9C).

e. Keep swinging the light source in this manner between the two eyes to look for any relative sluggishness of the reflex or paradoxical dilatation of the pupil of the illuminated eye (Fig. 7.9D).

Result

Paradoxical dilatation of the pupil when light is directed on it, signifying an optic nerve dysfunction in that eye (Fig. 7.9C).

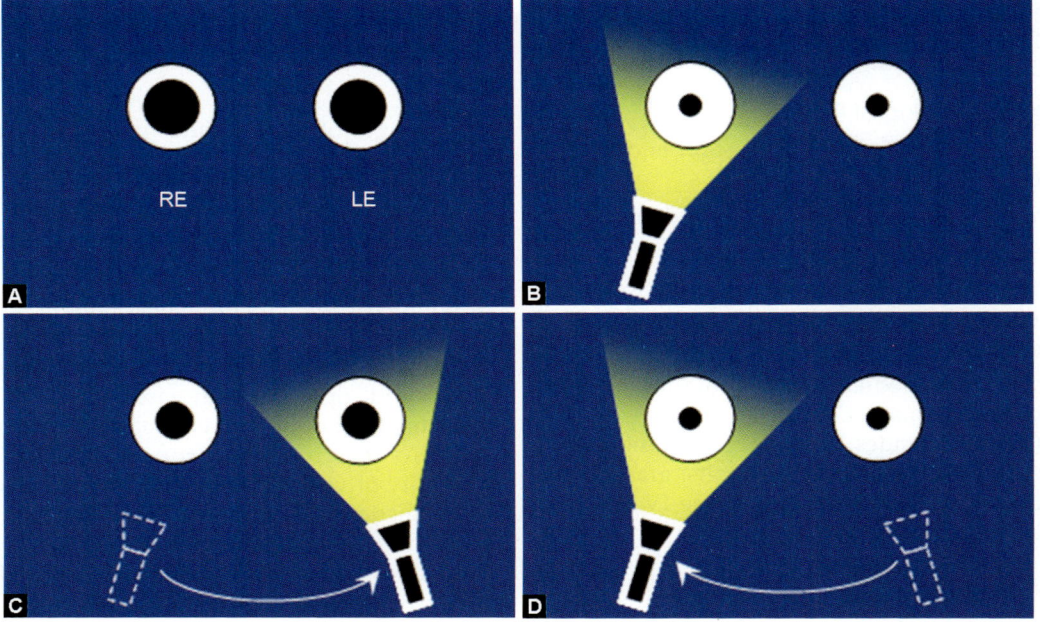

Fig. 7.9 *The swinging flashlight test: (A) Both pupils equally dilated in the dark; (B) Stimulus on RE produces visible R pupil constriction. Note that the unobserved L pupil constricts equally; (C) When the torch is swung to the LE, the left pupil paradoxically dilates. Note that the unobserved R pupil also "dilates" to the same size. Note also that compared to the pupil state in the dark in (A), the L pupil is actually constricting to light though not to the same degree as the R pupil in (B). (D) Swinging the torch back to the RE causes normal pupil constriction.* Inference: Left RAPD.

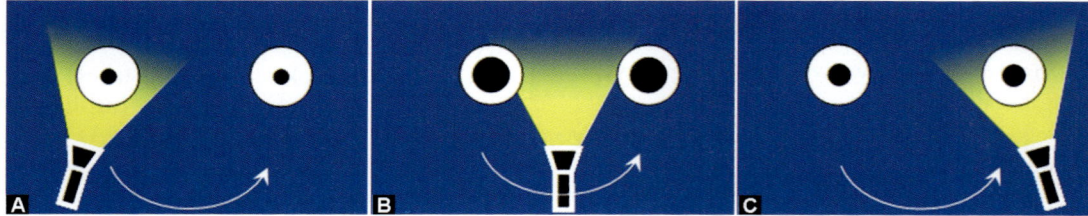

Fig. 7.10 *False Negative RAPD due to incorrect technique. The LE RAPD (B) is missed here. The L pupil in (C) constricts in light because the "swing" between the eyes is slow enough to allow dilatation in the dark (B). Although not observed by the examiner, the consensual reflex of the L pupil (A) is better than the direct reflex of the L pupil (C) indicating LE RAPD.*

The pupil is called the Marcus Gunn pupil indicating a relative afferent pupillary defect (RAPD) in that eye.

Note. It usually takes less than a second to swing the light source from one eye to another. Too great a time interval between stimulation of the eyes results in pupil dilatation in the intervening "dark period" causing a false negative test in eyes with mild optic nerve disease (Fig. 7.10). The swing between the two eyes should be reasonably rapid. This problem occurs less if the light source directly swings across the bridge of the nose as it passes from one eye to the other in a straight path.

Clinical grading of RAPD

Grade I: Weak initial constriction and greater redilatation.

Grade II: Initial stall and greater redilatation.

Grade III: Immediate pupil dilatation.

Grade IV: Immediate pupil dilatation following prolonged illumination of the good eye for 6 seconds

Grade V: Immediate pupil dilatation with no secondary constriction.

(The five grades have corresponding values in neutral density filter log units: grade I, 0.4; grade II, 0.7; grade III, 1.1; grade IV, 2.0; and grade V, infinity).

Quantifying RAPD

Equipment

- Neutral density (ND) filters (0.3, 0.6, 0.9, and 1.2 log units).
- (Cross polarizing lens filters and Bagolini striated lenses have also been used).

Principle

The filters degrade the intensity of the stimulus in the normal eye thus simulating an afferent defect in that eye. When this apparent defect balances the real afferent defect in the affected eye, the Marcus Gunn pupil disappears.

Method

- Perform swinging flashlight test to determine which eye has an RAPD.
- Place increasing log units of ND filters over the normal eye, while repeating the swinging flashlight test. The end point is reached when the Marcus Gunn pupil is abolished (Fig. 7.11).

Result

The strength of the ND filter placed over the normal eye at the end point quantifies the degree of RAPD (Fig. 7.11C).

Interpretation of RAPD

- RAPD will be present in unilateral or asymmetric bilateral optic nerve disease.
- RAPD will not be present in normals, and cannot be detected in patients with bilateral symmetric optic nerve disease.
- In unilateral optic nerve disease, the degree of RAPD is broadly proportional to the severity of visual loss caused by optic nerve dysfunction.
- Although the presence of RAPD usually indicates optic nerve disease, trace RAPD may be observed in dense amblyopia and significant macular disease—in these situations, the degree of visual acuity impairment will be far greater than the degree of RAPD.
- Significant cataract in one eye causes the stimulating light to scatter and increase the

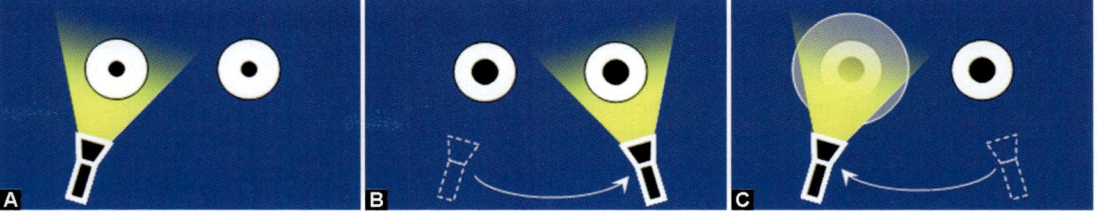

Fig. 7.11 *Quantifying RAPD with an ND filter (using the example of the L RAPD): (A) Bright light stimulus on RE produces visible R pupil constriction; (B) When the torch is swung to the LE, the left pupil paradoxically dilated indicating an RAPD; (C) An ND filter of appropriate strength reduces the intensity of light stimulus to the normal RE creating an artificial optic nerve dysfunction. Since both eyes are now equally "affected", swinging the torch back to the RE causes no pupil constriction. The L RAPD has been neutralized.*

pupillomotor "effectiveness" of the stimulus in that eye. This may induce an apparent RAPD in the opposite eye.

SWINGING FLASHLIGHT—SPECIAL SITUATIONS

Only one "normal" pupil

Common situations

- Sphincter damage (e.g. post intraocular surgery, acute angle closure glaucoma)
- Efferent defect (e.g. III nerve palsy with internal ophthalmoplegia)
- Poor visualization of the pupil (e.g. corneal opacity).

Method

It is based on the principle of the consensual reflex (Fig. 7.12):

- Use a second dim light source with just sufficient illumination to illuminate the normal pupil (Fig. 7.12A).
- Perform the test as described above, by swinging the bright stimulating light source between the two eyes but observe only the dimly illuminated normal pupil.

Result

- If there is optic nerve disease in either eye, the observed pupil will show Marcus Gunn features when the affected eye (irrespective of laterality) is stimulated (Fig. 7.12B).
- Remember the eye with RAPD is the eye being stimulated by the bright light source—this may or may not be the eye whose pupil is being observed.

Alternative method

If a second light source is unavailable perform the swinging flashlight test as usual but observe the normal pupil when it is illuminated by the stimulating light source.

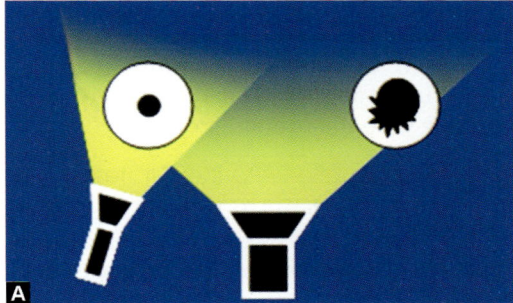

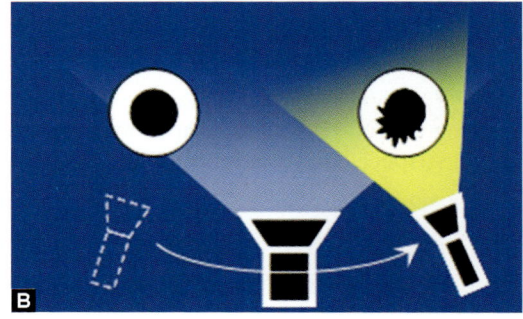

Fig. 7.12 *Testing RAPD with one reactive pupil - RE. The LE has traumatic sphincter tears rendering it unreliable for pupil reflex evaluation: (A) A diffuse dim illumination allows observation of the R pupil in the dark. The R pupil shows a brisk direct reflex; (B) With the stimulus over the LE, the L pupil is predictably immobile, but the R pupil dilates (by consensual reflex) indicating a L RAPD. (Compare this with the behaviour of the R pupil in Fig. 7.9C—the behaviour is the same, the only difference being that in this situation the R pupil is being observed.)*

Result

- *Same eye optic nerve affected*—RAPD directly observed.
- *Normal eyes*—equal optic nerve function— pupil remains steady or shows minimal constriction caused by the time lag of the swing.
- *Opposite eye optic nerve affected*—the amplitude of pupil constriction is exaggerated. Reason— owing to the relatively weaker consensual reflex, the normal pupil becomes relatively larger in size when the opposite eye with an afferent defected is stimulated. This is sometimes confusingly referred to as a "reverse" RAPD.

In strabismus

With large deviations an off-axis stimulation of the squinting eye may result in a suboptimal pupil response resulting in a false positive test in that eye (Fig. 7.13).

To avoid this ensure that the pupils of both eyes receive equal stimulating illumination by appropriately angulating the light source while swinging onto the squinting eye.

Uncovering a subtle RAPD the "Tilt" test

This refinement is useful when there is no "detectable" RAPD but clinical suspicion of unilateral optic nerve dysfunction exists.

Equipment

0.3 log unit ND filter.

Principle

A 0.3 log unit ND filter placed in front of an eye with a suspect RAPD heightens the inter-eye

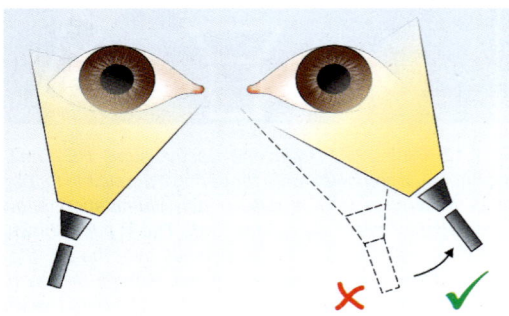

Fig. 7.13 *Exotropia LE - torch needs to be further out to allow maximal light stimulus to fall on the eye.*

0.3 log ND filter over	Total log defect OD	Total log defect OS	RAPD
OD	0.3	0.2	No RAPD
OS	0	0.5 (0.2+0.3)	L RAPD

Eg: 0.2 log clinically undetectable RAPD OS use 0.3 log ND filter for test

Fig 7.14 *The "Tilt test" for uncovering a subtle RAPD.*

difference in pupillomotor drive to a detectable level thus causing a Marcus Gunn pupil to become apparent.

Method (Fig. 7.14)

a. Place 0.3 log unit ND filter in front of one eye and perform the swinging flashlight test.

b. Repeat (a) with ND filter over fellow eye.

Result

Eye with subtle optic nerve dysfunction will show a demonstrable RAPD in the test when the 0.3 log ND filter is placed in front of it.

EDGE LIGHT PUPIL CYCLE TIME (ELPCT)

Equipment

- Slit lamp
- Stop watch

Method (Fig. 7.15)

a. Patient is seated at slit lamp in dark ambient illumination

b. Instruct patient to look at an imaginary distance target

c. Adjust slit beam to make it 0.5 mm thick and horizontally oriented.

d. The beam is focused on the inferior edge of the pupil such that half the thickness of the beam falls into the papillary aperture.

e. The pupil constriction that results from (d) causes the light stimulus to temporarily "shut off" as the entire thickness of the beam is on the iris below the inferior edge of the pupil.

f. The momentary loss of stimulus resulting from (e) causes pupil dilatation that cycles back to (d)

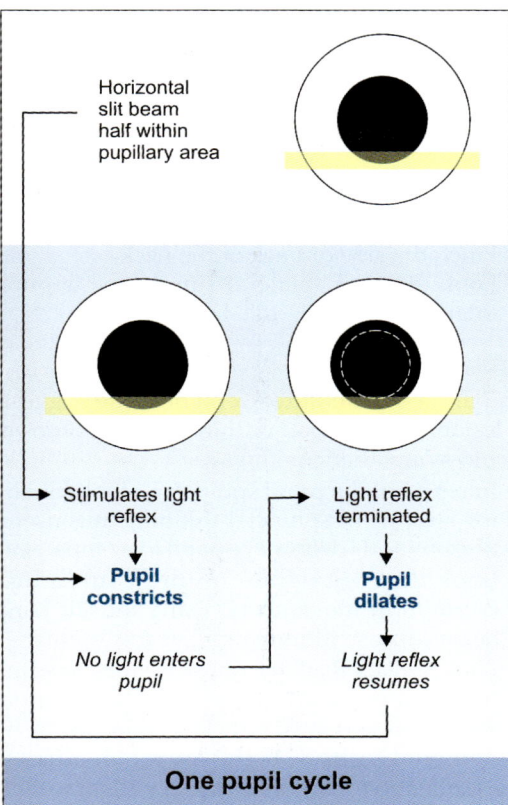

Horizontal slit beam half within pupillary area

Stimulates light reflex → Light reflex terminated

Pupil constricts → **Pupil dilates**

No light enters pupil → Light reflex resumes

One pupil cycle

Fig. 7.15 Edge light pupil cycle time.

g. Each constriction-dilatation is a cycle. With the stop watch measure the time for 30 cycles.

Result
- Repeat the test for five 30-cycle rounds and calculate the time taken for a single cycle.
- Total number of cycles = 30 × 5 = 150
- ELPCT (in ms) = Total time (in seconds) for 5 rounds × 1000/150
- Normal: 850–950 ms.

Note
- Test takes approximately 5 minutes.
- Requires concentration from patient and doctor.
- Best suited to evaluate mild to moderate optic nerve disease.
- Does not require a normal fellow eye for comparison.

NEAR REFLEX
Generally a pupil with a brisk, well-sustained direct reflex will have a normal near reflex.

Testing for the near reflex is therefore done when the direct reflex is suspect. There is no clinical condition in which the light reflex is present and the near response is absent.

Light-near dissociation: When near response tested in moderate light exceeds the best constriction that bright light can produce.

A positive near reflex in a blind individual is an indication of the integrity of the efferent pathway and the pupil sphincter.

Equipment
Any small accommodative target, which may sometimes include a Snellen optotype.

A light source such as a pen torch should not be used. Also avoid using your fingers as a near target.

Method
The ambient illumination should be moderate—sufficient enough for the patient to view the accommodative target.
a. Ask the patient to keep his eyes focused on a distant target
b. Bring the near target about 30 cm in front of the patient's eyes and positioned between and slightly below them.
c. Now instruct the patient to view the near target and observe the pupil constriction.

Note
- Keeping the near target too low causes the eyes to look down making it difficult to observe the pupils. Therefore keep the target only slightly below the level of the eyes so as not to obstruct the patient's view of the distance target.
- The near reflex may occur slowly in certain situations (such as in the tonic pupil). To avoid missing this finding, keep observing the pupil for at least 10 seconds.
- Observe degree of convergence as an indication of patient compliance—poor convergence indicates that the patient may not be trying enough to look at the near target, or that you are not holding the target near enough. This can result in an apparently poor near reflex.

- Never judge near response by adding a near stimulus to a bright light stimulus. This action almost always produces additional constriction leading to apparent light-near dissociation.

Testing near reflex in a blind individual

Methods

a. Observe pupil constriction while instructing patient to voluntarily cross his eyes. This action does not require vision.
b. Eye-closure pupil reaction—instruct patient to close his eyes while you keep the lids open—this produces a strong near response.

DILATATION LAG (DARK REFLEX)

Aim

To evaluate dilator pupillae.
Normal pupil dilatation = sphincter relaxation + dilator contraction

Method

a. Keep room illumination bright.
b. Use minimal illumination evenly over both eyes just sufficient to keep both pupils visible in the dark.
c. Switch off room illumination and observe dilatation of the pupils in the "dark".

Result

Normal dilator pupillae—both pupils should dilate equally in 2–4 seconds

(**Note.** The speed of the dilatation reflex is much slower than pupil constriction).

Weak dilator pupillae—A dilatation lag (an anisocoria developing after 2–4 seconds of dark) implies a sympathetic palsy (Horner's syndrome).

CILIOSPINAL REFLEX

The ciliospinal reflex (CSR) induces bilateral pupillary dilatation on nociceptive stimulation applied to the skin of the neck (afferent C2, C3).

The reflex is mainly mediated by second and third-order sympathetic nerves to the dilator muscle of the iris.

The CSR has been considered a useful tool in differentiating central from peripheral sympathetic dysfunction.

Method

a. Pinch the side or back of the neck.
b. Look for brisk bilateral simultaneous pupil dilatation.

Result

Impaired dilatation reflex on one side suggests a lesion of the second or third order neurons of oculo-sympathetic pathway.

- Integrity of the pupil sphincter—look for any iris atrophy or sphincter thinning. It is useful to examine the fellow eye pupil for comparison.
- Look for segmental pupil contraction (vermiform movements) using the slit lamp beam (diffuse illumination) as a stimulus.
- *Look for gaze dyskinesis.* In cases of suspected III nerve palsy with aberrant regeneration, subtle pupil-gaze dyskinesis may be detected—observe the pupil in diffuse illumination while instructing patient to shift gaze (abduction-adduction and elevation-depression).

BIBLIOGRAPHY

1. Bell RA, Waggoner PM, Boyd WM, et al. Clinical grading of relative afferent pupillary defects. 1: Arch Ophthalmol 1993;111(7):938–42.

2. Havelius U, Heuck M, Milos P, Hindfelt B, et al. Ciliospinal reflex response in cluster headache. Headache 1996;36(9):568–73.

3. Jacobson DM. A prospective evaluation of cholinergic supersensitivity of the iris sphincter in patients with oculomotor nerve palsies. Am J Ophthalmol 1994;118:377–83.

4. Miller SD, Thompson HS. Edge-light pupil cycle time. BJO 1978;62:495–500.

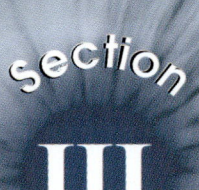

Section

III

Visual Pathways

8

ANATOMY OF VISUAL PATHWAY AND NEUROPHYSIOLOGY OF VISION

AK Khurana, Indu Khurana,
Aruj K Khurana, Bhawna Khurana

ANATOMY OF VISUAL PATHWAY
Anatomy of Different Components of Visual Pathway
• Optic chiasma
• Optic tracts
• Lateral geniculate body (LGB)
• Optic radiations
• Visual cortex
Arrangement of Nerve Fibers in Different Parts of the Visual Pathway
• In the retina
• In the optic nerve
• In the chiasma
• In the optic tract
• In the lateral geniculate body
• In the optic radiations
• In the visual cortex
Blood Supply of Optic Nerve
NEUROPHYSIOLOGY OF VISION
Genesis of Visual Impulse in the Photoreceptors
• Cone versus rod receptor potential

Processing and Transmission of Visual Impulse in the Retina
• Neurotransmitters in the retina
• Physiological activities in the retinal cells
Processing and Transmission of Visual Impulse in the Visual Pathway
• Optic nerve, chiasma and optic tract
• Lateral geniculate body
• Optic radiations
Analysis of Visual Impulse in the Visual Cortex
• Retinotopic organization
• Functional anatiomy and organization of the visual cortex
• Physiology of visual cortex
• Concept of receptive field of striate cortex
• Columnar organization of striate cortex
• Serial versus parallel analysis of visual image
• Role or extrastriate cortex (visual association cortex) in visual functions
• Psychophysiological aspect of visual functions
'Three-Part-System' Hypothesis of Visual Perceptions

ANATOMY OF VISUAL PATHWAY

Each eyeball acts as a camera; it perceives the images and relays the sensations to the brain (occipital cortex) via the visual pathway which comprises optic nerve, optic chiasma, optic tract, geniculate body and optic radiations. Anatomy of visual sensory system can be discussed under two main heads:
• Anatomy of different components of visual pathway
• Arrangement of visual fibers.

ANATOMY OF DIFFERENT COMPONENTS OF VISUAL PATHWAY

OPTIC NERVE

See Chapter 10 (page 129)

OPTIC CHIASMA

• It is a flattened structure measuring about 12 mm horizontally and 8 mm anteroposteriorly (Fig. 8.1).

• It is ensheathed by the pia and surrounded by cerebrospinal fluid. It lies over the diaphragma sellae and therefore presence of a visual field defect in a patient with a pituitary tumor indicates suprasellar extension.

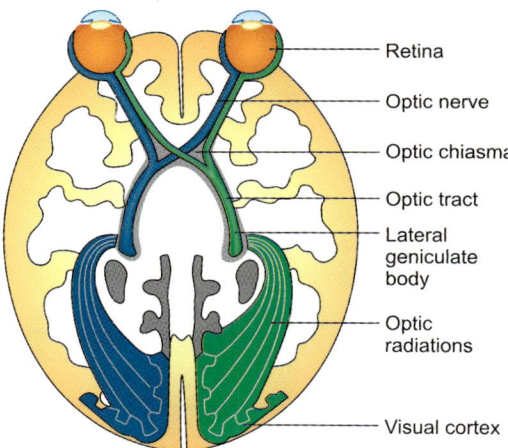

Retina

Optic nerve

Optic chiasma

Optic tract

Lateral geniculate body

Optic radiations

Visual cortex

Fig. 8.1 *Gross appearance of visual pathway.*

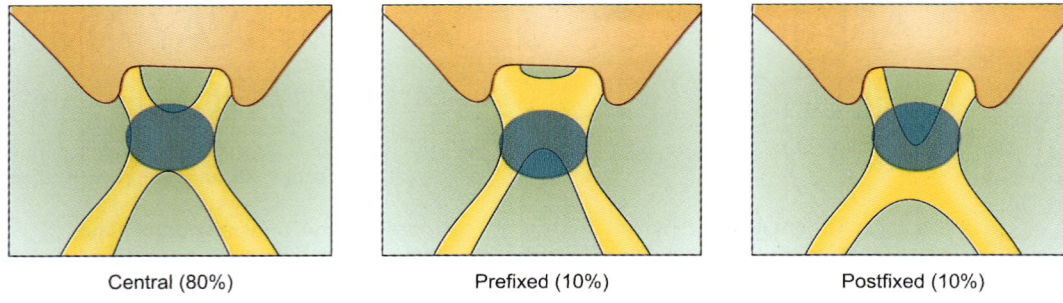

Central (80%)   Prefixed (10%)   Postfixed (10%)

Fig. 8.2 *Anatomical variations in the position of normal optic chiasma.*

- Posteriorly, the chiasma is continuous with the optic tracts and forms the anterior wall of the third ventricle.
- Nerve fibers arising from the nasal halves of the two retinae decussate at the chiasma.
- Variations in the location of the chiasma may have important clinical significance (Fig. 8.2) as follows:
  1. *Central chiasma* is present in about 80% of normal cases. It lies directly above the sella, so the expanding pituitary tumors involve the chiasma first.
  2. *Prefixed chiasma* is present in about 10% of normal cases. It is located more anteriorly over the tuberculum sellae. In such a situation, the pituitary tumor may involve the optic tracts first.

3. *Postfixed chiasma* is present in the remaining 10% of normal cases. It is located more posteriorly over the dorsum sellae so that pituitary tumors are apt to damage the optic nerve first.

Relations of the chiasma (Fig. 8.3)
- *Anterior:* Anterior cerebral arteries and their communicating arteries.
- *Posterior:* Tubercinereum, infundibulum (hypophyseal stalk), pituitary body, mammillary body and posterior perforated substance.
- *Superior* (above): Third ventricle.
- *Inferior* (below): Hypophysis.
- *Lateral:* Extracavernous part of the internal carotid artery and the anterior perforated substance.

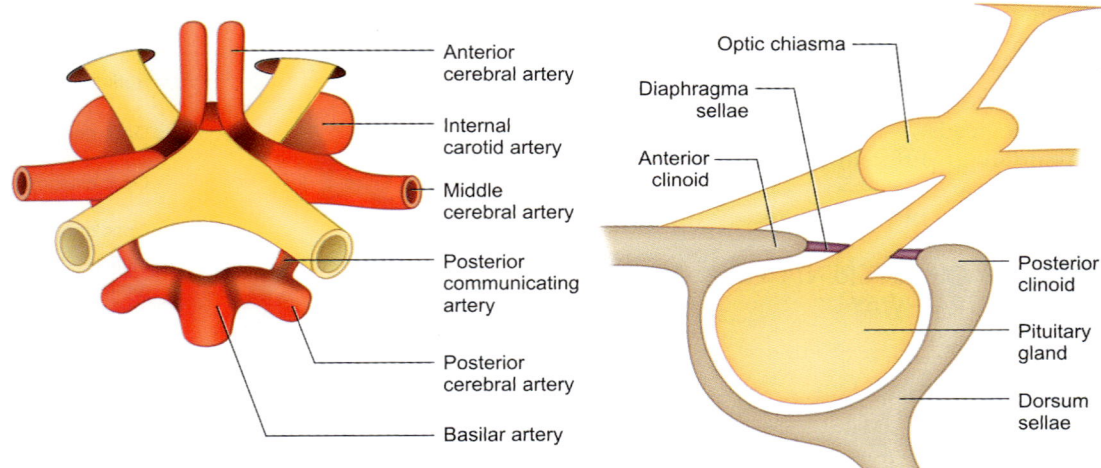

Anterior cerebral artery

Internal carotid artery

Middle cerebral artery

Posterior communicating artery

Posterior cerebral artery

Basilar artery

Optic chiasma

Diaphragma sellae

Anterior clinoid

Posterior clinoid

Pituitary gland

Dorsum sellae

Fig. 8.3 *Showing relations of optic chiasma.*

OPTIC TRACTS

- These are cylindrical bundles of nerve fibers running outwards and backwards from the posterolateral aspect of the optic chiasma, between the tuber cinereum and anterior perforated substance to unite with cerebral peduncles.
- Each optic tract consists of fibers from the temporal half of the retina of the same eye and the nasal half of the opposite eye.
- Posteriorly, each optic tract ends in the lateral geniculate body. The pupillary reflex fibers pass onto superior colliculi through the superior brachium.

LATERAL GENICULATE BODY (LGB)

- These are oval structures situated at the optic tracts.
- Each geniculate body consists of six layers of neurons (grey matter) alternating with white matter (formed by optic fibers). Fibers of second order neuron coming via optic tracts relay in these neurons.

OPTIC RADIATIONS

The optic radiations or geniculocalcarine pathway extend from the lateral geniculate body to the visual cortex (Fig. 8.4). They pass forwards and then laterally through the area of Wernicke as optic peduncles, anterior to lateral ventricle and traversing the retrolenticular part of internal capsule, behind the sensory fibers and medial to auditory tract.

- The fibers of optic radiations then spread out fanwise to form a medullary optic lamina. This is at first vertical but becomes horizontal near the visual cortex.
- The inferior fibers of the optic radiations, which subserve the upper visual fields, first sweep anteroinferiorly in Meyer's loop around the anterior tip of the temporal horn of the lateral ventricle, and into the temporal lobe.
- The superior fibers of the radiations, which subserve the inferior visual fields, proceed directly posteriorly through the parietal lobe to the visual cortex.

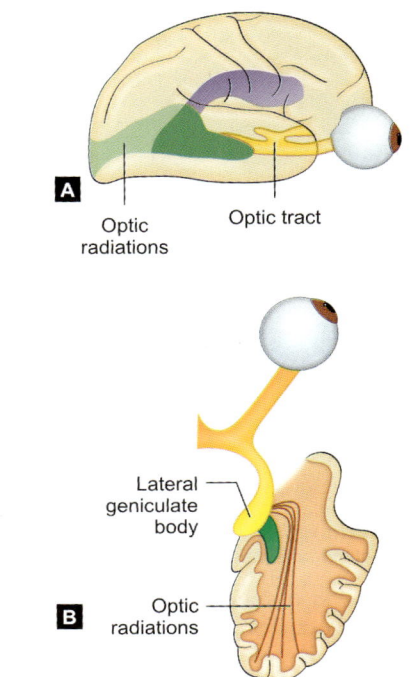

Fig. 8.4 *Optic radiations: (A) Lateral view; (B) Transverse section.*

VISUAL CORTEX

It is located on the medial aspect of the occipital lobe in and near the calcarine fissure. It may extend onto lateral aspect of the occipital lobe, but limited by a semilunar sulcus, the sulcus lumatus. The visual cotex is subdivided into the visuosensory area (striate area 17) that receives the fibers of the optic radiations, and the surrounding visuopsychic are (peristriate area 18 and parastriate area 19) (Fig. 8.5). Recently, a *modified nomenclature recongnizing five visual areas* has been described as follows:

1. First visual area (V1) in area 17.
2. Second visual area (V2) occupying the greater part of area 18, but not the whole of it.
3. Third visual area (V3) occupying a narrow strip over the anterior part of area 18.
4. Fourth visual area (V4) within area 19.
5. Fifth visual area (V5) at the posterior end of the superior temporal gyrus.

A section through the visual cortex of a fresh brain can be identified by naked eye, by the presence of a white line, the stria of Gennari

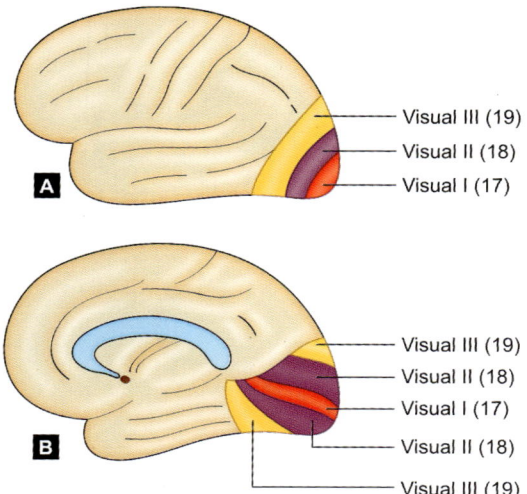

A

Visual III (19)
Visual II (18)
Visual I (17)

B

Visual III (19)
Visual II (18)
Visual I (17)
Visual II (18)
Visual III (19)

Fig. 8.5 *Location of visual cortex on superolateral: (A) Medial; (B) Surfaces of the cerebral hemisphere.*

(which is a layer of medullated fibers disposed in different structures).

The microscopic structure of the visual cortex is similar to other parts of cerebral cortex and consists of 6 layers, which from without inward are: plexiform layer, external granular layer, external pyramidal layer, internal granular layer, ganglionic layer and multiform layer (Fig. 8.6).

ARRANGEMENT OF NERVE FIBERS IN DIFFERENT PARTS OF THE VISUAL PATHWAY

IN THE RETINA

In contrast to the remaining fibers of the sensory retina, which course perpendicular to the surface of the retina, the fibers within the nerve fiber layer course parallel to the surface in the following manner (Fig. 8.7):

- Fibers from the nasal half of the retina come directly to the optic disc as superior and inferior radiating fibers (srf and irf).

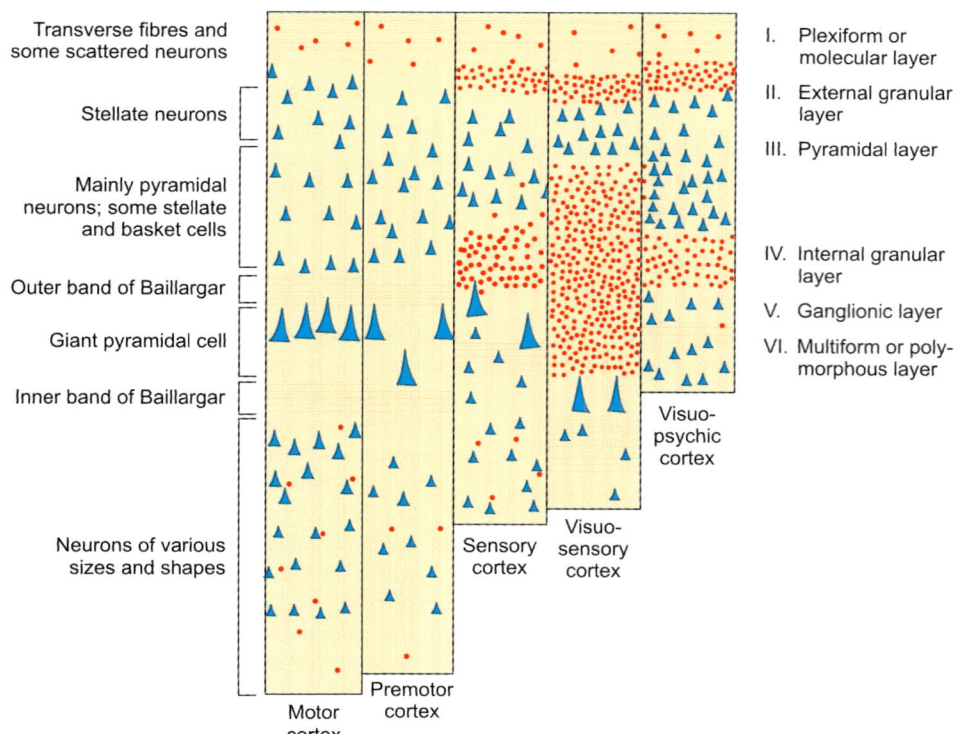

Fig. 8.6 *Microscopic structure of five different types of cerebral cortex.*

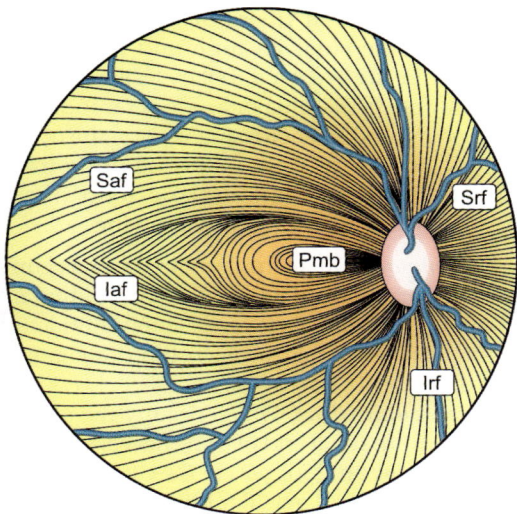

Fig. 8.7 *Arrangement of nerve fibres in the retina.*

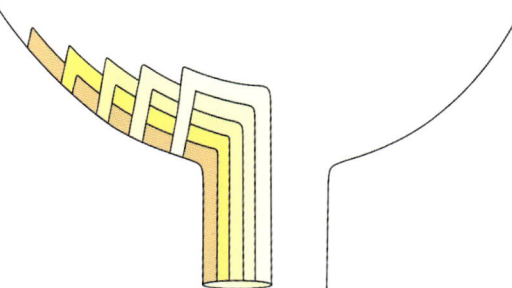

Fig. 8.8 *Arrangement of nerve fibres at the optic nerve head.*

- Fibers from the macular region pass straight in the temporal part of the disc as papillomacular bundle (pmb).
- Fibers from the temporal retina arch above and below the macular and papillomacular bundle (pmb).
- Fibers from the temporal retina arch above and below the macular and papillomacular bundle as superior and inferior arcuate fibers (saf and iaf) with a horizontal raphe in between.
- There occurs no overlap between the lower and upper halves of fibers of peripheral part of retina.
- Line dividing nasal and temporal fibers passes through the center of fovea. Hence, the temporal macular fibers remain on the same side, while the nasal ones cross.
- Upper temporal retinal fibers are separated from the lower by the macular fibers; an arrangement which holds throughout the central visual pathway.

IN THE OPTIC NERVE

(a) In the optic nerve head

Fibers from the peripheral part of the retina lie deep in the retina but occupy the most peripheral (superficial) part of the optic disc. While the fibers originating closer to the optic nerve head lie superficially in the retina and

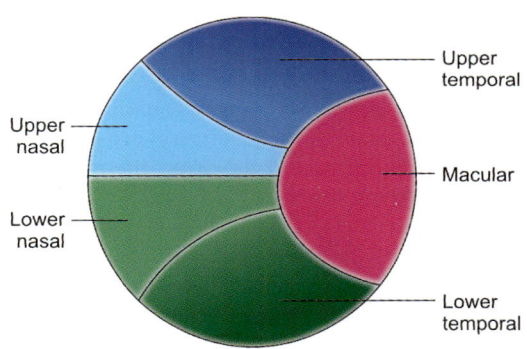

Fig. 8.9 *Arrangement of fibres in the distal region (behind the eyeball) of optic nerve.*

occupy a more central (deep) portion of the disc (Fig. 8.8).

Arrangement of nerve fibers in the optic nerve head is exactly same as in the retina (Fig. 8.9).

(b) In the distal region (behind the eye)

In the distal region of optic nerve, the nerve fibers are distributed exactly as in the retina, i.e. the upper temporal and lower temporal fibers are situated on the temporal half of the optic nerve and are separated from each other by a wedge-shaped area occupied by the papillo-macular bundle.

The upper nasal and lower nasal fibers are situated on the nasal side (Fig. 8.9).

(c) In the proximal region (near the chiasma)

In the proximal region of optic nerve, the macular fibers are centrally placed (Fig. 8.10).

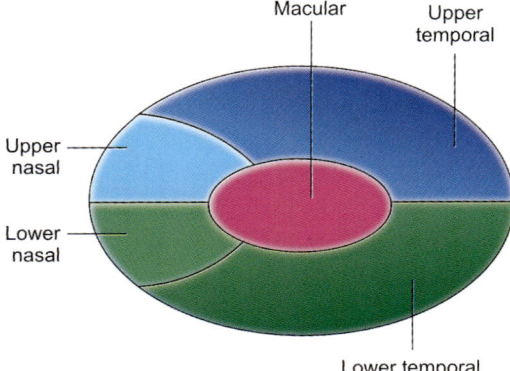

Fig. 8.10 *Arrangement of fibres in the proximal region of optic nerve. Note central position of papillomacular bundle.*

IN THE CHIASMA (Fig. 8.11)

1. The nasal peripheral fibers constitute about three-quarters of all the fibers and cross over to enter the medial part of the opposite optic tract in the following manner:

- The lower nasal fibers in the optic nerve, traverse the chiasma low and anteriorly (so are first affected in the tumors of pituitary body producing upper temporal quadrantic field defects). These fibers form convex loops in terminal part of the opposite optic nerve (therefore ipsilateral blindness due to lesions of the proximal most part of the optic nerve is associated with contralateral field defects) and then cross to the opposite tract and occupy its lower quadrant.

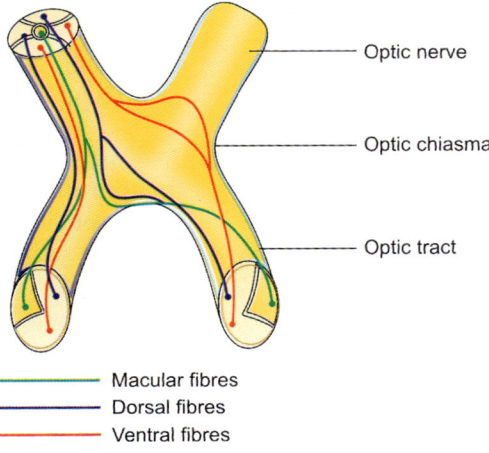

Fig. 8.11 *Decussation of fibres in the chiasma.*

Macular fibres
Dorsal fibres
Ventral fibres

- The upper nasal fibers of the optic nerve traverse the chiasma high and posteriorly (therefore are involved first by lesions coming from above the chiasma, e.g. craniopharyngiomas) and after crossing occupy the upper nasal quadrant of the opposite optic tract. Some of these fibers make a loop in the ipsilateral optic tract before crossing.

2. The temporal fibers from retina which occupy the temporal half of the optic nerves, remain uncrossed and run backwards in the lateral part of the optic chiasma to reach the dorsolateral part of the optic tract.

3. The macular fibers, which occupy the central part at the proximal end of optic nerve, keep this position in the anterior part of the chiasma. Then the crossing (nasal) macular fibers get separated from the uncrossed fibers and pass as a bundle obliquely backwards and upwards to decussate in the posterior most part of the chiasma, which is related to the supraoptic recess. Lesions here may produce central temporal hemianopic scotoma.

- **Other fibers.** In addition to the visual fibers, the optic chiasma also contains commissural fibers, pupillary fibers and fibers connecting the two medial geniculate bodies, the globus pallidus and the hypothalamus.

IN THE OPTIC TRACT

In the optic tract, the visual fibers are rearranged as follows (Fig. 8.12):

- *Macular fibers,* both uncrossed (temporal macular fibers from the ipsilateral retina) and crossed (nasal macular fibers from the opposite retina) occupy the dorsolateral aspect of the optic tract.
- *Upper peripheral fibers,* both uncrossed (from upper temporal part of lateral retina) and crossed (from upper nasal part of opposite retina) are situated medially in the optic tract.
- *Lower peripheral fibers,* both uncrossed (from lower temporal quadrant of ipsilateral retina) and crossed (from lower nasal quadrant of opposite retina) are situated laterally in the optic tracts.
- *Other fibers:* Besides the visual fibers, the optic tracts also contain the other fibers as described in optic chiasma.

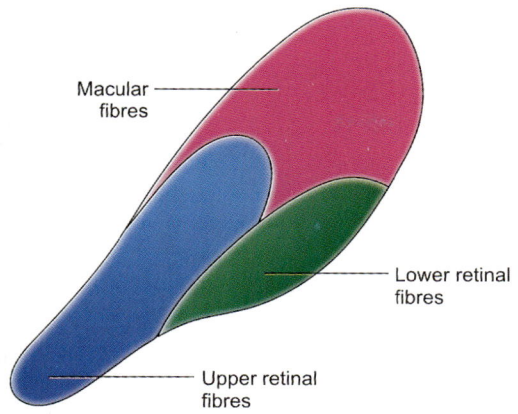

Macular fibres

Lower retinal fibres

Upper retinal fibres

Fig. 8.12 *Arrangement of fibres in optic tract.*

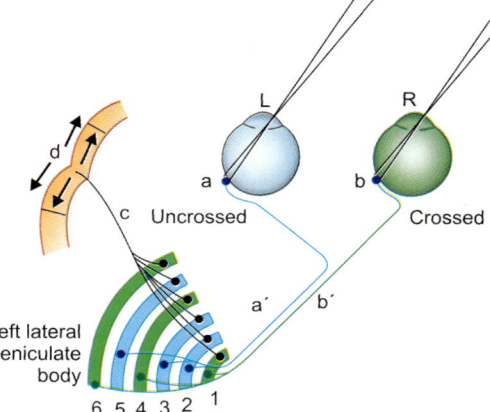

L   R

d

a   b

c   Uncrossed   Crossed

a'   b'

Left lateral geniculate body

6 5 4 3 2 1

Fig. 8.14 *Arrangement of termination of axons of ganglion cells (second order neurons of vision) of the two eyes in the lateral geniculate body. For explanation see text.*

IN THE LATERAL GENICULATE BODY

Position of visual fibers (Fig. 8.13)

- The *macular fibers* coming in the optic tract occupy the posterior two-thirds of the lateral geniculate body (LGB).
- The *upper retinal fibers* occupy the medial half of the anterior one-third of the LGB.
- The *lower retinal fibers* occupy the lateral half of the anterior one-third of the LGB.

Relay of second order neurons in LGB (Fig. 8.14)

The neurons of LGB from the third order neurons of the vision. The axons of the second order neurons (ganglion cells) synapse with the dendrites of the neurons of LGB. There is a regular point-to-point localization of the retina

in the lateral geniculate body nucleus which is also carried from the latter to the visual cortex. LGB has got 6 laminae (1 to 6). The crossed fibers end in the laminae 1, 4 and 6 while the uncrossed fibers end in the laminae 2, 3 and 5 in such a way that those from the corresponding parts of two retinae end in neighbouring parts of the adjacent laminae. Therefore, the smallest lesion of the retina results in degeneration of three laminae of the LGB in which the retinal fibers end. Hence, the conducting unit in optic nerve fibers is a 3 laminae unit. Since the optic radiations commence from all the six laminae (6 laminae unit), so a lesion in the visual cortex results in degeneration of all the 6 laminae of LGB.

IN THE OPTIC RADIATIONS

In the optic radiations, there occurs a temporal rotation of the fibers, thereby (Fig. 8.15):

- The *upper retinal fibers* occupy the upper part of the optic radiations.
- The *lower retinal fibers* occupy the lower part of the optic radiations.
- The *macular fibers* lie in the central part of optic radiations separating the upper retinal from the lower retinal fibers.
- *Other fibers:* Besides the visual fibers, the optic radiations also contain the fibers that pass from the cerebral cortex to LGB, to the superior colliculus and to the oculomotor nuclei.

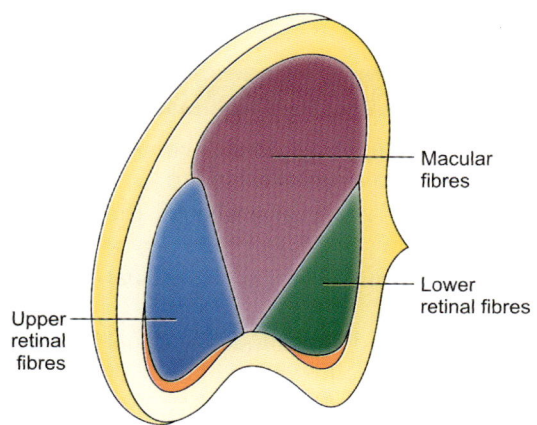

Macular fibres

Lower retinal fibres

Upper retinal fibres

Fig. 8.13 *Arrangement of fibres in the lateral geniculate body.*

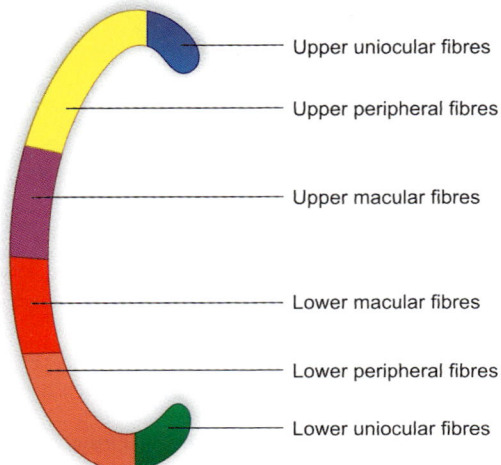

Upper uniocular fibres

Upper peripheral fibres

Upper macular fibres

Lower macular fibres

Lower peripheral fibres

Lower uniocular fibres

Fig. 8.15 *Arrangement of fibres in the optic radiations.*

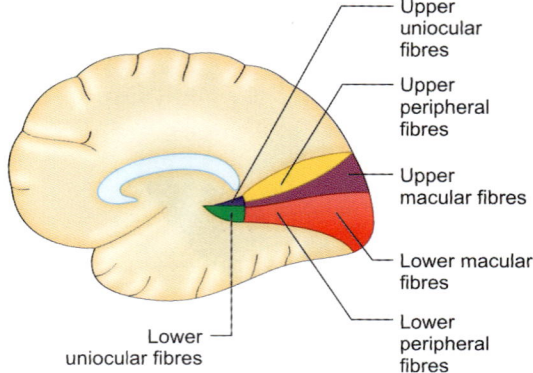

Upper uniocular fibres

Upper peripheral fibres

Upper macular fibres

Lower macular fibres

Lower peripheral fibres

Lower uniocular fibres

Fig. 8.16 *Arrangement of fibres in visual cortex.*

IN THE VISUAL CORTEX

- The visual cortex is also called the cortical retina, since a true copy of the retinal image is formed here. It is only in the visual cortex that the impulses originating from corresponding points of two retinae meet.
- There is a point-to-point projection of the retina in the visual cortex in such a way that the right visual cortex is concerned with perception of objects situated to the left of the vertical median line in the visual fields and left visual cortex with the objects situated to the right half. In other words, the right visual cortex receives impulses arising from the temporal half of right retina and nasal half of left retina; and the left visual cortex receives those arising from the temporal half of the left retina and nasal half of the right retina.
- The visual fibers contained in the optic radiations are relayed in the visual cortex in the following manner (Fig. 8.16):
  - Fibers from the macular area relay in an extensive area placed posteriorly in the visual cortex.
  - Fibers from the peripheral retinae end anterior to the macular fibers; those from the upper retinae above the calcarine sulcus.
- The visual areas give off efferent fibers also. These reach various parts of the cerebral cortex in both hemispheres. In particular, they reach the frontal eye field, which is concerned with eye movements.

Like other 'sensory' areas, the visual areas are, therefore, to be regarded as partly motor in function. This view is substantiated by the fact that movements of the eyeballs and head can be produced by stimulation of the areas 17 and 18, which constitute an occipital eye field. Efferents from the visual areas also reach the superior colliculus, the pretectal region, and the nuclei of the cranial nerves supplying muscles that move the eyeballs. There is physiological evidence of a corticogeniculate projection. Fibers also reach the thalamus (pulvinar).

BLOOD SUPPLY OF OPTIC NERVE

See Chapter 10 (page 132).

NEUROPHYSIOLOGY OF VISION

Neurophysiological processes concerned with vision can be discussed as under:
- Genesis of visual impulse in the photo-receptors.
- Processing and transmission of visual impulse in the retina.
- Processing and transmission of visual impulse in the visual pathway.
- Analysis of visual impulse in the visual cortex.
- A 3-part system hypothesis of visual perception.

GENESIS OF VISUAL IMPULSE IN THE PHOTORECEPTORS

As discussed earlier, the formation of metarhodopsin-II (also known as activated rhodopsin) triggers a cascade of biochemical reactions which results in reduction in the concentration of cyclic GMP in the photo-receptor; which in turn triggers the genesis of visual impulse by producing a generator potential in the photoreceptors. This process of translation of the information content of a light stimulus into electrical signals is known as transduction. The transduction process is highly quantum efficient, in that a single photon causes a response in the rod's membrane potential.

Normally, the inner segment of the photo-receptor continually pumps Na^+ from inside to outside, thereby creating a negative potential on the inside of entire cell. However, the Na^+ channels present in the cell membrane of the outer segment of photoreceptor are kept open by the cyclic GMP, in the dark. So, Na^+, from the extracellular fluid, flows inside the outer segment, i.e. in dark. As a result the cell mem-brane in the outer segment is hypopolarized with respect to the inner segment, i.e. the current flows from the inner to the outer segment (Fig. 8.17). Current also flows to the synaptic ending of the photoreceptor. This is called standing potential or dark current.

When light strikes the photoreceptor, the amount of cyclic GMP in the photoreceptor is reduced (as discussed in photochemistry of vision), so some of the Na^+ channels (which were kept open by cyclic GMP in dark) are closed, and the result is a hyperpolarizing receptor potential. Thus the photoreceptor potential is different from the receptor potentials in almost all other sensory receptors in that the excitation of photoreceptor causes increased negativity of the membrane potential (hyperpo-larization), rather than decreased negativity (depolarization) which is characteristic of all other receptors. Normally, in dark the electro-negativity inside the rod membrane is about 40 millivolts and after excitation it approaches about 70 to 80 millivolts. Further, the eye is unique in that the receptor potential of the photoreceptors is local graded potential, i.e. it

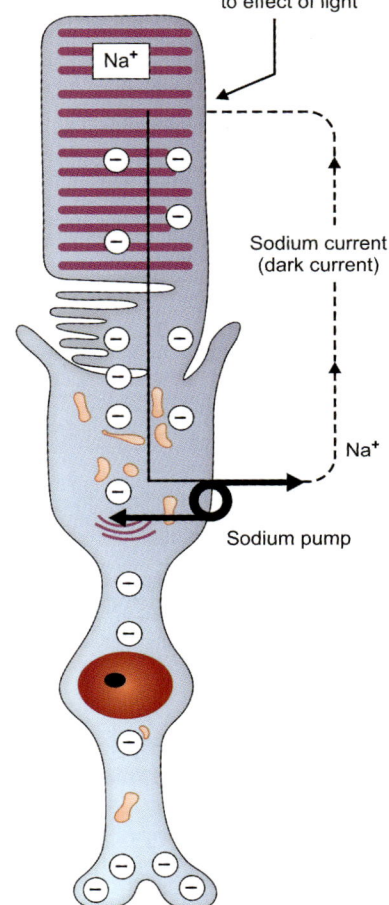

Leakage current decreased by decomposing rhodopsin due to effect of light

Sodium current (dark current)

Sodium pump

Fig. 8.17 *Basis of genesis of photoreceptor hyperpolari-zation.*

does not propagate and does not follow the 'all-or-none law'.

The sequence of events in photoreceptors by which incident light leads to production of a nerve impulse (*phototransduction*) is summarized in Fig. 8.18.

CONE VERSUS ROD RECEPTOR POTENTIAL

The cone receptor potential has a sharp onset and offset, whereas the rod receptor potential has a sharp onset and slow offset. The curve relating the amplitude of receptor potentials to stimulus intensity have similar shapes in rods and cones, but the rods are much more sensitive.

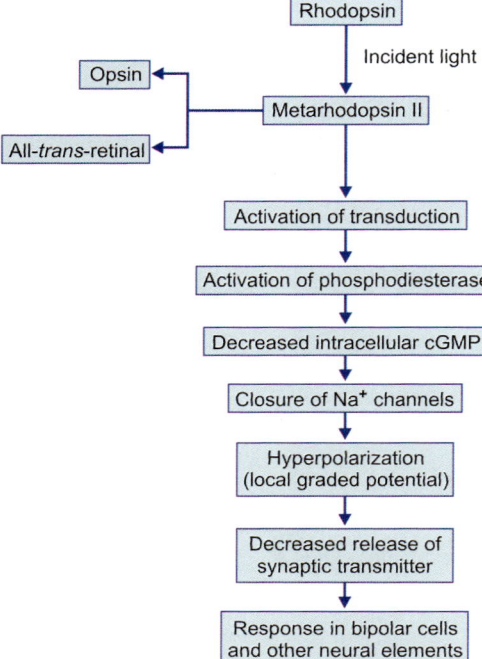

Fig. 8.18 *Sequence of events involved in phototransduction process in the photoreceptor.*

Therefore, rod responses are proportionate to stimulus intensity at levels of illumination that are below the threshold for cones. On the other hand, cone responses are proportionate to stimulus intensity at high levels of illumination when the rod responses are maximal and cannot change. That is why cones generate good response to change in light intensity above background but do not represent absolute illumination well, whereas rods detect absolute illumination.

PROCESSING AND TRANSMISSION OF VISUAL IMPULSE IN THE RETINA

The *receptor potential* generated in the photo-receptors (as discussed above) is transmitted by *electronic conduction* (i.e. direct flow of electric current, not action potential) to the other cells of the retina, viz. horizontal cells, bipolar cells, amacrine cells and ganglion cells. However, the ganglion cells transmit the visual signal by means of action potential.

NEUROTRANSMITTERS IN THE RETINA

Role of neurotransmitters employed for synaptic transmission in the retina still have not all been delineated clearly. However, a great variety of different synaptic transmitters are found in the retina. A few assumptions are as follows.

- *Glutamine,* an excitatory transmitter, is released by rods and cones at their synapses with bipolar and horizontal cells.
- *Amacrine cells* produce five different types of inhibitory transmitters. They include: gamma aminobutyric acid (GABA), glycine, dopamine, acetylcholine and indolamine.
- The transmitters of the bipolar cells and horizontal cells have still not been isolated.
- *Cholinesterase* has been found in the processes of Müller, horizontal, amacrine, and ganglion cells. In the human retina, only the true acetyl-cholinesterase has been found, suggesting that acetylcholine may be the dominant synaptic neurotransmitter in the human.
- *Carbonic anhydrase* has also been isolated from cones and RPE but not rods. Its exact role is also not clear.

PHYSIOLOGICAL ACTIVITIES IN THE RETINAL CELLS

The neurophysiological activities (concerned with the processing and transmission of visual signal) occurring in the different retinal cells can be summarized as follows.

Horizontal cells

Horizontal cells transmit signals horizontally in the outer plexiform layer from rods and cones to the bipolar cells. Their main function is *to enhance the visual contrast* by causing *lateral inhibitions.* This phenomenon of lateral inhibition has been observed by record of electrical activities occurring in the retina (Fig. 8.19), which shows that when a minute spot of light strikes the retina, the central most area is excited but the area around (called as surround) is inhibited. Thus, instead of the excitatory signal spreading widely in the retina because of the spreading dendritic and axonal trees in the plexiform layers, transmission through the horizontal cells puts a stop to this by providing lateral inhibition in the surrounding area. It has been found to be

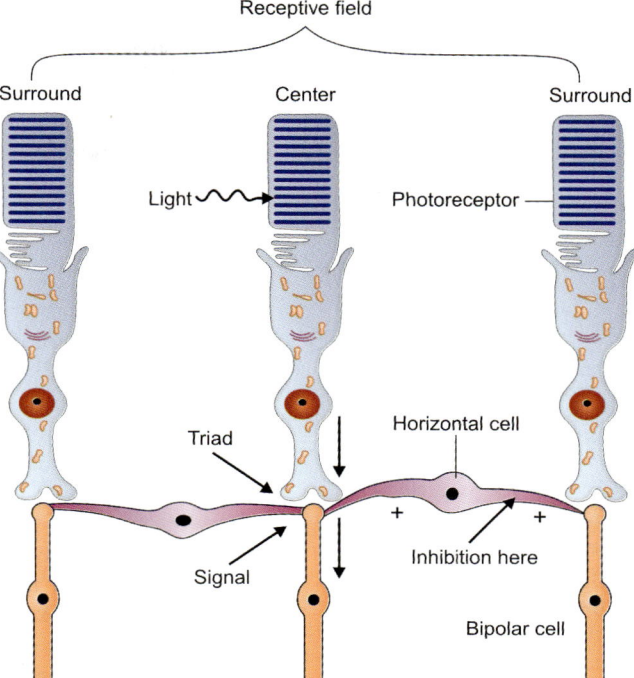

Fig. 8.19 *Showing phenomenon of lateral inhibition in the surround receptive plexiform layer. The central photoreceptor has been stimulated with light and the inner portion of the cell membrane has become more negative. The signal is transmitted upwards to the bipolar cell and also horizontally via the horizontal cells. This horizontal transmission results in inhibition of the photoreceptor—bipolar cell synapse of the neighbouring photoreceptor element. The stimulated bipolar cell may be hyperpolarized or depolarized.*

an essential mechanism which allows high visual accuracy in transmitting contrast borders in the visual image.

Thus, the principal purpose of the microcircuitry of the outer plexiform layer seems to be the processing of spatial information.

The concept of receptive field has been evolved to explain the processing of visual signal. In general sense, the receptive field is defined as the influence area of a sensory neuron. It is circular in configuration. It has been observed that receptive field of the horizontal cells is very large in contrast to the photoreceptor cell.

Bipolar cells

The bipolar cells are neurons of the first order of visual pathway. Their dendrites are stimulated by the light-induced hyperpolarization of the photoreceptors.

The important points delineated regarding the physiological activities concerning the bipolar cells are as follows:

- Some bipolar cells *depolarize* while others *hyperpolarize* (Figs 8.19 and 8.20) when the photoreceptors are excited, i.e. the two different types of bipolar cells provide opposing excitatory and inhibitory signals in the visual pathway. Two possible hypotheses put forward to explain this differential response are as follows:
  - Perhaps the *depolarizing bipolar cells* respond to the excitatory neurotransmitter, glutamate and the hyperpolarizing bipolar cells do not.
  - Perhaps some bipolar cells receive direct excitation from the photoreceptors, whereas the others receive the signal indirectly through the horizontal cells. Because horizontal cell is an inhibitory

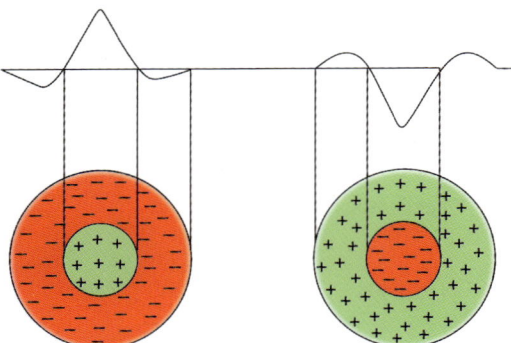

Fig. 8.20 *Showing the centre-surround response to light in 'on' or centre depolarizing bipolar cell (left) and 'off' or centre-hyperpolarizing bipolar cell (right). Plus signs indicate regions giving a depolarizing response, minus signs, a hyperpolarizing one.*

cell, this would reverse the polarity of the electrical response.

- *Receptive field* of the bipolar cell is also circular in configuration but has got a *center-surround antagonism*. As shown in Fig. 8.20 in case of center depolarizing cells (also called as 'on' cell) the light striking the center of receptive field activate and the light striking the 'surround' inhibits bipolar cell output. The reverse occurs in the center hyperpolarizing cell (also called as 'off cell'), i.e. the light striking the 'center' is inhibitory and the light striking the 'surround' is excitatory to bipolar cell output. The size of the center of the bipolar cell receptive field is determined by the reach of its dendrites and that of the much larger 'surround' is determined by the spread of interconnected horizontal cells.
- The importance of the above described reciprocal relationship between the depolarizing and hyperpolarizing bipolar cells is that it provides a second mechanism for lateral inhibition *(spatial information processing)* in addition to horizontal cell mechanism. Further, this reciprocal relationship allows half of the bipolar cells to transmit positive signals and the other half to transmit negative signals; both of these have a useful role in transmitting visual information to the brain.

Amacrine cells

- Amacrine cells receive information at the synapse of the bipolar cell axon with ganglion

cell dendrites (Fig. 8.21) and use this information for temporal processing at the other end of the bipolar cell. As shown in Fig. 8.21, at the synapse, the bipolar cells project onto both ganglion and amacrine cells. The amacrine cell then adjusts the bipolar cell in a *negative feedback arrangement* as to the subsequent response that will be projected onto the ganglion cell.

- Electrically, the amacrine cells produce *depolarizing potentials* and spikes that may act as generator potentials for the propagated spikes produced in the ganglion cells.
- Various types of amacrine cells have been identified by morphological or histochemical means. Functions of some of the types of amacrine cells have been characterized as below:
  - Some amacrine cells are part of the *direct pathway for rod vision*, i.e. the impulse travels from rod to bipolar cells to amacrine cell to ganglion cells.
  - Some amacrine cells respond very strongly at the onset of a visual signal, but the response dies out rapidly.

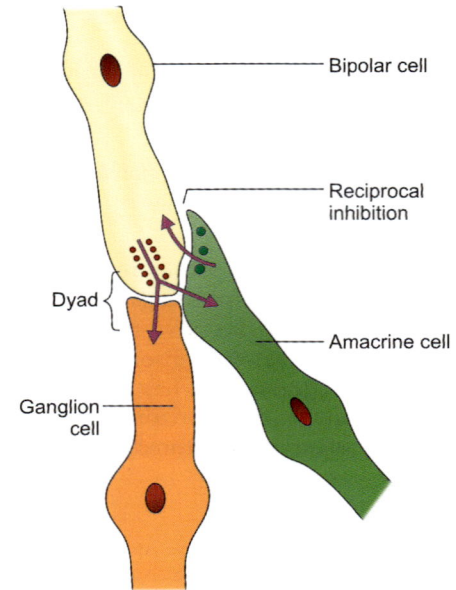

Fig. 8.21 *Showing the bipolar-amacrine-ganglion cell interaction. For explanation see text.*

- Other amacrine cells respond very strongly at the offset of the visual signal but again the response dies quickly.
- One type of amacrine cells respond both when a light is turned on or off signalling simply a change in illumination irrespective of direction.
- Another type of amacrine cells are direction sensitive and respond to movement of a spot across the retina in a specific direction. Thus the amacrine cells help in *temporal summation* and in the initial analysis of visual signals before they even leave the retina.

Ganglion cells

- The electrical response of bipolar cells (local graded potential) after modification by the amacrine cells is transmitted to the ganglion cells which in turn transmit their signals by means of action potential to the brain. Thus, the ganglion cell action potentials are similar to digital or frequency modulation (FM), while the slow graded potentials of the rest of retina are analogous to analog or amplitude modulation (AM) (Fig. 8.22).

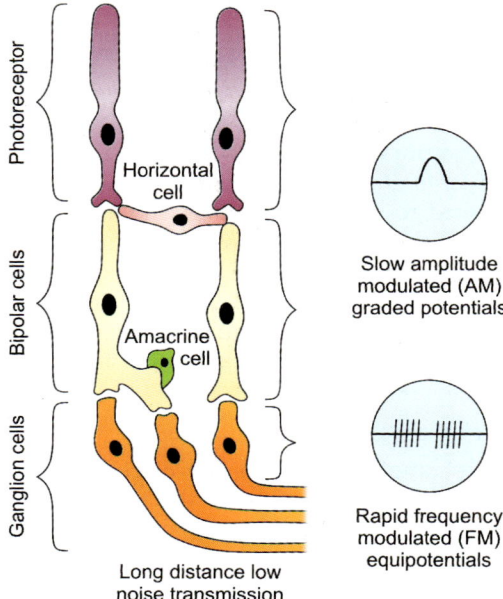

Fig. 8.22 *Showing the amplitude modulation (AM) and frequency modulation (FM), electrical responses from the retina. For explanation see text.*

- The ganglion cells which produce propagated spikes are of two types in terms of their center response: "on-center" cells that increase their discharge and "off-center" cells that decrease their discharge upon illumination of the center of their receptive fields.
- Three distinct groups of ganglion cells (W, X and Y) have been described depending upon the function they serve and are as follows:
  - *W-ganglion* cells are small (diameter >10 micrometre) and constitute about 40 percent of all the ganglion cells. Their dendrites spread widely in the inner plexiform layer and thus they have broad fields in the retina. These cells receive most of their excitation from rods, transmitted by way of small bipolar cells and amacrine cells and are thus important for much of our rod vision under dark conditions. These cells are also especially sensitive for detecting directional movements anywhere in the field of vision.
  - *X-ganglion cells:* Most numerous (55 per cent of total cells), are of medium diameter (between 10 and 15 micrometre). They have very small fields, because their dendrites do not spread widely. Thus, their signals represent discrete retinal locations and so the visual image is mainly transmitted through these cells. Further, since every X-ganglion cell receives input from at least one cone cell, so probably they are responsible for the color vision as well.
  - *Y-ganglion cells:* These are the fewest (5 per cent of total) and largest (up to 35 micrometer in diameter) of all the ganglion cells. However, they have a very broad dendritic field and are thus able to pick up signals from a widespread retinal area. They respond to rapid changes in visual image, either rapid movement or rapid change in the light intensity.

Cleland et al. described X-cells as *sustained cells* and Y-cells as *transient cells*. The studies performed while recording from optic nerve fibers identify transient units as type I and sustained units as type II. The response of Y-cells (type I fibers) is phasic, with a transient excitation to a spot stimulus that decays quickly

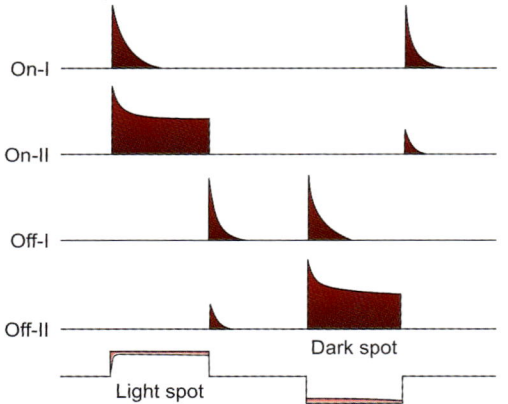

On-I

On-II

Off-I

Off-II

Dark spot

Light spot

Fig. 8.23 *Diagrammatic illustration of four types of responses to light and dark spot stimuli in the cat optic nerve. From Satio et al.*

(Fig. 8.23). The X-cell (type II fibers) response has a tonic sustained component to a spot stimulus.

Ganglion cells affect the relative sensitivity of different parts of the retina as follows:

- The number of ganglion cells in the center of fovea (about 35,000) is equal to the number of cones; this accounts for the high degree of visual acuity in the central retina in comparison with poorer acuity peripherally.

- Peripheral retina has much greater sensitivity to weak light than the central retina. This results partly from the fact that rods are about 300 times more sensitive to light than are cones, but it is further magnified by the fact that as many as 200 rods converge on the same optic nerve fiber in the peripheral retina.

PROCESSING AND TRANSMISSION OF VISUAL IMPULSE IN THE VISUAL PATHWAY

OPTIC NERVE, CHIASMA AND OPTIC TRACT

Optic nerve fibers are the axons of retinal ganglion cells and carry the total output of retina. Single optic nerve fiber can be excited only by a specific stimulus falling on a restricted area of the retina. This area is defined as the *receptive field* and is usually circular or elliptical in configuration.

The optic nerve fibers decussate partially at the *optic chiasma.* The fibers from the nasal half of the retina cross in the midline while the fibers from the temporal half of the retina remain uncrossed. This implies that the visual input from the temporal halves of the visual field goes to the opposite side while the input from the nasal halves of the visual field goes to the same side. Fibers from the fovea pass both ipsilaterally and contralaterally, leading to bilateral representation of the foveal visual field.

The crossed and uncrossed fibers beyond the optic chiasma constitute the *optic tract* of either side. The optic tracts end in the neurons of the lateral geniculate body (LGB).

LATERAL GENICULATE BODY

Functions

Lateral geniculate body (LGB) serves two principal functions:

1. *Relay station.* LGB serves as a relay station to relay visual information from the optic tract to the visual cortex by way of the geniculo-hypercalcarine tract. The relay function is very accurate, so much so that there is exact point-to-point transmission with a high degree of spatial fidelity all the way from the retina to visual cortex. The signals from the two eyes are kept apart in lateral geniculate body.

2. *To "gate" the transmission of signals.* The second major function of the LGB is to "gate" the transmission of signals to the visual cortex, that is, to control how much of the signals be allowed to pass to the cortex. LGB receives gating control signals from two major sources: (a) corticofugal fibers from the primary visual cortex, and (b) the reticular area of the mesencephalon. Both of these are inhibitory and thus control the visual information that is allowed to pass.

Retinotopic projection

- The ganglion cell axons project a detailed spatial representation of the retina on the lateral geniculate body, with precise point-to-point localization.
  Figure 8.13 shows the retinotopic projection on the LGB.
- As depicted in the anatomical description, the LGB contains 6 well-defined layers. On each

side layers 1, 4, 6 receive input from the contra-lateral eye, whereas layers 2, 3, and 5 receive input from the ipsilateral eye (Fig. 8.14). In each layer also there is a point-to-point representation of the retinal and all the six layers are in register, so that along a line perpendicular to the layer, the receptive fields of the cells in each layer are almost identical.

- The layers 1 and 2 of the LGB have large cells and are called *magnocellular*, whereas layers 3–6 have small cells and are called *parvocellular* (Fig. 8.24). *Magnocellular* layers receive their visual input almost entirely from the large Y-ganglion cells of the retina. The magnocellular system provides a very rapidly conducting pathway to the visual cortex, i.e. carry signals for detecion of movement and flicker. However, this system is 'color blind', i.e. transmits only black and white information, and also its point-to-point transmission is poor (because Y-ganglion cells are few in number and their dendrites spread widely in the retina).

- *Parvocellular layers* receive their input almost entirely from the X-ganglion cells and thus transmit color vision and also convey accurate point-to-point spatial information, for texture, shape and fine depth vision; but at only a moderate velocity of conduction rather than high velocity.

Electrophysiological properties of the LGB

- In many respects the electrophysiological properties including receptive fields of both P and I cells of LGB are similar to retinal ganglion cells and the optic nerve axons.

- Without exception, all geniculate receptive fields possess the familiar on-center/off-center configuration.

- The classification of receptive fields as sustained (X) and transient (Y) is maintained in the LGB.

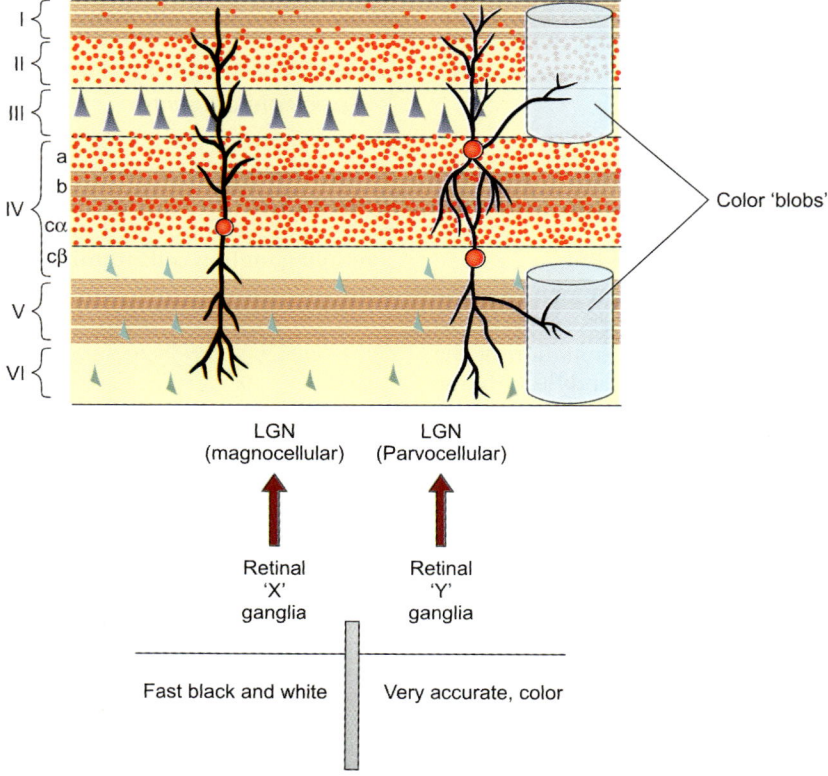

Fig. 8.24 *Cross section of the lateral geniculate body showing magnocellular (1 and 2) and parvocellular (3, 4, 5, 6) areas.*

- The receptive field organization of the geniculate cell differs from that of ganglion cell in the organization of its periphery. Hubel and Wiesel identified a high degree of peripheral suppression in geniculate receptive field. The larger 'off' periphery cancels the effects of an 'on' center. Thus, they are a little more sensitive in responding to spatial differences in retinal illumination rather than to the illumination itself. Thus the disparity between responses to small spot illumination of the entire retina is accentuated by the LGB neurons.
- The majority of geniculate relay cells have binocular receptive fields.

OPTIC RADIATIONS

- The optic radiations are composed of axons of lateral geniculate relay cells which project to the visual cortex on the same side.
- The optic radiations maintain a retinotopic organization in their passage to the visual cortex. The central portion contains macular fibers, while the dorsal fibers carry information from the upper parts of the retinae. The lower or ventral fibers represent lower retinal quadrants (Fig. 8.15).

ANALYSIS OF VISUAL IMPULSE IN THE VISUAL CORTEX

A. RETINOTOPIC ORGANIZATION

Visual cortex lies in the occipital lobe near the posterior pole. Just as the ganglion cell axons project a detailed spatial representation of the retina on the lateral geniculate body (LGB), the LGB projects a similar point-to-point representation on the visual cortex. Details of the anatomy of visual cortex and retinotopic organization of the visual cortex has been described on pages 87 and 92, respectively.

B. FUNCTIONAL ANATOMY AND ORGANIZATION OF THE VISUAL CORTEX

Types of visual cortex

It can be divided into a primary visual cortex and secondary visual cortex.

Primary visual cortex. It is also known as Brodmann's cortical area 17 or visual area I or simply VI. Still another name for primary visual cortex is the striate cortex, because this area has a grossly striated appearance. The axons from the lateral geniculate body end in primary visual cortex.

Secondary visual cortex. It includes visual association areas which lie anterior, superior and inferior to the primary visual cortex. Secondary signals are transmitted to these areas for further analysis of the visual meaning. The visual association areas include the Brodmann's area 18 or visual area II or simply V2; area 19 (visual area III or V3) and so on.

Layers of primary visual cortex

Primary visual cortex, like other portions of cerebral cortex, has six distinct layers (Fig. 8.25). Layers I, II and III are thin and contain pyramidal cells. Layer IV is thickest and contains stellate cells. Layer IV may be further subdivided into layers, a, b, ca and cb; layers IV a + b contain the white stripe of Gennari. Layer V and VI are again relatively thin.

Connections of primary visual cortex

1. Geniculate afferents

The axons from the lateral geniculate nucleus (the geniculocalcarine fibers) terminate mainly in layer IV.
- The rapidly conducted signals from the Y retinal ganglion cells terminate in layer IV ca

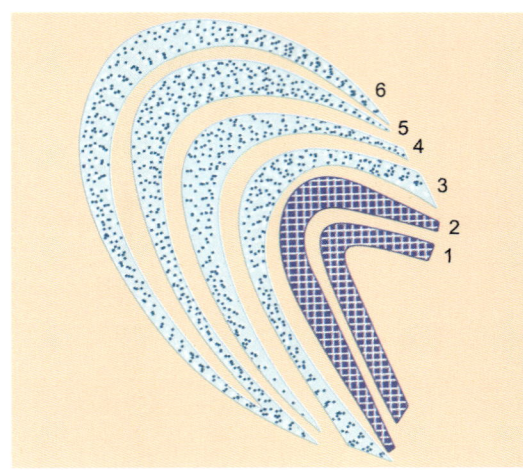

Fig. 8.25 *Layers of visual cortex vis-à-vis analysis of visual impulse in the visual cortex.*

and from here are relayed vertically both outwards toward the cortical surface and inwards toward deeper levels.

- The visual signals from the mediumsized optic nerve fibers derived from the X ganglion cells in the retina terminate in layers IVa and IVc (the shallowest and deepest portions of layer IV). From here these signals again are transmitted vertically both towards the surface of the cortex and to deeper layers. The X ganglion pathway transmits accurate point-to-point type of vision and also the color vision.

2. Subcortical connections

- The reciprocal connections returning from striate to LGB arise from the pyramidal cells of layer VI. Cells in the upper part of layer VI project primarily to magnocellular layers, while the projection to parvocellular layer arises mainly cells in the lower aspect of layer VI.
- Axons from pulvinar to striate cortex terminate among the dendrites of layers I and V whose axons project back to pulvinar and to superior colliculus.

3. Corticocortical connections

Striate cortex is extensively interconnected with other cortical regions. A few important ones are as follows:

- Fibers to extra-striate visual regions arise from the pyramidal cells of layers II and III of the striate cortex.
- Fibers to contralateral striate cortex, via corpus callosum also arise in layer III.
- Reciprocal connections from the extra-striate visual region and from contralateral striate cortex are made by the fibers that terminate predominantly in layers II and III of striate cortex.

C. PHYSIOLOGY OF VISUAL CORTEX

The present information available on physiology of the visual cortex is just the tip of iceberg. Thus, it is just not possible to construct a circuit diagram for the visual cortex with this little information about the enormous complexity of the interactions between the highly branched processes of cortical neurons. However, microelectrode recording and receptive field mapping

by various workers have led to a number of significant observations and to an interesting model for how cortical cells interact. Hubel and Wiesel showed that there are some peculiarities associated with the functions of striate cortex. They observed that unlike retinal ganglion cells and lateral geniculate neurons (which respond to both diffuse retinal stimulation and spot stimulus) the cortical neurons prefer stimuli in the form of straight line, bar or edge presented in the proper spatial orientation. thus, in visual cortex the orientation and configuration receptive field differ from those earlier points in the visual pathway.

Some of the aspects of physiology of visual cortex have been delineated, though incompletely, can be discussed under following headings:

- Concept of receptive field of striate cortex.
- Columnar organization of striate cortex.
- Serial versus parallel analysis of visual image.
- Role of extra-striate cortex in visual functions.
- Psychophysiological aspects of visual functions.

CONCEPT OF RECEPTIVE FIELD OF STRIATE CORTEX

Hubel and Wiesel (Nobel prize winners) were pioneers in this field. They identified and classified the cortical receptive fields of the cat and monkey. They named the cortical cells as three receptive field types—the simple, complex and hypercomplex. These are classical discoveries and form the basis on which a large portion of the visual processing theory is based.

Simple cells

Simple cells are found mainly in layer IV of the primary visual cortex (area 17) and form the first relay station within the visual cortex. These respond to bars of light, lines or edges, but only when they have a particular orientation. When, for example, a bar of light is rotated as little as 10 degrees from the preferred orientation, the firing rate of simple cells is decreased, and if stimulus is rotated much more, the response disappears. The orientation of a stimulus that is most effective in evoking a response is called *receptive field axis orientation*. The receptive field of simple cells can be mapped with small spots of light into 'on-areas' and 'off-areas', which like those of cells in the lateral geniculate body, are mutually antagonistic. However, unlike lateral geniculate neurons, the receptive fields of simple cells are arranged in parallel bands of 'on-areas' and 'off regions, rather than concentric center-surround arrangement of geniculate body (Figs 8.26A and B). Receptive fields of simple cells often have a central band that is either an 'on-region' or an 'off-region', with parallel flanking region on two sides that are opposite (Figs 8.26C to G).

Thus, the simple cell receptive fields play an important role not only in the detection of lines and borders in the different areas of retinal image, but also detects the orientation of each line or border—that is whether it is vertical, or horizontal or lies at some degree of inclination. It is assumed that for each such orientation of a line a specific neuronal simple cell is stimulated.

Complex cells

These cells are found in the cortical layers above and below layer IV of areas 17,18, and 19 of visual cortex, and only rarely in layer IV itself. They resemble simple cells in requiring a preferred orientation of a linear stimulus but are less dependent upon the location of a stimulus in the visual field than the simple cells. They often respond maximally when a linear stimulus is moved laterally without a change in its orientation (Fig. 8.27). Unlike simple cells, it is not possible to map out distinct antagonistic 'on' and 'off' region in the receptive fields of complex cells. Complex cells often receive input from both eyes and are thus called binocular. The receptive field of a given binocular complex cell are on corresponding parts of the two retinae and have identical receptive field properties.

Four types of complex cell receptive fields are described according to their preferred stimulus:

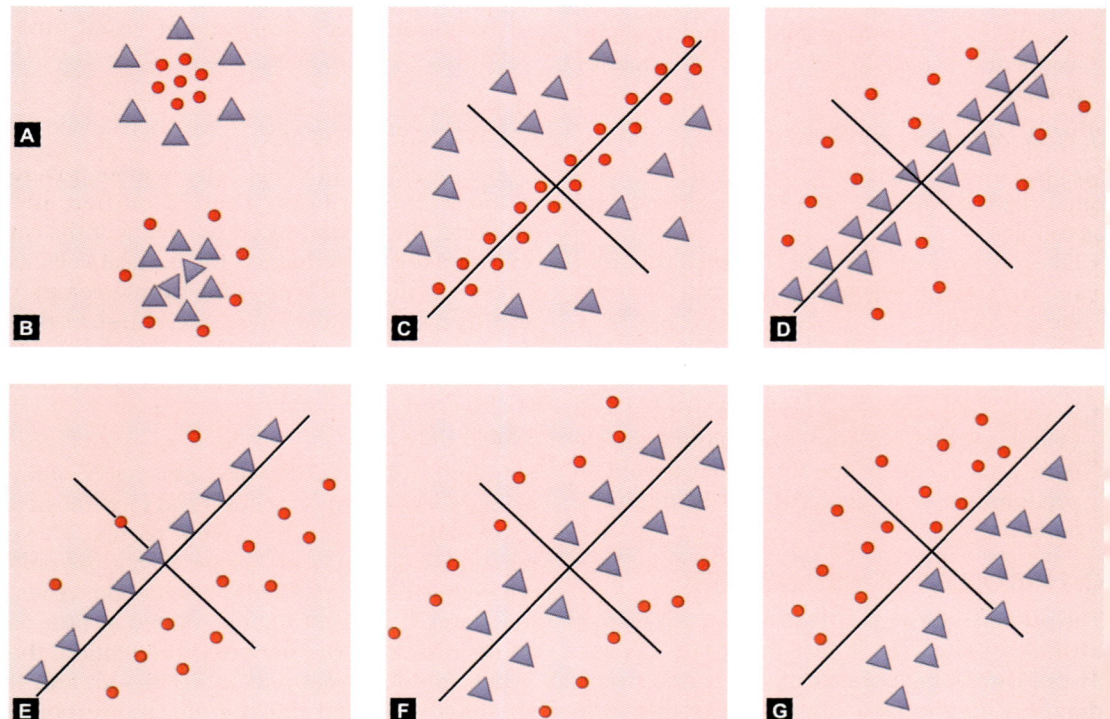

Fig. 8.26 *Showing arrangement of receptive fields of lateral geniculate body and primary visual cortex (area): (A) 'on-centre geniculate receptive field; (B) 'off-centre geniculate receptive field; (C to G) arrangement of receptive field of simple cortical cells. X, areas give excitatory responses (on-responses) and D areas give inhibitory responses (off-responses. Receptive field axes are shown by continuous lines through field centres. After Hubal and Wiesel.*

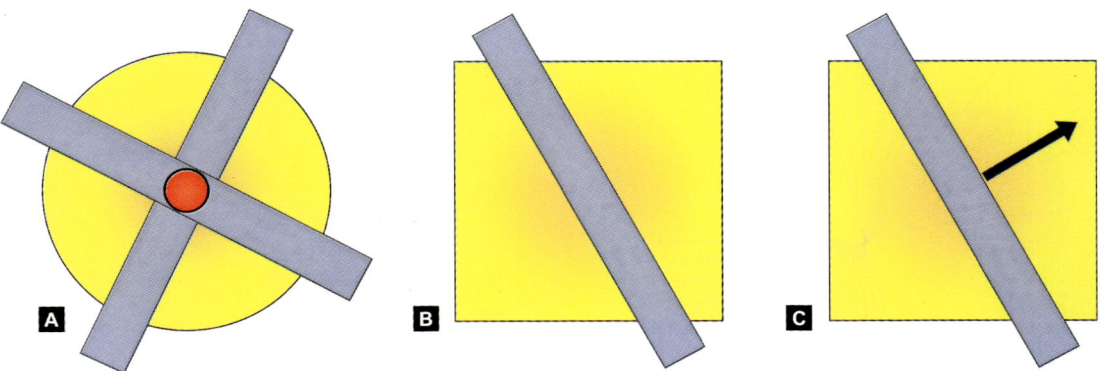

Fig. 8.27 *Showing receptive fields and stimuli: (A) For ganglion cells and lateral geniculate cells (receptive field is circular with an excitatory centre and an inhibitory surround or an inhibitory centre and an excitatory surround). There is no preferred orientation of a linear stimulus; (B) For simple cortical cells which respond best to a linear stimulus with a particular orientation in a particular part of the cell's receptive field; (C) For complex cortical cells which respond to linear stimuli with a particular orientation, but they are less selective in terms of location in the receptive field and often respond maximally when the stimulus is moved laterally, as indicated by the arrow. Modified from Hubel.*

- Activated by a slit—nonuniform field
- Activated by a slit—uniform field
- Activated by an edge
- Activated by a dark bar.

Thus, the complex cell receptive fields play an important role in the detection of lines, bars and edges and but especially so, when they are moving. In other words, by means of simple and complex cells, the person perceives the features, orientation, and movements of objects. Therefore, simple and complex cells together are known as 'feature detectors'.

Hypercomplex cells

These are found in cortical laysers II and III of the areas 17, 18, 19. These cells retain all the properties of complex cells but also have the added feature of requiring the line stimulus to be of a specific length.

The stimuli to which they respond vary greatly, as does their complexity.

Four types of 'lower' hypercomplex cells and two categories of 'higher' hypercomplex cells were described by Hubel and Wiesel. Dreher has classified hypercomplex cells into two types: I and II.

Thus, the hypercomplex cells play a role in the detection of lines of specific length, angles or other shapes.

COLUMNAR ORGANIZATION OF STRIATE CORTEX

Orientation columns

Hubel and Wiesel identified the orientation column as the unit of organization in the visual cortex, which can be defined as *'vertical grouping of cells with identical orientation specificity'*. The visual cortex is thus organized structurally into several million vertical columns of neuronal cells, each column having a diameter of 25–50 micrometers. Roughly, the number of neurons in each of the vertical column is around 1,00,000.

It has been observed that the orientation preferences of neighbouring column differ in a systematic way; as one moves from column to column across the cortex, there are sequential changes in orientation preference of 5–10 degrees (Fig. 8.28). Thus, it is possible to speculate that for each ganglion cell receptive field in the visual field, there is collection of column in a small area of visual cortex representing the possible preferred orientation at small intervals throughout the full 360 degrees.

The orientation columns can be mapped with the aid of radioactive 2-deoxyglucose. The uptake of this glucose derivative is proportionate to the activity of neurons.

Balkemore described two separate column systems for processing depth-perception information. One column system contains

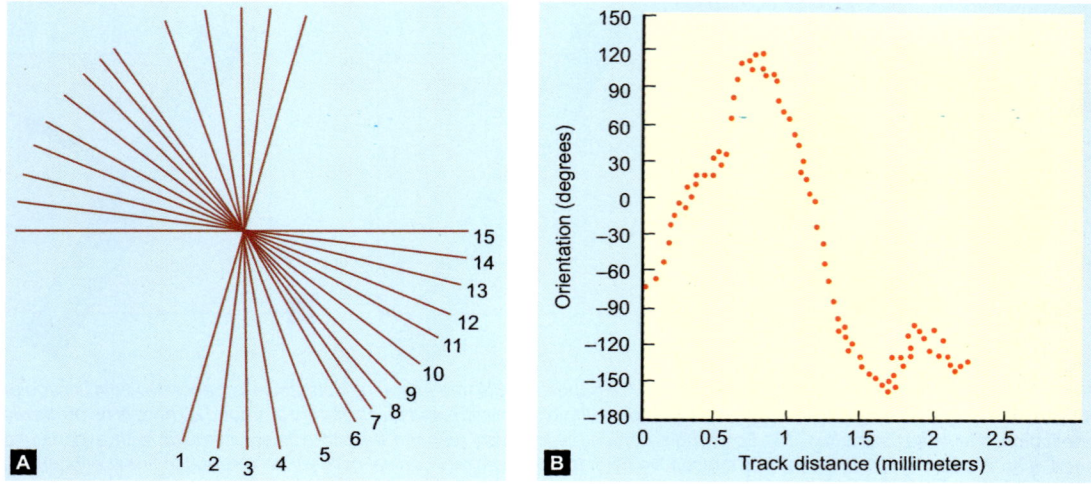

Fig. 8.28 *(A) Orientation preferences of 15 neurons encountered as a microelectrode penetrated the visual cortex obliquely. The preferred orientation changed steadily in a counterclockwise direction; (B) Results of a similar experiment plotted against distance the electrode travelled. In this case, there were a number of reversals in the direction of rotation modified from Hubel and Wiesel.*

binocular units with exactly the same retinal disparity for properly oriented stimuli (*constant depth column*). The second type is *constant direction columns* which view points perpendicular to the center of the contralateral eye. Together they localize points in three-dimensional space.

Ocular dominance columns

Ocular dominance columns refer to an independent system of columns which exist in the visual cortex with respect to the binocular input to cortical cells. As discussed earlier the simple cells in layer IV of striate cortex receive input from one eye only, whereas most complex and hypercomplex cells in layers above and below the layer IV receive input from both eyes. Although most cortical neurons are binocularly activated, there remains a strong monocular dominance. Neurons with receptive fields dominated by one eye are grouped alternately into left eye and right eye columns that are 0.25–0.5 mm in width.

The ocular dominance columns can be mapped by injecting a large amount of a radioactive amino acid into one eye. The amino acid is incorporated into protein and transported by axoplasmic flow to the ganglion cell terminals, across the geniculate synapses and along the geniculocalcarine fibers to the visual cortex. Layer IV becomes evenly labelled, but above and below this layer in the cortex, labelled columns alternate with unlabelled columns receiving input from the uninjected eye. The result is a vivid pattern of strips that covers much of the visual cortex (Fig. 8.27) and is separated from and independent of the grid of orientation columns.

Thus, a group of binocular complex and hypercomplex cells in layers II, III, V and VI that receive a stronger input from one of the two eyes, along with the cells in layer IV that receive input from the same eye, is called an ocular dominance column. There are other methods also to demonstrate ocular dominance columns.

The reason for the existence of rigorously ordered complex binocular input to some complex cells is unknown but may have something to do with *binocular stereoscopic vision*.

Color blobs

Interspersed among the primary visual columns are special column-like areas called *color blobs* (Fig. 8.29). These receive lateral signals from the adjacent visual column and respond specifically to color signals. Therefore, it is presumed that

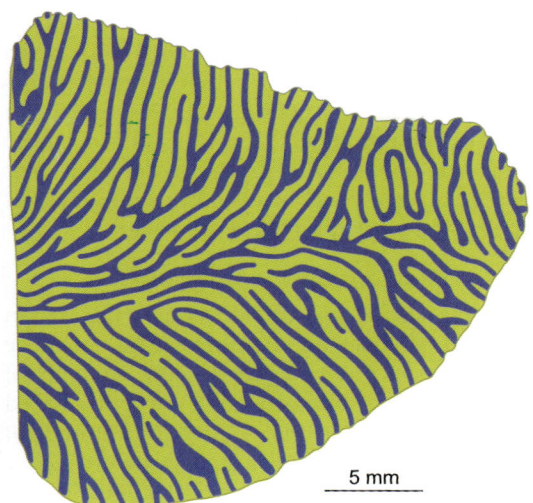

Fig. 8.29 *Representation of ocular dominance columns in a relatively large segment of monkey striate cortex of right occipital lobe. View is of layer IV C seen from above; ocular dominance columns for one eye are in black and those for the other eye in white. The foveal representation is to the right. From Levay et al. and Hubel and Wiesel.*

5 mm

SERIAL VERSUS PARALLEL ANALYSIS OF VISUAL IMAGE

Hubel and Wiesel, who first studied receptive fields of visual cortex and named those receptive field types as simple, complex and hypercomplex, have suggested a hierarchial model for cell inter-connection. The sequence for simple to complex to hypercomplex is *serial analysis* with more and more details being deciphered.

In the Hubel Wiesel model (Fig. 8.30), a complex cell is thought of as receiving input from several simple cells of the same orientation whose receptive fields are overlapping to produce the complex cell receptive field. This suggestion is strengthened by the observation that cells of the same orientation are located in the same cortical column and that a major feature of cortical anatomy is the wealth of vertical interconnections between cells. Since the complex cells are binocular and simple cells are mainly monocular, this adds support to the idea that complex cells are at a more advanced stage of processing.

these blobs are the primary areas for deci-phering color. Also in certain secondary visual areas additional color blobs are found, which presumably perform still higher levels of color deciphering.

Thus, an orderly process (serial system) for synthesizing increasing complex receptive fields has been clearly established, and there is no disagreement about the columnar organization of the cortex. There has been some controversy

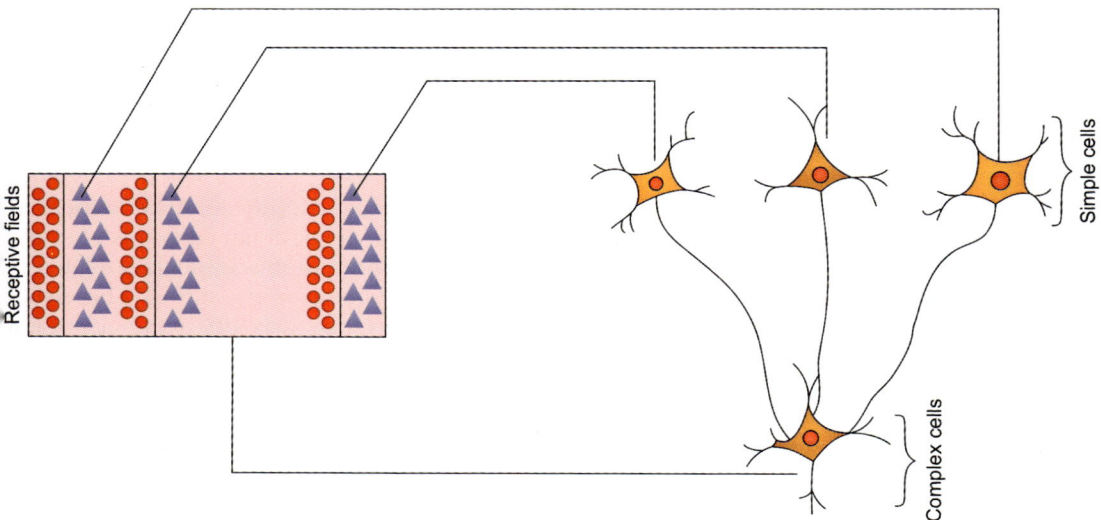

Fig. 8.30 *Hubel and Wiesel's model of serial pathway explaining the organization ot complex receptive fields. A number of cells with simple fields, of which three are shown schematically, are imagined to project to a single cortical cells of higher order. Areas marked with • represent the excitatory regions and those marked with Δ represent the inhibitory region.*

as to whether this serial mechanism of visual processing is the only process or whether information is also handled by means of parallel inputs. However, Hoffmann and Stone propose that the transmission of different types of visual information into different brain locations represents parallel processing systems.

From the foregoing discussion, it should by now be clear that the visual image is deciphered and analyzed by both serial and parallel pathways. It is the combination of both types of these analysis that gives one full interpretation of a visual scene. However, highest levels of analysis are still beyond the present physiological understanding.

ROLE OF EXTRASTRIATE CORTEX (VISUAL ASSOCIATION CORTEX) IN VISUAL FUNCTIONS

For many years, the traditional view of the organization of the visual system held that the striate cortex (area 17) and two "adjcent cortical zones in the occipital lobe (areas 18 and 19) were the only higher visual centers. However, recent advances in the technique of neuroanatomy and neurophysiology have led to many alterations and revisions in the old concepts and brought forward few new concepts.

It is now believed that from the neurons (simple, complex and hypercomplex) of striate cortex (area 17, or VI) information goes to neurons in area 18 (V2), area 19 (V2) and many more like V3, V4 and MT (Fig. 8.31). Fibers from these extrastriate areas go back to striate cortex, they are connected to each other and also receive visual input from the pulvinar. Such cells, which receive information from the feature detectors (simple and complex cells) and hypercomplex cells, are sometimes called *'pontifical cells'* (pontiff—Pope or Bishop, i.e. the highest master). It would appear from the present evidence that some of these regions are specialized for processing particular aspects of visual information. Some of the examples of functionally specialized areas are as follows.

Color processing area

V4 area in rhesus monkey shows group of clusters of opponent color cells. They are much less prevalent in the other extrastriate regions indicating that it forms a color detecting specialized area. This concept has been supplemented by the fact that a few patients have been reported with cortical lesions (at the level of extrastriate visual cortex at the occipital temporal junction) that produced deficient color vision; other aspects of visual function such as acuity and stereopsis were preserved.

Motion (movement) processing area

The extrastriate area called MT area (located in middle portion of temporal lobe) may be specialized in some way for the analysis of motion in the visual scene. This concept is based on the observation that a striking number of cells in this region show a strong preference for stimuli *moving in a* particular direction.

Stereoscopic depth perception area

The extrastriate cortex area V2 and probably also V3 may be processing information for stereoscopic depth perception, since, these cells (called as retinal disparity cells) respond poorly or not at all when the receptive field in one eye is stimulated alone, but respond quite well when both receptive fields are stimulated simultaneously. Cells having uncrossed retinal disparity and those having crossed retinal disparity are noted. Such units with binocular disparity in the receptive fields could thus be functioning in stereoscopic depth perception.

It is quite likely that eventually additional cortical areas will be discovered.

PSYCHOPHYSIOLOGICAL ASPECT OF VISUAL FUNCTIONS

The complex psychophysiological aspect of visual function can be assigned to specific areas of the brain since vision is intimately related in the verbal language and reading. The visual cortex connects, by way of its associational cortex, with tactile sensory motor auditory, olfactory and speech centers (Fig. 8.31). The corpus callosum connects the two hemisphere while other bundles of axons connect the cortical area of same hemisphere (Fig. 8.31). It is these interconnections that allow us to perceive *several* qualities simultaneously and to synthesize a unified picture for our minds' eye. For example, while walking into a room we do

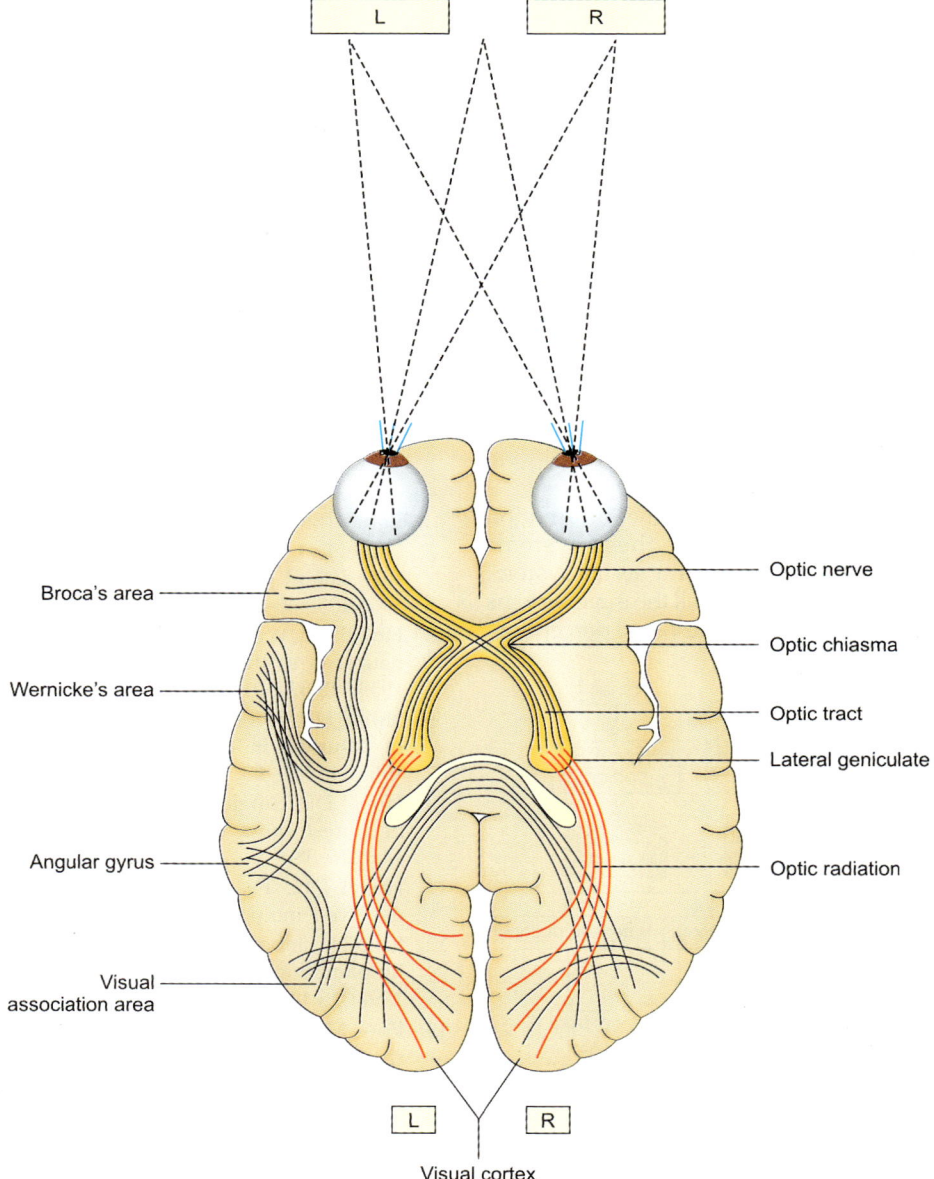

Fig. 8.31 *Showing visual pathway, visual cortex and connections with some of the visual association areas.*

not identify each object separately, but form an impression from its appearance, sound or orders. The brain's response to stimuli is not that of excitation to individual stimuli but is in the form of an overall gestalt, i.e. overall picture.

It has been observed that the angular gyrus (area 40) of the parietal lobe functions as the visual memory center for words by forming associations between visual and auditory centers.

'THREE-PART-SYSTEM' HYPOTHESIS OF VISUAL PERCEPTIONS

From the foregoing discussion on physiology of vision a hypothesis that a *'3-part-system'* is responsible for visual sensations can be well evolved from the data available till date. Although much is still unknown about the physiology of vision. The pathways involved in this 3-part-system are summarized in Fig. 8.32. The components of this 3-part-system are as follows:

- First system is concerned with the perception of movement, location and spatial organization (Fig. 8.32A).
- Second system is concerned with the perception of color (Fig. 8.32B), and
- Third system is concerned with the perception of shapes (Fig. 8.32C).

These three systems process the information as parallel systems. Each of these systems processes the information in a serial system. Ultimately, information from all the three systems is then integrated into a single visual perception.

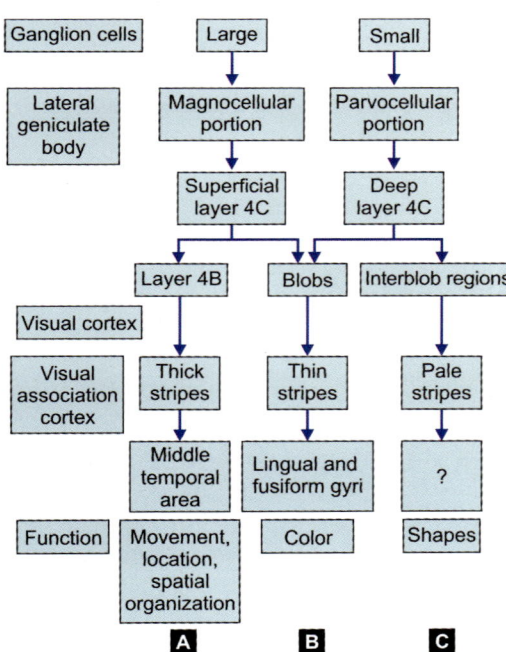

Fig. 8.32 *Organization of visual pathway into a three-part-system that processes information in parallel. Information from the system that detects movement, location and spatial organization (A); the system that detects color (B); and the system that detects shapes (C); is then integrated into single visual perception.*

BIBLIOGRAPHY

1. Arden GB. Receptor potentials. Br Med Bull 1970;26:125–9.
2. Burke W, Sefton AJ. Inhibitory mechanisms in lateral geniculate nucleus of rat. J Physiol (Long) 1966;187:231–46.
3. Curcio C.A., Sloan K.R., Kalina R.E., et al. Human photoreceptor topography. J. Comp. Neural 1990;292:497.
4. Dreher B. Hypercomplex cells in the cat's striate cortex. Invest Ophthalmol 1972;11:355–26.
5. Fukada Y. Receptive field organization of cat optic nerve fibres with special reference to conduction velocity, Vision Res 1971;11:209–26.
6. Garey LJ, Powell TPS. An experimental study of the termination of the lateral geniculo-cortical pathway in the cat and monkey, Proc. R. Soc. Lond. (Biol.) 1971;179:41.
7. Hubel DH, Wiesel TN. Integrative action in the cat's lateral geniculate body. J Physiol (Lond) 1961;155:385–98.
8. Hubel DH, Wiesel TN. Receptive fields of single neurones in the cat's striate cortex. J Physiol 1959;148:574–91.
9. Hubel DH, Wiesel TN. Shape and arrangement of columns in cat's striate cortex, J Physiol 1963;165:559–68.
10. Hubel DH. Single unit activity in striate cortex of unrestrained cats. J Physiol (Lond) 1959; 141:226–38.
11. Hubel DH. The visual cortex of normal and deprived monkey Am Sci, 1979;67:532.
12. Kolb H, Linberg KA, Fisher SK. Neurons of the human retina: Golgi study. J. Comp. Neural 1992;318:147.
13. Poo MN, Cone RA. Lateral diffusion of rhodopsin in necturus rods. Exp Eye Res 1973; 17:503–10.
14. Tripathi RC. Tripathi BJ. Anatomy of the human eye, orbit and adnexa. In 'The Eye', 3rd edition (Ed. H. Davson), Academic Press, London, 1984;145:40.
15. Walls GL. The lateral geniculate nucleus and visual histophysiology. UCLA Publ. Physiol. vol. 9, 1953.
16. Werblin FS. Control of retinal sensitivity. II, Lateral interactions at the outer plexiform Layer. J Gen Physiol 1974;63:62–81.
17. Werblin FS. Lateral interaction at inner plexiform layer of the vertebrate retina: antagonistic responses to change. Science 1972;175:1008–10.

9

LESIONS OF THE VISUAL PATHWAY

Aruj K Khurana, Bhawna Khurana, AK Khurana

OPTIC NERVE LESIONS
- Lesions of the distal optic nerve
- Lesions through proximal part of the optic nerve

CHIASMAL LESIONS
Chiasmal Syndrome
- Definition and types
- Etiology
- Clinical features
- Diagnosis
- Treatment

RETROCHIASMAL LESIONS
General Considerations
- Optic tract syndrome type I
- Optic tract syndrome type II
Lateral Geniculate Nucleus Lesions
- Common causes
- Characteristic features
Lesions of Optic Radiations
- Temporal lobe lesions
- Parietal lobe lesions
Lesions of Visual Cortex
- Visual field defects
- Other manifestations

OPTIC NERVE LESIONS

Salient features and important causes of lesions of the visual pathway at different levels (Fig. 9.1) are described briefly.

Lesions of optic nerve can be divied into:
- Lesions of the distal optic nerve, and
- Lesions through proximal part of the optic nerve.

Common causes of optic nerve lesions are: optic atrophy, traumatic avulsion of the optic nerve, indirect optic neuropathy, ischaemic optic neuropathy and acute optic neuritis.

LESIONS OF THE DISTAL OPTIC NERVE

Salient features include (Fig. 9.1)[1]:
- Marked loss of vision or complete blindness on the affected side,
- Abolition of the direct light reflex on the ipsilateral side and consensual on the contralateral side, and
- Near (accommodation) reflex is present.

LESIONS THROUGH PROXIMAL PART OF THE OPTIC NERVE

Salient features of such lesions are (Fig. 9.1[2]):
- Ipsilateral blindness,
- Contralateral hemianopia,
- Abolition of direct light reflex on the affected side and consensual on the contralateral side, and
- Intact near reflex.

Note. Optic nerve disorders are described in detail in Section IV.

CHIASMAL LESIONS

CHIASMAL SYNDROME
DEFINITION AND TYPES

Chiasmal syndrome refers to the set of signs and symptoms associated with lesions of optic chiasma. Chiasmal syndrome has been classified into three types:

I. *Anterior chiasmal syndrome* is produced by lesions that affect the ipsilateral optic nerve fibres and the contralateral inferonasal fibres

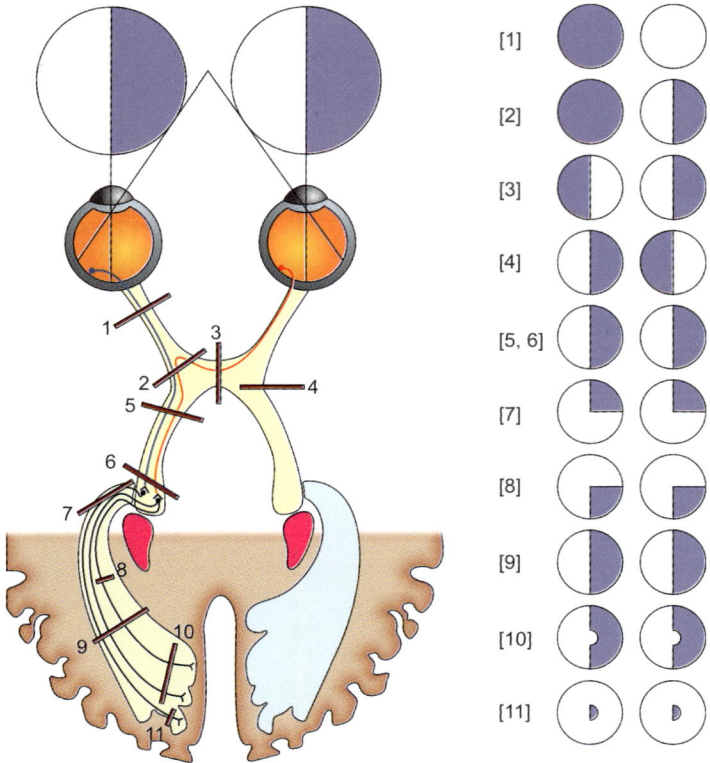

Fig. 9.1 *Lesions of the visual pathways at the level of : [1] optic nerve; [2] proximal part of optic nerve; [3] central chiasma; [4] lateral chiasma (both sides); [5] optic tract; [6] geniculate body; [7] part of optic radiations in temporal lobe; [8] part of optic radiations in parietal lobe; [9] optic radiations; [10] visual cortex sparing the macula; [11] visual cortex, only macula.*

located in the Wilbrand knee; typically producing the so-called junctional scotoma.

II. **Middle chiasmal syndrome** is produced by lesion involving the decussating fibres in the body of chiasma typically producing bitemporal hemianopia. Rarely the middle lesions can affect the uncrossed temporal fibres and produce nasal or binasal hemianopia.

III. **Posterior chiasmal syndrome** is produced by lesions affecting the caudal fibres in chiasma. Characteristic features are as below:

- *Paracentral bitemporal field defects* occur because macular fibres cross more posteriorly in the chiasma and are damaged in the posterior chiasmal lesions

- *Visual acuity and colour vision* may be preserved as temporal macular fibres are not damaged.

- *Homonymous hemianopia* on the contralateral side may occur when posterior chiasmal lesions involve the optic tract.

ETIOLOGY

I. **Intrinsic causes,** i.e. which produce thickening of chiasma itself include:

- Gliomas, and
- Multiple sclerosis

II. **Extrinsic causes,** i.e. compressive lesions are more common and include:

- Pituitary adenomas (most common cause)
- Craniopharyngiomas, and
- Meningiomas

III. **Other causes** of chiasmal syndrome (rare) include:

- Metabolic causes,

- Toxic causes,
- Traumatic, and
- Inflammatory conditions, e.g. lymphoid hypo-physitis, sarcoidosis

CLINICAL FEATURES

Chiasmal syndrome is characterised by following clinical features:

A. OCULAR FEATURES

I. Symptoms

1. **Visual loss.** Visual loss, especially of unexplained etiology should be suspected of a chiasmal syndrome and should warrant MRI of the brain. In some cases visual field defects may be present with normal visual acuity.

2. **Headache** may be associated with pituitary tumours and is usually due to stretching of meninges.

3. **Diplopia** may occur due to:

- *Misalignment of two eyes* occurring as a result of III, IV or VI cranial nerves due to extension of lesion into either or both cavernous sinuses.

- *Hemifield slide phenomenon* refers to diplopia in the absence of ocular misalignment seen in patients with bitemporal hemianopia. It occurs due to vertical slide of eyes in the absence of binocular area of overlapping or interlocking visual field.

4. **Photophobia** may be complained by some patients. Possibly it occurs due to hypersensitivity of trigeminal in patients with parasellar tumours.

5. **Postfixation blindness,** i.e. an area of blindness immediately beyond the point of fixation during near vision fixation. This occurs because of the fact that when eyes converge the area beyond the point of regard falls within the bitemporal hemianopic area.

6. **Difficulty in depth perception,** near work, or precision task may be encountered by many patients.

II. Signs

1. *RAPD*

- RAPD is usually present in patients with asymmetric or unilateral visual loss.

2. *Acquired colour vision defects*

Acquired dyschromatopsia in one or both eyes may be noted in patients with chiasmal syndrome.

3. *Optic disc changes*

- *Optic disc pallor* may be seen in patients with partial optic atrophy. A characteristic band atrophy of the optic disc is produced in patients with bitemporal hemianopia.
- *Papilledema,* i.e. disc oedema, though unusual, may be seen in some patients due to raised intracranial pressure especially with craniopharyngioma.

4. *Visual field defects*

Depending upon the location of lesion, following field defects can occur in chiasmal disorders:
- Junctional scotoma,
- Monocular temporal hemianopic defect,
- Bitemporal hemianopia,
- Homonymous hemianopia, and
- Binasal visual field defects.

i. *Junctional scotoma*

Junctional scotoma refers to a combination of central scotoma in one eye and temporal hemianopic defect in the other eye (Figs 9.1[2] and 9.2). Location of lesion in such cases is at the junction of optic nerve and chiasma on the side of scotoma (Figs 9.1[2] and 9.2).

ii. *Monocular temporal hemianopic defect*

Monocular temporal hemianopic visual field defects with no visual field loss in the contralateral eye (Fig. 9.3) can occur when the lesion involves only the crossing visual fibres at the anterior angle of the optic chiasma.

iii. *Bitemporal hemianopia*

- Bitemporal hemianopia (Fig. 9.1[3]) typically obeying the vertical meridian is a classical field defect noted in patients with sagittal (central) lesions of chiasma. The visual field defect may be complete or incomplete (Fig. 9.4). In many cases pure bitemporal hemianopic field may not occur. A central bitemporal field defect (Fig. 9.5) may occur in patients with prefixed chiasma or posterior growing tumours because macular fibres are located posteriorly.

- *Bitemporal hemianopic paralysis of pupillary reflex* is almost always associated with bitemporal hemianopic defects.

- *Partial descending optic atrophy* is usually produced by central chiasmal lesions.

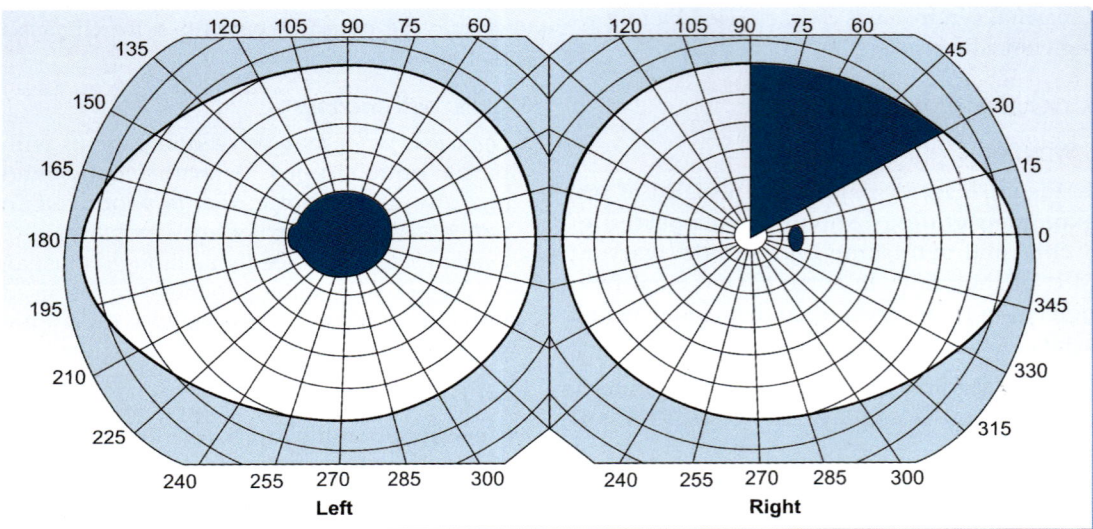

Fig. 9.2 *Junctional scotoma; pattern of field defects.*

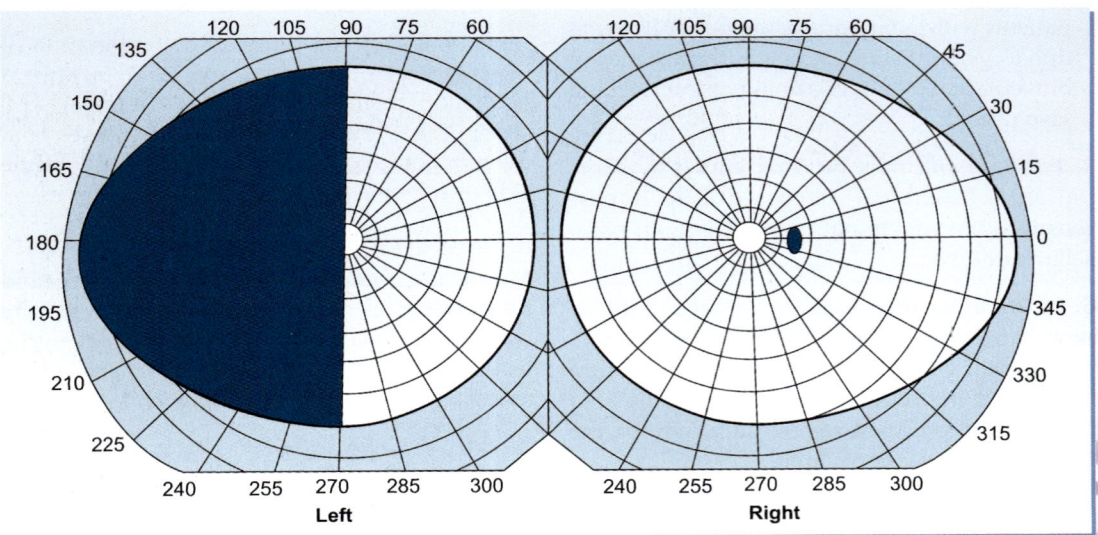

Fig. 9.3 *Monocular temporal hemianopic defect.*

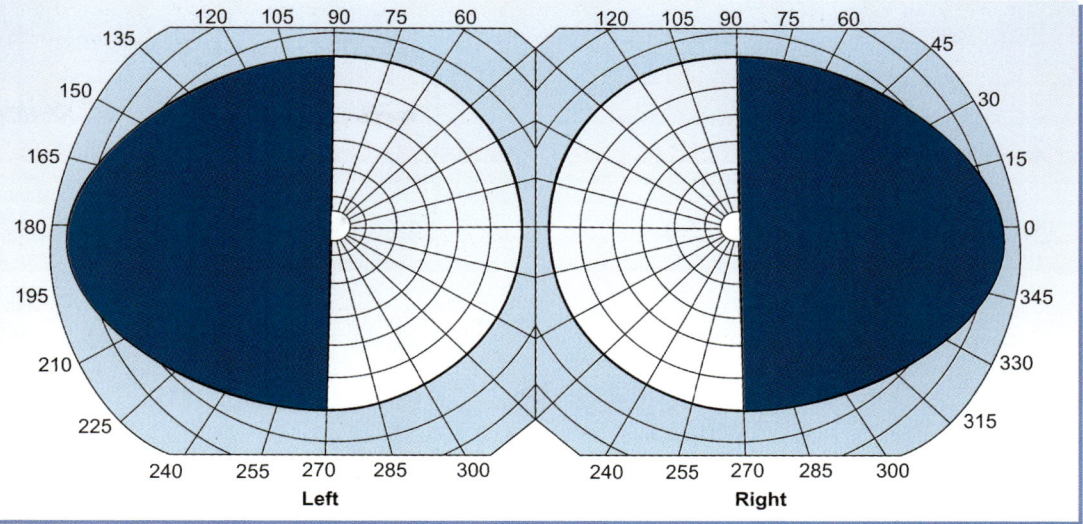

Fig. 9.4 *Bitemporal hemianopia.*

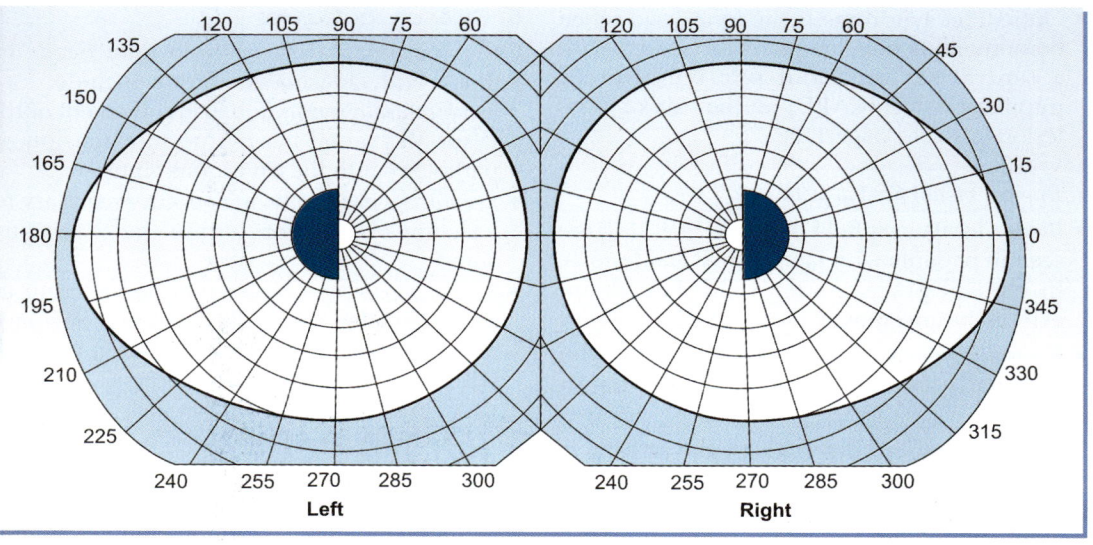

Fig. 9.5 *Central bitemporal hemianopia.*

Common causes of central chiasmal lesions include:
- *Pituitary adenoma* in 50–55% of cases
- Craniopharyngioma in 20–25% of cases
- Supracellar meningiomas in 10% of cases
- Glioma of third ventricle in 7% of cases
- Other rare causes include supracellar aneurysms, third ventricular dilatation due to obstructive hydrocephalous and chronic chiasmal arachnoiditis.

iv. *Homonymous hemianopia*
- Homonymous hemianopia, usually incongruous (Fig. 9.6), may occur due to involvement of optic tract in parasellar lesions.
- Circumstances in which parasellar chiasmal lesions produce homonymous hemianopia include:
  - Prefixed optic chiasma, and
  - Posteriorly directed mass lesions

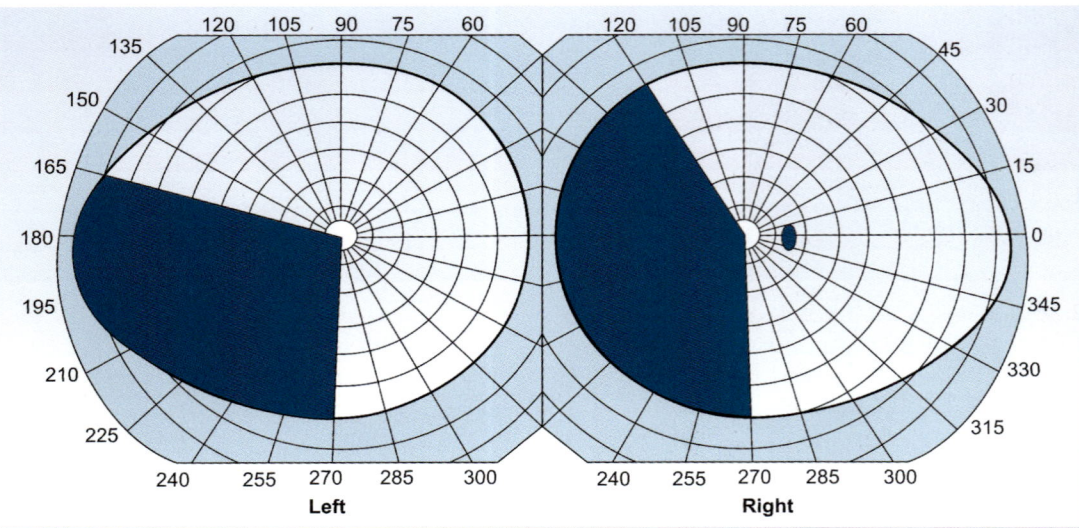

Fig. 9.6 *Incongruous homonymous hemianopia.*

- Optic tract syndrome is the term used when homonymous hemianopia is associated with a central scotoma and relative afferent pupillary defect (RAPD) on the side of mass lesion (also see page 116).

v. Binasal visual field defects
- *Binasal hemianopic* field defects (Fig. 9.1[4]) are seen in patients with lateral chiasmal lesions. In clinical practice such field defects are extremely uncommon.
- *Binasal hemianopic paralysis of pupillary reflex* is usually associated with binasal hemianopia.
- *Partial (temporal) descending optic atrophy* is usually produced by lateral chiasmal lesions.

Common causes of such lesions are:
- *Distention of third ventricle* causing pressure on each side of the chiasma.
- *Atheroma* of the carotids or posterior communicating arteries.
- *Post-fixed chiasma* with mass lesion located between both optic nerves along the anterior aspect of the chiasma displacing the optic nerves laterally against the supraclinoid internal carotid arteries or AI segments of the anterior cerebral arteries is a typical situation for such field defects.

5. *Other ocular features*

Other ocular features which may occur in patients with chiasmal syndrome include:
- *Ocular misalignment* due to involvement of III, IV or VI cranial nerve due to extension of pathology into the cavernous sinus.
- *Proptosis*, very rarely, may occur secondary to vascular obstruction within the cavernous sinus.
- *See-saw nystagmus* is also reported to occur in patients with parasellar lesions. See-saw nystagmus is frequently reported in patients with craniopharyngioma.

B. ENDOCRINAL SIGNS AND SYMPTOMS

Endocrinal signs and symptoms produced by tumours of pituitary gland are as below:
1. *Amenorrhoea-galactorrhoea syndrome in women* and *impotence in men* are produced by prolactin secreting tumours of pituitary gland.
2. *Acromegaly* is a manifestation of excessive secretion of growth hormone.
3. *Cushing syndrome*, characterised by obesity, centripetal fat deposition, proximal myopathy, moon facies, is a feature of tumour arising from ACTH producing cells.
4. *Hypopituitarism and hypothyroidism* are produced by endocrinologically inactive pituitary tumours.

5. *Pituitary apoplexy,* i.e. acute sudden hypo-pituitarism characterised by shock, coma, and even death, is a feature of haemorrhage into a pre-existing pituitary tumour.

DIAGNOSIS

1. *Visual fields* should be ordered in all patients presenting with unexplained visual loss. Visual field defects in chiasmal syndromes are described above.
2. *Neuroimaging.* MRI of the brain and sellar region with multiplanar thin sections is of critical importance in all suspected cases of chiasmal syndrome.
3. *Endocrinal assays* are useful in testing various associated endocrinal dysfunctions.
4. *Histopathological examinations* of pituitary tumour is critical in final diagnosis.

TREATMENT

1. *Medical treatment* may be indicated in endo-crinologically active tumours and patients should be referred to neurologist-endocrino-logist team.
2. *Surgical treatment* is required in most cases of pituitary adenomas, craniopharyngioma, meningioma and glioma and the patient should be referred to neurosurgeon.

ROLE OF OPHTHALMOLOGISTS

Role of ophthalmologists following treatment of pituitary tumour is as below:

i. Sequential visual field testing

Typical schedule for follow-up perimetry is as follows:
- First year—every 3 months
- Up to 5 years—annually, and
- After 5 years—every 2 years

Causes of deterioration in visual fields include:
- *Recurrence* of tumour
- *Radiation necrosis* of chiasma in patients treated with radiotherapy
- *Chiasmal prolapse* into empty sella
- *Arachnoiditis* following surgery

Post-treatment recovery in visual field. After successful surgical treatment of pituitary tumours, pattern of recovery in visual fields is as below:

- *Dramatic and rapid recovery* is noticed after 24 hours of surgery
- *Moderate continued recovery* occurs during the next six weeks
- *Slow recovery* is continued for a year or so.

ii. Retinal nerve fibre layer (RNFL) evaluation with OCT

Retinal nerve fibre layer (RNFL) evaluation with OCT is very useful in predicting the recovery of visual fields. Dramatic recovery in visual fields is reported in patients with RNFL thickness greater than 76 to 85 µm.

iii. Sequential MRI

Sequential MRI should also be performed to document early recurrences.

RETROCHIASMAL LESIONS

GENERAL CONSIDERATIONS

Retrochiasmal lesions include:
- Lesions of optic tract,
- Lesions of lateral geniculate nucleus,
- Lesions of optic radiations,
  - Temporal lobe lesions, and
  - Parietal lobe lesions
- Lesions of occipital lobe

Contralateral homonymous hemianopias of different forms (depending upon site of lesion) without loss of visual acuity is the predominant visual field defect of all the retrochiasmal lesions.
- *Incomplete homonymous hemianopia* can be congruous or incongruous. Congruous homo-nymous hemianopias are identical in shape, size, depth and slope of the margins. The con-gruousity of field defects increases from optic tracts to occipital cortex. This is because of the fact that as the visual fibres travel toward occipital lobe the corresponding retinal points lie adjacent to one another and hence visual field defects due to posterior lesions are more congruous. Thus, depending upon the incon-gruousity of field defect the site of lesion can be localised.
- *Complete homonymous hemianopia* cannot be categorized into congruous versus incon-gruous and then it is not possible to localise

the site of lesion. In such cases, the clinician must rely on other symptoms and signs of neurological disease or on neuroimaging.

Homonymous visual field defects in intra-cranial tumours versus in vascular lesions

In intracranial tumours, irrespective of the location, the homonymous visual field defects are characterised by:
- Slow progression
- Progression occurs from periphery to centre
- Defects appear early for coloured objects than for black and white objects
- After surgical decompression the recovery progresses from centre towards periphery

In vascular lesions such as haemorrhage or infarction the homonymous visual field defects are characterised by:
- Sudden onset with rapid progression, and
- Recovery occurs from centre towards periphery.

LESIONS OF OPTIC TRACT

The set of clinical features produced by lesions of optic tract are referred as 'optic tract syndrome', which are of two types: type I and type II.

OPTIC TRACT SYNDROME TYPE I

Etiology

Optic tract syndrome type I is caused by a large compressive mass lesion that involves the optic tract, optic chiasma and even the optic nerve. *Common causes* include:
- Craniopharyngioma (most common),
- Tumours of optic thalamus, and
- Large aneurysms of superior cerebellar or posterior cerebral arteries.

Characteristic features

Optic tract syndrome type I is characterised by following set of signs:
- *Visual acuity* is decreased ipsilaterally
- *Hemianopia.* Contralateral incongruous homonymous hemianopia (Fig. 9.6), since nerve fibres of corresponding retinal points from two eyes do not lie adjacent to each other in the optic tracts.
- *Pupillary reflex* defects may be any of the following:
  - *Ipsilateral RAPD,* i.e. relative afferent pupillary defect

  - *Wernicke's hemianopic pupil,* i.e. pupillary reflex is present when light is shown to normal halves of retina and absent when shown to blind halves of retinae.
- *Optic disc changes* include Bow-tie atrophy on the side contralateral to the side of lesion (the side with temporal field defect) and temporal pallor on the ipsilateral side.

OPTIC TRACT SYNDROME TYPE II

Etiology

Optic tract syndrome type II results from intrinsic lesions of optic tract produced by conditions like:
- Demyelinating diseases, and
- Infarction

Characteristic features

Characteristic features of optic tract syndrome type II include:
- *Visual acuity* is usually intact
- *Pupillary reflex defects* may be:
  - RAPD on the side opposite to lesion
  - Wernicke's hemianopic pupil
- Homonymous hemianopia is complete or nearly so (Figs 9.1[5] and 9.7)
- Optic disc changes are similar to optic tract syndrome type I

LESIONS OF LATERAL GENICULATE NUCLEUS

Lesions of lateral geniculate nucleus (LGN) are extremely rare. Characteristic features include:

Field defects of following types may occur:
- *Homonymous hemianopia is* incongruous similar to OTS type I (Fig. 9.6)
- *Homonymous horizontal sectoranopia* nearly congruous (Fig. 9.8), associated with sectorial optic atrophy may occur due to posterior choroidal artery infarction
- *Hourglass shaped visual field defects* due to infarction of anterior choroidal artery supplying ventral nucleus or *hourglass-preserved visual field defects* due to infarction of posterior choroidal artery supplying the dorsal nucleus may occur with bilateral LGN involvement.

Pupillary reflexes are normal

Optic disc pallor may occur

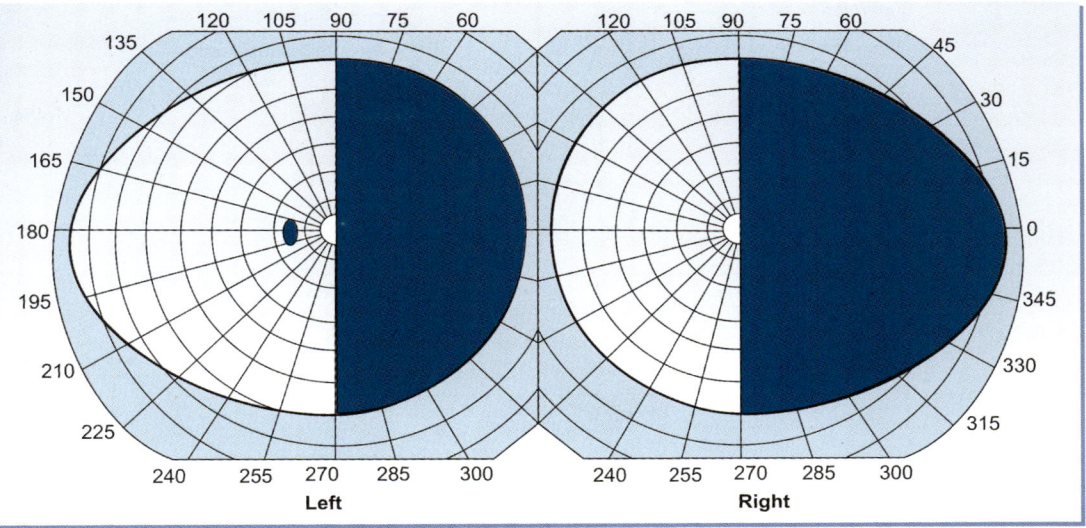

Fig. 9.7 *Complete homonymous hemianopia.*

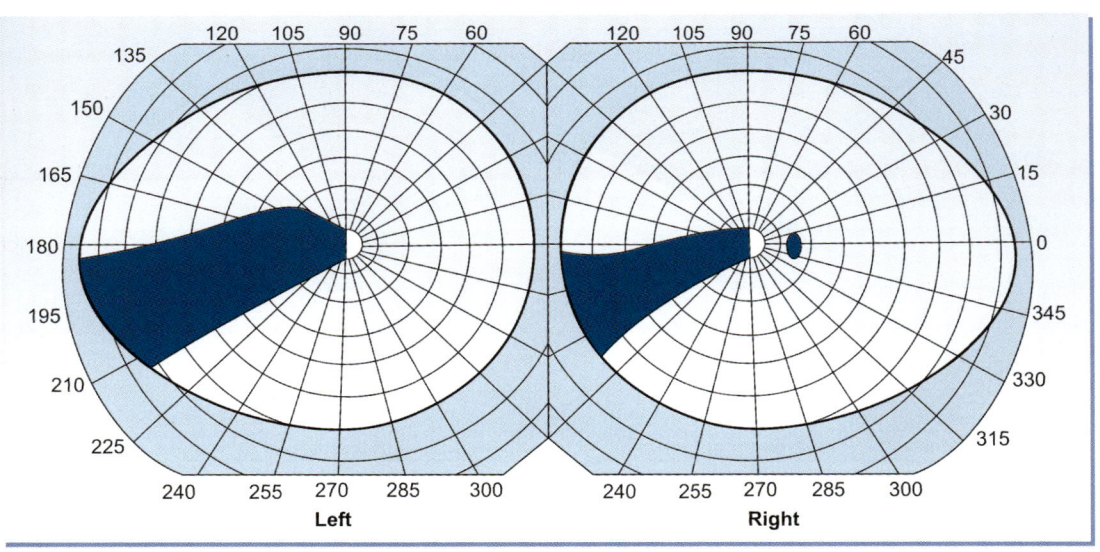

Fig. 9.8 *Homonymous horizontal sectoranopia.*

LESIONS OF OPTIC RADIATIONS

TEMPORAL LOBE LESIONS

Causes

Common causes of temporal lobe lesions are:
- Tumours,
- Temporal lobectomy for seizures, and
- Vascular occlusions

Visual features

Anterior temporal lobe lesions involving Meyer's loop, formed by anteroinferior sweeping of the inferior fibres of optic radiations (Fig. 9.9A), produce midperipheral and peripheral contralateral homonymous superior quadrantopia (pie-in-the-sky field defect) (Figs 9.1[7] and 9.9B).

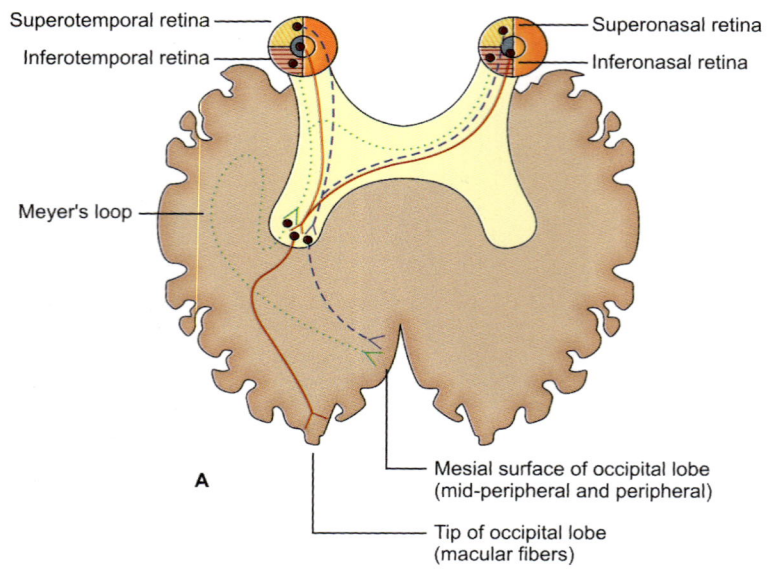

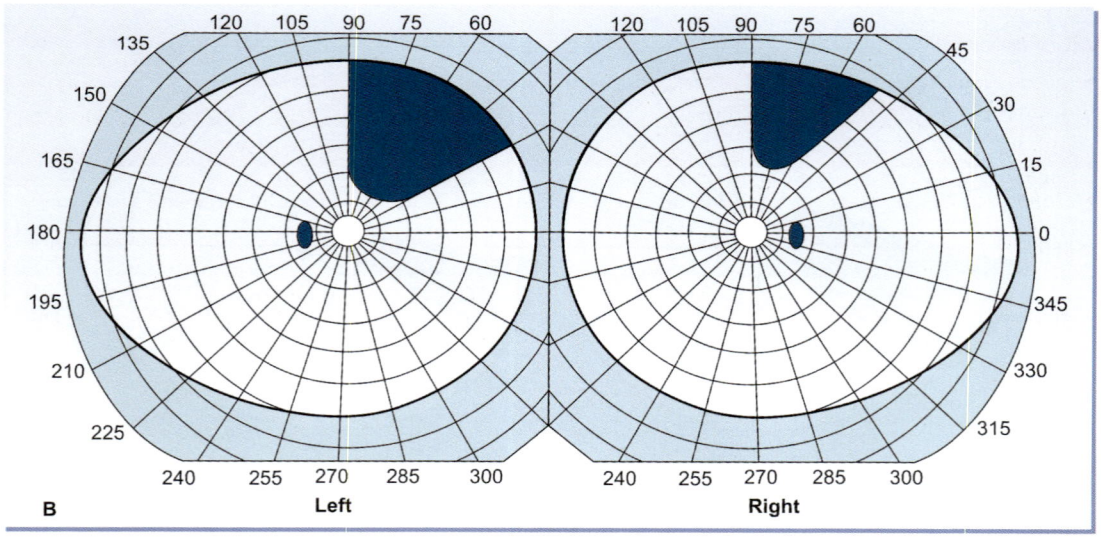

Fig. 9.9 *Anterior temporal lobe lesion involving inferior fibres of optic radiations forming Meyer's loop (A) and producing homonymous superior quadrantopia (B).*

More extensive temporal lobe lesions produce a homonymous hemianopia, but the field defect will be denser superiorly (Fig. 9.10).

Systemic features

Systemic features of temporal lobe tumours which may be associated with visual fields include:

- Headache
- Auditory hallucinations or illusions
- Memory disturbances
- Language disturbances, when dominant temporal lobe is involved
- Mood, emotion and behaviour changes
- Uncinate fits characterised by aura of unusual taste or smell followed by abnormal motor activity of the mouth and lips.

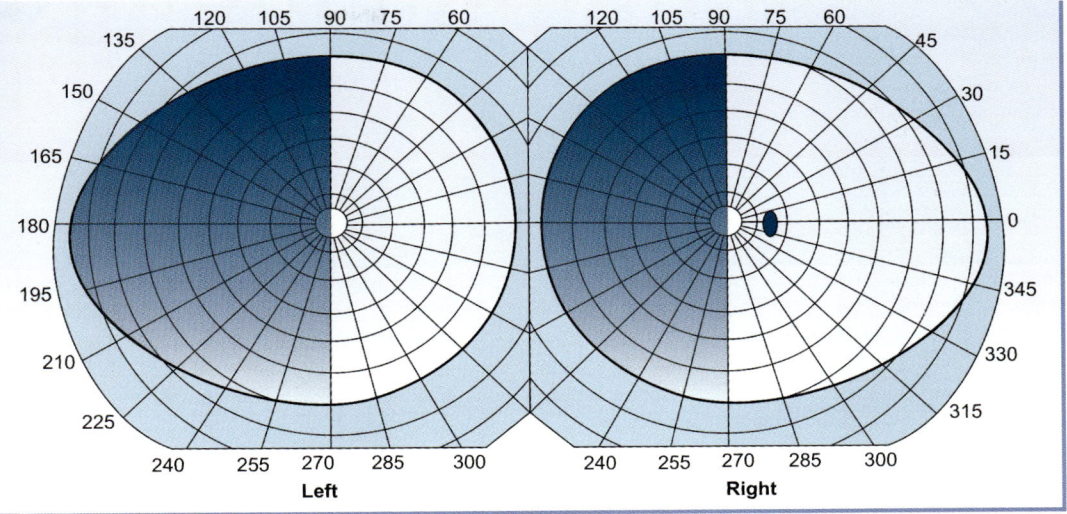

Fig. 9.10 *Homonymous hemianopia denser superiorly produced by extensively temporal lobe tumours.*

PARIETAL LOBE LESIONS

Visual field defects

- *Inferior quadrantic hemianopia, i.e. pie-in-the-floor* (Figs 9.1[8] and 9.11) occurs initially in the lesions of parietal lobe (containing superior fibres of optic radiations).
- *Homonymous hemianopia denser inferiorly* (Fig. 9.12) occurs with further extension of lesion.

Neuro-ophthalmic features

Neuro-ophthalmic features seen in parietal lobe tumours include:

- *Spasticity of conjugate gaze,* i.e. tonic deviation of eyes to the side opposite a parietal lesion during an attempt to produce Bell's phenomenon (i.e. during forced lid closure).
- *Asymmetric optokinetic nystagmus,* i.e. evoked nystagmus is dampened when stimuli are moved in the direction of the involved parietal lobe.

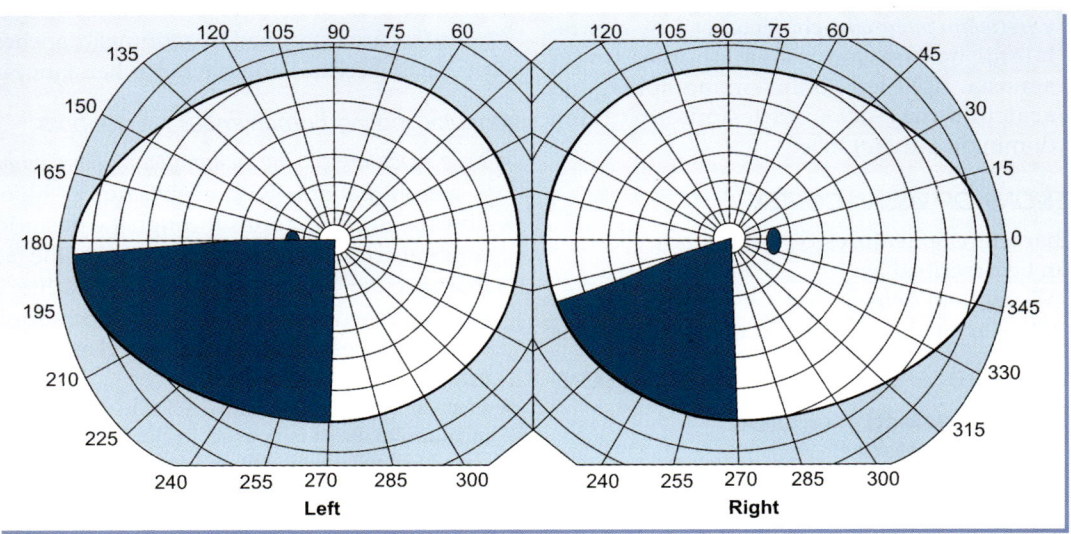

Fig. 9.11 *Inferior quadrantic hemianopia (pie-in-the-floor) produced by parietal lobe lesions involving superior fibres of optic radiations.*

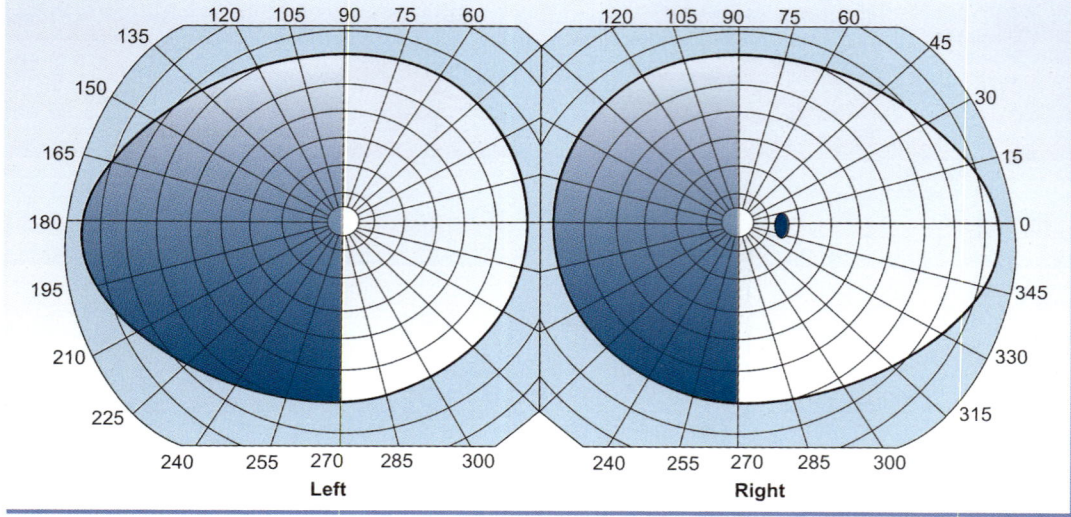

Fig. 9.12 *Homonymous hemianopia denser inferiorly produced by temporal lobe lesions.*

- *Deficient pursuit eye movements* to the side of lesion.

Neurologic features

Neurologic features associated with parietal lobe tumour include:

- Impairment of complex sensory integration
- Neglect of contralateral space and inattention may occur in patients with non-dominant parietal lobe lesions.
- *Gerstmann syndrome* characterised by contralateral homonymous hemianopia, finger agnosia, right-left confusion, agraphia, and acalculia may occur in lesions involving dominant parietal lobe.

LESIONS OF VISUAL CORTEX

Characteristic features of visual cortex lesions can be described as:

- Visual field defects, and
- Other manifestations of occipital lobe lesions

VISUAL FIELD DEFECTS IN OCCIPITAL LOBE LESIONS

Visual field defects in unilateral occipital lobe lesions

Different types of visual field defects occurring in occipital lobe lesions with their characteristic features and common causes are described below.

Central homonymous hemianopia

Central homonymous hemianopia is characterised by only loss of central halves of field of vision. Such field defects are exquisitely congruous (Figs 9.1[11] and 9.13).

Causes include:

- Lesions affecting tip of occipital lobe
- In generalised hypoperfusion state (e.g. intra-operative hypotension), the first area of the visual cortex to be affected is the watershed zone (i.e. area supplied by terminal branches) producing central homonymous hemianopia.

Macular sparing homonymous hemianopia

- *True macular sparing homonymous hemianopia* is seen in patients with obstruction of blood flow to the visual cortex through the posterior cerebral artery. This occurs because of the fact that macular area of the visual cortex lies in the watershed area, i.e. has dual blood supply from branches of posterior cerebral as well as middle cerebral arteries.
- *Macular sparing is labelled* when at least 5 degrees of macular field is spared in both eyes on the side of hemianopia (Figs 9.1[10] and 9.14).
- *False macular sparing* may sometimes be produced by an artefact of testing as a result of shifting fixation. The patient may shift fixation, anticipating the appearance of the test object.

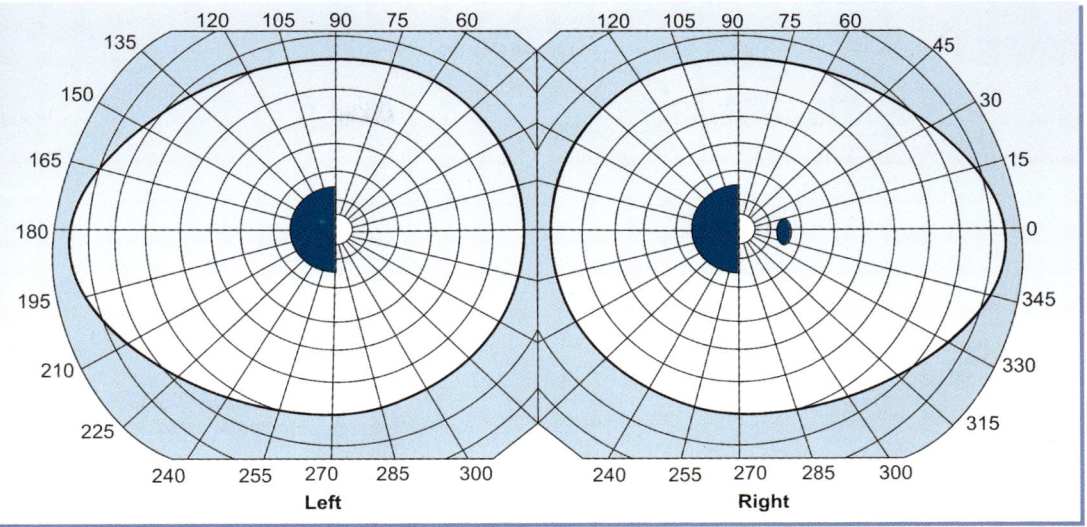

Fig. 9.13 *Central homonymous hemianopia seen in occipital lobe lesions.*

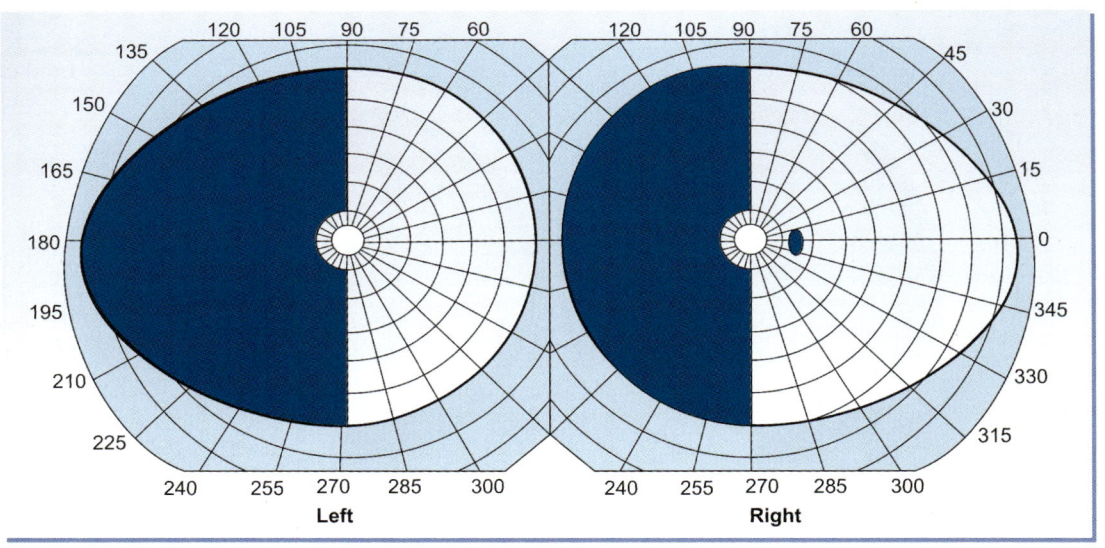

Fig. 9.14 *Macular sparing homonymous hemianopia.*

Homonymous hemianopia with sparing of temporal crescent

- *Temporal crescent of visual field* in each eye is produced by the nasal crescent of retina for which there is no corresponding visual points in the other eye (Fig. 9.15).
- *Homonymous hemianopia with sparing of temporal crescent* (Fig. 9.16) is characteristic of occipital lobe lesion since this is the only site

where the temporal crescent field fibres are separated from the other nasal retina fibres of the contralateral eye. Because of sparing of temporal crescent of field in one eye the homonymous hemianopia appears incongruous.

Temporal crescent field defect

- Temporal crescent field defect (Fig. 9.17) is produced due to lesion involving that area of

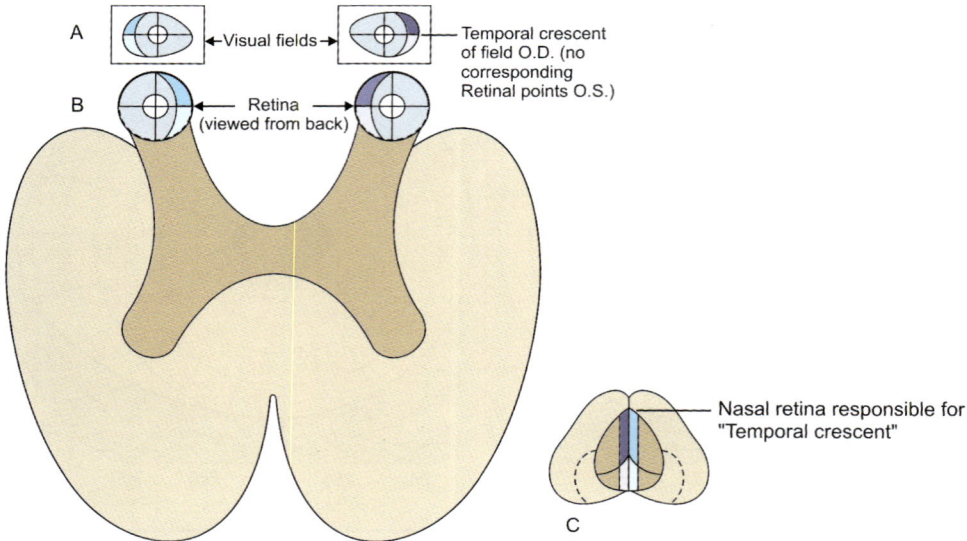

Fig. 9.15 *Temporal crescent of visual field (A), corresponding to crescent of extreme nasal retina (B), is projected to contralateral visual cortex (Anterior mesial surface) (C).*

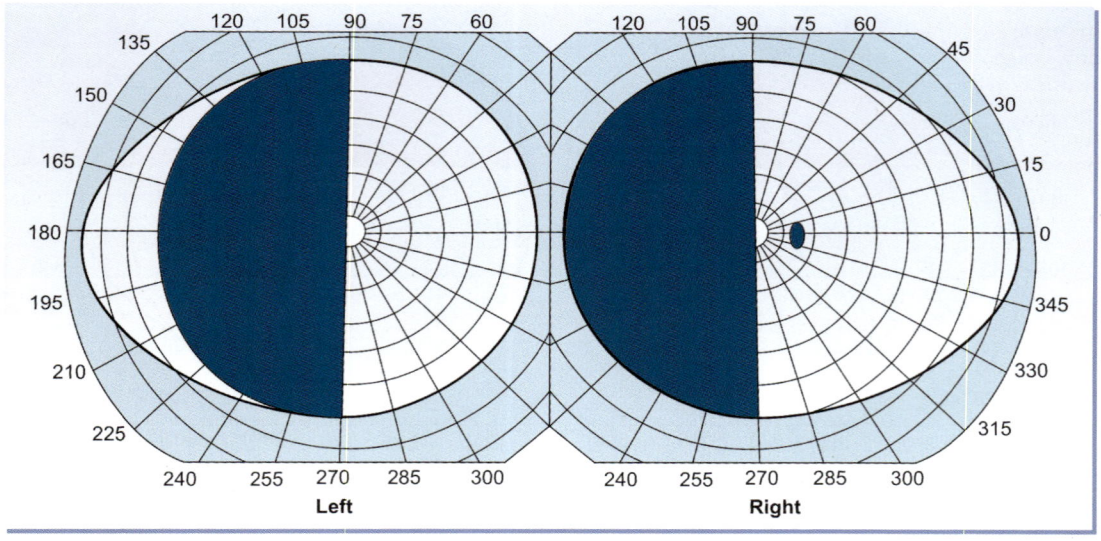

Fig. 9.16 *Left homonymous hemianopia with sparing of the temporal crescent of the left eye.*

visual cortex (Fig. 9.15C) which represents the nasal crescent of retina (Fig. 9.15B) for which there is no corresponding visual points on the contralateral retina. Therefore, this is the only area of the visual cortex which produces unilateral visual field defect. Representation of the temporal crescent occupies less than 10% of total surface area of striate cortex.

- Temporal crescent field defect (Fig. 9.17) has its widest extent in the horizontal meridian and extends from 60 to 90 degrees. It is important to note that standard automated static perimetry programs fail to detect this field defect because it is further in the peripheral field than these tests measure.

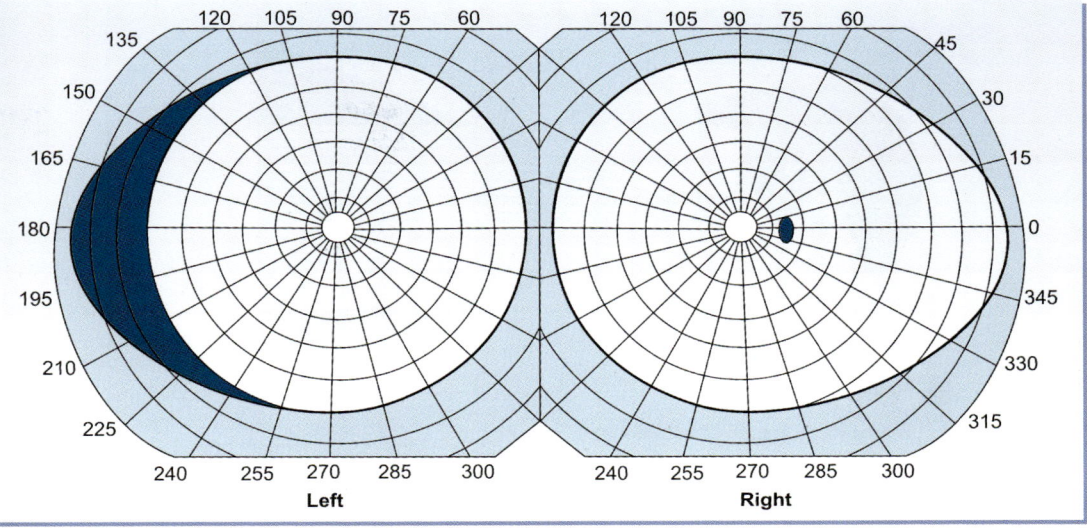

Fig. 9.17 *Temporal crescent field defect.*

VISUAL FIELD DEFECTS IN BILATERAL OCCIPITAL LOBE LESIONS

In bilateral occipital lobe lesions following field defects may occur:

1. *Bilateral homonymous hemianopia with macular sparing* produces a picture of ring scotoma (Fig. 9.18). Such field defects need to be differentiated from:

• Glaucomatous field defect
• Hysterical and malingering defects

• Field defects due to optic disc drusen
• Field defects in post-papilledemic optic atrophy
• Field defects in retinitis pigmentosa

Note. In all the above conditions except hysteria and malingering the typical fundus picture helps in making the diagnosis. Differentiation from hysteria and malingering requires visual field testing at the tangent screen at 1 and 2 metres (Fig. 9.19).

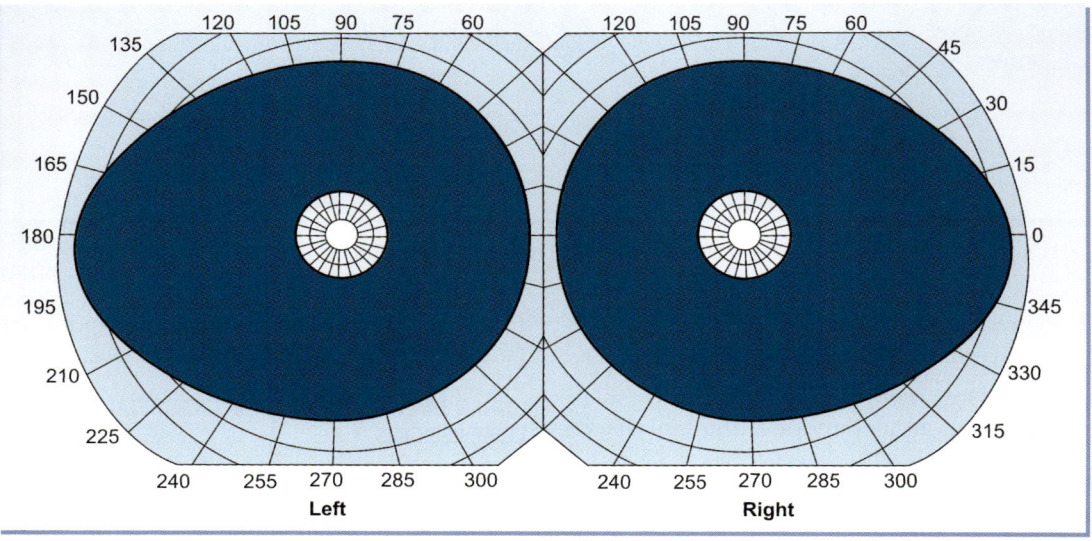

Fig. 9.18 *Bilateral homonymous hemianopia producing a picture of ring scotoma.*

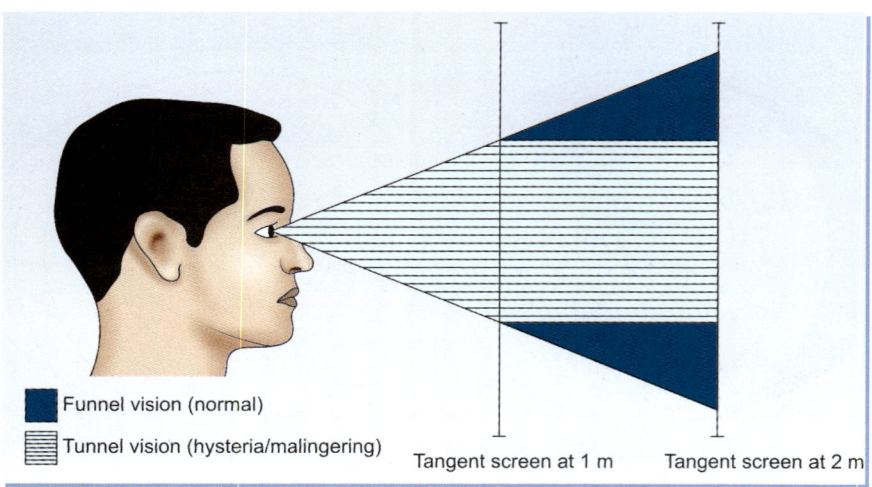

Funnel vision (normal)

Tunnel vision (hysteria/malingering)

Tangent screen at 1 m   Tangent screen at 2 m

Fig. 9.19 *Normal funnel vision versus tunnel vision seen in hysteria/malingering depicted on tangent screen at 1 and 2 meters.*

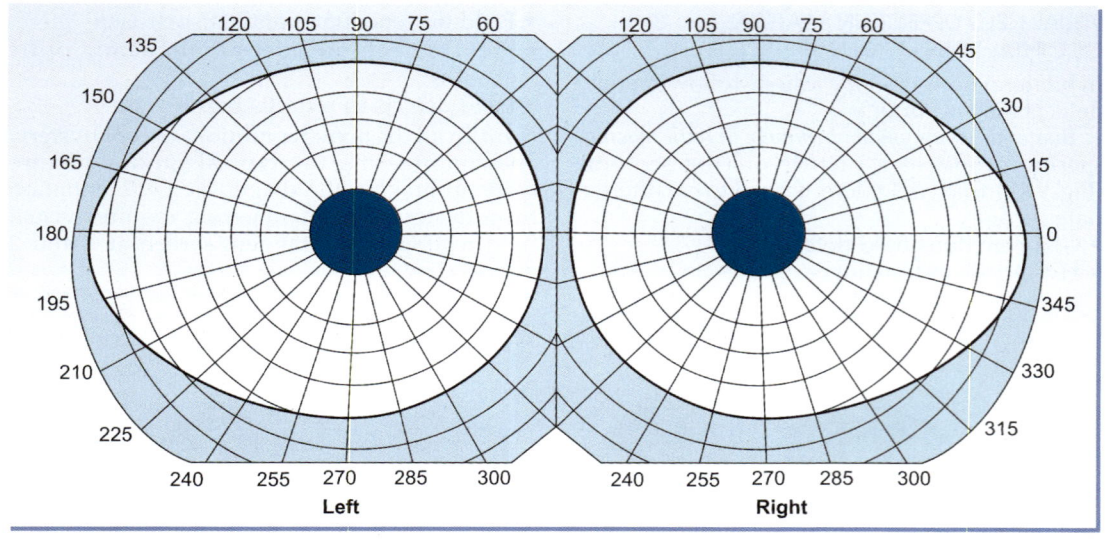

Left   Right

Fig. 9.20 *Bilateral central homonymous hemianopia.*

2. *Bilateral central homonymous hemianopia* presents like bilateral central scotoma (Fig. 9.20).

3. *Bilateral homonymous quadrantic defects* (usually inferior) present as inferior altitudinal defects (Fig. 9.21).

4. *Checker board field defects* or *crossed quadrantopia* (Fig. 9.22) is produced by lesions which affect the superior occipital lobe above the calcarine fissure on one side and the inferior occipital lobe below the calcarine fissure on the other side.

OTHER MANIFESTATIONS OF OCCIPITAL LOBE LESIONS

Manifestations of occipital lobe lesions other than the visual field defects include:

1. **Cortical blindness** can occur in bilateral occipital lobe lesions (*see* page 210).

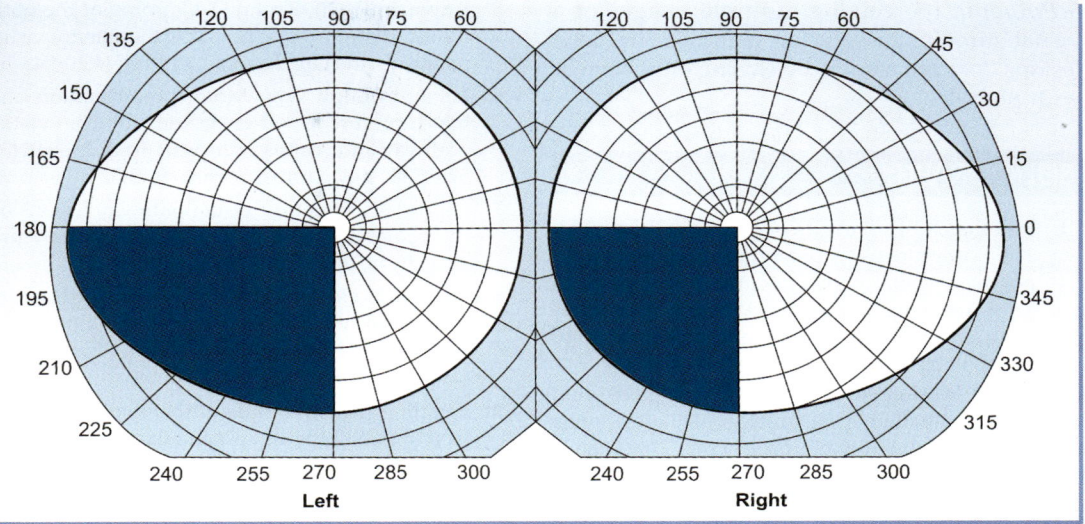

Fig. 9.21 *Bilateral homonymous quadrantic defects.*

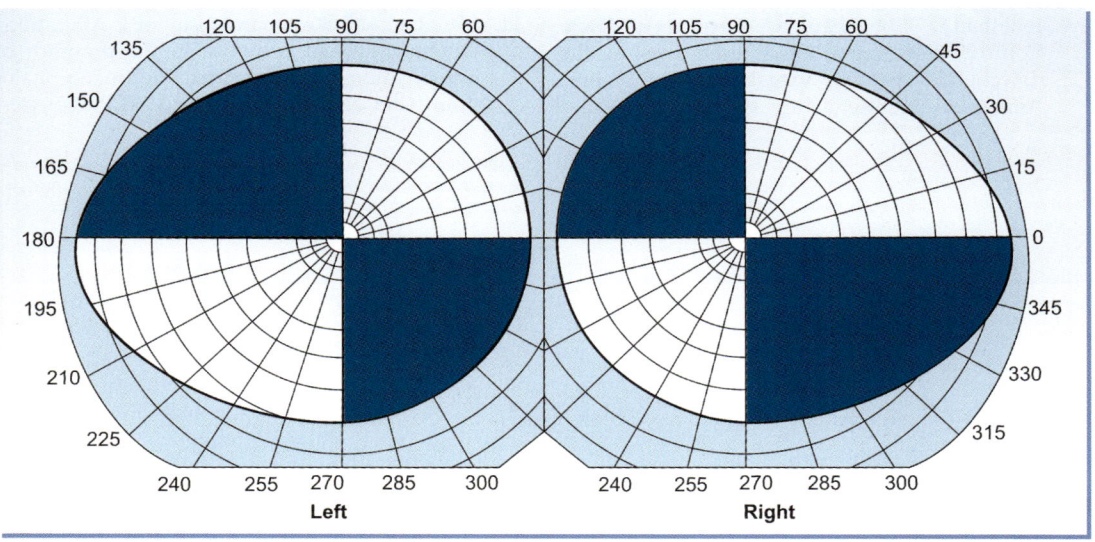

Fig. 9.22 *Checker-board field defects (crossed quadrantopia).*

2. *Dyschromatopsia.* Bilateral occipital lobe lesions can also produce acquired colour vision defects, i.e. dyschromatopsia (*see* page 194).

3. *Visual hallucinations* seen in occipital lobe lesions are unformed, while hallucinations seen in temporal lobe lesions are formed (*see* page 208).

4. *Palinopsia* refers to persistent or recurrent perception of a visual image after removal of the stimulus.

- It is typically seen following parietal or occipital lobe lesions in the non-dominant hemisphere.
- Palinopsia is usually associated with homonymous hemianopia.

5. *Visual allesthesia* is characterised by transposition of visual stimuli from one hemifield to another. It is known to occur most commonly with parieto-occipital lesions.

6. *Polyopia* (perceiving multiple images of a visual stimulus) associated with occipital lobe lesions does not resolve by closing either eye or with pinhole.

BIBLIOGRAPHY

1. Blumhardt LD, Barrett G, Kiss A, Halliday AM: The pattern-evoked potential in lesions of the posterior visual pathways, Annals of the New York Academy of Sciences. Aerosols: Anthropogenic and Natural, Sources and Transport May 1980;338:265–89.

2. Blythe IM, Kennard C, Ruddock KH. Residual vision in patients with retrogeniculate lesions of the visual pathways, Brain 1987; 110 (4):887–905.doi: 10.1093/brain/110.4.887.

3. Garey LJ, Jones EG, and Powell TP: Interrelationships of striate and extrastriate cortex with the primary relay sites of the visual pathway. J Neurol Neurosurg Psychiatry. April 1968;31(2):135–57.

4. Jonathan D. Trobe, Paulo C. Acosta. et al. Trick: Confrontation visual field techniques in the detection of anterior visual pathway lesions, Annals of Neurology July 1981;10(1):28–34.

5. Kupersmith MJ, Krohn D. Cupping of the optic disc with compressive lesions of the anterior visual pathway, Ann Ophthalmol. Oct 1984; 16(10):948–53.

6. Lehman Ralph AW. Motor co-ordination and hand preference after lesions of the visual pathway and corpus callosum, Brain 1968;91(3):525–538. doi: 10.1093/brain/91.3.525.

7. Lepore FE: Effects of visual pathway lesions on the visual aura of migraine, Cephalalgia April 2009;29:4430–35.

8. Regan D, Heron JR. Clinical investigation of lesions of visual pathway: a new objective technique. J Neurol Neurosurg Psychiatry. October 1969;32(5):479–83.

9. Spalding JMK. Wounds of the visual pathway, J Neurol Neurosurg Psychiatry. August 1952; 15(3):169–83.

10. Vaphiades MS, Celesia GG, Brigell MG. Positive spontaneous visual phenomena limited to the hemianopic field in lesions of central visual pathways, Neurology August 1996; 47(2): 408–17.

11. Vaughan HG, Katzman R, Taylor J. Alterations of visual-evoked response in the presence of homonymous visual defects. Electroencephalogram Clin Neurophysiol Oct 1963;15:737–46.

10 | ANATOMY AND BLOOD SUPPLY OF OPTIC NERVE

AK Khurana, Aruj K Khurana, Bhawna Khurana

ANATOMY OF OPTIC NERVE
Parts of the Optic Nerve
- Intraocular part
- Intraorbital part
- Intracanalicular part
- Intracranical part

Meningeal Sheaths of Optic Nerve
- Dura mater
- Arachnoid layer
- Pia mater

BLOOD SUPPLY OF OPTIC NERVE
Arterial Supply
- Blood supply of intraocular part
- Blood supply of intraorbital part
- Blood supply of intracanalicular part
- Blood supply of intracranial part

Venous Drainage
- Venous drainage of orbital part
- Venous drainage of intracranial part

ANATOMY OF OPTIC NERVE

Each optic nerve (second cranial nerve) starts from the optic disc and extends up to the optic chiasma, where the two nerves meet (Fig. 10.1). It is the backward continuation of the nerve fiber layer of the retina which consists of the axons originating from the ganglion cells. It also contains the afferent fibers of light reflex and some centrifugal fibers.

Morphologically and embryologically, the optic nerve is comparable to a sensory tract (white matter) of the brain, because of the following points:

- The optic nerve is an outgrowth of the brain.
- Unlike peripheral nerves, it is not covered by neurilemma (so it does not regenerate when cut).
- The fibers of optic nerve numbering about a million, are very fine, 2–10 μm in diameter as compared to 20 μm in sensory nerves.
- The optic nerve is surrounded by meninges.
- Both the primary and secondary sensory neurons are in the retina.

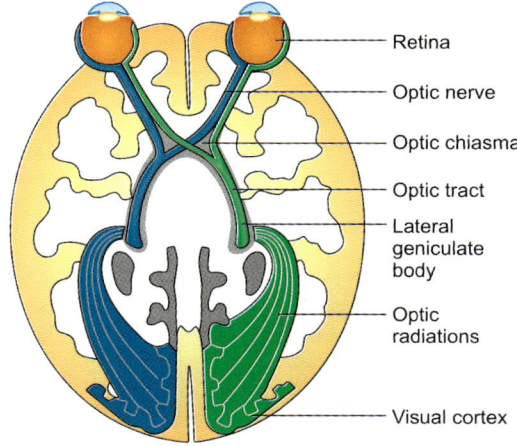

Fig. 10.1 *Visual pathways.*

PARTS OF THE OPTIC NERVE

The optic nerve is about 47–50 mm in length and can be divided into 4 parts: intraocular (1 mm), intraorbital (30 mm), intracanalicular (6–9 mm) and intracranial (10 mm).

129

INTRAOCULAR PART

This part passes through sclera, choroid and finally appears in the eye as optic disc (Fig. 10.2). The intraocular portion of the optic nerve head has an average diameter of 1.5 mm, which expands to approximately 3 mm just behind the sclera, where the neurons acquire a myelin sheath. The optic nerve head may be arbitrarily divided into the following four portions from anterior to posterior.

1. Surface nerve fiber layer

This part is essentially composed of axonal bundles, i.e. nerve fibers of the retina (94%) which converge on the optic disc and astrocytes (5%). The optic disc is covered by a thin layer of astrocytes, the internal limiting membrane of Elschnig, which separates it from the vitreous and is continuous with the internal limiting membrane of the retina. When the central portion of this membrane is thickened, it is referred to as the central meniscus of Kuhnt.

All the layers of retina, apart from nerve fiber layer, near the optic nerve, are separated from it by a partial rim of glial tissue called the intermediate tissue of Kuhnt.

2. Prelaminar region

The predominant structures at this level are neurons and a significantly increased quantity of astroglial tissue. The border tissue of Jcoby (a cuff of astrocytes) separates the nerve from the choroid.

3. Lamina cribrosa

It is a fibrillar sieve-like structure made up of fenestrated sheets of scleral connective tissue lined by glial tissue. It bridges the posterior scleral foramina or the scleral canal. The bundles of optic nerve fibers leave the eye through these fenestrations. A rim of collagenous connective tissue with some admixture of glial cells which intervenes between the choroid and sclera and optic nerve fibers is called the border tissue of Elschnig. The lamina cribrosa gets its rich blood supply from the circle of Zinn.

4. Retrolaminar region

This area is characterised by a decrease in astrocytes and the acquisition of myelin that is supplied by oligodendrocytes. The addition of myelin sheath nearly doubles the diameter of the optic nerve (from 1.5 to 3.0 mm) as it passes through the sclera. The axonal bundles are surrounded by connective tissue septa. The posterior extent of the retrolaminar region is not clearly defined.

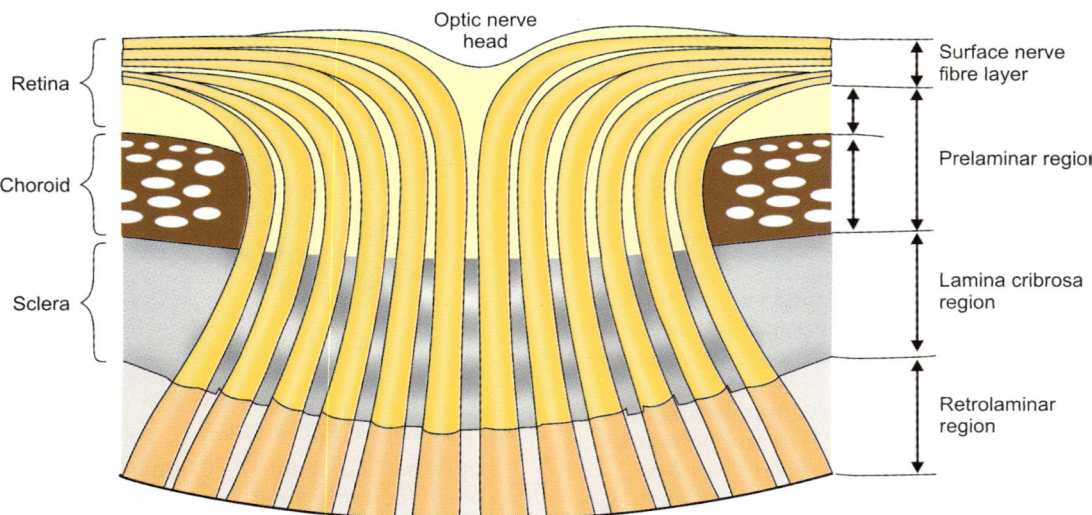

Fig. 10.2 *Schematic drawing of optic nerve head.*

INTRAORBITAL PART

Intraorbital part of the optic nerve extends from back of the eyeball to the optic foramina. This part is slightly sinuous to give play for the eye movements. Important relations of this part are as follows (Fig. 10.3):

- The optic nerve in the orbit is covered by dura, arachnoid and pia. The pial sheath contains capillaries and sends septa to divide the nerve into fasciculi. The subarachnoid space containing cerebrospinal fluid ends blindly at the sclera but continues intracranially.
- The central retinal artery along with the accompanying vein crosses the subarachnoid space to enter the nerve on its inferomedial aspect about 10 mm from the eyeball.
- Posteriorly, near the optic foramina, the optic nerve is closely surrounded by the annulus of Zinn and the origin of the four rectus muscles (Fig. 10.4). Some fibers of the superior rectus muscle and medial rectus muscle are adherent to its sheath here and account for the painful ocular movements seen in retrobulbar neuritis.
- Anteriorly, the nerve is separated from the extraocular muscles by the orbital fat.
- The long and short ciliary nerves and arteries surround the optic nerve before these enter the eyeball.
- Between the optic nerve and lateral rectus muscle are situated the ciliary ganglion, divisions of the oculomotor nerve, the nasociliary nerve, the sympathetic and the abducent nerve (Fig. 10.3).

The ophthalmic artery, superior ophthalmic vein and the nasociliary nerve cross the optic nerve superiorly from the lateral to medial side.

INTRACANALICULAR PART

- This part (Fig. 10.4) is closely related to the ophthalmic artery which crosses the nerve inferiorly from medial to lateral side in the dural sheath and then leaves the sheath at the orbital end of the canal.
- Sphenoid and posterior ethmoidal sinuses lie medial to it and are separated by a thin bony lamina. This relation accounts for retrobulbar neuritis following infection of the sinuses.

INTRACRANIAL PART

- This part of the optic nerve, about 1 cm in length, lies above the cavernous sinus and converges with its fellow (over the diaphragma sellae) to form the chiasma.
- It is ensheathed in pia mater, but receives arachnoid and dural sheaths at the point of its entry into the optic canal.
- The internal carotid artery runs, at first below and then lateral to it. The ophthalmic artery arises from the internal carotid artery below the optic nerve at about its middle.

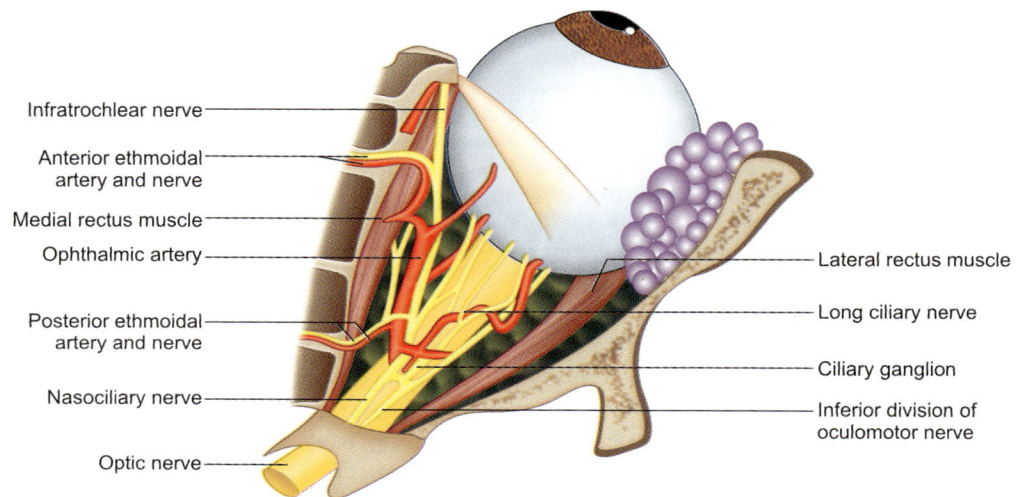

Fig. 10.3 *Relations of intraorbital part of optic nerve.*

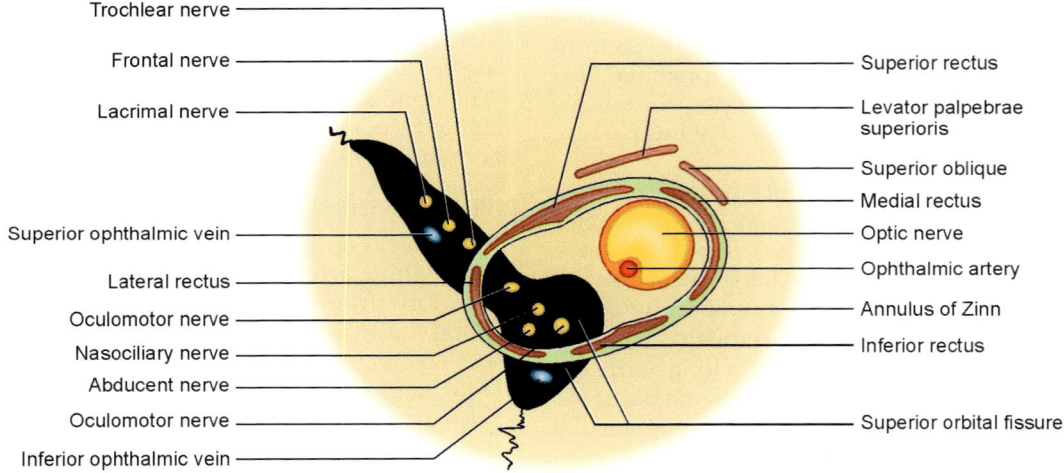

Fig. 10.4 *Relations of intracanalicular part of optic nerve.*

• The anterior perforated substance, the medial root of the olfactory tract and the anterior cerebral artery lie above this part of the optic nerve.

MENINGEAL SHEATHS OF OPTIC NERVE

• The intracranial part of the optic nerve is covered by pia only, while the intracanalicular and intraorbital parts of the nerve have three coverings: the pia, arachnoid and dura.

• The meningeal sheaths and the subarachnoid and the subdural spaces around the optic nerve are continuous with those of the brain.

• Anteriorly, all the three meningeal sheaths terminate by becoming continuous with the sclera.

• *Dura mater.* At the apex of the orbit, the dura splits into layers, the outer is continuous with the periosteum of the orbit while the inner forms the dural sheath of the optic nerve.

• *Arachnoid layer* is connected to pia with numerous trabeculae. These connections have led to the concept of a compound *pia-arachnoid meninx*, containing cerebrospinal fluid.

• *Pia mater* sends numerous septa into the optic nerve, dividing its fibers into fascicles. In fact, these septa are admixture of pia and glial tissue, leading to the term 'pia-glia'.

BLOOD SUPPLY OF THE OPTIC NERVE

ARTERIAL SUPPLY

1. Blood supply of intraocular part (optic nerve head) (Fig. 10.5)

a. *The surface nerve fiber layer* is mainly supplied by the capillaries derived from the retinal arterioles, which anastomose with vessels of the prelaminar region. Occasionally a ciliary-derived vessel from the prelaminar region may enlarge to form the cilioretinal artery.

b. *The prelaminar region* is supplied by vessels of ciliary region. There is lack of agreement as to whether these vessels are derived primarily from the peripapillary choroidal system or from separate branches of the short posterior ciliary arteries.

c. *The lamina cribrosa region* is also supplied by the ciliary vessels which are derived from the short posterior ciliary arteries and arterial circle of Zinn-Haller.

d. *The retrolaminar region* is supplied by both the ciliary and retinal circulation with the former coming from recurrent pial vessels. The central retinal artery provides centripetal branches from the pial plexus and also centrifugal branches.

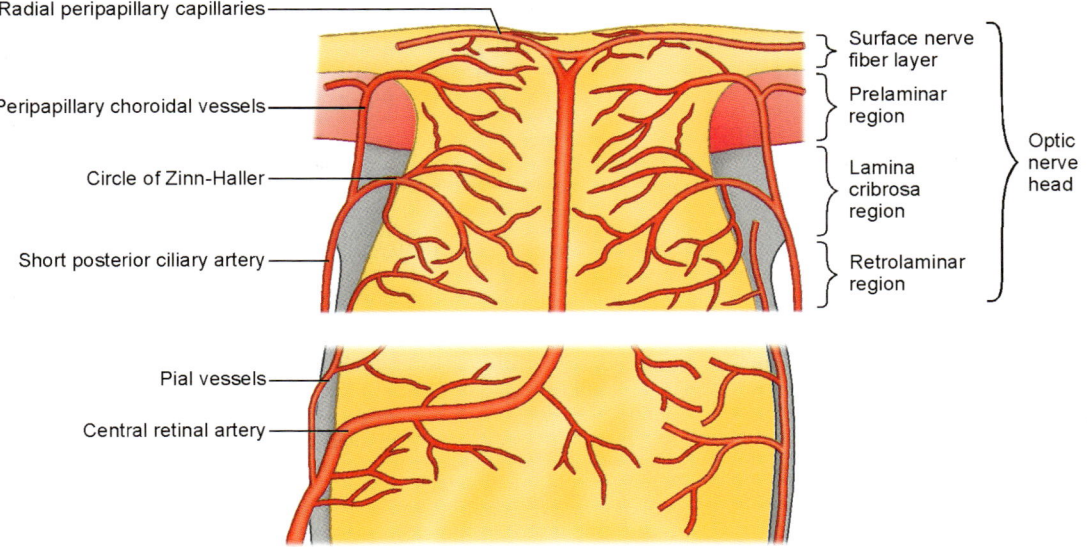

Radial peripapillary capillaries

Peripapillary choroidal vessels

Circle of Zinn-Haller

Short posterior ciliary artery

Pial vessels

Central retinal artery

Surface nerve fiber layer

Prelaminar region

Lamina cribrosa region

Retrolaminar region

Optic nerve head

Fig. 10.5 *Blood supply of the optic nerve head.*

2. Blood supply of the intraorbital part (Fig. 10.6)

The intraorbital part of optic nerve is supplied by two systems of vessels—a periaxial and an axial:

a. *The periaxial system* of vessels supplying this part of optic nerve is derived from the six branches of internal carotid artery namely: ophthalmic artery, long posterior ciliary

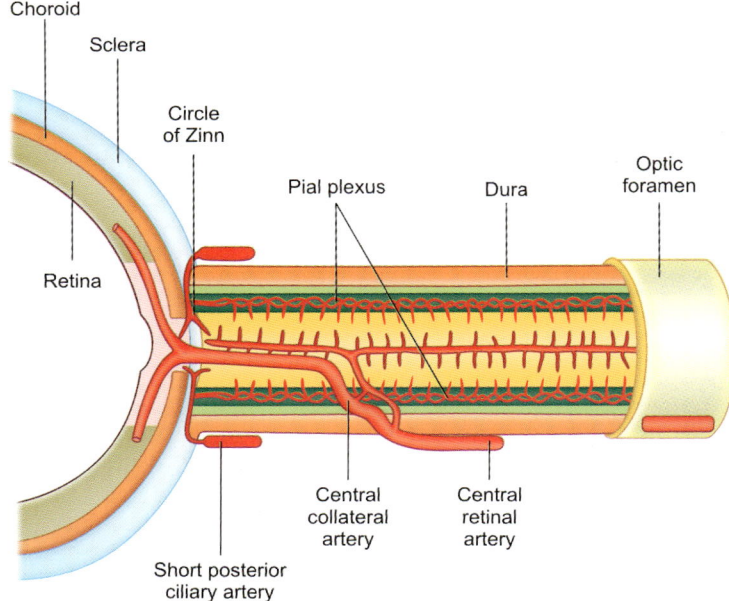

Choroid

Sclera

Circle of Zinn

Pial plexus

Dura

Optic foramen

Retina

Short posterior ciliary artery

Central collateral artery

Central retinal artery

Fig. 10.6 *Blood supply of the optic nerve.*

arteries, short posterior ciliary arteries, lacrimal artery and central artery of retina before it enters the optic nerve and circle of Zinn.

b. *The axial system of vessels* supplying the axial part of the optic nerve is derived from (i) the intraneural branches of the central retinal artery, (ii) central collateral arteries which come off from the central retinal artery before it pierces the nerve, and (iii) central artery of optic nerve.

The capillary network for the optic nerve is derived from both the systems. Anastomosis between the two systems has also been demonstrated.

3. Blood supply of the intracanalicular part

The nerve within the optic canal is supplied only by the periaxial system of vessels. The pial plexus in this part is fed mainly by branches from the ophthalmic artery.

4. Blood supply of the intracranial part

This part of the optic nerve is exclusively supplied from the periaxial system of vessels. The pial plexus here is contributed by four sources: (i) branches from the internal carotid artery either directly or through the recurrent branch of anterior superior hypophyseal artery (supply the inferior aspect of the optic nerve containing lower retinal fibers), (ii) branches from anterior cerebral artery (supply the superior aspect of the optic nerve containing upper retinal fibers), (iii) small recurrent branches from the ophthalmic artery, and (iv) the twigs from the anterior communicating artery.

VENOUS DRAINAGE

The venous return in the optic nerve head is primarily by the central retinal vein.

Venous drainage of orbital part

The orbital part is drained by peripheral pial plexus and also by central retinal vein in the distal part.

Venous drainage of intracranial part

The intracranial part is drained by the pial plexus which ends in anterior cerebral and basal vein.

BIBLIOGRAPHY

1. Kolb H, Linberg KA, Fisher SK. Neurons of the human retina: Golgi study. J. Comp. Neural, 1992;318:147.
2. Khurana AK, Khurana Indu. Anatomy and Physiology of Eye, 2nd edition, CBS Publishers and Distributors, 2006;152–5.
3. Tripathi RC, Tripathi BJ. Anatomy of the human eye, orbit and adnexa. In 'The Eye', 3rd edition (Ed, H. Davson), Academic Press, London 1984; 145:40.

11

CONGENITAL ANOMALIES OF OPTIC NERVE

Ashwin Gupta, Ramesh Kekunnaya

INTRODUCTION

COMMON CONGENITAL ANOMALIES OF OPTIC NERVE
- Optic nerve hypoplasia (ONH)
- Optic disc coloboma
- Morning glory disc anomaly

- Peripapillary staphyloma
- Optic disc pit
- Megalopapilla
- Congenital tilted disc syndrome
- Optic disc drusen
- Myelinated fibers
- Congenital optic disc pigmentation

INTRODUCTION

Congenital anomalies of the optic nerve are rare. Evaluation of patients with these abnormalities is challenging and needs a detailed understanding of the disease—etiology, pathophysiology, other associations and any further evaluation if required. Accurate diagnosis and management of these conditions is of utmost importance.

These disorders can be both unilateral and bilateral. Children with unilateral involvement usually present with sensory strabismus while those with bilateral affection present with poor vision and nystagmus. Color vision is usually normal in children with congenital abnormality of optic disc compared to those with acquired optic disc abnormalities. Many of these disorders have associated neurologic and systemic abnormalities. Fundus evaluation, neuro-imaging and genetic testing are helpful in the further management. Thus, ophthalmologist plays a crucial role in recognizing patients who require further evaluation.

COMMON CONGENITAL ANOMALIES OF OPTIC NERVE

OPTIC NERVE HYPOPLASIA (ONH)

It is the most common congenital optic nerve anomaly encountered in clinical practice. Ophthalmoscopically, it appears as a small optic nerve head with the distance between the disc and fovea exceeding 3 disc diameters. It may appear gray or pale in color and is often surrounded by a yellowish mottled peripapillary halo, bordered by a ring of increased or decreased pigmentation, i.e. the double ring sign (Fig. 11.1). Anomalous retinal vessel morphology may also be associated (Fig. 11.2). It is unilateral in 15–25% of the patients.

Visual acuity varies from 20/20 to perception of light. There may be associated nerve fiber bundle defects. Astigmatism is known to be associated with ONH. Other signs include relative afferent pupillary defect, visual field loss, abnormal VEP and ERG.

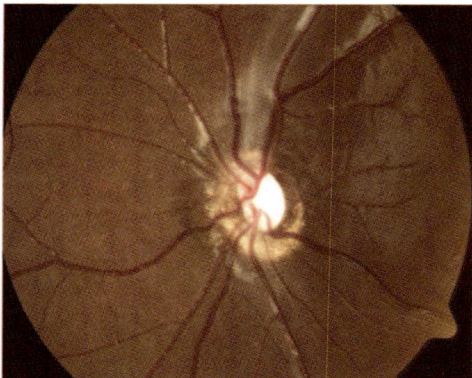

Fig. 11.1 *ONH with double ring sign.*

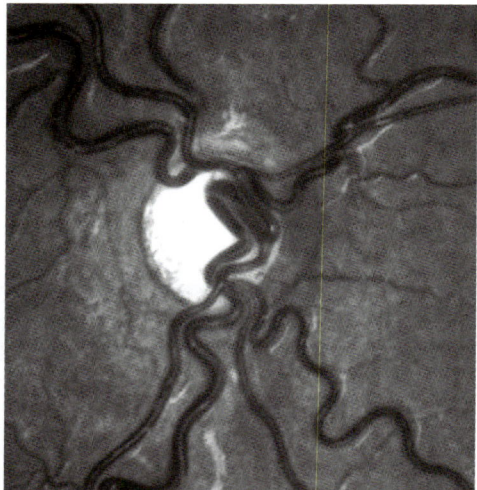

Fig. 11.2 *ONH with abnormal retinal vessels.*

- *Supranormal regression of axons* in the optic nerve is thought to be the principal mechanism of development of ONH. Most cases occur sporadically.
- *Risk factors* for ONH include young maternal age, first parity, maternal smoking, preterm birth and its complications, fetal alcohol syndrome, maternal diabetes mellitus, anticonvulsant therapy, valproic toxicity, Aicardi syndrome, CHARGE syndrome, Phace (S) syndrome and other chromosomal abnormalities. Periventricular leucomalacia (PVL) is associated with ONH in patients with early onset pathology.

Clinical Features

- *A pathognomonic superior segmental hypoplasia* with an inferior visual field defect occurs in some children of insulin-dependent diabetic mothers. OCT and HRT aid in the diagnosis of these segmental abnormalities.

Associated Features

Structural brain malformation like absence of septum pellucidum, agenesis of corpus callosum (Fig. 11.4), porencephaly, schizencephaly, arachnoid cysts, encephalomalacia and leukomalacia. Septo optic dysplasia (de Morsier syndrome) comprises ONH, pituitary gland hypoplasia and midline facial abnormalities are near in up to 60% of patients.

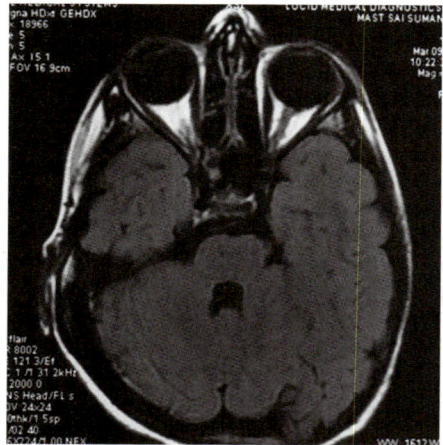

Fig. 11.3 *Optic disc hypoplasia.*

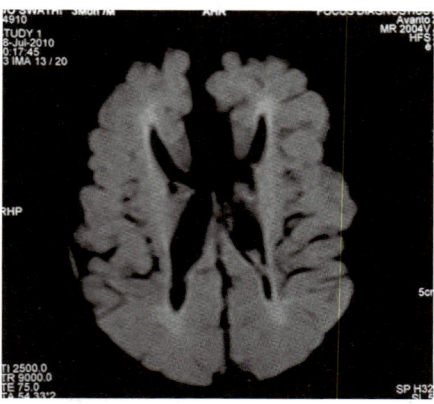

Fig. 11.4 *Absent corpus callosum.*

- *Endocrinal abnormalities* are known to be associated with ONH. MRI of the neurohypophysis predicts the risk of congenital hypopituitarism in association with ONH.
- *Developmental delay* is another known association of ONH.

Management

Appropriate refractive correction and amblyopia therapy in unilateral cases forms the mainstay of ophthalmological management. Pituitary hormone replacement in children with endocrinal deficiency helps in amelioration of complications of hypopituitarism.

OPTIC DISC COLOBOMA

Optic nerve colobomas are congenital excavations of the optic disc that typically involve the inferior portion of the nerve and can extend inferiorly into the adjacent retina and choroid. It is usually associated with a larger optic disc. Inferior neuroretinal rim is thin or absent while the superior neuroretinal rim is usually spared (Fig. 11.5). It may occur unilaterally or bilaterally. Visual loss is variable in these cases depending upon the extent of involvement of papillomacular bundle. It may co-exist with iris colobomas, microphthalmia, microcornea, lens notching, orbital cysts and retinal venous malformations.

Patients have an increased risk of serous retinal detachment due to intercommunication between vitreous cavity, subarachnoid and subretinal spaces. They also have higher chances of macular hole and choroidal neovascular membrane.

These colobomas result from incomplete closure of the proximal part of optic fissure. Most cases are sporadic and up to 20% of patients have an autosomal dominant inheritance pattern. It has been recently shown to be associated with PAX2 gene mutations as part of the renal-coloboma syndrome. Charge (coloboma, congenital heart disease, choanal atresia, mental retardation, genital hypoplasia and ear anomalies), Walker-Wardberg syndrome, Goltz focal dermal hypoplasia, Aicardi syndrome, Goldenhar syndrome and linear sebaceous naevus syndrome and Dandy-Walker malformation are some of the known multisystem associations.

Treatment may be required for the associated complications if any.

MORNING GLORY DISC ANOMALY

It is a congenital round optic disc anomaly with a central glial tuft and the retinal vessels exit in a radial fashion from the enlarged posterior scleral opening (Fig. 11.6). There is an associated peripapillary pigment. The term reflects the morphological similarity to the flower of the morning glory plant. It is usually unilateral. The visual loss is variable. Serous retinal detachments are seen in one-third of cases. Subretinal neovascularization is another known association.

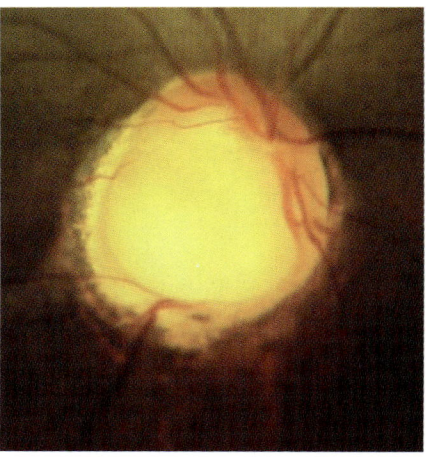

Fig. 11.5 *Optic disc coloboma.*

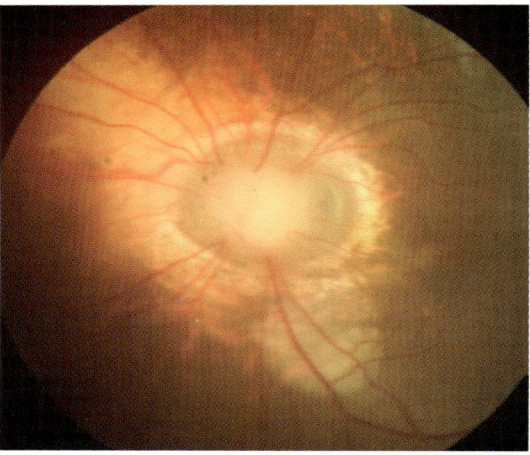

Fig. 11.6 *Morning glory disc.*

It is usually sporadic in nature. It is more common in females. Some hypotheses described by few authors are failure of the closure of foetal fissure and primary mesenchymal abnormality, dysgenesis of the terminal optic stalk and primary neuro-ectodermal dysgenesis.

The association of morning glory disc anomaly with the trans-sphenoidal form of basal encephalocele and panhypopituitarism is well established. Infants with morning glory disc anomaly should therefore be considered at increased risk of respiratory and endocrinological problems. Midfacial anomalies are common in this group of patients. Contractility of the posterior defect in these cases is thought to be due to presence of myofibroblasts in the papilla. Neuroimaging is usually recommended for patients with this anomaly.

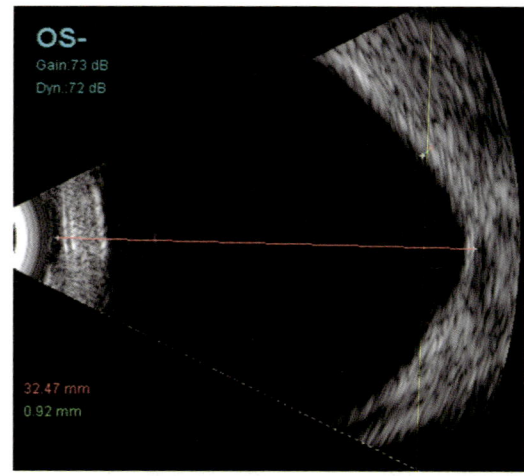

Fig. 11.8 *USG of peripapillary staphyloma.*

PERIPAPILLARY STAPHYLOMA

It appears as a deep, cup-shaped excavation with a relatively normal, well-formed optic disc with some temporal pallor but otherwise normal disc conformation and normal blood vessels (Figs 11.7 and 11.8). In this condition, the disc is seen at the bottom of the excavated defect and may appear normal or shows temporal pallor. Unlike the morning glory anomaly, there is no central glial tuft overlying the disc and the retinal vascular pattern remains normal. Visual acuity is usually markedly reduced.

The condition is sporadic and the etiology is unknown. It appears as a sequel to the disturbance of the scleral development at about 20 weeks of gestation. It is known to be associated with basal encephalocele. Other ocular associations may be high myopia, microphthalmia, congenital cataract, persistent pupillary membrane, retinal detachment.

OPTIC DISC PIT

An optic pit is an oval, gray white or yellowish depression in the optic disc (Fig. 11.9). Optic pits commonly involve the temporal optic disc, but may be situated in any sector. Although optic pits are typically unilateral, bilateral pits are seen in 15% of cases. The incidence is 1 in 11,000. Visual acuity is typically normal in the absence of sub-retinal fluid. Visual field defects are

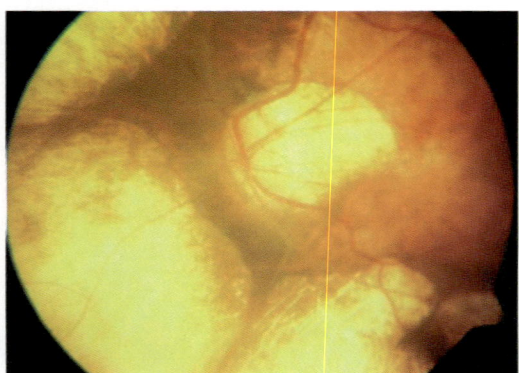

Fig. 11.7 *Peripapillary staphyloma.*

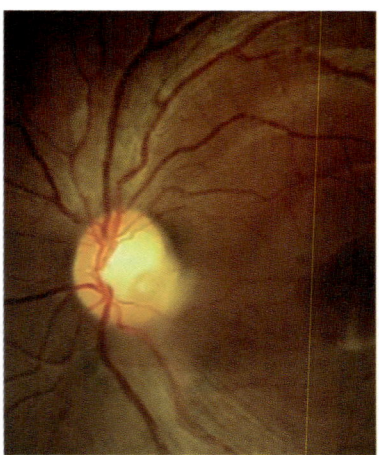

Fig. 11.9 *Optic disc pit.*

variable, the most common being paracentral arcuate scotoma connected to the enlarged blind spot. In affected discs the size of the disc is larger than the other normal disc. Patients with optic pit do not have additional CNS malformations.

In approximately half of the patients, serous retinal detachment may be seen in the 2nd or 3rd decade of life. A proposed mechanism for this detachment is fluid entering the optic disc pit and leading to schisis between inner and outer retina.

MEGALOPAPILLA

Megalopapilla is a condition in which the optic disc diameter is abnormally large (more than 2.1 mm). It is commonly associated with increased cup disc ratio. Visual acuity and visual fields are usually normal in this condition. There is no neurological association with this abnormality and thus neuroimaging is unwarranted.

CONGENITAL TILTED DISC SYNDROME

It consists of inferonasal rotation of the optic disc, usually with a contiguous inferonasal crescent (conus), thinning or atrophy of the RPE and choroid, posterior staphyloma of the affected area, and situs inversus of the retinal vessels (Fig. 11.10).

Visual sequelae described with tilted optic discs include myopia, astigmatism, visual field loss, deficient color vision and retinal abnormalities. The anomalous optic disc appearance is secondary to a posterior ectasia of the inferonasal fundus and the optic disc.

OPTIC DISC DRUSEN

Buried disc drusen is the most common cause of pseudopapilledema in children. They consist of calcified, acellular concretions within the substance of the optic nerve head (Fig. 11.11) and are often associated with visual field defects. Surface drusens are usually yellow and can be translucent or reflective. Optic disc drusen are associated with retinal hemorrhages, subretinal hemorrhages, and peripapillary CNV.

The current theory for the pathogenesis of optic disc drusen states that an abnormally narrow aperture of the scleral canal leads to axonal crowding and resultant slow degeneration of axons over years. Drusens are thought to be byproducts of degenerate axons.

The prevalence of optic disc drusen ranges from 0.34 to 2.0% (US), although it is rare in black populations. Family members of patients with disc drusen are 10 times more likely to have the condition than the general population. It is usually bilateral.

Several conditions have been associated with optic disc drusen: pseudoxanthoma elasticum, retinitis pigmentosa, megalencephaly, choroidal neovasculization, and migraine.

B-scan ultrasonography (Fig. 11.12), computed tomography, autofluorescence studies, and fluorescein angiogram help to confirm the diagnosis. The angiogram is characterized by hyperfluorescence of the drusen starting in the arteriovenous phase, and staining without leakage in late frames.

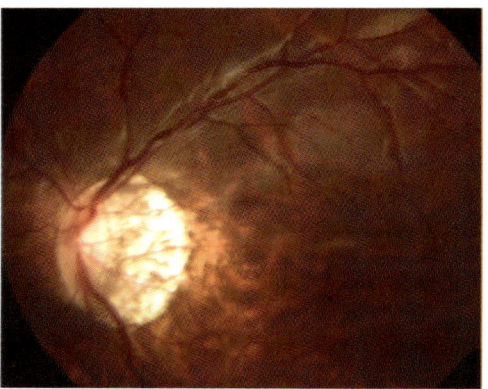

Fig. 11.10 *Tilted disc syndrome.*

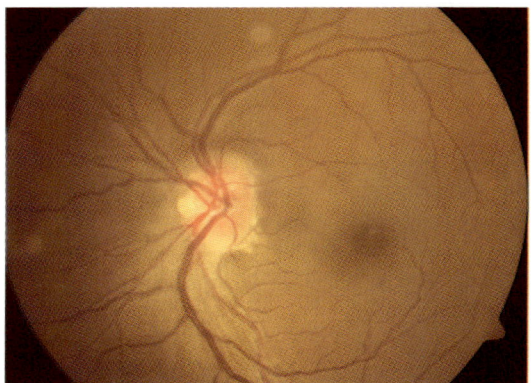

Fig. 11.11 *Optic disc drusen.*

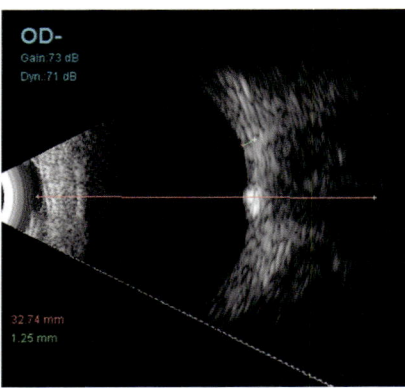

Fig. 11.12 *Scan of optic disc drusen.*

MYELINATED FIBERS

Myelinated retinal nerve fibers are a developmental anomaly, which may be continuous or discontinuous with the optic nerve head (Fig. 11.13). They are reported to occur in 0.57 to 0.98% of ophthalmic patients. The pathogenesis has not been established. Myelinated retinal nerve fibers are clinically conspicuous. Although they are generally believed to be benign lesions, they are occasionally associated with ocular complications such as myopia.

CONGENITAL OPTIC DISC PIGMENTATION

Melanin deposition anterior or within the lamina cribrosa imparts a gray appearance to

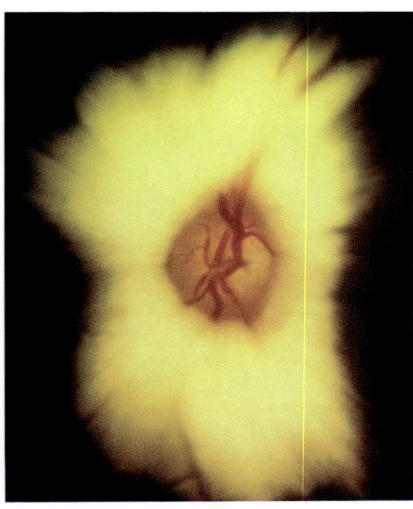

Fig. 11.13 *Myelinated nerve fiber.*

the optic disc. Fortunately, visual acuity remains unaffected in all except when associated with coexistent optic disc anomalies. Children with Aicardi syndrome and interstitial deletion of chromosome 17 are known to have optic disc pigmentation.

BIBLIOGRAPHY

1. Alvarez E, Wakakura M, Khan Z, et al. The disc-macula distance to disc diameter ratio: a new test for confirming optic nerve hypoplasia in young children. J Pediatr Ophthalmol Strabismus 1988;25:151–4.
2. Brodsky MC, Schroeder GT, Ford R. Superior segmental optic hypoplasia in identical twins. J Clin Neuro-ophthalmol 1993;13:152–4.
3. Brodsky MC. Congenital optic disk anomalies. Survey of Ophthalmol 1994;39(2):89–112.
4. Brown G, Tasman W. Congenital anomalies of optic disc. New York Grune and Stratton, 1983: 31–215.
5. Brown GC, Shield JA, Goldberg RE. Congenital pits of the optic nerve head II. Clinical studies in humans. Ophthalmol 1980;87:51–65.
6. Capo H, Repka MX, Edmond JC, et al. Optic nerve abnormalities in children: A practical approach. J AAPOS. 2011 Jun;15(3):281–90.
7. Eccles MR, Schimmenti LA. Renal-coloboma syndrome: a multisystem developmental disorder caused by PAX2 mutations. Clin Genet 1999;56:1–9.
8. Franceschetti A, Bock RH. Megalopapilla. A new congenital anomaly. Am J Ophthalmol 1950;33:227–35.
9. Friedman AH, Gartner S, Modi SS. Drusen of the optic disc: a retrospective study in cadaver eyes. Br J Ophthalmol 1975;59:413–21.
10. GarciaML, Ty EB, TabanM, et al. Systemic and ocular findings in 100 patients with optic nerve hypoplasia. J Child Neurol 2006;21:949–56.
11. Golnik K. Cavitary anomalies of the optic disc: Neurologic significance. Curr Neurol Neurosci Rep 2008;8:409–13.
12. Hellstrom A, Wiklund LM, Svensson E. The clinical and morphologic spectrum of optic nerve hypoplasia. JAAPOS 1999;29:212–20.
13. Jacobson L, Hellstrom A, Flodmark O. Large cups in normal-sized optic discs: a variant of optic nerve hypoplasia in children with periventricular leukomalacia. Arch Ophthalmol 1997;115:1263–9.

14. Kim SH, et al. Peripapillary staphyloma: clinical features and visual outcome in 19 cases. Arch Ophthalmol 2005;123:1371–6.

15. Kranenburg EW. Crater-like holes in the optic disc and central serous retinopathy. Arch Ophthalmol 1960;64:912–24.

16. Lambert SR, Hoyt CS, Narahara MH. Optic Nerve Hypoplasia. Surv Ophthalmol 1987;32:1–9.

17. Lorentzen SE. Drusen of the optic disk, an irregularly dominant hereditary affection. Acta Ophthalmol (Copenh) 1961;39:626–43.

18. Nicholson B, Ahmad B, Sears JE. Congenital optic nerve malformations. IOC 2011;51(1): 49–76.

19. Optical coherence tomography and Heidelberg retina tomography for superior segmental optic hypoplasia. Lee HJ, Kee C. Br J Ophthalmol 2009;93(11):1468–73.

20. Pollock S. The morning glory disc anomaly: contractile movement, classification and embryogenesis. Doc Ophthalmol 1987;65:439–60.

21. Savino PJ, Glaser JS, Rosenberg MA. A clinical analysis of pseudopapilledema. II: visual field defects. Arch Ophthalmol 1979;97:71–5.

22. Traboulsi E. Morning glory disk anomaly-more than meets the eye. J AAPOS 2009;13:333–4.

23. Velasque L, Mortemosque B Myelinated retinal nerve fibers. Review of the literature. J Fr Ophthalmol 2000;23(9):892–6.

24. Witmer MT, Margo CE, Drucker M. Tilted optic discs. Survey of Ophthalmol 2010;55(5): 403–28.

25. Yamashita T, Kawano K, Ohba N. Autosomal dominantly inherited optic nerve coloboma. Ophthalmic Paediatr Genet 1988;9:17–24.

26. Zeki SM. Optic nerve hypoplasia and astigmatism: a new association. Br J Ophthalmol 1990;74(5):297–9.

12 OPTIC NEURITIS

Rohit Saxena, Swati Phuljhele, Vimla Menon

OPTIC NEURITIS: CLINICO-ETIOLOGICAL PROFILE
- Etiology
- Clinical features
Typical Versus Atypical Optic Neuritis
INVESTIGATIVE PROFILE
- Ophthalmic investigations
- Systemic investigations
- Recommendation for MRI

DIFFERENTIAL DIAGNOSIS AND MANAGEMENT
Differential Diagnosis
Management
- Optic neuritis treatment trial
- Controlled high-risk subjects Avonex multiple sclerosis prevention study
- PRISMS trial
- BENEFIT study

OPTIC NEURITIS: CLINICO-ETIOLOGICAL PROFILE

Optic neuritis is an acute inflammation of the optic nerve. Although it has been reported from almost all parts of the world, regions with the highest incidence include Northern Europe, Southern Australia and Central North America.

ETIOLOGY

Optic nuritis can occur due to demyelinating, infective or autoimmune diseases. Most of the cases, however, are idiopathic. Multiple sclerosis is reported to be the most common etiology in Western literature. The inflammation may be due to the direct involvement of the optic nerve; or secondary to the contagious spread of inflammation from the orbit, sinuses or meninges; or may be associated with the intraocular inflammation of the retina and the uvea. Common causes of optic neuritis are listed as follows:

1. *Demyelinating causes*
   - Multiple sclerosis
   - Neuromyelitis optica
   - Schilder's disease
   - Encephalitis periaxialis concentrica
   - Acute demyelinating encephalopathy

2. *Infectious and para-infectious causes*
   - Viral (adenovirus, coxsackievirus, measles, mumps, rubella, varicella-zoster)
   - Bacterial (syphilis, tuberculosis, Lyme disease, cat-scratch disease, β-hemolytic streptococcal infection, brucellosis, typhoid fever, meningococcal infection, Whipple's disease)
   - Nematode infection
   - Post-vaccination

3. *Autoimmune disorders*
   - Sarcoidosis
   - Systemic lupus erythematosus
   - Polyarteritis nodosa
   - Guillain-Barré syndrome
   - Wegner's granulomatosis

CLINICAL FEATURES

There is a female preponderance, with most patients presenting between 20 and 45 years of age. The clinical features of the typical optic neuritis are listed below.

- Young adult patient typically in 3rd and 4th decade, but can present at any age
- Acute onset of unilateral loss of vision progressing over a few days (2 weeks-peak loss)
- Visual loss varies from subtle subclinical involvement to no perception of light
- Often accompanied with retrobulbar pain which worsens on eye movement
- Exacerbation of symptoms with increased body temperature (Uhthoff's phenomenon)
- Presence of relative afferent pupillary defect (RAPD)
- Fundus is normal in a case of retrobulbar neuritis (RBN) or disc edema may be present in a case of papillitis (Fig. 12.1)
- Recovery of vision usually begins after 2 weeks.

The above mentioned features though are characteristic of optic neuritis, they are not sacrosanct. There may be variations in clinical features depending upon the etiology and type of the optic neuritis. Twenty percent of adult cases can present with bilateral involvement which is more common in children. Although RBN is reported to be the predominant type in Western literature, 60% of the patients from this part of the world present with disc oedema. Minimal vitritis can be associated with optic neuritis, however, the presence of active inflammation in the anterior or the posterior chamber should arouse the suspicion of co-existing uveitis. It has been reported that retinal venous sheathing associated with the optic neuritis indicates increased risk of developing of MS. In 80% of the patients, visual recovery may occur by 3 weeks. Improvement may continue after this, especially in patients with poor vision, up to a period of 12 months. Though good functional visual recovery is seen in most of the patients, around 5 to 10% of the patients fail to recover fully. Fellow eye involvement may be seen in the form of reduced contrast sensitivity, defective color vision and/or increased latency on visually evoked potential.

Typical versus atypical optic neuritis

Traditionally, a *typical optic neuritis* is classified as one associated with demyelination, particularly MS and presents with above mentioned clinical features. Nonetheless the presentation and the prognosis may vary when the optic neuritis is secondary to causes other than demyelination, and is considered as *atypical optic neuritis*. Atypical features include absence of pain; marked swelling of the nerve with retinal exudates and peripapillary hemorrhages; severe visual loss to no light perception; progression of visual loss or pain for more than 2 weeks; and lack of recovery after 3 weeks. Patients with atypical optic neuritis are at lower risk of developing MS and should be extensively evaluated for other causes of optic neuropathy.

Opticospinal form of MS (OSMS), which is characterized by high incidence of visual involvement at onset and recurrent acute transverse myelitis is prevalent in Asian region and has a high degree of overlap with neuron myelitis optica (NMO).

INVESTIGATIVE PROFILE

OPHTHALMIC INVESTIGATIONS

The diagnosis of optic neuritis is based on the clinical presentation. Investigations are ancillary

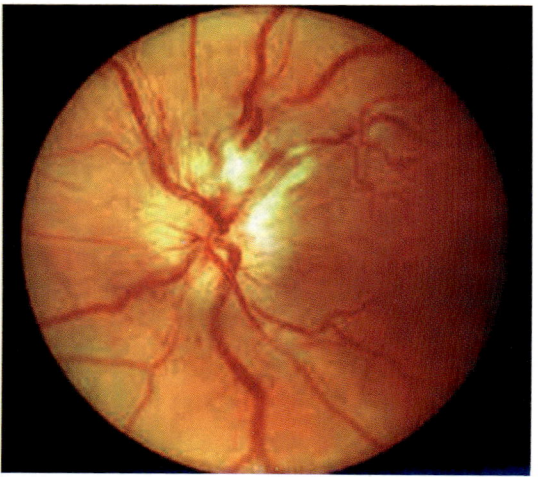

Fig. 12.1 *Papillitis.*

and can be used to identify sub-clinical involvement of the fellow eye and to monitor the prognosis of the disease.

All the patients suffering from the optic nerve disorder would have subnormal contrast sensitivity and defective color vision. A patient with optic neuritis may show almost any variety of *visual field defects*, most common being central or centrocecal scotoma. On *visually evoked* potential examination there is increased latency of P1 wave.

Fundus fluorescein angiography (FFA) may be helpful in differentiating it from the other causes of optic neuropathy as well as to rule out the retinal pathology. The disc shows mild-to-moderate leak in early phase which increases with the time.

Recently, studies have evaluated the role of *optical coherence tomography* in the demyelinating disorders, particularly in MS. It has been seen that the patients of MS who have never had an episode of optic neuritis during their disease course show reduced retinal nerve fiber layer (RNFL) thickness as compared to the normals; similarly, the fellow eyes of patients of optic neuritis with MS also show thinning of RNFL. Thus, thinning of RNFL layer on OCT may be used to prognosticate the disease burden. However, role of OCT in cases of optic neuritis without any associated demyelinating disorders is controversial.

SYSTEMIC INVESTIGATIONS

The diagnosis of optic neuritis is a clinical one, made in a patient of appropriate age with the clinical features mentioned above. Although no investigations are necessary for confirming the diagnosis, investigations are needed to assess the risk of developing MS and to rule out other disorders. In atypical cases, e.g. patients older than 50 years, or cases with a history suggestive of a secondary etiology, an additional work up to identify etiology should be considered. Since *tuberculosis* is common in our country, a baseline chest X-ray is done in all the patients prior to starting treatment with the steroids. *Serology* for syphilis, bartonella and toxoplasmosis; Mantoux test; blood culture; cerebrospinal fluid (CSF) examination; and blood tests should be done to rule out infective and inflammatory causes.

Specialized tests, e.g. toxin screens and serum B_{12} for toxic optic neuropathy; markers for autoimmune diseases; antibody to aquaporin-4 and *MRI spine* in NMO; *genetic analysis* for mitochondrial mutation in cases of Leber's hereditary optic neuropathy, are required in suspected conditions.

RECOMMENDATIONS FOR MRI

In populations with a high incidence of MS, all patients with an acute monosymptomatic demyelinating optic neuritis should undergo gadolinium-enhanced MRI of the brain and spine to determine if they are at a high-risk for the subsequent development of clinically definite multiple sclerosis (CDMS). MRI imaging becomes essential in recurrent optic neuritis, in patients keen to know about the long-term prognosis, in patients with a history or evidence of other neurological involvement, in atypical cases and in acute optic neuritis in children. The presence of demyelinating lesions on brain MRI at the time of clinical presentation is the strongest predictor for developing CDMS (Figs 12.2 and 12.3). MRI showing ≥2 white matter lesions (≥3 mm in diameter, at least 1 lesion periventricular or ovoid) indicates a high-risk for CDMS.

DIFFERENTIAL DIAGNOSIS AND MANAGEMENT

DIFFERENTIAL DIAGNOSIS

In a patient of optic neuritis it is important to differentiate various etiologies as listed above.

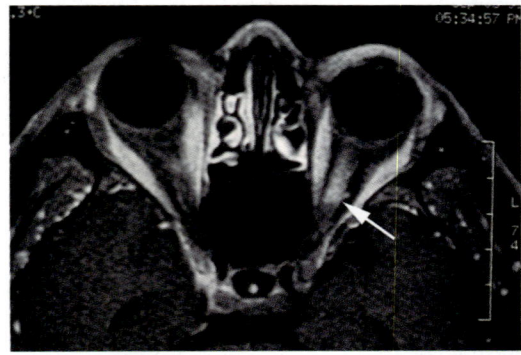

Fig. 12.2 *Axial section of MRI showing hyperintensity along optic nerve in optic neuritis.*

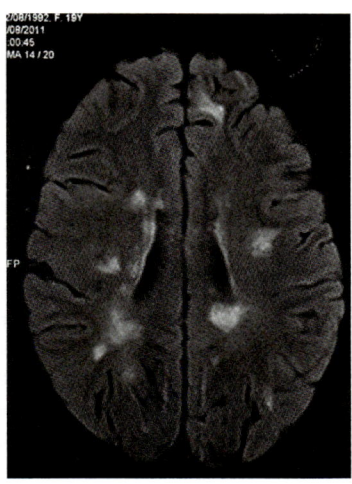

Fig. 12.3 *MRI showing white matter lesions and plaques in a case of multiple sclerosis.*

The above mentioned systemic investigations are required to distinguish inflammatory, infective and other pathology. The other conditions that can simulate the clinical picture of optic neuritis include; ischemic optic neuropathies, Leber's hereditary optic neuropathy and papilledema. Table 12.1 shows salient differentiating features.

MANAGEMENT

Before discussing the management of optic neuritis it is pertinent to understand the natural history of the typical demyelinating optic neuritis.

Optic Neuritis Treatment Trial (ONTT) is a pioneering study that has shaped our understanding about the demyelinating optic neuritis.

		Table 12.1 *Differential diagnosis of optic neuritis*		
	Optic neuritis	*Papilledema*	*Ischemic optic neuropathy*	*Leber's hereditary optic neuropathy*
Age at presentation	2nd to 4th decade of life	Any age	Usually above 40 years of age	Usually in 20–30 years of age group
Laterality	Usually unilateral (20% of cases may be bilateral)	Bilateral	Unilateral	Either bilateral or sequential involvement of both the eyes
Visual acuity	Vary from subclinical involvement to no PL	Preserved in early stages	Varies from no PL (AAION) mild loss of vision	<20/200
Pain	Present in majority of cases	Severe headache associated with nausea	Severe headache or jaw claudication in cases of AAION	Painless
Disc edema	Present in cases of papillitis	Always present	Sectoral disc oedema pallor may be present in arteritic cases	Present in all cases
Visual field defect	Any type (centrocecal is most common)	Enlargement of blind spot	Altitudinal field defect	Centrocecal field defect
FFA	Mild to moderate disc leak from early phase	Profuse disc leak	Choroidal delay and delayed filling of the disc especially in arteritic cases	No disc leak, however presence of telangiectatic vessels on disc can be seen
Association	MS	Any ICSOL or BIH	DM, HTN, dyslipidemia, GCA	Mitochondrial disease, other members of family may be affected

AAION—arteritic ischemic optic neuropathy, DM—diabetes mellitus, HTN—hypertension, GCA—giant cell arteritis, ICSOL—intracranial space occupying lesion, BIH—benign intracranial hypertension

ONTT was a multi-centered randomized trial involving 454 patients from 1988 to 2006. The main objective of the study was to evaluate the efficacy of corticosteroid in treatment for acute optic neuritis and to investigate the relationship between optic neuritis and MS. The cases included in the study had a clinical picture consistent with unilateral optic neuritis, visual loss lasting 8 days or less with no previous episodes of optic neuritis in the affected eye, no previous steroid treatment for MS or optic neuritis and no other systemic disease except MS as a cause of optic neuritis. The patients were randomized into 3 different treatment groups: oral placebo for 14 days; intravenous methyl-prednisolone (250 mg, 6 hourly) for 3 days, followed by oral prednisolone (1 mg/kg/day) for 11 days and a 3-day tapering of prednisolone thereafter; oral prednisolone (1 mg/kg/day) for 14 days, followed by a 3-day tapering.

The results showed that the intravenous steroid group recovered vision faster compared to those treated with oral administration or placebo. Intravenous steroids afforded a short-term but statistically significant benefit in visual functions but not in visual acuity at 6 months. At the 1-year follow-up, there was no statistically significant difference in visual function among the groups. The interesting finding was that the patients with oral regimen had a two fold greater rate of recurrent optic neuritis. Of the patients treated with oral steroids, 30% experienced a recurrence, either in the fellow eye or in the affected eye in the first 2 years of follow-up, compared to only 13% in the intravenous steroid group and 16% in the placebo group. At 2 years, 8% of the patients treated with intravenous steroids had clinically definite MS, whereas 18% of the placebo group and 16% of the oral steroid group developed MS. The 15 years result of the study are now available and it is reported that 72% of the eyes affected with optic neuritis had visual acuity of ≥20/20, and 66% of the patients had ≥20/20 acuity in both eyes.

ONTT also identified the characteristics associated with low conversion rate; male gender and optic disc swelling were associated with a lower risk of MS, and presence of the following atypical features like no light perception vision; absence of pain; and presence of peripapillary hemorr-hages, or retinal exudates.

Based on the findings of the ONTT it can now be concluded that a typical case of demyelinating optic neuritis does not necessitate any systemic investigations including lumbar puncture. The treatment with oral prednisolone in conventional doses alone is absolutely contra-indicated. Treatment with intravenous steroids should be considered to reduce 2-year risk of developing MS in cases where 3 or more signal abnormalities are present on the MRI, or in the patients requiring expedited recovery of vision (i.e. monocular patients, employment demands, bilateral involvement and patients desiring intervention).

Studies have been done to evaluate and compare the efficacy of intravenous dexamethasone vis-à-vis intravenous mega-dose methyl-prednisolone. Intravenous dexamethasone was found to be as effective as mega-dose intravenous methylprednisolone therapy recommended by the ONTT study, with the added advantage of being easier to administer and less costly (costing one sixth of injection methylprednisolone).

Controlled High-risk Subjects Avonex Multiple Sclerosis Prevention Study (CHAMPS) was a randomized, double-blind trial in the patients of acute monosymptomatic demyelinating event and at least 2 silent T2 lesions on brain MRI in which role of immunomodulators in form of interferons have been evaluated in delaying the progression and preventing the relapses in MS. The patients were randomized to weekly intramuscular interferon β-1a (Avonex®, Biogen Idec) or placebo. The treatment group experienced a 44% reduction in the rate of development of CDMS compared with the placebo group over 3 years of follow-up. There were statistically significant beneficial effects on all MRI parameters for the treatment group, including decrease in T2 lesion development, gadolinium-enhancing lesions and T2 lesion volume. The 10-year follow-up showed that patients treated immediately after their first episode had a significantly lesser chance of experiencing a second attack compared to those who had delayed treatment.

Prevention of Relapses and Disability by Interferon β-1a Subcutaneously in Multiple Sclerosis (PRISMS) Trial assessed efficacy of interferon (IFN)β-1a in dosages of 22 μg and 44 μg s.c. given subcutaneously compared to placebo in relapsing-remitting multiple sclerosis patients, and it was seen that both the treatment groups had fewer relapses.

Likewise interferon β-1b was studied in *betaferon in newly emerging multiple sclerosis for initial treatment (BENEFIT)* study, which included patients with a single neurologic event and at least 2 clinically silent MRI lesions. In a 24-month study period it was seen to reduce the risk of MS by 50%.

However, the rationale of initiating immunomodulator therapy in patients of optic neuritis with MS should be based on the fact that the prevalence of MS is low in Asian countries and the treatment is expensive with unknown long-term benefits.

The management of optic neuritis that is not associated with MS depends upon the etiological cause. Therefore, it becomes extremely important to thoroughly investigate the patients who do not fit in the diagnosis of typical optic neuritis, such as; failure of spontaneous visual recovery, relapse on stopping the corticosteroids. These patients should be investigated to rule out any infective or autoimmune pathology. Moreover the diagnosis of NMO should be kept in mind in cases where the visual recovery is poor or the patient develops lower limb paraplegia, and should be treated accordingly.

BIBLIOGRAPHY

1. Balcer LJ. Optic Neuritis. Curr Treat Options Neurol 2001;3:389–98.
2. Beck RW, Arrington J, Murtagh FR, Cleary PA, Kaufman DI. Brain MRI in acute optic neuritis. Experience of the Optic Neuritis Study Group. Arch Neurol 1993;50:841–6.
3. Beck RW, Cleary PA, Backlund JC. The course of visual recovery after optic neuritis. Experience of the Optic Neuritis Treatment Trial. Ophthalmology 1994;101:1771–8.
4. Beck RW, Trobe JD. What we have learned from Optic Neuritis Treatment Trial. Ophthalmology 1995;102:1504–8.
5. Chong HT, Li P, Ong B, et al. Severe cord involvement is a universal feature of Asians with multiple sclerosis: A joint Asian study. Neurol J Southeast Asia 2002;7:35–40.
6. Cleary PA, Beck RW, Anderson MM, et al. Optic Neuritis Study Group: Design, methods and conduct of the Optic Neuritis Treatment Trial. Control Clin Trials 1993;14:123–42.
7. Ebers GC. Optic neuritis and multiple sclerosis. Arch Neurol 1985;42:702–4.
8. Jacobs LD, Beck RW, Simon JH, et al. Intramuscular interferon beta-1a therapy initiated during a first demyelinating event in multiple sclerosis. CHAMPS Study Group. N Engl J Med 2000;343:898–904.
9. Kappos L, Polman CH, Freedman MS, et al. Treatment with interferon beta-1b delays conversion to clinically definite and McDonald MS in patients with clinically isolated syndromes. Neurology 2006;67:1242–9.
10. Kuroiwa Y, Shibashaki H, Tabira T. Clinical picture of multiple sclerosis in Asia. In: Kuroiwa Y, Kurland LT (Eds). Multiple sclerosis-East and West. Japan: Kyushu University Press, Fukuoka 1982;43–7.
11. Lightman S, McDonald WI, Bird AC, Francis DA, Hoskins A, Batchelor JR, Halliday AM. Retinal venous sheathing in optic neuritis. Its significance for the pathogenesis of multiple sclerosis. Brain 1987;110:405–14.
12. Lim S A, Goh K Y, Tow S, et al. Optic neuritis in Singapore. Singapore Med J 2008;49:667–71.
13. Menon V, Mehrotra A, Saxena R, et al. Comparative evaluation of megadose methylprednisolone with dexamethasone for treatment of primary typical optic neuritis. Indian J Ophthalmol 2007; 55:355–9.
14. Optic Neuritis Study Group. The clinical profile of optic neuritis. Experience of the Optic Neuritis Treatment Trial. Arch Ophthalmol 1991;109: 1673–6.
15. Optic Neuritis Study Group. Visual function 15 years after optic neuritis: a final follow-up report from the Optic Neuritis Treatment Trial Ophthalmology. Ophthalmology 2008;115: 1079–82.
16. Optical coherence tomography and disease subtype in multiple sclerosis. Pulicken M, Gordon-Lipkin E, Balcer LJ, et al. Neurology 2007 27;(69): 2085–92.
17. Pugliatti M, Sotgiu S, Rosati G. The worldwide prevalence of multiple sclerosis. Clin Neurol Neurosurg 2002;104:182-91.

18. Rosati G. The prevalence of multiple sclerosis in the world: an update. Neurol Sci 2001;22: 117–39.

19. Sethi HS, Menon V, Sharma P, et al. Visual outcome after intravenous dexamethasone therapy for idiopathic optic neuritis in an Indian population: A clinical case series. Indian J Ophthalmol 2006;54:177–83.

20. Siger M, Dziegielewski K, Jasek L, et al. Optical coherence tomography in multiple sclerosis: thickness of the retinal nerve fiber layer as a potential measure of axonal loss and brain atrophy. J Neurol 2008;255:1555–60.

21. Simon JH, Li D, Traboulsee A, et al. Standardized MR imaging protocol for multiple sclerosis: Consortium of MS Centers consensus guidelines. Am J Neuroradiol 2006;27:455–61.

22. The PRISMS (Prevention of Relapses and Disability by Interferon β-1a Subcutaneously in Multiple Sclerosis Study) Group and University of British Columbia MS/MRI Analysis Goup: PRISMS-4: Long term efficacy of interferon beta-1a in relapsing MS. Neurology 2001;56:1628–36.

23. Wang JC, Tow S, Aung T, et al. The presentation, aetiology, management and outcome of optic neuritis in an Asian population. Clin Experiment Ophthalmol 2001;29:312–5.

24. Wilejto M, Shroff M, Buncic JR, et al. The clinical features, MRI findings, and outcome of optic neuritis in children. Neurology 2006;67:258–62.

13 | ISCHAEMIC OPTIC NEUROPATHIES

Virendra Sachdeva

INTRODUCTION AND CLASSIFICATION

INTRODUCTION

The term ischaemic optic neruopathies refers to a group of diseases characterized by a sudden reduction in the blood supply to the optic nerve causing an infarction. Ischaemic optic neuropathies are one of the common causes of sudden onset decrease in vision usually in the elderly patients, however, the condition can sometimes present in the young and middle aged adults as well. In some patients, the disease may be a result of some underlying systemic diseases such as hypertension, diabetes mellitus, dyslipidemia, coronary artery diseases, while in a few others it may result from a severe inflammation of blood vessels (giant cell arteritis) affecting the optic nerve circulation.

As non-arteritic ischaemic optic neuropathy has been reported in the young population these days, role of possible further systemic risk factors is speculated. Although there is no known treatment for non-arteritic ischaemic optic neuropathy, updated knowledge of the possible risk factors and pathophysiology helps to develop an approach to the management of this condition. In this chapter, we attempt to develop a proper understanding of the condition, its classification, pathophysiology, treatment options and visual outcomes.

CLASSIFICATION

According to the underlying pathophysiology

The disease process can be sub-classified according to the underlying cause as:
- Arteritic (resulting from a necrotising vasculitis of the blood vessels)
- Non-arteritic type (resulting from a dysregulation of the circulation in the optic nerve).

According to the location of the disease process

Ischaemic optic neuropathy can affect result from an infarction of the optic nerve head (optic disc), immediate retrolaminar portion or uncommonly in the intraorbital, intracanalicular and intracranial part.

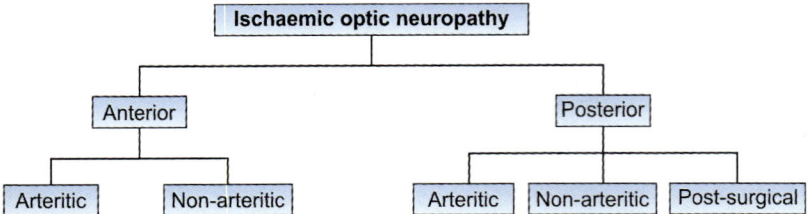

Fig. 13.1. *Classification of ischaemic optic neuropathy.*

Thus, the spectrum encompasses both anterior and posterior ischaemic optic neuropathy depending upon the location of ischemia.

Clinical classification

Clinically, acute ischemia of the optic nerve results in two very distinct types of neuropathy:

a. *Anterior ischaemic optic neuropathy (AION)* involving the optic nerve head. It is characterized by a disc swelling and blurring of disc margins with a segmental disc pallor characteristically termed **Pallid disc edema**.

b. *Posterior ischaemic optic neuropathy (PION)* involving a segment of the retrobulbar part of optic nerve. It is characterized usually by a profound loss of vision while the fundus appears normal. However, later on mild disc pallor may set in.

Classification of ischaemic optic neuropathy is summarized in Fig. 13.1.

EPIDEMIOLOGY AND PATHOGENESIS

EPIDEMIOLOGY

Primary ischaemic neuropathy is the most common cause of disc swelling in people older than 50 years of age in USA. The estimated annual incidence of non-arteritic ischaemic optic neuropathy is 2.3–10.2/100,000 and 0.36/100,000 of arteritic type.

Although both arteritic and non-arteritic ischaemic optic neuropathy present in middle aged and elderly patients, the two diseases present significant differences in epidemiology.

According to the available data from ischaemic optic neuropathy decompression trial (ONDT), peak incidence of non-arteritic ischaemic optic neuropathy (NA-ION) ranges from 60 to 69 years, with a peak at 66 years of age. However, in the recent years, as reported by Kawasaki et al. NA-ION has been reported in the younger population and NA-ION occurring in patients less than 50 years of age is defined as *NA-ION in young.*

Arteritic AION on the other hand presents in patients aged 55 years and older. It is rare to have arteritic AION in patients less than 50 years of age.

In addition, arteritic AION is almost three times more common in women than in men while *non-arteritic AION* usually affects men and women almost equally.

RELEVANT ANATOMY AND ETIOPATHOGENESIS

To understand the pathogenesis completely, it is useful to review the vascular supply of optic nerve. Hayreh in his pioneering work described in great detail the blood supply of the visual pathways.

BLOOD SUPPLY TO THE OPTIC NERVE

Main source of blood supply to the optic nerve is the posterior ciliary artery (PCA) circulation via the peripapillary choroid and the short PCAs (or the circle of Zinn and Haller). Posterior ciliary arteries may supply the prelaminar and laminar portions of the optic nerve via the circle of Zinn (or Haller, when present) or may supply directly in cases these do not form the anastomotic circle of Haller. In addition, the PCAs give recurrent pial branches that run along the retrolaminar portion of the optic nerve and give centripetal branches that supply the central trunk of the optic nerve.

Ancillary sources of the blood supply to various parts of the optic nerve are:

Table 13.1 *Summary of blood supply of optic nerve*

Portion of the optic nerve	Chief source of blood supply	Other sources of blood supply	Remarks
Optic nerve head: Surface nerve fiber Layer	Retinal arterioles	PCA circulation; cilioretinal artery when present	
Prelaminar region	Centripetal branches from peripapillary choroid		
Lamina cribrosa	Centripetal branches from peripapillary choroid	Anastomotic circle of Haller when present	Central retinal artery does not give any branches here
Retrolaminar region	1. Centripetal branches from pial branches of ophthalmic artery 2. Centrifugal branches from central retinal artery		Centrifugal system is not constantly present but PCA circulation is the main source of blood supply
Posterior portion of the optic nerve	1. Centripetal branches from the recurrent branches of ophthalmic artery and its intraorbital branches 2. Centrifugal branches from central retinal artery		Supply from central retinal artery may extend 1–4 mm behind the site of penetration of the central retinal artery into the optic nerve

- *The retinal arterioles* that may form additional blood supply to the surface nerve fiber layer of the optic nerve head.
- *Central retinal artery* that supplies the retro-laminar portion of the optic nerve (Table 13.1).

To summarise, the blood supply of the optic nerve can be subdivided into the following parts, according to the different regions of the optic nerve.

A. Arterial blood supply of the anterior part of the optic nerve (ONH) (Fig. 13.2)

The ONH consists of, from front to back (i) surface nerve fiber layer, (ii) prelaminar region, (iii) lamina cribrosa region, and (iv) retrolaminar region (Fig. 13.2A).

B. Segmental distribution

Fluorescein angiographic studies by Hayreh SS et al. have shown a sectoral blood supply in the ONH, which goes along with the overall segmental distribution of the PCA circulation. This helps explain the segmental visual loss in AION.

C. Inter-individual variation in the blood supply of the optic nerve head

Pattern of blood supply of the ONH is not identical in all eyes as is generally thought of and all ischaemic lesions cannot be explained by one standard vascular pattern. Hayreh et al. have clearly shown marked inter-individual variation in vascular supply of optic nerve head which is produced by variations in the number of the posterior ciliary vessels, patterns of distribution of the PCA circulation:

1. Variations in the anatomical pattern of the arterial supply

The usual pattern of vascular supply is described above. However, there are tremendous variations in the anatomical pattern.

2. Variations in the pattern of PCA circulation

The PCAs show marked inter-individual variation, which must profoundly influence the blood supply pattern of the ONH. A brief review of the work by Hayreh et al. is detailed as follows:

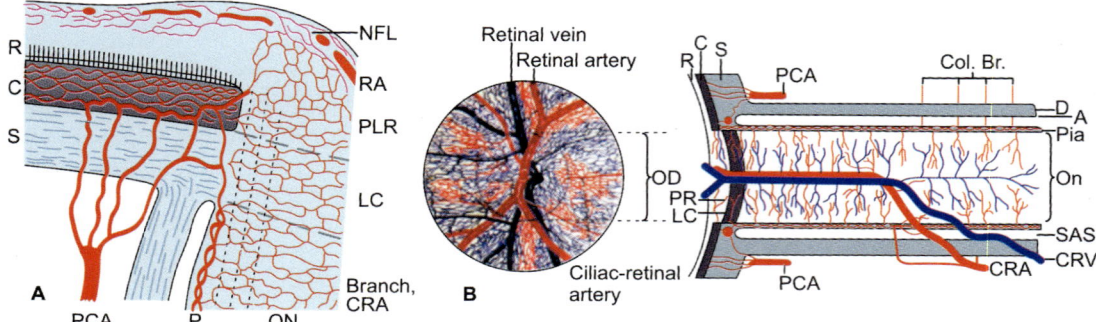

Fig. 13.2 *Schematic representation of blood supply of: (A) the optic nerve head and (B) the optic nerve modified from Hayreh SS (1974) Irans. AM. Acad. Ophthalmol itikartbgik 78. OP2 40–OP254. A reproduced from Hayreh 1978a. Abbreviations: A—arachnoid; Ant. sup. Hyp. Art.—anterior superior hypophyseal artery; C—cgiriud; CAR and CAR—central retinal artery; Col Br.—collateral branches; CRV—central retinal vein; CZ—circle of Zinn and Haller; D—dura; ICA—internal carotid artery; LC—lamina cribrosa; LPCA—lateral posterior ciliary artery; MMA—medial muscular artery; MPCA—medial posterior ciliary artery; NFL—surface nerve fiber layer of the disc; OA—ophthalmic artery; OD—optic disc; ON—optic nerve; P—pia; PCA—posterior ciliary artery; PR and PLR—preliminary region; R—retina; RA—retinal arteriole; Rec Hr CZ—recurrent pial branches from peripapillary choroid/CZ; S—sclera; SAS—subarachnoid space.*

a. *There may be variations in number of PCAs supplying an eye.* Usually, 2 or 3 PCAs supply the optic nerve but they may be 1–5 in number. The PCAs enter the eyeball usually medial and lateral to the optic nerve and hence are called medial and lateral PCAs.

b. *Variations in the in vivo supply by the PCAs.* Hayreh, et al.[11] have shown that PCAs and their branches have a segmental distribution *in vivo*, in the choroid as well as in the ONH. The lateral and medial PCAs supply the corresponding parts of the choroid. However, there is marked inter-individual variation in the area supplied by the PCAs in humans, both in the choroid and in the ONH.

Numerous variations may exist in the distribution of the area of the blood supply by the PCAs. The inter-individual variation in number and distribution by the various PCAs produces an extremely variable pattern of distribution by the PCAs in the ONH—this may explain the various patterns of the optic disc pallor and visual field disturbances that occur in patients with NA-ION.

c. *Watershed zones in the PCA distribution and their location.* Watershed zones are the areas of the comparatively poor vascularisation in the border zone between the territories of distribution of any two end-arteries.

They are most vulnerable to ischemia in the event of a fall in the perfusion pressure in the vascular bed of one or more of the end-arteries. Since PCAs and their subdivisions are end-arteries *in vivo*, they have watershed zones between them. But the exact location of the watershed zones can differ according to the anatomy of the PCA circulation as regards the number of the PCAs and their distribution.

The location of the watershed zones in relation to the ONH is important. This is because in the event of fall of perfusion pressure in the PCAs or their branches, the part of the ONH located in the watershed zone becomes vulnerable to ischemia.

d. *Difference in blood flow in various PCAs as well as short PCAs.* Clinical and experimental studies by Hayreh et al. have indicated that the mean blood pressure (BP) in the various PCAs may be different in health and in disease.

In the event of a fall of perfusion pressure, the vascular bed supplied by one artery may be affected earlier and more than the others.

PATHOGENESIS

NA-AION is caused most commonly by transient non-perfusion or hypoperfusion of ONH circulation. It may rarely be caused by embolism to the arterioles feeding the ONH.

Points to Remember...

1. Posterior ciliary artery is the chief source of the blood supply to optic nerve head and immediate retrolaminar portion of the optic nerve.
2. Considerable variation exists in the number of the posterior ciliary artery (PCA) circulation as regards the number of PCAs and distribution.
3. PCAs are end-arteries with watershed zones between them and also show a segmental distribution of the blood supply to the choroid and disc.
4. The area of the optic nerve head that may be supplied by a given branch of PCA varies according to the number of PCAs and their distribution.

A. NA-AION DUE TO HYPOPERFUSION OF ONH CIRCULATION

The blood flow in the optic nerve head depends upon several factors, the most important of which is the blood pressure in its vessels. Hayreh, et al. have done pioneering work on the dynamics of the blood circulation in the ONH.

The blood flow in the ONH is calculated by using the following formula (Hayreh et al.)

Perfusion pressure = Mean BP – intraocular pressure (IOP).

Mean BP = Diastolic BP + 1/3 (systolic minus diastolic BP).

From this formula, it is evident that the blood flow depends upon (a) resistance to blood flow, (b) BP and (c) IOP.

Therefore, a reduction in blood flow may develop consequent to alterations in one of these three factors.

Hayreh et al. have shown that transient poor circulation or loss of circulation in the optic nerve head can occur due to a transient fall of blood pressure below a critical level in its vessels, which in turn, in susceptible persons, would produce AION. In this mode of development of AION there is no actual blockage of the posterior ciliary arteries, rather it results from a fall of the blood pressure below the critical level in the capillaries of the optic nerve head that may be caused either by a marked fall in blood pressure or by a rise in the eye pressure, or a combination of these factors.

Autoregulation in optic nerve circulation

Normally, an autoregulation mechanism operates like in many body parts even in the optic nerve as well and therefore, helps compensate for any decrease in the blood flow however, in relation to the optic nerve head this autoregulation operates only over a critical range of perfusion pressure, so that with a rise or fall of perfusion pressure beyond the critical range, the autoregulation becomes ineffective and breaks down.

Derangement of the autoregulation in the ONH may be caused by many factors. Some of these factors have a proven association with NA-AION while some others have presumed to be associated with NA-AION.

A. *Systemic factors believed to cause dysregulation are* ageing process, arterial hypertension, diabetes mellitus, marked arterial hypotension from any cause, hypercholesterolemia and hyperhomocysteinemia.

B. *Local factors believed to cause dysregulation.* Absent or small cup in the optic disc, location of the watershed zone of the PCAs in the relation to the optic disc and vascular disorders in the nutrient vessels of the ONH.

C. *Precipitating factors.* In a given patient predisposed to dysregulation of autoregulation, some precipitating factors which may act as final insult leading to infarction of ONH, thereby NA-AION.

These include nocturnal arterial hypotension especially in hypertensive patients on antihypertensive therapy.

B. NA-AION DUE TO EMBOLISM

NA-AION may rarely occur as a result of embolism arising from optic nerve head circulation. ONH damage is usually severe and permanent depending upon area of nerve supplied by occluded artery.

Role of systemic factors in leading to NA-ION

Although many systemic factors have been implicated from time-to-time, not all have withstood the test of the controlled trials in the recent past.

1. A dysfunction of normal autoregulation may cause a significant ischemia of the optic nerve head.
2. NA-AION usually results from an ischemia of the optic nerve in a compromised circulation and rarely a result of acute embolism.
3. This may result from many systemic and local factors that affect the systemic blood pressure, increased intraocular pressure and increased resistance to blood flow.

Hayreh et al. have suggested various risk factors may be important in pathogenesis of NA-ION:

Hypertension, diabetes mellitus, hypercholesterolemia—all age groups:

Ischaemic heart disease and hyperthyroidism—Middle aged population

Young patients—An association may exist with increased ESR, CRP, antiphospholipid antibody syndrome.

They also reported a possible association with hematological disorders and collagen vascular diseases.

Solomon et al. further investigated the role of other procoagulant risk factors and found that if diabetes, hypertension and hypercholestrolemia are excluded, only identifiable significant risk factor is hyperhomocysteinemia.

CLINICAL TYPES OF ISCHAEMIC OPTIC NEUROPATHIES

ANTERIOR ISCHAEMIC OPTIC NEUROPATHY (AION)

Clinically, based on its cause, AION is of two types:

• Non-arteritic AION
• Arteritic AION

NON-ARTERITIC AION (NA-AION)

This is more common variety seen in clinics, and results from causes other than those due to giant cell arteritis.

As described above, systemic, local vascular alone or in combination cause insufficiency of the optic disc circulation, exacerbated by ocular factors like structural crowding of nerve fibers and supporting structures at the nerve head, eventually reaches a point at which inadequate oxygenation produces ischemia and swelling of the disc. Impairment of blood flow occurs possibly at the level of paraoptic branches that supply the optic nerve head directly.

Histopathologically, cavernous degeneration is noted within ischaemic regions of the optic nerve head, with distortion of adjacent axons.

Clinical features

Symptoms

Non-arteritic AION typically presents with:

1. *Loss of vision*

Typically sudden onset and painless deterioration of vision, which may progress rapidly over few hours to days.

It is usually discovered on waking in the morning and involves the lower part of the visual field in one eye.

Visual acuity is variable ranging from better than 20/20 (6/6) to no perception of light, depending upon the area of the optic nerve involved by the AION.

2. *Visual field loss*

Sometimes patients may present with loss of visual field rather than a decrease in vision especially if it involves the inferior half of visual field.

3. *Intermittent visual loss*

In eyes where the visual field defect bisects the fixation point, the patient may complain of intermittent blurred vision because of unconscious shifting fixation between the seeing and the blind areas near the fixation.

Ophthalmoscopy

Classically NA-ION presents with:
1. A sector of optic disc hyperemia, disc elevation and edema.
2. Usually there is a visible pallor of a small part of the disc—hence, the term **pallid disc edema**
3. Attenuation of blood vessels

4. Hemorrhages over the disc margin and peri-papillary area.

5. Some patients may have presence of hard exudates and cotton wool spots.

6. There may be changes of associated hypertensive or diabetic retinopathy when present.

Although classically described as a segmental disc edema, it may be diffuse, and the disc pallor may not always be visible in all the patients.

Another usually noted finding is a small sized optic disc which is usually bilateral and is believed to predispose to the development of NA-ION as it leads to crowding of the nerve fibers and thus may increase impedance to the blood flow in PCA circulation.

Since such an optic disc in the other eye is at a risk of NA-ION in future, it is called as disc at risk.

Changes in disc morphology with time

In addition, in patients with NA-ION, optic discs undergo evolutionary changes in the first 2–3 months and the findings vary according to the stage at which a particular eye is seen; in the initial phases the disc may be edematous which may be more marked in one part of the disc than the other but does not show any evidence of disc pallor. Frequently there are splinter hemorrhages at the disc margin. After a few days the entire disc may show generalized edema (this may or may not occur). However,

Points to Remember...

The optic disc becomes visibly atrophic, usually within 6 to 8 weeks. Persistence of edema past this point should prompt consideration of an alternate diagnosis.

Points to Remember...

1. Classically, NA-ION leads to segmental optic disc edema with disc pallor.
2. However, optic disc edema in NA-ION may be diffuse or segmental, hyperemic or pale, but pallor occurs less frequently than in the arteritic form.
3. Classically, NA-ION presents with inferior altitudinal field loss but it can be any pattern, diffuse or localized.
4. Frequently, there is little or no relationship between the extent and severity of optic disc pallor and the severity of visual loss.

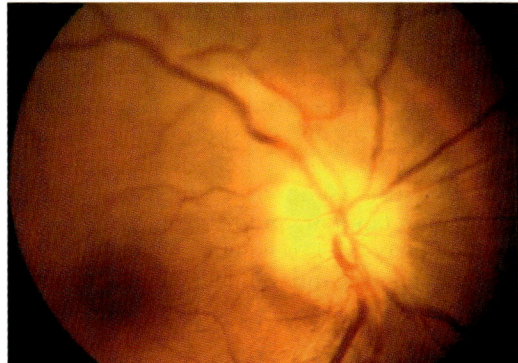

Fig. 13.3 *Acute onset ischaemic optic neuropathy showing presence of a superior disc edema with a segmental pallor of the superior portion of the optic disc and a more hyperemic inferior disc (luxury perfusion).*

later on as the optic disc edema resolves spontaneously, disc pallor may become obvious.

Perimetry

Classically, NA-ION is associated with an inferior altitudinal field loss. However, it may be variable. Perimetry usually shows complete or partial loss of vision which may be sectoral, altitudinal, central scotoma or any other possible pattern—most common being the inferonasal sectoral defect which may be relative or absolute.

Fundus fluorescein angiography

In non-arteritic AION, during the very early stages of the disease, angiography may show filling defects in the optic disc. In contrast, peripapillary choroidal filling is not delayed.

Clinical course

Untreated, NA-ION generally remains stable, most cases showing no significant improvement or deterioration over time and deterioration after reaching the low point of visual function within 1–2 months (i.e. at the time when optic atrophy sets in) is rare.

In addition, spontaneous improvement of visual acuity is not unusual. Recovery of at least 3 Snellen acuity lines has been reported in up to 42.7% patients (in the IONDT).

Eventual involvement of the contralateral eye has been reported in 40% of the eyes over a follow-up period of about 3 years.

ARTERITIC AION (AAION)

This is considered as one of the ophthalmic emergency and occurs due to giant cell arteritis.

AAION results from infarction of ONH secondary to vasculitis of short posterior ciliary artery (SPCA). Histopathologically, optic disc edema with ischaemic necrosis of the prelaminar, laminar, and retrolaminar portions of the optic nerve is seen with an infiltration of SPCA by chronic inflammatory cells.

Clinical features

In arteritic AION, AION usually occurs in association with other systemic symptoms of the disease.

The common presenting signs and symptoms of the Giant cell arteritis are:
• Headache
• Scalp tenderness
• Jaw claudication
• Myalgia

Other symptoms can be ear pain, fever, malaise, anorexia, and weight loss.

Headache is the most common symptom, while jaw claudication and temporal artery or scalp tenderness are the most specific for the disorder.

Patients may complain of intermittent episodes of transient blurring of vision or loss of vision in the involved eye before permanent loss of vision.

Unlike NA-AION, loss of vision can occur at any time of the day, although more often during the night. In addition, visual loss in NA-ION usually is much worse, so that a high proportion of the eyes are either completely blind or have extremely poor vision.

Ophthalmoscopy

Ophthalmoscopic examination during the initial stages reveals sectoral disc edema which may be diffuse or segmental and may/may not be associated with peripapillary splinter hemorrhages.

According to a study by Hayreh et al. they found that in 69% of arteritic AION eyes, the optic disc swelling has a characteristic chalky white appearance. Within 2–3 months the optic disc swelling resolves spontaneously and the disc becomes pale either in only one region or all over unlike NA-AION, fellow eye has normal disc and cup in A-AION.

Fundus fluorescein angiography

In arteritic AION, both the choroid and the optic disc in the area supplied by the involved posterior ciliary artery do not fill. FFA is a useful tool for confirming the diagnosis of AION.

Arteritic versus non-arteritic ischaemic optic neuropathy

Since, arteritic and non-arteritic forms of the ischaemic optic neuropathy differ in the underlying risk factors, it is extremely important to distinguish between the two forms of the disease. These are summarised in Table 13.2.

Table 13.2 *Differentiating features between arteritic and non-arteritic forms of ischaemic optic neuropathy*

	NAAION	AAION
Laterality†	Usually unilateral (second eye involvement may occur later on)	Unilateral or bilateral
Age	5th–6th decade	7th–8th decade
Gender	60% male	Female : male : 3 : 1 to 4 : 1
Visual dysfunction	Minimal to severe	Usually severe
Involvement of 2nd eye	Approximately 40%	Approximately 70%
Fundus	Swollen disc, often segmental	Swollen disc with marked pallor and attenuated vessels
Systemic association	Hypertension 50%	Malaise, weight loss, fever, headache
ESR	Within normal range (<40 mm Hg)	50–120 mm
CRP	Normal	Usually raised
Temporal artery biopsy	Not required	Diagnostic

† Simultaneous bilateral involvement is uncommon in the non-arteritic form of the disease, it may however, very rarely occur in the settings of massive blood loss, spine surgery or cardiovascular surgery under hypotensive anesthesia, hemodialysis)

Clinical course

If untreated, AAION results in severe damage of the affected optic nerve. Recovery of useful vision after initial involvement is unusual, even with prompt therapy. In cases with unilateral presentation, an estimate for development of AAION in the fellow eye without therapy is 70%.

DIFFERENTIAL DIAGNOSIS

Major differential diagnoses of ischaemic optic neuropathies are papillitis, papilledema, diabetic papillopathy, hypertensive optic neuropathy and compressive optic neuropathy.

Hypertensive optic neuropathy

Differentiating points are:

1. Bilateral involvement is very common
2. Arterial attenuation (on contrary, in acute stages, AION is usually associated with characteristic prominent, dilated and frequently telangiectatic vessels over the disc)
3. Presence of diffuse hemorrhages over the posterior pole and mid-periphery
4. Presence of arteriovenous cross over changes
5. Disc edema tends to be diffuse, unlike NA-ION where it tends to be segmental
6. Disc pallor is absent
7. Visual fields show presence of an enlargement of blind spot rather than dense scotomas resembling inferior altitudinal field loss or other scotomas.

Compressive optic neuropathy

It tends to present with:

- Gradual onset
- Associated history of headaches or neurological dysfunction
- Visual field loss varying according to the etiology and severity
- Relapsing nature of disease even after steroid treatment.

Papillitis and popilledema

The rest two major conditions which can be of diagnostic dilemma are optic neuritis and papilledema. The chief differentiating features between ischaemic optic neuropathy, papillitis and papilledema are summarized in Table 13.3.

Although in classical cases it may be easy to distinguish between the three disease entities, however, at times it may be difficult to distinguish between these; especially optic neuritis and ischaemic optic neuropathy. In those cases, a clue may be obtained by keeping in view the overall picture of the patient. It is however, imperative to distinguish between them because the treatment options and management implications are strikingly different for them.

POSTERIOR ISCHAEMIC OPTIC NEUROPATHY

Ischemia can independently affect the posterior portion of the optic nerve because of the distinct and separate arterial supplies of the anterior and posterior portions of the optic nerve.

Posterior ischaemic optic neuropathy (PION) is a syndrome of acute visual loss with characteristics of optic neuropathy without initial disc edema and marked by the subsequent development of optic atrophy.

The diagnosis of PION is most often made in one of the following settings:

- Arteritic: Mostly GCA
- Nonarteritic: PION in a population of patients with similar demographics to those patients with NA-ION
- Related to surgery (coronary artery bypass and lumbar spine procedures most frequently reported), or severe bleeding, or hypotension.

MANAGEMENT OF AION AND COMPLICATIONS

MANAGEMENT

Management of AION varies whether it is arteritic or non-arteritic in origin. While arteritic AION is associated with GCA and is an ophthalmic emergency necessitating early immunosuppressive treatment with high dose steroids. If delayed it can proceed to second eye involvement and bilateral visual loss.

On the other hand, there are no clear cut guidelines for the management of NA-AION. Management of NA-ION on the other hand revolves primarily around the control of various systemic risk factors and control of inflammation with systemic steroids.

Table 13.3 *Chief differentiating features between ischaemic optic neuropathy, papillitis and papilledema*

Characteristic	Optic neuritis	Papilledema	Ischaemic optic neuropathy
Age	Most common in middle aged, can occur at any age	Any age	Any age, peak in 6th decade
Gender	Female > Male (2:1 to 6:1)	None	Males > Females (3:2)
Symptoms			
Visual loss	Rapidly progressive loss of vision	Only transient obscurations of vision, visual acuity stable in acute disease	Acute onset visual loss in a field of vision, variable loss of visual acuity
Accompanying signs	Pain on ocular movements	Headaches, nausea, vomiting	Previous episodes of transient obscuration of vision
Bilaterality	Uncommon in adults, possible in children	Usually bilateral	Typically unilateral, however, second eye may get involved, very rarely bilateral involvement may occur
Signs			
Pupil	Affected eye shows sluggish reactions, RAPD	Pupillary reactions are usually normal unless there is asymmetric optic atrophy or patient is semiconscious	Affected eye shows sluggish reactions, RAPD may or may not be present
Acuity	Variable diminution of vision, from 6/6 to PL	Normal acuity	Variable acuity; from 6/6 to PL
Fundus	Disc edema with blurred margins in papillitis Normal in Retrobulbar neuritis	Variable degree of disc edema, hemorrhages	Usually segmental pallid disc edema, with few flame shaped hemorrhages, attenuation of vessels
Visual fields	Variable, most common generalized depression of sensitivity, others, centrocecal scotoma, etc.	Enlargement of blind spot, generalized constriction of blood vessels	Classically, altitudinal field defects, however, any kind of field defects including centrocecal scotoma possible
Visual-evoked potential	Classically, in acute episode reduced amplitudes with delayed latency	Classically, normal with acute episode	Classically, reduced amplitudes or extinguished with normal implicit times
Visual prognosis	Vision usually returns to normal or functional levels	If underlying cause is taken care of in time, good prognosis can be expected	Poor, second eye involvement likely in one-third of cases

Unfortunately, visual prognosis for patients with ischaemic optic neuropathy does not change much with any forms of treatment. Optic nerve decompression was once believed to be useful in NA-AION patients; however ischaemic optic neuropathy decompression trial (IONDT) clearly showed that there was no significant benefit of the same.

The role of systemic steroids is also not clearly established. However, most physicians like to give a trial of systemic steroids in patients with acute presentation of NA-AION.

However, prognosis for visual recovery remains in general poor, although occasionally patients may show a good visual recovery also but that is due to steroid treatment or natural course of disease, is not proved.

On the contrary, in patients with giant cell arteritis, the mainstay of the treatment is in form of high dose systemic steroids.

In the wake of the above findings, goals of management in patients with ischaemic optic neuropathy are:

- To establish the diagnosis
- To distinguish between arteritic and non-arteritic forms of the disease (Table 13.2).

Role of ESR and CRP in distinguishing NA-AION form A-AION

Most authorities routinely recommend investigating all patients presenting with ischaemic optic neuropathy with ESR and CRP. Miller and Green have shown that ESR tends to increase with age. They provided the following rule for calculation of maximal normal ESR at a given age:

Men: Age in years/2

Women: Age in years + 10/2

According to a study by Hayreh et al. cut-off criteria of 33 mm/1st hr in men and 35 mm/1st hr in women may provide a sensitivity and specificity of 92%.

Same study also showed that C-reactive protein (CRP) is elevated along with ESR in patients with giant cell arteritis but not in control subjects with an elevated ESR. Therefore, CRP assumes more importance in such cases.

Role of temporal artery biopsy in arteritic AION

Temporal artery biopsy is considered the gold standard in the diagnosis of temporal artery biopsy. The reported specificity of temporal artery biopsy is 100%. In a patient with active disease, temporal artery biopsy shows the presence of a necrotizing vasculitis, with marked thickening and edema of the tunica intima, disruption/loss of internal elastic lamina, presence of inflammatory infiltrates with lymphocytes, macrophages, and giant cells that may be present at all levels of vessel wall.

However, one should understand that temporal artery biopsy also has its own limitations.

1. Temporal artery biopsy tends to be positive in only 15–40% of patients.

2. Since the disease may affect segments of blood vessels with intervening areas being spared of the condition, there may be skip lesions, i.e. areas being free of the disease, hence in case the biopsy has been done from the area where the skip lesions are present, we may have a false negative results.

3. In addition, in about 5% of the patients where a unilateral temporal artery biopsy was negative, doing the temporal artery biopsy on the other side may give positive results. However, most studies in literature show that in cases of negative results of an adequate temporal artery biopsy on one side, doing the temporal artery biopsy on the other side may not increase yield by 3%.

4. In certain patients, systemic condition may preclude an immediate temporal artery biopsy:

Patients with bleeding diathesis, patients on anti-coagulants, patients with an imminent scalp ischemia, patients with a large amount of subcutaneous fat.

DIAGNOSIS OF GIANT CELL ARTERITIS

To aid in the diagnosis of temporal arteritis, both clinical diagnostic criteria and laboratory tests are useful.

In 1990, the American College of Rheumatology (ACR) analyzed 214 patients with temporal arteritis (196 proven by positive temporal artery biopsy) and compared them with 593 patients with other forms of vasculitis.

Based on this study, they established the following diagnostic criteria for giant cell arteritis:

- Age ≥ 50 years
- New-onset localized headache
- Temporal artery abnormality (such as tenderness/beading of temporal artery or loss of pulsation)
- Increased erythrocyte sedimentation rate, and a positive temporal artery biopsy
- With this classification, fulfilment of three or more criteria is 93% sensitive and 91% specific for the diagnosis

Of the 33 criteria analyzed they found that highest sensitivity criteria were:

1. Age over 50 years (mean age, 69 years and 90% over 60 years)
2. Westergren erythrocyte sedimentation rate (ESR) 50 mm/hr
3. Abnormal temporal artery biopsy.

Lee et al. have defined the presence of any one of the following as a high-risk criteria in a patients with age >50 years and elevated ESR >50 mm 1st hour.

1. Jaw or tongue claudication
2. Visual abnormalities (for example, anterior ischaemic optic neuropathy, amaurosis fugax, and optic atrophy)
3. Temporal artery abnormalities (for example, decreased pulse, tenderness, or nodules).

These were the highest specificity criteria for temporal arteritis in the original study by ACR.

They also defined high suspicion if three of the following four were met and intermediate suspicion if two of the following were met.

1. New headache (localized)
2. Temporal artery abnormality (decreased pulse, tenderness, or nodules)
3. Elevated ESR (>50 mm/hr)
4. Abnormal temporal artery biopsy (for example, necrotizing arteritis, multinucleated giant cells).

Thus, a diagnosis of temporal arteritis can be made in the presence of diagnostic criteria other than positive temporal artery biopsy. Most authorities recommend that presence of strong clinical suspicion is adequate to make a diagnosis of temporal arteritis and immediate treatment with corticosteroids can be started while waiting to arrange for temporal artery biopsy or if it is negative.

SYSTEMIC CORTICOSTEROID THERAPY

Arteritic ischaemic optic neuropathy

Immediate initiation of treatment with systemic steroids is essential in management of giant cell arteritis. since patients with giant cell arteritis are in danger of bilateral total blindness. Blindness is almost always preventable with aggressive treatment.

Points to Remember...

1. Giant cell arteritis related arteritic ischaemic optic neuropathy is a true ophthalmic emergency.
2. Arteritic ischaemic optic neuropathy can be diagnosed by presence of multiple clinical and laboratory criteria.
3. Temporal artery biopsy though is highly specific it may be false negative in a large number of patients.
4. Treatment with corticosteroids can be started while awaiting the results of temporal artery biopsy.
5. A biopsy may still show signs of positive temporal arteritis even when carried out 14 days after starting of corticosteroid treatment.

The primary objective of treatment is to prevent loss of vision in the fellow eye.

Recommendations

It is recommended to start with high-dose corticosteroid therapy (80–120 mg of prednisone orally daily) keeping in mind that this aggressive treatment cannot provide a cure, but can prevent any further visual loss. Some authorities like to use high doses of intravenous methyl prednisolone (IVMP) in these cases in doses of 1–2 g/per day followed by oral steroids. All patients are maintained at the high dose of prednisone till both the ESR and CRP have stabilized at low levels (that usually takes 2–3 weeks—CRP comes down much faster than ESR, with gradual tapering of prednisone, guided by the ESR and CRP levels only. It is recommended that high dose of steroid should be maintained for 4 to 8 weeks and then tapered as long as the patient remains symptom free and the ESR is below 40 mm/1st hour.

Systemic immunosuppressives

Immunosuppression may be augmented by other antimetabolites, such as azathioprine or methotrexate in cases who are intolerant to steroids or steroid dependant. It is also important to remember the complications of long-term usage of steroids which include: gastric ulcers, myopathies, aseptic necrosis of femur, osteoporosis, worsening of diabetes mellitus etc. Keeping these in view it may be useful to seek the involvement of a rheumatologist while the patient is on long-term steroid therapy.

Non-arteritis anterior ischaemic optic neuropathy

Steroids in NA-AION

Unlike giant cell arteritis, there is NO established treatment for non-arteritic AION. It is well known that 'a disease which has no treatment has many treatments'.

a. *Systemic corticosteroids:* There is a definite evidence of significant visual improvement with steroids in a small group of patients, particularly those with incipient non-arteritic AION, if treated early.

However, whether the visual improvement is such cases is a result of systemic steroids or natural course of disease is controversial.

In addition, many of such patients are diabetic and hypertensive so there is an added risk of worsening of diabetes control and systemic complications in such cases.

Hence, though most authorities agree to give steroids, caution should be exercised in such cases.

Thus, patients who shall definitely be given treatment are:
- Those with incipient NA-ION
- Those patients with a second eye involvement
- One eyed patients
- Those patients presenting early within one week of onset of disease.

Steroids should be avoided in patients with systemic contraindications and those presenting late (especially more than one month duration) as these are unlikely to benefit from systemic steroid therapy.

Aspirin

It is now believed that there is no role of aspirin as non-arteritic AION is NOT an embolic disorder but mainly a hypotensive disorder, as discussed above. Aspirin is indicated only occasionally when there is a definite evidence that AION is embolic in nature.

The most important aspect of management of a patient with NA-ION revolves around the identification of the possible risk factors in the given patient as this may help reduce the risk of recurrent NA-AION and second eye involvement. Thus, a careful history taking and appropriate investigations should be done to

Points to Remember...

While systemic corticosteroids (and immuno-suppressive agents) are mandatory in the treatment of giant cell arteritis, role of same in treatment of NA-AION is inconclusive and needs to weighed against the risk of complications that can arise out of systemic treatment with steroids.

elucidate all possible risk factors for the development of NA-ION.

In our settings, we routinely investigate our patients for the risk factors:
- Complete hemogram with ESR
- C-reactive protein
- Blood sugar
- Serum lipid profile
- Serum homocysteine (in young patients)
- Carotid Doppler

In case, there is evidence for any other risk factor which can be found, appropriate measures are taken, such as institution of the lipid lowering drugs, combination of the vitamin B_{12}, folic acid and thiamine in patients with elevated serum homocysteine levels.

COMPLICATIONS

- Other than *visual loss in the second eye*, which may occur simultaneously with that in the first eye, few ocular complications accompany AION.
- *Ocular palsies* in the arteritic form of the disease and
- *Ischemia of the entire globe* have been reported.
- Rarely, *scalp necrosis* can occur.

Thus it is clear from the above mentioned discussion, though ischaemic optic neuropathies constitute a heterogeneous group of diseases that differ in their etiopathogenesis, and have some understood pathogenetic mechanisms. Over the last few years a lot has been understood regarding the pathophysiology and management of the disease still a lot remains to be understood. Also, over the past few years, many controversies have surrounded the management of ischaemic optic neuropathies, most of which have been covered in this chapter. However, for a detailed discussion of the same the interested readers are referred to the most recent major review on the topic by Hayreh.

Acknowledgements

Authors gratefully acknowledge the permission given by Hayreh SS to use the diagrams and figures to illustrate the various aspects of the disease. Authors also acknowledge the constant guidance and encouragement provided by him for the same.

BIBLIOGRAPHY

1. Arnold AC, Hepler RS. Natural history of non-arteritic anterior ischaemic optic neuropathy. J Neuro-ophthalmol 1994;14:66–69.

2. Beck RW, Servais GE, Hayreh SS. Anterior ischaemic optic neuropathy-IX. Cup-to-disc ratio and its role in pathogenesis. Ophthalmology 1987;94: 1503–8.

3. Burke A, Virmani R. Temporal artery biopsy of giant cell arteritis. Pathol Case Rev 2001;6:265–73.

4. Diaz VA, DeBroff BM, Sinard J. Comparison of histopathological features, clinical symptoms, and erythrocyte sedimentation rates in biopsy-positive temporal arteritis. Ophthalmol 2005; 12:1293–8.

5. Glaser JE. The ischaemic optic neuropahties in Albert Jackobiec. Principles and practice of Ophthalmology, 2nd edition. WB Saunders Company, Philadelphia 2002;5:4138–49.

6. Hayreh SS, Joos KM, et al. Systemic diseases associated with NA-ION: Am J ophthalmol 1994;118:766–80.

7. Hayreh SS, Podhajsky P. Visual field defects in anterior ischaemic optic neuropathy. Doc Ophthalmol Proc Ser 1979;19:53–71

8. Hayreh SS, Podhajsky PA, Raman R, et al. Giant cell arteritis: Validity and reliability of various diagnostic criteria. Am J Ophthalmol 1997; 123:285–96.

9. Hayreh SS, Podhajsky PA, Raman R, et al. Giant cell arteritis: Validity and reliability of various diagnostic criteria. Am J Ophthalmol 123;285:1997.

10. Hayreh SS, Podhajsky PA, Zimmerman B. Non-arteritic anterior ischaemic optic neuropathy-Time of onset of visual loss. Am J Ophthalmol 1997;124:641–7.

11. Hayreh SS, Podhajsky PA, Zimmerman B. Ocular manifestations of giant cell arteritis. Am J Ophthalmol 1998;125:509–20.

12. Hayreh SS, Podhajsky PA, Zimmerman B. Ocular manifestations of giant cell arteritis. Am J Ophthalmol 1998;125:509–20.

13. Hayreh SS. Acute ischaemic disorders of the optic nerve: Pathogenesis, Clinical Manifestations and Management. Ophthalmol Clin North Am 1996;9:407–42.

14. Hayreh SS. Anterior ischaemic optic neuropathy IV. Occurrence after cataract extraction. Arch Ophthalmol 1980;98:1410–6.

15. Hayreh SS. Anterior ischaemic optic neuropathy: Differentiation of arteritic from non-arteritic type and its management. Eye 1990;4:25–41.

16. Hayreh SS. Blood supply and vascular disorders of the optic nerve. An Inst Barraquer 1963; 4:7–109.

17. Hayreh SS. Blood supply of the optic nerve head and its role in optic atrophy, glaucoma and oedema of the optic disc. Br J Ophthalmol 1969;53:721–48.

18. Hayreh SS. Inter-individual variation in blood supply of the optic nerve head. Its importance in various ischaemic disorders of the optic nerve head, and glaucoma, low-tension glaucoma and allied disorders. Doc Ophthalmol 1985;59:217–46.

19. Hayreh SS. Ischaemic Optic Neuropathies. Review. Progress in Retinal and Eye Research 28 (2009); 34–62.

20. Hayreh SS. Ischaemic optic neuropathy. Review article. Indian J Ophthalmol 2000;48:171.

21. Hayreh SS. Structure and blood supply of the optic nerve. In: Heilmann K, Richardson KT (Eds): Glaucoma. Conceptions of a Disease. Pathogenesis, Diagnosis, and Therapy. Stuttgart, Thieme 1978;78–96.

22. Hayreh SS. The optic nerve head circulation in health and disease. Exp Eye Res 1995;61:259–72.

23. Hayreh SS. The optic nerve head circulation in health and disease. Exp Eye Res 1995;61:257–72.

24. Hunder GG, Bloch DA, Michel BA, et al. The American College of Rheumatology 1990 criteria for the classification of giant cell arteritis. Arthritis Rheum 1990;33:1122–8.

25. Ischaemic Optic Neuropathy Decompression Trial Research Group, Arch. Ophthalmol 1996; 1336–42.

26. Ischaemic Optic Neuropathy Decompression Trial Research Group. Optic nerve decompression surgery for nonarteritic anterior ischaemic optic neuropathy (NA-ION) is not effective and may be harmful. JAMA 1995;273:625–32.

27. Ischaemic Optic Neuropathy Decompression Trial. Incidence of nonarteritic anterior ischaemic optic neuropathy. Am J Ophthalmol 1997;123(1):103–7.

28. Kawasaki A, et al. Hyperhomocysteinemia in NA-ION in Young patients: Br J Ophthalmol 1999;83:1287–90.

29. Kline LB. Progression of visual defects in ischaemic optic neuropathy. Am J Ophthalmol 1988;106:19–203.

30. Lee AG, Brazes PW. Temporal arteritis: a clinical approach. J Am Geriatr Soc 1999;47:1364–70.

31. Lee AG. Efficacy of unilateral vs. bilateral temporal artery biopsies for the diagnosis of giant cell arteritis (letter to editor). Am J Ophthalmol 2000;129:118–9.

32. McDonnell PJ, Moore W, Miller NR, et al. Temporal arteritis: a clinicopathologic study. Ophthalmology 1986;93:518–30.

33. Miller A, Green M. Simple rule for calculating normal erythrocyte sedimentation rate. Br Med J 1983;286:266.

34. Mizener JB, Podhajsky P, Hayreh SS. Ocular ischaemic syndrome. Ophthalmology 1997;104:859-64.

35. Roth AM, Milsow L, Keltner JL. The ultimate diagnoses of patients undergoing temporal artery biopsies. Arch Ophthalmol 1984;102:901–3.

36. Solomon O, Baron RA. Analysis of prothrombotic and vascular risk factors in patients with NA-ION: Ophthalmology 1999;106:739–42.

14

TRAUMATIC OPTIC NEUROPATHY

Akshay Gopinathan Nair, Rashmin A Gandhi

INTRODUCTION AND APPLIED ANATOMY
- Introduction
- Applied anatomy

PRESENTATION AND EVALUATION

Presentation Evaluation
- Check list for evaluation
- Brief comments on evaluation
- Examination of eye and adnexa
- Electrophysiological tests
- Neuroimaging

PATHOPHYSIOLOGY OF TRAUMATIC OPTIC NEUROPATHY

Direct Traumatic Optic Neuropathy

Indirect Traumatic Optic Neuropathy
- Primary mechanisms
- Secondary mechanisms

TREATMENT OF TRAUMATIC OPTIC NEUROPATHY
- Role of steroids
- Surgical management
- Recent advances and current research

INTRODUCTION AND APPLIED ANATOMY

INTRODUCTION

Traumatic optic neuropathy is a controversial yet enigmatic entity in neuro-ophthalmology. It is a rare but devastating cause of partial or complete visual loss caused by deformational forces that injure the optic nerve. Injuries can be broadly classified as direct or indirect. Direct injuries usually involve direct anatomical disruption of the optic nerve caused by injuries to the head, face and orbit due to projectiles. Indirect injuries result from deforming forces applied to the bony orbit, or by motion of the globe, where the optic nerve absorbs energy concentrated at the orbital apex. These injuries are seen in the absence of open wounds but with a positive history of blunt frontal trauma. Incidence of traumatic optic neuropathy in facial trauma is 0.7 to 5 percent. Causes of traumatic optic neuropathy can be as varied as motor injuries, falls; falling debris; assaults trivial causes such as weightlifting as well as following endoscopic sinus surgery.

APPLIED ANATOMY

The optic nerve is the neural conduit linking inputs received from the retina to the brain (consisting of approximately 1.2 million axons) originating from the retinal ganglion cells. The nerve also contains oligodendrocytes which provide axonal myelination; microglia which are immunocompetent phagocytic cells and modulate apoptosis; and astrocytes. The nerve is enclosed within all three meningeal coats—a perineural sheath from the pia mater which also contains the blood vessels, an intermediate sheath from the arachnoid, and an outer sheath from the dura mater, which is also connected with the periosteum as it passes through the optic foramen. Optic nerve fenestration involves incision of the outer two coats surrounding the optic nerve. The total length is about 50 mm in length and is anatomically divided into:
- Intraocular (about 1 mm)
- Intraorbital (20–30 mm)

- Intracanalicular (5–11 mm)
- Intracranial (316 mm)

The optic nerve travels superomedially and passes through the annulus of Zinn to the entrance of the optic canal at the optic ring, which is located medial to the superior orbital fissure. The canal lies within the lesser wing of the sphenoid bone and is approximately 9 mm in length. The intraorbital portion of the nerve extends 18 mm from the posterior aspect of the globe to the orbital apex. The nerve measures between 20 and 30 mm, and therefore, takes a sinuous course, allowing for a range of movements by the eye. However, as the nerve enters the optic foramen its dural sheath becomes continuous with that lining the orbit and the optic foramen, rendering it immobile. This portion of the nerve, is the focus of forces encountered in head trauma and is the most common site of optic nerve injury. The intracranial portion of the optic nerve may suffer trauma when it is displaced superiorly against the sharp edge of the falciform dural fold. In addition, the anterior clinoid process lies lateral to the nerve, and when fractured, it can crush the nerve.

PRESENTATION AND EVALUATION

PRESENTATION

Traumatic optic neuropathy is a clinical diagnosis and it usually follows head trauma with or without a history of loss of consciousness. Patients of traumatic optic neuropathy usually present with reduced visual acuity which may be as profound as only light perception or even no light perception. In patients with relatively better visual acuity on presentation, loss of color vision is a common finding.

EVALUATION

Check list for evaluation

Check list for examing a patient with suspected traumatic optic neuropathy includes:
- Vision check
- Color vision (if vision permits)
- Pupillary evaluation
- Check for globe rupture, IOFB, fracture

- Fundus examination
- VEP
- ERG
- Neuroimaging (in case of suspected fracture)

Brief comments on evaluation

Patients who have suffered extensive head trauma must be neurologically examined and an ophthalmological examination should be performed only after stabilizing the patient.

Examiantion of eye and adnexa

The eye and the adnexa must be examined looking specifically for globe rupture, foreign bodies and fractures.

- *Pupillary reflexes* should be evaluated. The presence of an afferent papillary defect (APD) indicates the possibility of unilateral traumatic optic neuropathy.
- *Ocular motility* and *visual fields* should be evaluated, as possible.
- *Fundus examination* typically reveals a disc of normal appearance unless an avulsion or an anterior optic neuropathy is present. Furthermore, a ring of hemorrhage at the site of injury is indicative of partial or complete avulsion of the optic nerve head. Optic atrophy ensues usually after a period of 2 weeks to 3 months.

Electrophysiological tests

Visual-evoked potential

In comatose on unresponsive patients, a visual-evoked potentials (VEDP) may be needed in diagnosing traumatic optic neuropathy, especially when pupillary evaluation is not helpful, as in bilateral traumatic optic neuropathy.

In unilateral traumatic optic neuropathy, flash VEP amplitudes that are at least 50% of the normal eye are critical for a good visual outcome. An absent VEP response indicates that visual loss is complete, and recovery of vision may be unlikely, although reports have shown that patients with persistently negative VEPs may also show visual improvement.

Electroretinography

An absent electroretinogram (ERG) is associated with a poor potential for visual recovery.

Neuroimaging

A CT scan of the brain with fine cuts (axial sections of 1 to 1.5 mm) through the orbits should be sought. Coronal images are necessary to evaluate the optic canal properly and rule out a fracture. In patients with traumatic optic neuropathy, orbital fractures especially canal fractures have been associated with poorer visual acuity and a poor prognosis. MRI of the orbit may reveal focal edema of the optic nerve or optic nerve sheath enhancement with gadolinium.

PATHOPHYSIOLOGY OF TRAUMATIC OPTIC NEUROPATHY

Direct traumatic optic neuropathy

This is less common because the laxity of the intraorbital optic nerve allows for both absorption and deflection of the penetrating object. The resilience of the dura to penetration also offers further protection.

Indirect traumatic optic neuropathy

In more common and is believed to be caused by a primary and secondary mechanism of injury.

Primary mechanism While the optic nerve can be injured anywhere along its course, the most common site of injury is the intracanalicular part followed by the intracranial portion. Blunt trauma to the frontal bone result in forces being transmitted to the fixed intracanalicular segment of the optic nerve which can result in a fracture of the optic canal. As mentioned earlier, the tight adherence of the optic nerve's dural sheath to the periosteum within the optic canal causes the optic nerve to be vulnerable to the impact of skull injuries. Hemorrhage—either within the optic nerve sheath or in the orbital cavity can cause loss of optic nerve function. Mechanical forces are considered to be the primary mechanism of injury. These forces cause lacerations, partial or complete avulsion of the retrobulbar nerve (Fig. 14.1), contusion necrosis, and disruption of the nerve's vascular supply, resulting in hemorrhages, and thereby cause permanent damage.

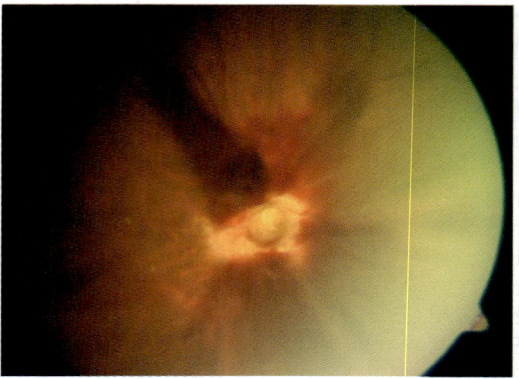

Fig. 14.1 *Fundus photography of a patient with optic nerve avulsion.*

Secondary mechanism. Once the vascularity of the optic nerve is disturbed, the secondary mechanisms of injury come into play. Edema sets in soon after and this in turn further compromises the vascular supply by causing a rise in intraluminal pressure. Secondary mechanisms that have been studied include numerous pathways for the generation of free radicals and arachidonic acids, lipid peroxidation, production of inflammatory mediators such as bradykinin, loss of calcium homeostasis with disruption of cellular function, glutamate-induced excitotoxicity, cell-mediated inflammation, and initiation of neuronal apoptosis. Most treatment modalities revolve around limiting the secondary injury with the hope of rescuing those axons which have survived the initial trauma.

TREATMENT OF TRAUMATIC OPTIC NEUROPATHY

Management of traumatic optic neuropathy remains controversial owing to a general lack of understanding of the pathophysiology involved and uncertainty about clinical results after therapeutic intervention. Three major therapeutic options for traumatic optic neuropathy exist:

• Corticosteroids

• Surgical optic nerve decompression

• Combination of the two.

ROLE OF STEROIDS

The use of systemic corticosteroids in traumatic optic neuropathy is currently thought to be the best form of treatment as opposed to none at all. It is hypothesized pathologic free radical reactions are initiated following major central nervous system trauma and that very high doses of corticosteroid functioned as antioxidants to inhibit free radical damage. Steroids as a form of therapy for traumatic optic neuropathy has been accepted after the results of National Acute Spinal Cord Injury Study (NASCIS 2) which showed positive results when systemic corticosteroids were used in patients of acute spinal cord trauma. NASCIS 2 was a multicenter, randomized, double-blind, placebo-controlled study involving patients with acute spinal cord injury, patients. These patients were randomly assigned to receive placebo, naloxone, or methylprednisolone within 12 hours of spinal injury. Intravenous methylprednisolone was given as an initial dose of 30 mg/kg followed by a continuous infusion of 5.4 mg/kg/h. When compared with placebo, treatment with methylprednisolone within 8 hours of injury resulted in a significant improvement in motor and sensory function.

However, whether the results of NASCIS can be extrapolated to justify the use of systemic corticosteroids in traumatic optic neuropathy needs to be further investigated. The International Optic Nerve Trauma Study, in which visual outcomes were compared with patients following observation alone, high dose steroids given within 7 days of the injury, and optic canal decompression with or without corticosteroids and performed within 7 days of the injury; showed no clear benefit for either corticosteroids or optic canal decompression in patients of traumatic optic neuropathy.

Other recent studies have also shown that there is no difference in visual acuity improvement between intravenous high-dose corticosteroids and placebo in treatment of recent traumatic optic neuropathy. Most recently, the corticosteroid randomization after significant head (CRASH) injury trial, a large randomized, placebo-controlled study, evaluated the effect of early administration of 48 hours infusion of methylprednisolone on the risk of death and disability after head injury. The investigators found a small but statistically significant increase in the risk of death within 2 weeks after head injury in the group allocated to corticosteroids compared with placebo. Furthermore, recently a Cochrane systematic review in 2007 critically analyzed the available evidence for the role of systemic steroids in traumatic optic neuropathy and showed that there were no convincing data of additional benefits of steroids over observation alone. The spontaneous improvement seen in many patients makes it difficult to assess the efficacy of any treatment method. Thus the use of corticosteroids in traumatic optic neuropathy continues to be a controversy.

SURGICAL MANAGEMENT

Optic canal decompression surgery has a limited role in the management of traumatic optic neuropathy. This treatment is based on the hypothesis that swelling in the optic canal may lead to a compartment syndrome. The increasing edema would decrease tissue perfusion to cause more postinjury ischemia to the optic nerve. This decompression procedure is believed to decrease edematous pressure in the optic canal to reverse ischemia and axonal conduction block, which can result in irreversible axonal degeneration. A variety of approaches have been described, including transfrontal craniotomy, and transethmoidal, transantral ethmoidal, sphenoethmoidal, and endoscopic decompression. The surgical approach should be based on the location of the pathology as visualized by CT scanning. The goal of optic nerve decompression is to provide surgical relief of pressure on the intracanalicular segment of the optic nerve. Nerve sheath hemorrhage occurs rarely and the images must be looked at together by an experienced neuroradiologist and clinician to avoid calling peri-sheath blood an intrasheath hemorrhage. If intrasheath blood is convincingly demonstrated, optic nerve sheath fenestration is indicated.

The corticosteroid randomization for acute head trauma study is immediately relevant to the treatment of traumatic optic neuropathy as individuals with traumatic optic neuropathy often have concomitant head trauma. However, it must be borne in mind that high-dose corticosteroids for traumatic optic neuropathy will result in a measurable loss of life in patients who also have a brain injury. Death has never been an endpoint for traumatic optic neuropathy studies. There is a school of thought that believes that since there is no class I evidence in its favor, corticosteroids should not be used to treat traumatic optic neuropathy. Optic canal decompression too has not established its usefulness unequivocally. Although significant advances have been made in the understanding of neuronal damage and repair, there is still no consensus among practitioners regarding the protocol for managing traumatic optic neuropathy. The diagnosis of traumatic optic neuropathy remains a clinical one. Clinicians must use their discretion to decide with the patient or family whether the implementation of medical or surgical intervention outweighs the risks.

RECENT ADVANCES AND CURRENT RESEARCH

It has been shown that the innate adaptive T cell mediated immune response directed against self-antigens located at the site of damage can be neuroprotective after optic nerve or injury. By augmenting this response in individuals who spontaneously manifest it and by inducing this autoimmune response in those incapable of manifesting it, optimal neurological functional recovery was attained. Research on neuritogenic and neurotropic agents such as monosial-ogangliosides and neurotropic growth factors has had promising results. Gene transfer of anti-inflammatory cytokines may help prevent neurodegeneration. Also, a new family of corticosteroids known as lazaroids or 21-amino-steroids provide the free radical-inhibiting properties of corticosteroids without their glucocorticoid activity.

BIBLIOGRAPHY

1. Agarwal A, Mahapatra AK. Visual outcome in optic nerve injury patients without initial light perception. Indian J Ophthalmol 1999;47(4): 233–6.

2. Bracken MB, Shepard MJ, Collins WF, et al. A randomized, controlled trial of methylpredniso-lone or naloxone in the treatment of acute spinal cord injury: Results of the Second National Acute Spinal Cord Injury Study. N Engl J Med 1999; 322:1405.

3. Bracken MB. CRASH (Corticosteroid Rando-mization after Significant Head Injury Trial): Landmark and storm warning. Neurosurgery 2005;57(6):1300–2.

4. Cornelius CP, Altenmuller E, Ehrenfeld M. The use of flash visual-evoked potentials in the early diagnosis of suspected optic nerve lesions due to craniofacial trauma. J Craniomaxillofac Surg 1996;24(1):1–11.

5. Entezari M, Rajavi Z, Sedighi N, et al. M. High-dose intravenous methylprednisolone in recent traumatic optic neuropathy: A randomized double-masked placebo-controlled clinical trial. Graefes Arch Clin Exp Ophthalmol 2007;245(9): 1267–71.

6. Gossman MD, Roberts DM, Barr CC. Ophthalmic aspects of orbital injury. Clin Plast Surg 1992;19(71):71–6.

7. Holmes MD, Sires BS. Flash visual-evoked potentials predict visual outcome in traumatic optic neuropathy. Ophthalmic Plast Reconstr Surg 2004;20(5):342–6.

8. Hughes B. Indirect injury of the optic nerve and chiasm. Bull Johns Hopkins Hospital 1962; 111(98):98–126.

9. Jayle GE, Tassy AF. Prognostic value of the electroretinogram in severe recent ocular trauma. Br J Ophthalmol 1970;54(1):51–8.

10. Kanski JJ. Clinical Ophthalmology: A Systemic Approach. Butterworth Heinemann, 6th, 2007; 786.

11. Kipnis J, Yoles E, Porat Z, et al. T cell immunity to copolymer 1 confers neuroprotection on the damaged optic nerve: possible therapy for optic neuropathies. Proc Natl Acad Sci USA 2000; 97(13):7446–51.

12. Koeberle PD, Gauldie J, Ball AK. Effects of adenoviral-mediated gene transfer of interleukin-10, interleukin-4 and transforming growth factor-beta on the survival of axotomized retinal ganglion cells. Neuroscience 2004;125(903): 903–20.

13. Levin LA, Baker RS. Management of traumatic optic neuropathy. J Neuro-ophthalmol 2003; 23(1):72–5.

14. Levin LA, Beck RW, Joseph MP, et al. The treatment of traumatic optic neuropathy: the International Optic Nerve Trauma Study. Ophthalmology 1999;106(7):1268–77.

15. Lindqvist N, Peinado-Ramónn P, Vidal-Sanz M, et al. GDNF, Ret, GFR alpha1 and 2 in the adult rat retino-tectal system after optic nerve transection. Exp Neurol 2004;187(2):487–99.

16. Steinsapir KD, Goldberg RA. Traumatic optic neuropathy: an evolving understanding. Am J Ophthalmol. 2nd edn. June 2011;151(6):928–33.

17. Steinsapir KD. Traumatic optic neuropathy. Curr Opin Ophthalmol 1999;10(5):340–2.

18. Steinsapir KD. Treatment of traumatic optic neuropathy with high-dose corticosteroid. J Neuro-ophthalmol 2006;26(1):65–7.

19. Vagefi MR, Seiff SR. Traumatic optic neuropathy. Contem Ophthal 2005;4(14):1–7.

20. Villa RF, Gorini A. Pharmacology of lazaroids and brain energy metabolism: A review. Pharmacol Rev 1997;49(1):99–136.

21. Wang BH, Robertson BC, Girotto JA, Liem A, Miller NR, Iliff N, Manson PN. Traumatic optic neuropathy: A review of 61 patients. Plast Reconstr Surg 2001;107(7):1655–64.

22. Yu-Wai-Man P, Griffiths PG. Steroids for traumatic optic neuropathy. Cochrane Database Syst Rev 2007;17(4):CD006032.

15 PAPILLEDEMA

Vijay Ananth

DEFINITION AND PATHOGENESIS

DEFINITION

Stauungspapille was the term used by Albrecht von Graefe in 1860 after his observation in four patients with brain tumor and swelling of the optic nerve head. Parsons was the person who coined the English term papilledema in 1908. **Papilledema is the bilateral optic disc edema that has been caused by elevated intracranial pressure**. Papilledema is an important physical sign and may be considered as a medical emergency. Papilledema the term should be not used for other forms of disc swelling caused by local or systemic processes like ischemic, compressive or inflammatory causes. They should be called as optic disc edema with reference to the etiology like anterior ischemic optic neuropathy, optic nerve meningioma, etc.

PATHOGENESIS

Papilledema is caused by intrinsic swelling of the ganglion cell axons because of stasis of axoplasmic flow in the prelaminar optic nerve (Fig. 15.1). High ICP causes this axoplasmic stasis, by direct compression of axons (mechanical theory) or by reduced perfusion of axons (ischemic theory). This explains why atrophic optic discs cannot swell when intracranial pressure is elevated. Hayreh in his experiments revealed that merely decompressing the nerve would reduce the disc edema even when the intracranial pressure was not reduced. This suggested that the intracranial pressure rather than the subarachnoid fluid was transmitted.

Development and resolution of papilledema

The rapidity of developing papilledema depends to a large extent on the etiology and degree of the increased ICP. Experimental models using inflatable balloons in the subarachnoid space of monkeys showed papilledema in 30% of the animals in 24 hours, in 50% after 2 days, and in 90% after 5 days. Clinical experience with humans suggests that the largest study investigating this process was performed in 37 patients with acutely elevated ICP from cerebral

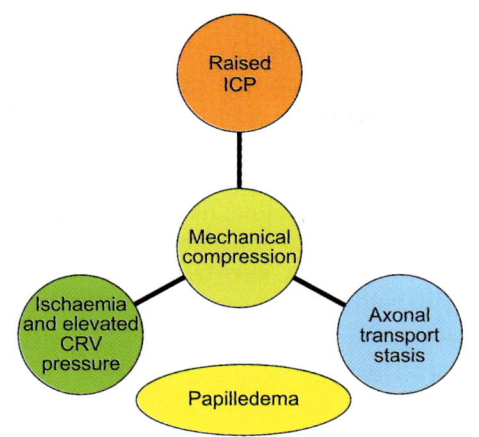

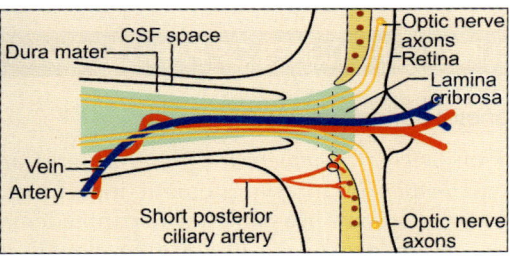

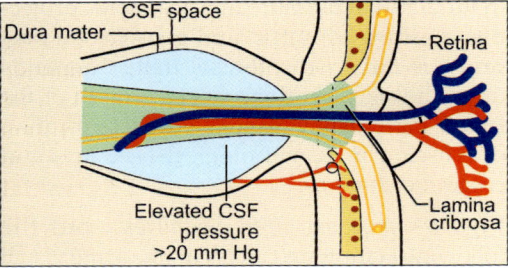

Fig. 15.1 *Pathogenesis of papilledema.*

successful treatment), none of 17 patients had papilledema. This experience suggests that clinically detectable papilledema is not usually present with acute elevations of ICP, and may take over a week to develop.

Fully developed papilledema may resolve completely within hours, days, or weeks, depending on the way in which ICP is lowered. In monkeys with experimental intracranial hypertension produced by an inflatable balloon, papilledema disappeared within 2 weeks after the intracranial pressure was abruptly normalized. In humans, papilledema can resolve 6–8 weeks after a successful craniotomy to remove a brain tumor or after subtemporal decompression for Idiopathic intracranial hypertension IIH. Optic disc edema may improve in less than a week following optic nerve sheath decompression surgery, but the time course to complete resolution is uncertain. Papilledema from IIH generally takes two or more months to resolve.

In most cases, retinal venous as well as disc capillary dilations begins to regress as soon as ICP is lowered to a normal level. During the next few days to weeks, presumably because of the change in hemodynamics at the disc, new hemorrhages may appear; however, these are of no significance and they disappear within a short time. Gradually, disc hyperemia and elevation resolve. The last abnormalities to disappear are blurring of the disc margins and abnormalities of the peripapillary retinal nerve fiber layer.

The unilateral finding is rare. However, well-documented cases of unilateral papilledema have been described and it is thought that the mechanism is one of, sheltering the uninvolved eye from the elevated pressure—due to an absence of the perineural subarachnoid space around the anterior portion of the optic nerve. This could be either developmental or acquired because of inflammatory scarring. When it is encountered, MRI scanning of the optic nerves is necessary to rule out other causes.

Causes of papilledema

Any elevation of intracranial pressure can result in papilledema. In this connection, it should be clear that spinal tumors can also cause papill-

hemorrhage or trauma receiving continuous ICP monitoring. Using both direct and indirect ophthalmoscopy, no papilledema was observed in the 13 patients with mildly elevated ICP and only two patients had venous congestion by day six. In seven patients with ICP ranging from 30 to 70 mm Hg, papilledema developed in one patient with a subarachnoid hemorrhage who developed fatal cerebral edema and carotid artery distribution infarction. No optic disc or fundus abnormalities were seen in the other six patients. Within the first three days of developing transient increased ICP (prior to

Table 15.1 *Common causes of papilledema*

Primary causes	*Secondary causes*
• Idiopathic intracranial pressure (IIH)	• Intracranial mass lesions • Obstruction of the path of cerebrospinal fluid (CSF) flow by a mass, stenosis, or other cause • Limitation of intracranial space by deformities of the skull • Cerebral edema caused by tumors, inflammation or toxic disorders • Increased rates of CSF production associated with tumors or inflammatory disorders • Impaired outflow of CSF, e.g. caused by increased viscosity of the CSF, due to protein formation by a tumor or inflammation • Elevated pressure in the venous sinuses that drain the CSF

edema. Common causes of papilledema are listed in Table 15.1.

Idiopathic intracranial hypertension (IIH)

The diagnostic criteria of idiopathic intracranial hypertension (IIH) according to the modified Dandy criteria, include symptoms of elevated ICP such as headache, signs of elevated ICP such as papilledema, confirmation of an elevated opening pressure (at least 250 mm H_2O) by lumbar puncture with normal CSF contents, absence of localizing neurological signs (with the exception of an abducens paresis and occasionally a fourth nerve paresis), and normal neuro-imaging—apart from signs consistent with elevated intracranial pressure, like an empty sella turcica.

Risk factors of IIH

Risk factors for IIH are listed below:
- Idiopathic
- Obesity

- Pregnancy and postpartum period without sinus thrombosis (20%)
- Endocrine disorders, e.g. (Addison's disease, Cushing's syndrome, corticosteroid withdrawal, hypothyroidism, hypo or hyperparathyroidism, Turner's syndrome, adrenal adenoma)
- Drugs, e.g. tetracycline, nalidixic acid, nitrofurantoin, penicillin, amiodarone, non-steroidal anti-inflammatory agents, lithium, corticosteroids both in high doses and on withdrawal])
- Hypervitaminoses
- Associated hematologic disorders (chronic myeloid leukemia, polycythemia, iron deficiency anemia)

CLINICAL FEATURES OF PAPILLEDEMA

General considerations

- *Papilledema is sometimes found at routine examination* in an asymptomatic individual. Most symptoms in a patient with papilledema are secondary to the underlying elevation in intracranial pressure like headache, projectile vomiting, tinnitus, and mass lesion may produce focal neurological defect depends upon the size, location, rate of growth of the lesion. Patient may present with deterioration of consciousness, neurological—seizures and cognitive changes.

- *Visual symptoms often are absent,* but the following symptoms can occur like acute visual disturbance, transient visual obscuration, field defect, gradual peripheral visual loss and diplopia.

Headache

Headaches caused by stretching of pain sensitive intracranial structure, like dura and proximal part of large pial vessels. The typical feature of headache in patient with raised ICT are headache that is worst upon awakening and increased with Valsalva's maneuver where as tension headaches are not affected at all. A study showed that morning headache is only present in about one-third of patients with tumors and this is specific for feature of raised ICT.

Visual complaints

Transient visual obscuration (TVO)

As papilledema worsens, patients may experience brief, transient obscurations of vision. During these episodes, vision may vary from mild blurring to complete blindness. Some patients describe a rapid gray-out of vision, whereas others experience positive visual phenomena, such as photopsias and phosphenes that obscure their vision. In all cases, however, recovery of vision is invariably rapid and complete. The obscurations may affect either eye or both eyes simultaneously. They usually last only a few seconds, although attacks lasting several hours rarely occur. The episodes may occur up to 20 to 30 times a day, and are often precipitated by changes in posture, particularly from a bent-over position. The proposed mechanism for this symptom could be due to chiasmal compression by expanding III ventricle, increased ICP which alters orbital blood flow, optic nerve head ischemia or occipital ischemia due to uncal herniation.

Optic nerve functions like vision, color vision and fields are usually well preserved with acute papilledema and this one of the main differentiating factor from the other optic neuropathies. In late stages, visual functions are compromised due to chronic papilledema—the axon no longer receives its nourishment from the axoplasmic flow and dies. The result is loss of neural function and optic atrophy sets in.

In acute stage of papilledema, visual disturbance like visual reduction and metamorphopsia can happen secondary to macular exudation or optic nerve head ischemia (Fig. 15.2).

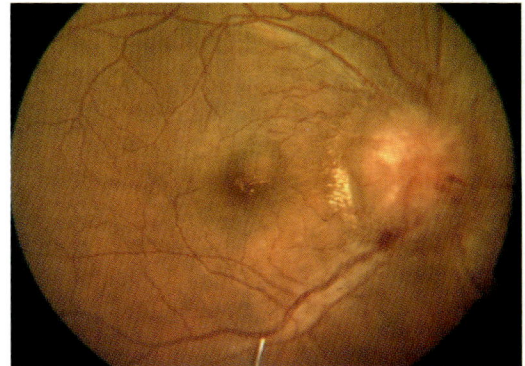

Fig. 15.2 *Acute visual loss in papilledema.*

Diplopia/False localizing sign

The most common cause of diplopia from increased ICP is lateral rectus palsy, as one or both abducens nerves are compressed against one of the transverse branches of the basilar artery at the base of the skull. Infrequently, III and IV palsies occur in patients with increased ICP, presumably from compression of either the dorsal midbrain or the nerves themselves.

Disc findings

Early stage of papilledema (Fig. 15.3)

There is blurring of the disc margin and elevation of the disc in the nasal half. Capillary ectasias are visible on the surface of the disc, and the peripapillary nerve fiber layer has lost its clarity, consistent with the fact that the "edema" is intrinsic to the nerve fibers themselves. Small hemorrhages can be present.

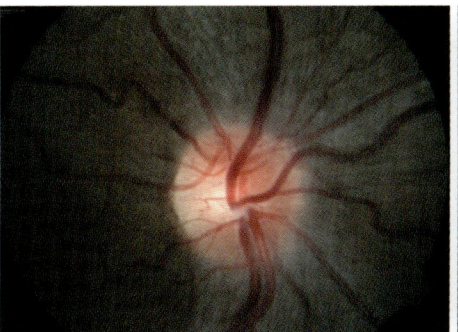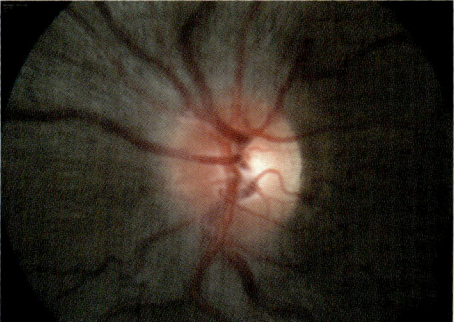

Fig. 15.3 *Early papilledema.*

Fully developed papilledema (Fig. 15.4)

Elevation, blurring, and hemorrhages have worsened, and exudates are now visible. The physiologic cup is usually preserved.

Chronic papilledema (Fig. 15.5)

The hemorrhages and exudates have subsided, being replaced by small glistening deposits. The physiologic cup has disappeared. Cilioretinal collateral vessels can appear at this stage. Small, concentric, retinal folds can appear in the peripapillary fundus (Paton's lines).

Atrophic papilledema (Fig. 15.6)

Peripapillary retinal vessels are attenuated and sheathing dirty white appearance due to gliosis secondary optic atrophy.

Recognition of Paton's lines is difficult only because it is a subtle sign that will probably be missed if the observer does not specifically check for it. It is one of the surest signs of true disc edema. The lines appear on the temporal side of the disc and are in a vertical direction concentric with the disc (Fig. 15.6).

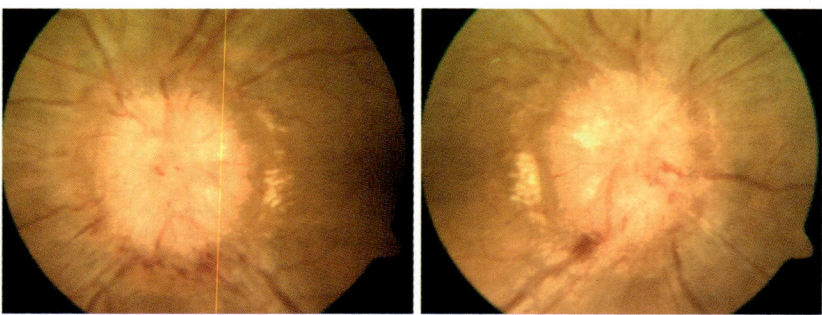

Fig. 15.4 *Established stage.*

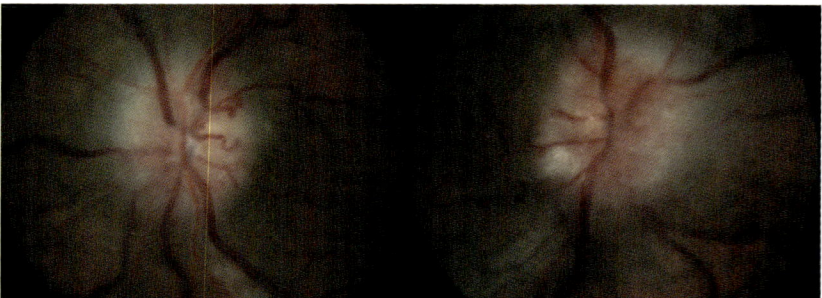

Fig. 15.5 *Chronic stage.*

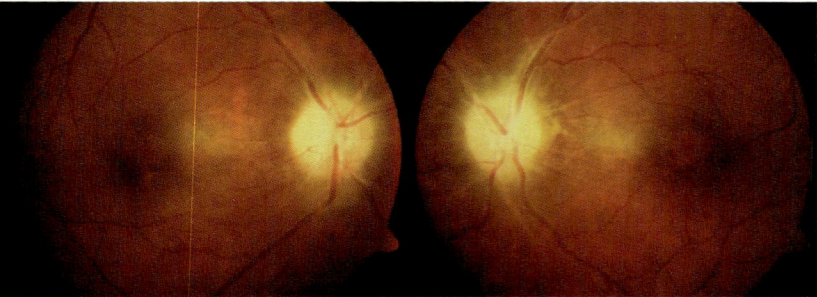

Fig. 15.6 *Atrophic papilledema.*

As the disc swells, a slight displacement of the retina away from the temporal edge of the disc occurs, causing the retina to fold on itself, or corrugate. This folding, in turn, causes a variation of the reflection from the internal limiting membrane, which is seen as Paton's lines. As the edema increases, this area becomes edematous and Paton's lines are no longer seen. Any cause of edema can produce Paton's lines, so that their presence signifies only edema.

Spontaneous venous pulses are an important diagnostic criterion. It is always absent in the presence of papilledema. If it is visible, it is a reliable sign that intracranial pressure (ICP) is normal. The presence of venous pulses is a good sign, since it rules out elevated pressure *at the time of the examination*, but it does not exclude the possibility of there being intermittent elevations in ICP. The absence of spontaneous venous pulses is of no help, since at least 20% of healthy people do not show venous pulsations.

Field defects

Concentric enlargement of the blind spot is the most common and frequently the only visual field defect in patients with papilledema, (Fig. 15.7). Compression, detachment, and lateral displacement of the peripapillary retina appear to be the major reasons that the blind spot increases in size in patients with papilledema. In this setting, the enlarged blind spot represents a refractive scotoma caused by acquired peripapillary hyperopia. In chronic papilledema, the inferior nasal quadrant is most often affected can produce central and arcuate scotoma (Fig. 15.7), and may progress to form ring scotomas. Visual acuity usually deteriorates late in the course of the disease. The defects can be reversed if ICP is lowered before chronic

papilledema develops. As with loss of visual acuity, loss of visual field is usually slow and progressive. Sudden loss of visual field suggests a superimposed local cause such as ischemia.

MANAGEMENT OF PIPILLEDEMA

Management of pipilledema includes:
- Differential diagnosis,
- Investigations, and
- Treatment

DIFFERENTIAL DIAGNOSIS

Papilledema need to be differentiated from following conditions:
- Anomalously elevated optic disc
  - With and without buried drusen
  - Tilted optic disc
  - Hypoplastic optic disc
- Intraocular inflammation
- Asymptomatic non-arteritic anterior ischemic optic neuropathy
- Hypertensive disc edema and optic neuritis, optic perineuritis (perioptic neuritis)
- Infiltrative optic neuropathy (e.g. from leukemia)
- Compressive optic neuropathy (e.g. from optic nerve sheath meningioma)

INVESTIGATIONS

Papilledema is a medical emergency that requires immediate attention. Documentation of the pupillary findings, oculomotor function, and visual field examination should be completed as soon as possible. At the same time it is very important to the ophthalmologist to rule out pseudopapilledema. Noninvasive refined methods like proper disc examination, ultrasound eye, OCT investigation will help to rule out anomalous elevated optic disc prior to referral of patients for potentially hazardous and often unnecessary neuroradiological investigations.

When trying to differentiate papilledema from buried ONH drusen ultrasound and CT scan are useful tools that can demonstrate calcification.

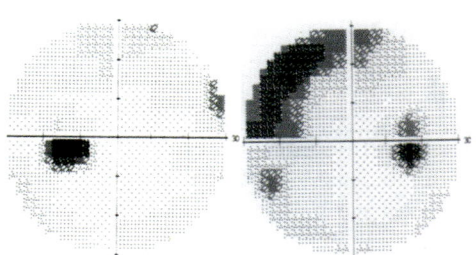

Fig. 15.7 *Common field defects in papilledema.*

Fundus fluorescein angiography

Fundus fluorescein angiography (FFA) is not indicated in papilledema may helpful in differentiating from pseudopapilledema like autofluorescence—seen disc drusen.

FFA in papilledema

- *A-V phase*—shows dilated capillaries, micro-aneureysms on the surface disc
- *Venous phase*—leak from superficial dilated capillaries
- *Late phase*—hyperfluorescence of the superficial and deep portions of the optic disc

Optical coherence tomography

Role of optical coherence tomography (OCT) in papilledema is not well established but studies has shown that it can help to differentiate from pseudopapilledema. Johnson et al. evaluated OCT scans using time domain—OCT from 20 patients with papilledema, 20 patients with nerve head drusen, and 20 control subjects were used to identify qualitative and quantitative features. Quantitatively, the mean RNFL thickness was significantly greater in patients with papilledema compared with those who had pseudopapilledema and controls.

Neuroimaging

Neuroimaging should initially be focused on ruling out evidence of intracranial disease, such as mass lesions or hydrocephalus. Magnetic resonance imaging (MRI) and magnetic resonance venography (MRV) are, at present, the imaging studies of choice for detecting IIH. MRI is superior to computed tomography (CT) scan in detecting a sinus or venous thrombosis, certain malignancies, gliomatosis cerebri, and meningeal abnormalities.

In atypical patients (slim patients, children, and men), MRV should be considered. Neuroimaging results should be normal in IIH except for signs of ICP. The ventricles should be of normal to small size, and the following signs of raised ICP may be found: flattening of the posterior sclera empty sella distention of the perioptic subarachnoidal space enhancement of the prelaminar optic nerve and intraocular protrusion of the prelaminar optic nerve.

Lumbar puncture

If the scan is normal, the next step is a lumbar puncture to determine the CSF pressure and confirm normal CSF chemistry (no protein elevation, no pleocytosis). Normal cerebrospinal fluid (CSF) pressure in adults, measured by lumbar puncture with the patient in the lateral decubitus position, varies between 80 and 200 mm of water. Contrary to popular belief, CSF pressure is not dependent on weight or height although pressure readings may be spuriously elevated when the patient coughs, strains, or holds his or her breath during the procedure. Measurements between 201 and 249 mm water are not diagnostic and those greater than 250 mm water are elevated. Normal values have not been well established in children but are generally accepted to be 200 mm water or less. If these conditions are met, one is dealing with IIH.

TREATMENT

Management should be focused upon the primary cause specific therapy should be directed to the underlying mass lesion if present. Management of IIH is determined by the degree of vision loss and the progression of visual dysfunction as assessed primarily by visual acuity and visual field examinations. Lowering the CSF pressure, whether by medical or surgical means, to protect vision by averting a potentially blinding optic neuropathy.

Medical treatment

Acetazolamide, a sulfa-derived diuretic and carbonic anhydrase inhibitor, that reduces CSF production, often is used as the first-line therapeutic agent for IIH. The starting dose recommended in adults 250 mg DID and in children is 25 mg/kg per day, which may be increased to 100 mg/kg per day (maximum, 2 g/d). Well-recognized adverse effects of acetazolamide include gastrointestinal upset, metallic taste, tingling of the lips and digits, loss of appetite, electrolyte imbalances, metabolic acidosis, and nephrocalcinosis. Acetazolamide is contraindicated in the presence of sulfonamide allergy and significant renal or liver disease.

Furosemide, a loop diuretic, can be used in combination with or as an alternative to aceta-zolamide if there is an intolerance of or contraindication to this drug. The effect of furosemide on CSF production is weaker than that of acetazolamide. The most common adverse effects are electrolyte imbalances, dehydration, and hypotension. The risk of hypokalemia increases when diuretics are combined. The suggested dose of furosemide is 1 mg/kg per day. Weight loss is advised for obese patients based on retrospective analyses indicating that a modest degree of weight loss (approximately 6% of body weight) correlates with a reduction in papilledema. Weight reduction should be considered a long-term management solution and is not useful as a sole treatment modality for patients with acute visual loss.

Surgical treatment

If the CSF pressure cannot be controlled quickly by medications, immediate surgical intervention should be considered. No randomized controlled studies have compared CSF diversion procedures to optic nerve sheath decompression. The choice of procedures depends largely on personal experience and the availability of resources. Both types of surgery appear to be effective. Lumboperitoneal and ventriculo-peritoneal shunts have been recommended in the treatment of IIH. No strong evidence supports one procedure over the other. Recently published data suggests that the choice of shunting procedure depends on the surgeon's preference.

Follow-up

Recovery of the optic disc appearance after correction of the elevated intracranial pressure can take many weeks.

The subjective evaluation of the optic nerve head appearance is an important factor that is used in the consideration of the success or failure of medical therapy. Although the degree of disc edema cannot be used to predict the extent of vision loss, higher-grade papilledema does correlate with an increased risk for more profound loss of central acuity and visual field.

Patients with chronic papilledema require regular ophthalmic follow-up examinations to monitor their vision, including careful perimetry and to rule out signs of impending destruction of the optic nerve. The effectiveness of OCT as a quantitative measure that may be used to reflect the severity of disease and the response to treatment in IIH has been described. The highly quantitative measurements also make it possible to judge the effect of treatment along with subjectively interpreting the funduscopic appearance of the optic nerve heads.

Although few longitudinal studies of patients with IIH have been published to date, it appears that there may be a correlation between RNFL thickness and visual function. With the new spectral domain OCT, additional parameters of the optic nerve imaging, including volume and height measurements, might provide greater sensitivity of the response to treatment and the long-term visual outcome in patients with IIH. Proper early diagnosis of papilledema may be a life and vision saving and excluding the diagnosis of papilledema helps needless investigation and surgical procedure.

BIBLIOGRAPHY

1. Bettman JW (Jr), Daroff RB, Sanders MD, et al. Papilledema and symptomatic intracranial hypertension in systemic lupus erythematosus. Arch Ophthalmol 1968;80:180–93.
2. Bird AC, Sanders MD. Choroidal folds in association with papilledema. Br J Ophthalmol 1973;57:89–97.
3. Brodsky MC, Vaphiades M. Magnetic resonance imaging in pseudotumor cerebri. Ophthalmol 1998;105:1686–93.
4. Cobbs WH, Schatz NJ, Savino PJ. Midbrain eye signs in hydrocephalus. Ann Neurol 1978;4:172.
5. Corbett JJ, Jacobson DM, Mauer RC, et al. Enlargement of the blind spot caused by papilledema. Am J Ophthalmol 1988;105:261–5.
6. Corbett JJ, Mehta MP. Cerebrospinal fluid pressure in normal obese subjects and patients with pseudotumor cerebri. Neurology 1983; 33:1386–8.
7. Forsyth PA, Posner JB. Headaches in patients with brain tumors: A study of 111 patients. Neurology 1993;43:1678–83.
8. Friedman DI, Jacobson DM. Diagnostic criteria for idiopathic intracranial hypertension. Neurology 2002;59:1492–5.
9. Grehn F, Knorr-Held S, Kommerell G. Glaucomatous-like visual field defects in chronic papilledema. Graefe's Arch Ophthalmol 1981;21:99–109.

10. Halpern JI, Gordon WH (Jr). Trochlear nerve palsy as a false localizing sign. Ann Ophthalmol 1981;12:53–6.

11. Hamed LM, Tse DT, Glaser JS, et al. Neuro-imaging of the optic nerve after fenestration for management of pseudotumor cerebri. Arch Ophthalmol 1992;110d:636–9.

12. Hayreh MS, Hayreh SS. Optic disc edema in raised intracranial pressure I. Evolution and resolution. Arch Ophthalmol 1977;95:1237–44.

13. Hayreh SS, Hayreh MS. Optic disc edema in raised intracranial presure II. Early detection with fluorescein fundus angiography and stereoscopic color photography. Arch Ophthalmol 1977;95:1245–54.

14. Hayreh SS. Pathogenesis of oedema of the optic disc (Papilledema). Br J Ophthalmol 1964; 48:522–43.

15. Huna-Baron R, Landau K, Rosenberg M, et al. Unilateral swollen disc due to increased intracranial pressure. Neurology 2001;56(11):1588–90.

16. Johnson LN, Diehl ML, Hamm CW, et al. Differentiating optic disc edema from optic nerve head drusen on optical coherence tomography. Arch Ophthalmol 2009;127:45–9.

17. Johnson LN, Krohel GB, Madsen RW, March GA. The role of weight loss and acetazolamide in the treatment of idiopathic intracranial hypertension (pseudotumor cerebri). Ophthalmology 1998;105:2313–7.

18. Lueck C, McIlwaine G. Interventions for idiopathic intracranial hypertension. Cochrane Database Syst Rev 2002.

19. Parsons JH. The pathology of the eye. New York, Putnam 1908; 4:1349–64.

20. Paton L. Optic neuritis in cerebral tumours. Trans Ophthalmol Soc UK 1908;28.

21. Shoeman JF. Childhood pseudotumor cerebri: clinical and intracranial pressure response to acetazolamide and furosemide treatment in case series. J Child Neurol 1994;9:130–4.

22. Steffen H, Eifert B, Aschoff A, et al. The diagnostic value of optic disc evaluation in acute elevated intracranial pressure. Ophthalmology 1996;103:1229–323.

23. Use of Optical Coherence Tomography to Evaluate Papilledema and Pseudopapilledema. Gena Heidary and Joseph F. Rizzo Seminars in Ophthalmology 2010;25(5-6):198–205.

24. Walsh and Hoyt Clinical neuro-ophthalmology 6th edition; 236–91.

16 OPTIC ATROPHY

Devendra V Venkatramani, Rashmin A Gandhi

DEFINITION AND EPIDEMIOLOGY
- Definition
- Epidemiology

ETIOPATHOLOGICAL PROFILE
- Etiology
- Histopathological changes

CLINICAL PROFILE
Clinical Features
Ophthalmoscopic Features
- Disc pallor
- Other disc features
- Other fundus findings

INVESTIGATIVE PROFILE
- Perimetry
- Neuroimaging
- Electrodiagnostic tests
- Second line tests

PROGNOSIS AND MANAGEMENT
- Treatment of underlying cause
- Neuroprotective agents
- Stem cell therapy
- Rehabilitation

DEFINITION AND EPIDEMIOLOGY

DEFINITION

The term optic atrophy denotes a clinico-pathological entity characterized by a change in color and structure of the optic disc associated with impaired optic nerve function. Optic atrophy, is therefore, a sign of (underlying or past) disease affecting the optic nerve, and is not a diagnosis in itself.

Some authors believe that the term 'atrophy' should be reserved for tissues that have a potential for regeneration, and hence strictly may not be applied to the optic nerve; however, the term is firmly entrenched in medical parlance.

The visual pathway begins with the photo-receptors, from where impulses travel via the bipolar cells to the ganglion cells. The axons of the ganglion cells, through the retinal nerve fiber layer, converge from all quadrants in a specific topographic manner to the optic nerve head. These fibers form the optic nerve and lead all the way up to the lateral geniculate bodies (*retinogeniculate pathway*). The optic nerve contains approximately 1.2 million such axons, which possess a myelin sheath and do not regenerate once damaged. Optic atrophy is the end result of any disease that causes degeneration of axons of the ganglion cells.

Anterograde degeneration (Wallerian degeneration) begins in the retina and proceeds toward the lateral geniculate body (e.g. toxic retinopathy, chronic simple glaucoma). Retrograde degeneration proceeds toward the optic disc from further down in the course of the optic nerve (e.g. optic nerve compression by intracranial tumor). It is important to note that postgeniculate lesions of the visual pathway do not result in optic atrophy.

EPIDEMIOLOGY

Optic atrophy can occur at any age group and affects both sexes. Population-based studies have found the prevalence of optic atrophy in bilaterally blind adults to be 3.42 to 8%.

ETIOPATHOLOGICAL PROFILE

ETIOLOGY

As mentioned, a plethora of diseases can result in optic atrophy (Table 16.1).

HISTOPATHOLOGIC CHANGES IN OPTIC ATROPHY

Notable histopathologic findings include deepening of the disc cup with baring of the lamina cribrosa, loss of both myelin and axons, glial cell proliferation, and widening of the subarachnoid space with redundant dura.

Table 16.1 *Causes of optic atrophy*	
Inflammatory	Demyelinating Post-viral illness Auto-immune
Ischemic	Non-arteritic Arteritic
Infiltrative	(Sarcoidosis, Systemic malignancy, Leukemia)
Post-papilledema	Including idiopathic intracranial hypertension (IIH)
Compressive	
Traumatic	
Toxic/Nutritional	Tobacco-alcohol amblyopia Drugs and medication
Hereditary	Mendelian (autosomal dominant, autosomal recessive) Mitochondrial (Leber hereditary optic neuropathy)
Miscellaneous optic nerve diseases	Radiation induced, para-neoplastic syndrome
Retinal pathology	Long-standing retinal detachment Post pan-retinal photo-coagulation Retinal degenerations Vascular occlusions
Glaucoma	

CLINICAL PROFILE

CLINICAL FEATURES

- *Visual acuity* is reduced, occasionally to no light perception.
- *Color vision* is also likely to be abnormal, red-green defects seen in neuropathies and blue-yellow defects in retinopathies (Kollner's rule), a notable exception being glaucoma.
- *Relative afferent pupillary defect* (RAPD) is a hallmark of unilateral or asymmetric afferent sensory abnormality. Occasionally it is the only objective sign elicited. RAPD can be quantitatively graded by balancing the defect using neutral density filters or can be graded clinically.
- *Extraocular movements* may show limitation in cases with compressive neuropathy due to an orbital mass, or in superior orbital fissure syndrome due to compression of ocular motor nerves and the optic nerve. Neighbouring cranial nerve examination may localize a compressive lesion.
- *Confrontation testing* is a good method of assessing the visual field. Desaturation of a red target within the visual field may be more sensitive to pick up localized areas of dysfunction (relative scotoma).
- *Other special tests* include contrast sensitivity (by Pelli-Robson chart or the Vistech chart), and Pulfrich phenomenon (a pendulum oscillating in a plane perpendicular to the visual axes appears to move in an elliptical path rather than in a flat plane).

OPHTHALMOSCOPIC FEATURES

Disc pallor

When light falls on the retinal nerve fibers, it undergoes total internal reflection, followed by reflection from optic disc surface capillaries. This is responsible for the orange-pink color of the normal optic disc. There are two postulated reasons for disc pallor in optic atrophy; one, the loss of the optical properties due to axonal degeneration, and two, an actual reduction in the capillary density of the optic nerve head. The Kestenbaum sign is a clinical indicator of optic nerve damage. It is the number of capillaries that can be counted on the optic disc surface. The normal number is around 10; less than 6 indicates optic atrophy.

- *Band-shaped or bow-tie atrophy* occurs due to damage to the contralateral optic tract. It is seen as a pale, horizontal, central strip along the superior and inferior poles of the optic disc. The other eye (ipsilateral to the lesion) may show temporal pallor, complete loss of the nasal hemifield, and an afferent pupillary defect.

- *Temporal pallor of the disc* may be physiological, when it appears to blend in with the surrounding areas. A more wedge-shaped segment of temporal pallor is seen if afflictions of the papillomacular bundle, such as toxic/nutritional neuropathy, optic neuritis, and hereditary optic neuropathy.

- *Segmental pallor of the optic disc* is common in ischemic neuropathy (non-arteritic), reflecting the segmental nature of vascular supply. In arteritic anterior ischemic optic neuropathy the disc appears chalky white.

Other disc features

'Primary' optic atrophy occurs without antecedent disc swelling or inflammation. There is a more organized manner of neuronal loss, with an orderly replacement with glial cells. There is no major change in the nerve head architecture. Importantly, disc margins are well demarcated, and retinal vessels are normal (Fig. 16.1A). Causes include compressive lesions like pituitary and optic nerve tumors, and traumatic optic neuropathy.

Secondary optic atrophy occurs subsequent to disc swelling. It is characterized by prolifera-

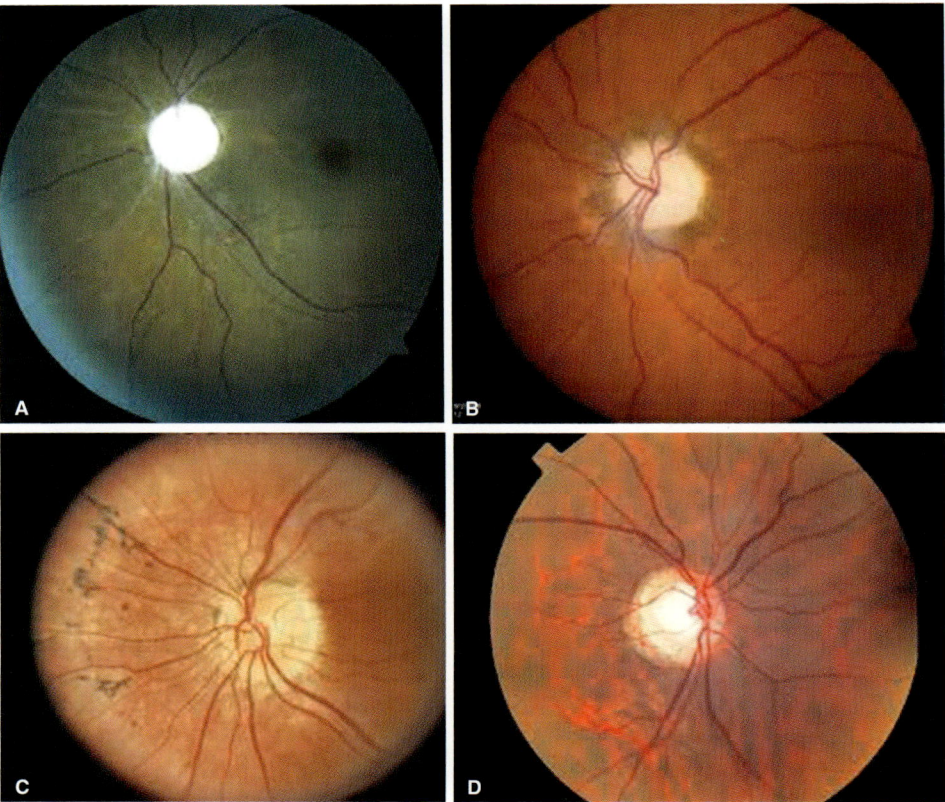

Fig. 16.1 *Ophthalmoscopic features of: (A) Primary optic atrophy; (B) Secondary optic atropy; (C) Consecutive optic atrophy; and (D) Glaucomatous optic atrophy.*

tion of glial tissue, which causes obscuration of the disc margins, the lamina cribrosa, and imparts a dirty grey color to the disc (Fig. 16.1B). Causes include post-papilledema atrophy, and papillitis.

Consecutive optic atrophy sets in as a consequence of retinal pathology. Features include waxy pallor of the disc, arteriolar attenuation, and a normal physiological cup and disc margins (Fig. 16.1C). Important causes are retinitis pigmentosa, retinal vascular occlusions, post pan-retinal photocoagulation, and pathological myopia.

Glaucomatous ('cavernous') optic atrophy shows marked cupping along with vertical enlargement of cup, exposure of lamina cribrosa pores, bayoneting and nasal shifting of the retinal vessel, and peripapillary atrophy (Fig. 16.1D). Severe atrophy is called bean-pot cupping, due to the cross-sectional appearance.

Other fundus findings

One should look for retinal nerve fiber layer defects, peripapillary atrophy (beta zone), and the caliber and tortuosity of blood vessels.

INVESTIGATIVE PROFILE

Perimetry

Visual field changes can include enlargement of the blind spot, central and caecocentral scotomata, altitudinal defects, and constricted fields in chronic papilledema.

Neuroimaging

In selected cases imaging may be indicated.
- *Orbital ultrasonography* is a simple and inexpensive technique in cases of suspected compression.
- *Non-contrast computerized tomography* (CT) scan is recommended in suspected orbital tumors and traumatic neuropathy.
- *Gadolinium-enhanced magnetic resonance imaging* (MRI) or utilizing a fluid-attenuated inversion recovery (FLAIR) sequence is useful to detect hyperintense foci of demyelinating plaques. In patients with demyelinating disease.

Electrodiagnostic tests

- *Electroretinogram* (ERG) is indicated in suspected retinal pathologies such as retinitis pigmentosa and vascular occlusions. The pattern ERG helps to distinguish between optic neuropathy and a maculopathy.
- *Visual-evoked potential* (VEP) in eyes with optic neuritis shows an increased latency of the P100 wave which persists even after visual recovery.
- *Multifocal testing strategies* provide a topographical representation of dysfunction.

Second-line tests

- Unexplained optic atrophy should be investigated to detect a potentially life-threatening disease.
- These tests include blood pressure, cardiovascular examination, blood glucose levels, carotid Doppler ultrasound study, serological tests for syphilis, serum vitamin B_{12} levels, anti-nuclear antibody levels, tests for sarcoidosis (serum angiotensin converting enzyme, serum lysozyme, serum calcium), antiphospholipid antibodies, and plasma homocysteine.
- In selected cases, enzyme-linked assays for toxoplasmosis, rubella, cytomegalovirus, herpes simplex virus (TORCH panel) may be carried out.

PROGNOSIS AND MANAGEMENT

- *No specific treatment* exists for optic atrophy as neuronal tissue cannot regenerate once damaged.
- *Treatment of underlying cause.* Focus of diagnosis is to detect a specific underlying cause which may be treatable, e.g. autoimmune disease. Optic atrophy may be the presenting sign of life-threatening illness such as an intracranial tumor. In some instances treatment is aimed at preventing similar vision loss in the other eye, for example, arteritic anterior ischemic optic neuropathy associated with giant cell arteritis. There may be some recovery of visual function in

patients with compressive and toxic neuro-pathies.

- *Neuroprotective agents* like ginkgo biloba have been tried with anecdotal success. Often, vitamin supplementation in the form of vitamins B_1 (thiamine), B_6 (pyridoxine), and B_{12} (cyanocobalamine) are prescribed empiri-cally.
- *Stem-cell therapy* may allow optic nerve regeneration in the not-too-distant future.
- *Rehabilitation.* Patient counseling, vocational training, and low-vision aids should be considered for rehabilitation.

BIBLIOGRAPHY

1. Kerr NM, Chew SSL, Eady EK, et al. Diagnostic accuracy of confrontation visual field tests. Neurology 2010; 74:1184–90.

2. Kestenbaum A. Clinical Methods of Neuro-ophthalmologic Examination: New York. Grune & Stratton 1946;81.

3. N. Accornero N, Rinalduzzi S, Capozza M, et al. Computerized color perimetry in multiple sclerosis. Multiple Sclerosis 1998;4:79–84.

4. Sadun A, Agarwal MR. Topical Diagnosis of Acquired Optic Nerve Disorders. In: Walsh & Hoyt's Clinical Neuro-ophthalmology. Miller NR, Newman NJ (Eds). 6th edn. Philadelphia: JB Lippincott; pp 208–18.

5. Thulasiraj RD, Nirmalan PK, Ramakrishnan R, et al. Blindness and Vision Impairment in a Rural South Indian Population: The Aravind Comprehensive Eye Survey. Ophthalmology 2003;110:1491–8.

6. Vijaya L, George R, Arvind H, et al. Prevalence and causes of blindness in the rural population of the Chennai Glaucoma Study. Br J Ophthalmol 2006;90:407–10.

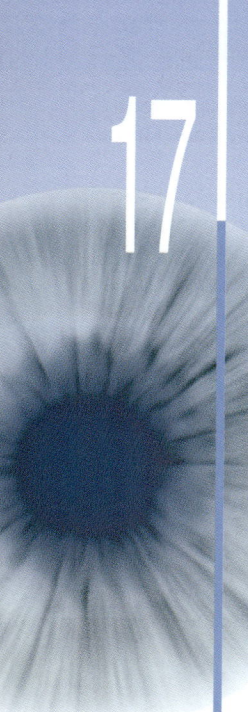

17 | TUMORS OF OPTIC NERVE

Akshay G Nair, Rashmin A Gandhi

INTRODUCTION

Optic nerve tumors are classified into those arising from the optic nerve matter and those arising from the surrounding sheath. These tumors are difficult to treat and manage owing to the high risk of damage to the optic nerve itself.

CLASSIFICATION

Primary tumors of the optic nerve
• Benign optic nerve glioma
• Malignant optic nerve glioma
• Ganglioglioma
• Medulloepithelioma
• Haemangioblastoma

Tumors of the optic nerve sheath
• Optic nerve sheath meningioma
  – Primary
  – Secondary
• Schwannoma
• Hemangiopericytoma
  More than 90% of primary optic nerve tumors are either benign gliomas of childhood or optic

nerve sheath meningiomas. These two commonly seen tumors will be discussed in this chapter.

Optic nerve gliomas comprise about 1% of all intracranial tumors. Optic nerve gliomas are of two different types—one being the juvenile benign pilocytic astrocytoma and the other being the malignant glioblastoma of adulthood.

OPTIC NERVE GLIOMAS

BENIGN OPTIC NERVE GLIOMA

These benign tumors usually present in the first decade of life. They are almost always unilateral and occur more frequently in females than in males. While the incidence may be sporadic or sometimes familial; most of the patients presenting with optic nerve gliomas have neurofibromatosis (NF) type 1. Reports have shown varying levels of incidence of NF1 among patients of optic nerve glioma: 10 to 70%; where as the incidence of optic nerve glioma in patients with NF1 varies from 8 to 31%.

Clinical features

1. **Proptosis.** Proptosis is usually gradual, often associated with infradisplacement of the globe caused by the fusiform from tumour (Fig. 17.1).

2. **Pain.** Optic nerve gliomas are usually painless. However, on rare occasions, a patient may present with acute loss of vision. This is associated with development or worsening of proptosis which results from hemorrhage into the tumor.

3. **Fundus findings.** Optic disc swelling or pallor, visual acuity loss, visual field loss and relative afferent pupillary defect are seen due to compressive effects of the tumor. The tumor eventually causes optic nerve atrophy because of pressure effects on the nerve fibers as well as the nutrient arteries.

4. **Strabismus**—both primary and secondary are seen, along with restriction of extraocular muscle motility. Also dissociated vertical nystagmus may be seen in suprasellar extending lesions.

5. **Compressive optic neuropathy.** Chronic compression of the central retinal vein can cause central retinal vein occlusion. As a result, venous stasis retinopathy, optociliary shunt vessels are seen. Furthermore this may lead to rubeosis irides and even neovascular glaucoma.

Diagnosis

Gliomas that are limited to only one optic nerve do not cause bilateral blindness and are not life-threatening. The prognosis for life and vision worsens once the optic chiasm is involved. Nearly 75% of the tumors involve both chiasm and one or both optic nerves, and half of those extending to the chiasm also involve the hypo-thalamus.[7] Therefore, early diagnosis and management is of important in these cases.

Magnetic resonance imaging (MRI) and computer tomographic (CT) scans are useful in the diagnosis of neurofibromatosis (Fig. 17.2). MR imaging can also show extension of tumor and tumor-associated changes beyond the optic nerve into the chiasm, findings that may not be apparent on CT scanning.

The appearance of the tumor is known to vary in those with NF1 and those without a fusiform enlargement of the optic nerve with a clearcut margin produced by the intact dural sheath is seen in the presence of NF1. However, the nerve is more irregular and tends to show both kinking and buckling, as well as low-density areas within the nerve in patients without NF1.

MR imaging typically shows gliomas to be hypo- to isointense on T1-weighted images and mildly to strongly hyperintense on proton density- and T2-weighted images. Some amount of contrast enhancement may also be appreciated in what has been suggested to be metabolically active areas within the tumor.

Treatment

As discussed earlier, optic nerve gliomas may sometimes involve the chiasm and cause visual symptoms in the contralateral eye as well. This occurrence however is very rare. The treatment of optic nerve gliomas consists of a multi-disciplinary approach.

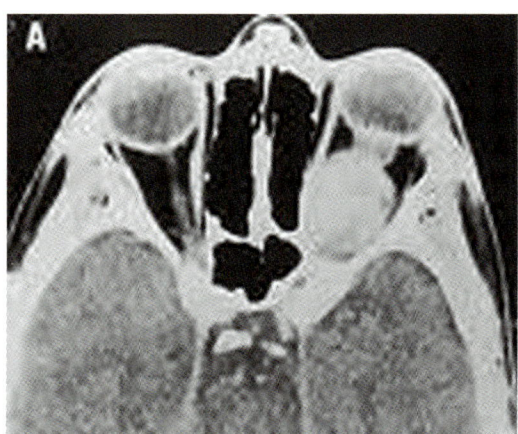

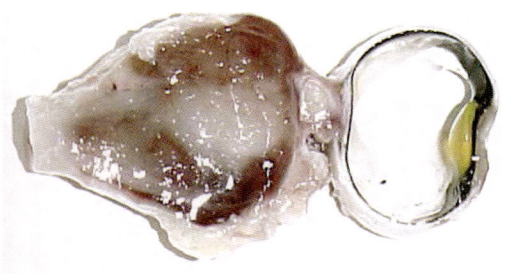

Fig. 17.1 *Gross specimen showing fusiform glioma of optic nerve (Courtesy: Kaustubh Mulay and Santosh Honavar).*

Fig. 17.2 *Axial CT scan of orbit showing optic nerve glioma.*

1. *Observation.* The natural history of optic nerve gliomas is almost always benign. Most grow slowly in a self-limited manner and some even spontaneously regress. Long-term studies indicate that patients who are not treated usually retain excellent, or at least have stable, visual function. It has been recommended that most patients with unilateral optic nerve gliomas, particularly those with NF1, be followed at regular intervals both clinically and with neuroimaging without intervention.

2. *Surgical excision.* Only if there is cosmetically unacceptable proptosis, progressive deterioration of visual function, evidence by MR imaging of definite tumor enlargement or extension but not to the optic chiasm, or a combination of these, should surgical excision of the lesion be considered. Either an orbital approach or a craniotomy may be performed to excise the tumor.

3. *Radiotherapy.* It has been seen that radiotherapy is effective in achieving functional improvement and stabilizing disease even with conventional techniques. In a retrospective analysis, early radiotherapy had a positive influence on progression-free survival. However, radiotherapy must be employed with caution as cerebral radiotherapy increases the risk for developmental abnormalities of the brain, including hearing and visual loss, and for tumors later in life.

4. *Chemotherapy.* To delay radiotherapy, chemotherapy has been attempted in young children with optic gliomas. Vincristine and carboplatin proved to be effective, with mild toxicity.

MALIGNANT OPTIC NERVE GLIOMA

Optic nerve gliomas are usually histologically benign and have a fairly predictable course as discussed above. However, rarely malignant astrocytomas that involve the anterior visual system are known to occur. These malignant tumors are known to have a rapid clinical course, characterized by progressive visual loss, neurologic deficits, and, eventually, death. The age of presentation varies from the second to the eighth decade and there is no specific sex predilection.

Clinical features and diagnosis

The clinical features depend on the site of the tumor. Patients with tumors in the proximal part of the optic nerve present with unilateral blurring of vision, posterior pole hemorrhages— resembling an ischaemic CRVO, and neovascular glaucoma may develop. This does not remain, however, a monocular disease. Within 5–6 weeks, both eyes become affected, and the patient soon becomes completely blind. Hypothalamic dysfunction, hemiparesis, and other neurologic deficits develop in the latter stages of the disease, and death usually occurs in less than 1 year. Because of the acute visual loss, it may be confused with optic neuritis or anterior ischemic optic neuropathy. In contrast to ischemic disease, marked enhancement of the optic nerve is seen on MRI.

Patients with tumors in the distal portion of the optic nerve present with progressive unilateral visual loss, neurologic symptoms, and death; however, the visual loss in these patients is associated with a normal—appearing optic disc that eventually becomes pale.

The histopathology of this tumor is completely different from that of the typical optic nerve glioma, being characterized by extreme cellular pleomorphism, nuclear hyperchromaticity, and scattered mitoses.

Treatment

No therapy seems to be able to stop the tumor; radiation is only palliative. Short-term successes have been seen with a combination of chemotherapy and radiation.

GANGLIOGLIOMA

Ganglioglioma of the optic nerve is rare. The clinical presentation is similar to that of an optic nerve glioma. The diagnosis is usually confirmed on histopathological examination of what is assumed, otherwise to be an optic nerve glioma. The tumor is composed of numerous ganglion cells, separated by connective tissue that is abundant in some areas and sparse in others.

TUMORS OF THE OPTIC NERVE SHEATH

OPTIC NERVE SHEATH MENINGIOMA

Optic nerve sheath meningioma (ONSM) is a term which indicates both primary and secondary meningiomas of the optic nerve. Optic nerve sheath meningiomas (ONSMs) account for one-third of primary optic nerve tumors, are the second most common optic nerve tumors after gliomas, and are the most common tumors of the optic nerve sheath. ONSMs also constitute 5% to 10% of all orbital tumors.

Primary ONSM represents a neoplasia of meningothelial cap cells of arachnoid villi and can develop anywhere along the course of the optic nerve, from globe to pre-chiasmal intracisternal optic nerve. Lesions may be unilateral, bilateral, or multifocal, with the latter two subgroups occurring most commonly in patients with type 2 neurofibromatosis. Meningiomas extending from other locations and involving the optic nerve are secondary and may arise from the cavernous sinus, falciform ligament, clinoid, sphenoid wing, pituitary fossa, planum sphenoidale, frontal-parietal area, or olfactory groove.

Approximately, 4 to 7% of ONSMs occur in childhood. Childhood OSNMs are known to have a more aggressive course and often show bilateral involvement. Unlike ONSMs that occur in adults, there is no gender predilection, and they are often associated with neurofibromatosis type 2.

Clinical features

1. *Loss of vision.* ONSMs spread around the optic nerve through the subdural and subarachnoid spaces, following pathways of least resistance such as vessels and dural septa. During the course of their growth and spread, they compromise the function of the nerve by impairing blood supply to the nerve and also by interfering with axon transport causing visual loss as well as disc edema. Patients may present with slowly progressive optic neuropathy characterized by a variable loss of visual acuity. The visual loss may be as profound as hand movements. In cases where visual acuity is relatively good, there may be defects in color vision and field defects. A relative afferent pupillary defect is seen in those with optic neuropathy.

2. *Fundus findings.* As discussed above, disc edema is commonly seen in ONSMs. However, The optic disc may be pale, with no prior swelling observed, when the meningioma is at the apex or within the optic canal.

3. *Other features* include macular swelling contiguous with a swollen optic disc, choroidal folds, and acquired retinochoroidal shunt vessels. The classically described triad of visual loss, optic atrophy and retinochoroidal shunts occur much later in the course of the disease.

4. *Proptosis.* Gradually progressive, non-pulsatile, proptosis is seen patients with ONSMs. Occasionally it may be painful and associated with mechanical restriction of ocular motility.

5. *Hyperostosis.* As the ONSM spreads, it may rarely, infiltrate the dura and spread beyond the confines of the nerve to infiltrate adjacent orbital structures, including fat, extraocular muscles, and bone. When the tumor spreads to adjacent bone, it may enter the Haversian canal system, inciting hyperostosis and bone proliferation, which are evident clinically and on radiological imaging.

Diagnosis

A detailed clinical examination may give important clues to the diagnosis of ONSM. Imaging modalities have however helped in the diagnosis, prognostication and management of ONSMs significantly.

1. *Ultrasonography.* Prior to computed tomography (CT) scans and magnetic resonance imaging (MRI), ultrasonography, both A and B scans were used to diagnose ONSMs. With ultrasonography, the tumor typically is revealed as an enlargement of the nerve sheath signal, with medium to high internal reflectivity. In addition, the nerve sheath diameter remains constant when measured from the perpendicular and 30 degree angle to the visual axis. In contrast, a 30-degree test is positive when a difference in the nerve sheath diameter is

detected with an increased cerebrospinal fluid space, typically accompanied by increased intracranial pressure.

2. *CT scans.* ONSMs have three main morphologic patterns on imaging: Tubular, fusiform, and globular. Thin sections (1–1.5 mm thin) of the orbit reveal irregular thickening of the meninges, which may enhance on injection of contrast. Classically, on axial cuts, hyperdense meningeal thickening is seen around a hypodense optic nerve (tram track sign). The thickness of the meninges (Fig. 17.3) and the optic nerve must be compared to the contralateral normal side. Sometimes calcification may be seen surrounding the optic nerve and the presence of such calcifications is thought to indicate slow growth.

3. *MRI.* Although MRI is less sensitive than CT in the recognition of calcification, it currently remains the procedure of choice for diagnosis of ONSM. ONSMs are typically isointense or slightly hypointense to brain and optic nerve tissue on T1-weighted images. ONSMs are typically hyperintense on T2-weighted images but may also be hypointense. In addition, the presence of enlarged, aerated posterior ethmoid and sphenoid sinuses, a condition known as *pneumosinus dilatans*, is thought by some authors to be pathognomonic of a meningioma.

4. *Histopathology.* Two histological patterns are seen in ONSMs. In the meningothelial or syncytial pattern, polygonal cells are seen arranged in sheets separated by vascular trabecular with uncommon mitotic figures. The other pattern is the transitional pattern where spindle or oval cells are arranged in whorls (Fig. 17.4). Further more, Psammoma bodies are also seen, more commonly in the transitional pattern.

Treatment

The natural history of visual function in ONSM has only recently been elaborated on. Studies have documented slow, progressive visual loss and tumor growth over years in the affected eye. However, some patients remain stable for many years, while others develop 'aggressive' periods with rapid decrease in visual loss with or without increase in tumor size. Also, cases of spontaneous regression have also been reported. ONSMs are compatible with good vision for many years, are not life threatening, and are unlikely to spread intracranially to the extent that they produce neurologic dysfunction. Spread to the contralateral optic nerve is a rare occurrence.

Observation. It has been recommended that patients of OSNMs with good and stable visual acuity be periodically followed. Only when there occurs a progressive visual loss should stereotactic or conformal fractionated

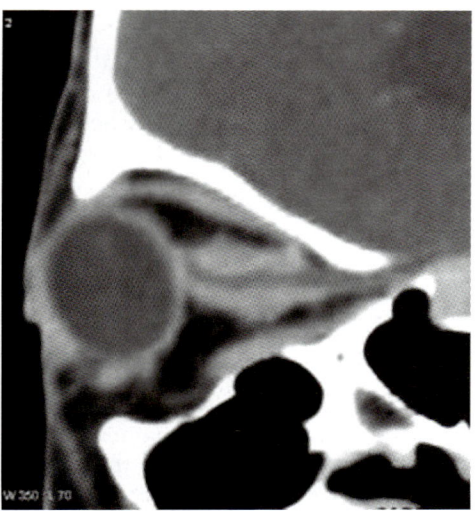

Fig 17.3 *Sagittal CT scan of orbit showing optic nerve sheath meningioma.*

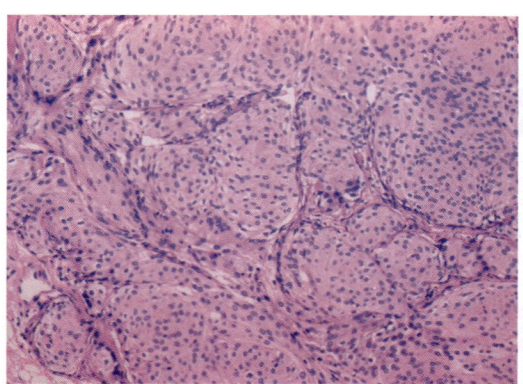

Fig. 17.4 *Histopathological picture of meningioma of the optic nerve showing ovoid to spindle shaped cells arranged in whorls (H&E, X100) (Courtesy: Kaustubh Mulay and Santosh Honavar).*

radiation therapy be instituted. Patients who present with significant visual loss should be given the option to undergo radiation therapy immediately.

Radiation therapy. Radiation is found to be effective in stopping the progressive visual loss. After radiation, tumor size is only mildly reduced on MRI follow-up despite marked functional improvement.

Surgery. Deterioration of vision is very rare. Given that the tumor mass and the optic nerve are virtually indistinguishable, any attempt to surgically excise the tumor may result in loss of residual vision as a result of damage to the pial circulation. Surgery in the treatment of ONSMs has a very small role, limited to obtaining biopsy material in atypical cases as well as radical surgery where visual prognosis is poor and intracranial extension is noted. Furthermore, surgery is advocated in cases of disfiguring proptosis.

Chemotherapy has no proven role in the management of ONSMs, although some authors have suggested the use of chemotherapeutic agents to treat unresectable meningiomas or to deal with failures of previous therapeutic attempts.

Summary. To summarize, although visual loss will generally occur in untreated eyes with ONSM, it typically occurs slowly, is limited to the affected eye, and is not associated with mortality. Therefore, treatments must take these natural history data and side effects into account when visual preservation is the primary goal.

OTHER TUMORS OF OPTIC NERVE

Other rare tumors of the optic nerve include: *Schwannoma* and *hemangiopericytoma*. The treatment of choice for both these tumors is surgical resection.

SUMMARY

* *Diagnosis of optic nerve tumors* is based on clinical presentation and imaging. Most tumors present with progressive visual loss and variable proptosis.

* *Role of neuroimaging.* Neuroimaging helps in diagnostic dilemmas such as differentiation between meningiomas and gliomas; and diagnosing infiltrative optic neuropathies such as leukemia or lymphoma.

* *Visual outcome and management* differ on the nature of the tumor.

BIBLIOGRAPHY

1. Alper MG. Management of primary optic meningiomas. Current status therapy in controversy. J Clin Neuro-ophthalmol 1981;1:101–17.
2. Balcer LJ, Liu GT, Heller G, et al. Visual loss in children with neurofibromatosis type 1 and optic pathway gliomas: relation to tumor location by magnetic resonance imaging. Am J Ophthalmol 2001;131:442–5.
3. Berman D, Miller NR. New concepts in the management of optic nerve sheath meningiomas. Ann Acad Med, Singapore 2006;35(3):168–74.
4. Brodovsky S, ten Hove MW, Pinkerton RM, et al. An enhancing optic nerve lesion: Malignant glioma of adulthood. Can J Ophthalmol 1997; 32:409–13.
5. Byrne SF, Green RL. Ultrasound of the Eye and Orbit. St. Louis, Mo: Mosby; 2002.
6. Cummings TJ, Provenzale JM, Hunter SB, et al. Gliomas of the optic nerve: histological, immunohistochemical (MIB-1 and p53), and MRI analysis. Acta Neuropathol 2000;99:563–70.
7. Danesh-Meyer HV, Savino PJ, Bilyk JR, et al. Aggressive glioma of adulthood simulating ischemic optic neuropathy. Arch Ophthalmol 2005;123:694–700.
8. Dutton JJ. Gliomas of the anterior visual pathway. Surv Ophthalmol 1994;38:427–52.
9. Dutton JJ. Optic nerve gliomas and meningiomas. Neurol Clin 1991;9:163–77.
10. Egan RA, Lessell S. A contribution to the natural history of optic nerve sheath meningiomas. Arch Ophthalmol 2002;120:1505–08.
11. Fouladi M, Wallace D, Langston JW, et al. Survival and functional outcome of children with hypothalamic/chiasmatic tumors. Cancer 2003;97:1084–92.
12. Gandhi RA, Nair AG. Role of imaging in the management of neuro-ophthalmic disorders. Indian J Ophthalmol 2011;59(2):111–6.
13. Grill J, Bhangoo R. Recent development in chemotherapy of paediatric brain tumors. Curr Opin Oncol 2007;19:612–5.

14. Hirst LW, Miller NRM, Hodges III FJ, et al. Sphenoid pneumosinus dilatans: A sign of meningioma originating in the optic canal. Neuroradiology 1982;22:207–10.

15. Karp LA, Zimmerman LE, Borit A, et al. Primary intraorbital meningiomas. Arch Ophthalmol 1974;91:24–8.

16. Knight CL, Hoyt WF, Wilson CB. Syndrome of incipient prechiasmal optic nerve compression. Progress toward early diagnosis and surgical management. Arch Ophthalmol 1972;87:1–11.

17. Kortmann RD, Timmermann B, Taylor RE, et al. Current and future strategies in radiotherapy of childhood low-grade glioma of the brain. Part I: Treatment modalities of radiation therapy. Strahlenther Onkol 2003;179:509–20.

18. Miller NR. Primary tumors of the optic nerve and its sheath. Eye (Lond) 2004;18(11):1026–37.

19. Probst C, Gessaga E, Leuenberger AE. Primary meningioma of the optic nerve sheaths: case report. Ophthalmologica 1985;190:83–90.

20. Saeed P, Rootman J, Nugent RA, et al. Optic nerve sheath meningiomas. Ophthalmology 2003;110: 2019–30.

21. Sharma A, Mohan K, Saini JS. Haemorrhagic changes in pilocytic astrocytoma of the optic nerve. Orbit 1990;9:29–33.

22. Spoor TC, Kennerdell JS, Martinez Z, et al. Malignant gliomas of the optic nerve pathways. Am J Ophthalmol 1980;89:284–92.

23. Turbin RE, Pokorny K. Diagnosis and treatment of orbital optic nerve sheath meningioma. Cancer Control 2004;11(5):334–41.

24. Wilhelm H. Primary optic nerve tumors. Curr Opin Neurol 2009;22(1):11–8.

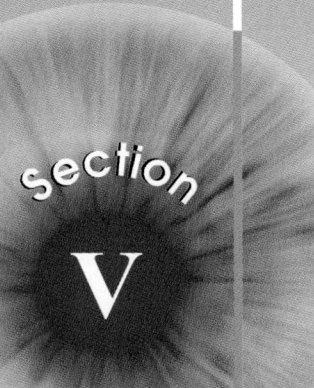

Section

V

Symptomatic Disturbances of Vision

18 | COLOR VISION DEFECTS

Nikhil Choudhari

COLOR VISION
- History aspects
- Theories of color vision
- Molecular genetics

COLOR VISION DEFECTS
Congenital Color Vision Defects

Acquired Color Vision Defects
- Etiological profile

- Congenital versus acquired defects
- Clinical evaluation

TESTS FOR COLOR VISION
- Plate tests
- Arrangement tests
- Anamaloscopes
- Lantern tests

COLOR VISION

Color vision is the ability to discriminate a light stimulus as a function of its wavelength. The visible spectrum consists of electromagnetic energy between approximately 380 and 760 nm and causes photoreactions on the human retina, which leads to the experience of vision.

HISTORICAL ASPECTS

The human eye differentiates colors according to wavelength of the corresponding color, the brightness and the saturation. Many great philosophers and scientists have written on theories of color vision and color sense and have provided a rich literature on the subject. Isaac Newton's (1642–1727) pioneering work with prisms transformed the science of color from study of objects to the study of light. Thomas Young (1773–1829) proposed a theory on three receptors in the retina that are sensitive to different spectral regions. The term 'color blindness' was coined by David Brewster (1781–

1868), which was formerly known as *Daltonism*, after John Dalton (1766–1844), who described in detail his inability to distinguish the color red. von Helmholtz (1821–1894) extended Young's hypothesis and devised spectral absorption curves for three visual photoreceptors. Herman Rudolf Aubert (1826–1892) demonstrated that color perception was largely restricted to the foveal region and depended on context in other parts of the retina. James Clerk Maxwell (1831–1879) devised methods to study color mixing and color defective subjects and developed many classifications that are still in use today.

THEORIES OF COLOR VISION

In the initial step of color perception, light must be converted into a neurochemical signal by photoreceptor cells. Rod cells primarily mediate scotopic (dim light) vision. Rods differentiate light intensity with a maximum response at approximately 510 nm. Cone photoreceptor cells are responsible for photopic (bright light) color vision. Cones are significantly less sensitive than rods, but they mediate differentiation of colors.

The human retinal fovea contains a high density of cones but essentially no rods.

The most salient feature of normal human color vision is that it is **trichromatic.** The three physiologic detection systems are the three classes of photoreceptor cells—each class containing a different photoreceptor pigment molecule—those being blue or short (S) wavelength sensitive, or the middle (M) sensitive, and red or long (L) sensitive cones. The three human cone types represent the three additive primary colors: blue, green and red.

The **Young-Helmholtz theory** of color vision emphasizes trichromacy and was essentially confirmed by three cone photoreceptor systems. Karl Hering (1834–1918) developed the **opponent theory** of color vision based on the hypothetical existence of three oppositional color pigment pairs. It is now known that oppositional pairs do not exist, but Hering's theory was correct in the sense that the signals from the three cones are combined, not at the pigment level as he had suggested but at the level of neurons to produce opposing pairs of red-green, blue-yellow and black-white. Later work confirmed the opposing excitatory and inhibitory interactions in color perception.

Several additional phenomena occur at the level of retina and influence color perception, including optical mixing of small surfaces. Optical mixing is also exploited in glowing television and computer screens that consist of points of blue, green and red light that mix to form a grey background. As intensities of the points change, all other colors are created.

MOLECULAR GENETICS

The molecular genetics of human color vision is complex because one of three distinct genes has to be expressed in a particular cone cell that is otherwise identical to its neighboring cones. The complexity arises in part because M- and L-sensitive genes, which are approximately 98% identical, are juxtaposed on the X chromosome. Recent advances in molecular biology have allowed remarkable parallel advances in understanding the molecular basis for color perception. The most reasonable hypothesis that links genotype to clinical phenotype is the spectral proximity hypothesis, which states that

red-green color discrimination is a function of the difference between the wavelengths of maximal absorption of the M- and L-sensitive pigments. An optimal separation might be approximately 30 nm.

COLOR VISION DEFECTS

CONGENITAL COLOR VISION DEFECTS

Color vision deficiency (CVD) is a common functional disorder of vision affecting 8% males and 0.4% females in Caucasian societies. The classification system for congenital color vision dates back to the nomenclature introduced by von Kries in 1875. This system describes congenital defects by the Greek terms protan (Ist), deutan (second), and tritan (third), referring to red, green, and blue deficiencies, respectively. Table 18.1 summarizes the various forms of abnormal congenital color vision defects.

ACQUIRED COLOR VISION DEFECTS

Etiological profile

Special consideration should be given to the study of acquired color vision defects. These defects are the secondary features of a variety of pathological states. The category of acquired defects includes changes in pre-receptor, receptor, and post-receptor mechanisms that affect the perception of light stimuli. Thus, age-related deterioration of the lens, the toxic effects of anti-epileptic therapy, macular degeneration, and optic neuritis are all pathological states that impact the perception of color.

Congenital versus acquired defects

Acquired color vision defects differ from congenital defects in fundamental ways, although it is not always easy to distinguish the two clinically. Acquired defects begin after birth. Unlike congenital defects, they may fluctuate in severity and type. Individuals with acquired defects often have an associated decrease in visual acuity and visual field loss. In congenital deficiency, except for the monochromatic variety, it is not common to find these

Table 18.1 *Types of congenital defective color vision*

Classification	Mechanism	Characteristics
Monochromasy		
Typical monochromasy	Once thought to be due to an absence of cones or to cones being filled with rhodopsin but now proposed to be the result of mutation of genes encoding the cone-specific alpha and beta sub-units of the cation channel	Color blind. No perception of colors Colors distinguished by brightness differences only. Very insensitive to red light Nystagmus. Low visual acuity 6/36 to 6/60. Painless photophobia
Blue cone mono-chromasy	S (Blue) cone pigment only. No L (red) or M (green) cone pigment	Color blind. Colors distinguished by brightness differences only. Rudimentary color vision in mesopic vision from red and blue cone activation. Very insensitive to red light
	Nystagmus. Low visual acuity 6/12 to 6/24. Painless photophobia	
Dichromasy		
Protanopia	Absence of L (red) cone pigment	Very reduced ability to identify colors. Confuse red, yellow and green, white and green, and blue and purple. Reduced sensitivity to red light
Deuteranopia	Absence of M (green) cone pigment	Very reduced ability to identify colors. Confuse red, yellow and green, and white and green
Tritanopia	Absence of S (blue) cone pigment	Very reduced ability to identify colors. Confuse blue with blue-green and green, and white with yellow
Anomalous trichromasy		
Protanomaly	L (red) cone pigment absorption spectrum shifted to shorter wavelengths of light	May confuse white with green and confuse reds, yellows and greens but loss of color discrimination varies greatly between individuals. Reduced sensitivity to red light. Make abnormal color matches: For example will add excess red in the color match $R + G = Y$
Deuteranomaly	M (green) cone pigment absorption spectrum shifted to longer wavelengths of light	May confuse white with green and confuse reds, yellows and greens but loss of color discrimination varies greatly between individuals. Make abnormal color matches: For example will add excess green in the color match $R + G = Y$
Tritanomaly	Partial loss of S (blue) cone pigment	Loss of color discrimination for blues, blue-greens, and greens

This table is adapted from Table 18.1 in International Recommendations for Color Vision Requirements for Transport. CIE Technical Report 143. Vienna; CIE: 2001.

symptoms. Congenital defects are easier to classify by type into precise categories of protan, deutan, or tritan. Acquired defects are often hard to classify and may be a combination of types. Congenital defects usually affect both eyes equally. Acquired defects are frequently monocular. Congenital defects are most commonly protan or deutan and rarely tritan. In contrast, acquired defects most commonly affect the short-wave spectrum (blue-yellow defect; Kollner's rule). Congenital defects are predominantly X-linked, and therefore, usually found in men. Acquired defects result from disease, aging, or drugs, processes that affect men and women equally.

Clinical evaluation

It is preferable that both an anomaloscope and a test of chromatic discrimination such as the FM 100-hue test are used. Tests for blue-color defects are also necessary. Each eye should be examined separately and testing must take into account factors such as reduced visual acuity and visual field defects. In older individuals, short-wavelength defects may be a part of the aging process and it may be difficult to sort out the effects of disease pathology. Pseudo-isochromatic tests, especially tritan plates, can be an important screening tool. However, individuals with acquired defects may not give the expected readings. The lines of color confusion are often different for individuals with acquired defects than those expected for congenital defects. Thus, for example, a patient with an acquired defect may miss both classification numerals meant to distinguish protan from deutan defects. Before using isochromatic plates, the visual acuity of the patient should be checked.

TESTS FOR COLOR VISION

It is useful to group these tests into several different categories based on design. Pseudo-isochromatic plates, arrangement tests, anomaloscopes, and lanterns represent the most widely used designs. Different tests are appropriate for different circumstances (Table 18.2).

Plate tests

J. Stilling Ist introduced pseudoisochromatic designs in 1873. Today, they are the most commonly used screening tests for color deficiency in clinical practice. These tests are inexpensive, durable, and readily available. Most tests provide very efficient (90–95%) screening of congenital red-green defects. On the other hand, the tests have distinct limitations. They must be administered under the standard viewing conditions for which they were designed. They are not effective in grading the severity of the color defect and thus tell us limited information about the extent or type of deficiency. In short, plate tests are best used as screening tools.

Plate tests come in several forms; however, the principle of construction is the same. Ishihara test is the prototype of this category. The test consists of a series of cards on which a figure is printed in multiple colors against a multicolored background. The figure is recognizable to normal trichromats, but camouaged to those with color defects. The figure used in the test is usually an easily identifiable number, letter, or shape. Figures and background are drawn in dots. The size of the dots used in plate design can be varied or uniform; however, the only difference between the figure and the background is the color. Saturation and lightness are accounted for, such that detection of the figure in ways other than hue is unlikely.

The Ishihara test is published in a full 38-plate edition, an abridged 24-plate edition and a 14-plate edition for quick screening. Scoring instructions for the Ishihara plates accompany each test. In the 38-plate edition, for example, a normal score permits four or fewer errors. In the 24-plate edition, two errors or less are considered normal. The 16-plate edition also puts two

Table 18.2 *Categories of color vision tests*		
Test type	*Function*	*Example*
Screening tests	Quick diagnosis	Pseudoisochromatic plates, e.g. Ishihara test
Grading tests	Assess severity of the defect	FM 100-hue test
Diagnostic tests	Precisely classify a defect	Anomaloscope
Vocational tests	Simulate environment encountered on the job	Lantern test

Interesting facts

The Ishihara test was designed by Shinobu Ishihara (1879–1963), who was a surgeon in the Japanese army before specializing in ophthalmology. Some of his research was on the selection of soldiers and he was asked to devise a test to screen military recruits for color vision deficiency. He was helped by a color-blind physician who tested the plates, which were originally painted in water colors and used hirangana symbols. The Ist edition using Arabic numerals was published in 1917 but few were sold until 1929 when the International Congress of Ophthalmology in Holland recommended its use for testing military personnel. In 1958, it was adopted in Japan as the official test for school children when a law was introduced to require color vision testing in schools as part of a general medical assessment. The Ishihara test is not the first pseudoisochromatic test of color vision. The German ophthalmologist Jakob Stilling had devised his test in 1878 but the Ishihara test has proved to have the best sensitivity and specificity of all the pseudoisochromatic tests.

errors or less in the normal range. It does not matter which edition is used because the fail criterion is three or five errors and total number of errors has no diagnostic significance. The Ishihara can be used in children as young as 5 years. The color differences between the figure and the background are chosen to separate normal trichromats from mild anomalous trichromats. If the differences in color are too large, anomalous trichromats will be able to identify the hidden figure. Small differences may cause normal trichromats to fail some screening plates.

Arrangement tests

Modern arrangement tests were first put into popular use in the 1940s and 1950s by Dean Farnsworth. Farnsworth originally designed the Farnsworth-Munsell 100-hue test (FM 100-hue test) and the Farnsworth Dichotomous test for color blindness (Farnsworth Panel D-15). The principle of design for these tests is colored caps of fixed chroma and value selected from the hue circle. The patient is asked to arrange randomly placed caps in what he/she perceives to be a natural order. The color differences between adjacent caps on the FM 100-hue test were designed to be very small. Good color vision as well as chromatic discrimination ability is needed to perform well on this test. Farnsworth Panel D-15 was designed to have larger color differences, but, unlike the FM 100-hue test, only one box containing 15 caps is presented to the patient.

Anomaloscopes

An anomaloscope is an instrument that uses the principle of color matching to test color vision. It serves as a clinical standard for diagnosing and classifying congenital color deficiency. The use and maintenance of an anomaloscope can be challenging and requires the expertise of a trained technician. For this reason, anomaloscopes are not used as frequently as other clinical tests.

The Nagel (model I) anomaloscope is the most common and accurate of these and uses the Rayleigh equation to diagnose red-green color vision defects. The subject views a circular field through a telescopic barrel. This field is divided into two parts, each of which is filled with light of different spectral wavelengths. The lower half of the field is filled with spectral yellow at 589 nm. According to the Rayleigh match, the subject should be able to match the 'color' of the upper to the lower field by adjusting the mixture of red and green light. The luminance knob is particularly useful in distinguishing deutan from protan defects. The subject is asked to comment on whether the upper and lower fields are the same color. Normal and dichromatic individuals will accept this as a normal or near-normal match. Deuteranomalous trichromats will state that the upper field is too red and protanomalous trichromats will state that the upper field is too green. Scoring of an anomaloscope examination begins by recording the values at which a match was made.

Lantern tests

Lantern tests are simple devices geared towards measuring a subject's competency to perform a specific task, namely recognize colored light signals. Lanterns are used in the maritime, air, and railway industries to screen employees. The subject is asked to name the colors of the light signals that are presented to him. Two types of lanterns exist: those that present single colors and those that present pairs of lights together. The speed and sequence of color presentation is important to the efficacy of the test. Individuals with defective color vision make characteristic mistakes in naming the colors presented to them; however, most lantern tests are not meant to screen or categorize color defectives for clinical purposes.

BIBLIOGRAPHY

1. Birch J. A practical guide for color vision examination: report of the Standardization Committee of the International Research Group on Color Vision Deficiencies. Ophthalmol Physiol Opt 1985;5:265–85.
2. Birch J. Efficiency of the Ishihara test for identifying red-green color deficiency. Ophthalmic Physiol Opt 1997;17:403–8.
3. Cole BL. Assessment of inherited color vision defects in clinical practice. Clin Exp Optom 2007;90(3):157–75.
4. Committee on Vision, Assembly of Behavioral and Social Sciences, National Research Council. Procedures for Testing Color Vision, Report of Working Group 41.Washington, DC: National Academy Press, 1981.
5. Jameson D, Hurvich LM. Some quantitative aspects of an opponent colors theory I. Chromatic responses and spectral saturation. J Opt Soc Am 1955;45:546–52.
6. Neitz M, Neitz J. Molecular genetics of color vision and color vision defects. Arch Ophthalmol 2000;118:691–700.
7. Pokorny J, Smith VC. Eye disease and color defects. Vision Res 1986;26:1573–84.
8. Rayleigh Lord. Experiments on color. Nature 1881;25:64–7.
9. Swanson WH. Color vision: assessment and clinical relevance. In: Fuller DG, Birch DG (Eds). Ophthalmology clinics of North America. Philadelphia: WB Saunders Co., 1989; 391–413.
10. von Kreis J. Uber Farbensysteme. Z Psychol Physiol Sinnesorg 1897;13:241–324.

19 FUNCTIONAL VISUAL LOSS

Devendra V Venkatramani

FUNCTIONAL DISORDERS

A functional (non-organic) disorder is one in which the symptoms have no detectable underlying organic basis, either by clinical examination or by specialized testing. The symptoms are believed to be produced by internal conflict, rather than a specific tissue pathology.

Conversion disorder

Conversion disorder (also known as hysteria, or hysterical neurosis) is defined as a mental disorder whose central feature is the appearance of symptoms affecting the patient's senses or voluntary movements that suggest a neurological or general medical disease or condition. Conversion disorder are classified as a somatoform disorders; these are characterized by persistent physical symptoms that cannot be fully explained by a medical condition, substance abuse, or other mental disorder, and seem to stem from psychological issues or conflicts. The symptoms are not willfully produced, and appear to correspond to the patient's concept of the disease. Additionally, the patient is not unduly disturbed by the severity of the symptoms (la belle indifference), although this finding probably has poor discriminating value.

Malingering

Malingering is defined as the intentional production of false or grossly exaggerated physical or psychological symptoms, motivated by external incentives such as avoiding military duty, avoiding work, obtaining financial compensation, evading criminal prosecution, or obtaining drugs'. Thus, the deliberate falsification of symptoms is done with a view to receive external gratification (secondary gain). Symptoms may be fabricated, exaggerated, or even down-played (negative malingering, in an attempt to appear healthier than one actually is). Malingering, however, is not considered a mental illness.

Incidence

It is very difficult to calculate the incidence of functional visual loss. Retrospective studies have suggested a relatively high incidence, especially in children. Conversely, there appears to be a high prevalence of psychosocial disturbance in children with functional visual loss. The incidence of malingering is higher in patients with insurance claims or compensation.

CLINICO-INVESTIGATIVE PROFILE

CLINICAL FEATURES AND TESTING

Malingering is a diagnosis of exclusion, which requires a high index of suspicion. Indicators include medicolegal disputes, litigation, or insurance claims, inconsistencies between the clinical history and ocular findings, frequent amendments to the clinical history, and when patients are uncooperative. Ultimately, the only true test is when the patient is caught-out in an outright lie. However, a simple clinical examination is sufficient in most cases.

Malingerers are usually adolescents or young adults who face mental stress at home or in the workplace, or who have sustained a trivial ocular or head injury. Functional disorders can produce a variety of ocular symptoms (Table 19.1).

Ocular symptoms. Relationship of symptoms with functional disorders is depicted in Fig. 19.1.

Table 19.1 *Functional ocular symptoms*

Afferent system
  Total blindness (binocular or monocular)
  Diminished vision (binocular or monocular)
  Visual field defects (binocular or monocular)
  Night blindness
Efferent system
  Diplopia (binocular or monocular)
  Accommodative spasm
  Voluntary nystagmus
  Gaze palsy
Disorders of eyelid function
  Blepharospasm
  Ptosis
Disturbances of lacrimation

A variety of clinical tests have been described. One needs to adapt the examination depending on the presenting symptoms and response. Algorithm for testing a patient with afferent system symptoms are shown in Fig. 19.2.

The pupillary light reflex is perhaps the single-most informative test. It is most useful in patients with severe unilateral or asymmetric visual loss, where the absence of relative afferent pupillary defect almost excludes an organic cause. However, the pupillary reflexes may be normal in patients with cortical blindness, and are confounded by the concealed application of mydriatics or miotics.

BINOCULAR PROFOUND VISUAL LOSS

Observation. In a patient with binocular profound vision loss, observing how he or she

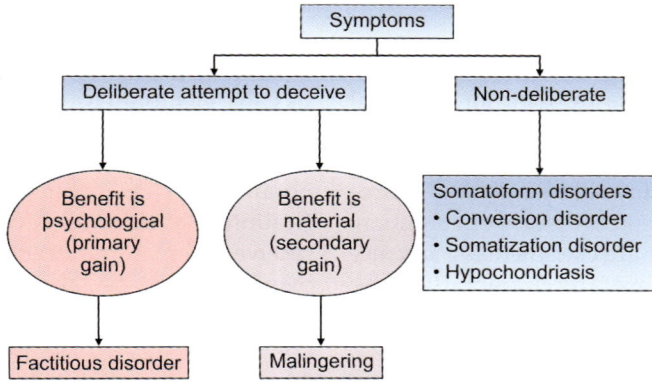

Fig. 19.1 *The relationship between functional disorders.*

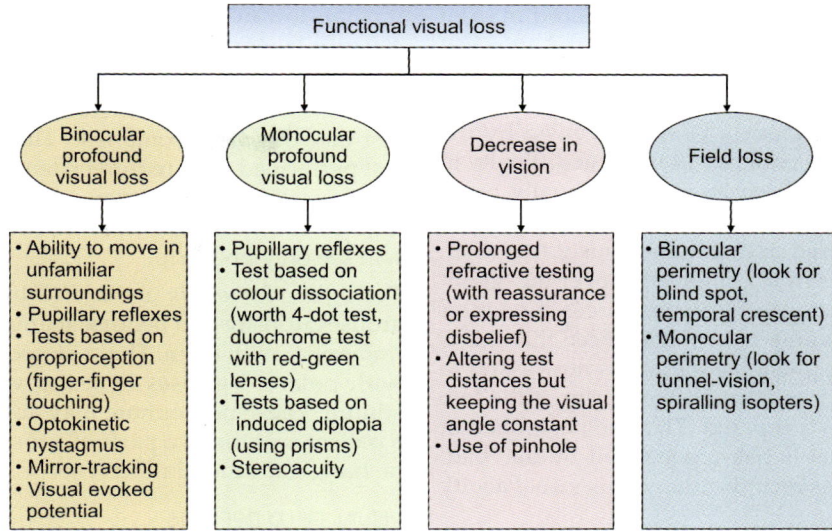

Fig. 19.2 *Algorithm for testing a patient with afferent system symptoms.*

negotiates unfamiliar surroundings can be revealing.

- A truly blind person moves around carefully, whereas a malingerer appears to deliberately walk into obstacles.

- *Wearing of sunglasses* by a patient who has no obvious ophthalmic reason to, is a sign found to have a surprisingly association with non-organic visual loss.

The menace reflex may also be used in this situation, but may produce false-positive as well as false-negative results. Shining an intense light produces reflex tearing which is difficult to suppress.

Tests based on proprioception are normal even in bilateral blindness. These include asking the patient to look at his own outstretched hand, or to touch the index fingers of his two hands together. A malingerer will fail to perform these satisfactorily. Similarly, a person with acute onset of bilateral blindness can sign his or her name accurately, whereas a malingerer may either claim inability to or produce an illegible scrawl.

Optokinetic nystagmus can be elicited using the OKN drum. The fast phase (refixation movement) is opposite to the direction of rotation of the drum. Using stripes of varying widths, one can even estimate the grating acuity. In the mirror test, one elicits a nystagmoid movement when rotating or tilting a mirror from side to side in front of the patient.

The visual-evoked potential is an objective method to assess the integrity of the visual pathway. A normal pattern VEP is highly suggestive of functional visual loss, especially if small check sizes are used. Malingerers have been shown to suppress the VEP response by defocusing the pattern by convergence or concentrating beyond the plane of the checks. The P300 response, however, is more robust, and not amenable to voluntary suppression.

MONOCULAR PROFOUND VISUAL LOSS

A complaint of total blindness in one eye is far commoner, especially in malingerers. The tests described for bilateral blindness can be performed monocularly in these patients, by covering the alleged 'good' eye.

A common principle while evaluating a patient with alleged monocular blindness is to dissociate the eyes, but making sure that both eyes are kept open throughout the test. Dissociation can be produced using prisms or colored lenses.

A 4 prism-dioptre prism can be placed in front of the 'good' eye with its base up and apex just bisecting the pupil, after occluding the 'bad' eye. This results in monocular diplopia. As both images are obviously being perceived by the 'good' eye, the patient will have no difficulty in admitting that both images are equally clear. Emphasis is laid on this fact. The other eye is then uncovered and simultaneously the prism is slipped down to completely cover the 'good' eye. The patient now experiences binocular diplopia, but may remain convinced that this is a monocular phenomenon. He is now asked to read letters in a line, and the clarity of the two lines may be compared. The line positioned at a higher level is being perceived by the 'bad' eye, and gives an indication of his visual acuity in that eye.

An 8 prism-diopter prism placed in front of the allegedly blind eye will cause difficulty in climbing up or down a flight of stairs with both eyes open.

Physiological diplopia occurs due to biretinal disparity when an object falls outside Panum's fusional area. When the patient fixates at a distant object and a finger is suddenly interposed, appreciation of two fingers indicates binocularity.

Lenses can also be used to fog the apparently good eye. With the trial frame in place, the patient is asked to read with both eyes open. A strong convex (or concave) lens is placed in front of the good eye. If the patient continues to read,

it points towards functional visual loss. This test can also be performed using a pinhole in front of the 'good' eye.

Color dissociation tests include the worth 4-dot test and the duochrome test. The duochrome test performed with red-green lenses in front of the eyes allows a binocular subject to see both letter strips, whereas a truly monocular patient will see only one strip.

Tests for stereopsis are useful because they arouse curiosity and because many subjects are unfamiliar with them. These dissociate the eyes with polaroid glasses or using vectographic stimuli. The synoptophore may also be used; if a patient sees the two parts of a fusion test pair, he has good vision in each eye.

VISUAL FIELD DEFECTS

The classic functional visual field defect is contraction of the visual field, either in one or in both eyes. The differential diagnosis for this pattern includes glaucoma, retinitis pigmentosa, post pan-retinal photocoagulation, and chronic papilledema, disorders that can generally be excluded by fundus examination. A point of interest is that patients with functional field loss demonstrate 'tunnel vision' rather than 'funnel vision', seen in organic disorders. If the tangent screen is moved away from the patient and a proportionately larger target is used, the absolute size of the field remains the same in functional loss, rather than increasing (the angle subtended remaining the same) in organic visual loss (*see* Fig. 9.19).

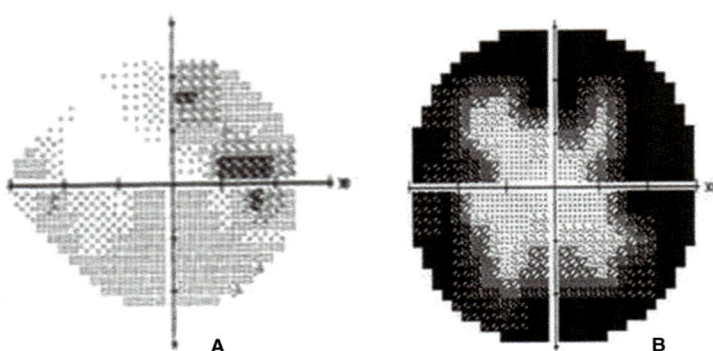

Fig. 19.3 *Visual fields showing (A) 'white' scotoma in a patient with high false-positive errors, and (B) clover-leaf pattern in an inattentive subject.*

The visual field in functional loss is ideally tested using manual perimeters like the Goldmann perimeter. Characteristic patterns in patients with conversion disorder include spiralling of the isopters, crossing isopters, and star-shaped fields. Other functional field defects described are unilateral or bilateral central scotomata, unilateral hemianopia, bitemporal hemianopia, and binasal hemianopia.

Binocular field testing in patients with true monocular visual loss shows absence of the corresponding temporal crescent, and a visible blind spot of the normal eye. In patients with functional loss these findings are absent.

Suggestive features on automated perimetry are 'squaring' of the visual field, a clover-leaf pattern, or 'white' scotomas due to responses to sub-threshold stimuli (high false-positive errors) (Fig. 19.3).

Field defects in malingerers tend to be highly inconsistent and variable, whereas those in patients with both organic field loss and conversion disorder are consistent over repeated testing.

DIFFERENTIAL DIAGNOSIS AND MANAGEMENT

DIFFERENTIAL DIAGNOSIS

Organic conditions can sometimes be mis-diagnosed as functional disorders. Ocular disorders that need to be excluded are retinal diseases such as heredomacular degenerations (e.g. Stargardt disease), juvenile X-linked retinoschisis, central serous retinopathy, retinitis pigmentosa sine pigmento, corneal disorders *especially keratoconus, and amblyopia. Efferent symptoms* may need to be differentiated from disorders like myasthenia gravis and convergence insufficiency.

Electrophysiological tests. In selected cases, ancillary testing in the form of electrophysiological test may be needed.

MANAGEMENT AND PROGNOSIS

Patients with functional visual loss need to be approached with great tact.

Conversion disorder generally has a very good prognosis. The physician should reassure the patient that the visual system is healthy, and that a full recovery is anticipated. Use of medication, drugs, glasses, or other orthoptic devices should be discouraged. Ultimately, the patient and his family need to work towards relieving the underlying stressor, so as to prevent another somatoform reaction.

Malingerers also need to be informed of the findings of the ocular examination in a non-confrontational manner. For medicolegal purposes, however, detailed documentation of the clinical history, examination findings and investigations is paramount.

Follow-up. All patients with functional disorder need to be followed up carefully. There may be a missed underlying organic disease, or serious psychiatric illness with suicidal tendency.

BIBLIOGRAPHY

1. American Psychiatric Association. Diagnostic and Statistical Manual of Mental Disorders, 4th edn, text revised. Washington, DC: American Psychiatric Association, 2000.

2. Bengtzen R, Woodward M, Lynn MJ, et al. The "sunglasses sign" predicts nonorganic visual loss in neuro-ophthalmologic practice. Neurology 2008;15:70(3):218–21.

3. Han SB, Han ER, Hyon JY, et al. Measurement of distance objective visual acuity with the computerized optokinetic nystagmus test in patients with ocular diseases. Graefe's Arch Clin Exp Ophthalmol 2011 May 21. [Epub ahead of print.]

4. Keane JR. Pattern of hysterical hemianopia. Neurology 1998;51:1230–1.

5. Keane JR. Pattern of hysterical hemianopia. Neurology 1998;51:1230–1.

6. Kline LB, Bajandas FJ. Neuro-ophthalmology Review Manual. 5th ed. Thorofare, NJ: Slack Incorporated 2004;209–20.

7. Miller BW. A review of practical tests for ocular malingering and hysteria. Surv Ophthalmol 1973;17(4):241–6.

8. Miller NR. Walsh and Hoyts Clinical Neuro-Ophthalmology. Philadelphia, Pa: Lippincott Williams & Wilkins 2004;1:1317–35.

9. Muñ oz-Herná ndez AM, Santos-Bueso E, Sá enz-Francés F, et al. Nonorganic visual loss and associated psychopathology in children. Eur J Ophthalmol. 2011 May 27. pii: C6E157EC-62D3-4136-9581-C5B9841B2A16. doi: 10.5301/ EJO.2011.8378. [Epub ahead of print]

10. Ohkubo H. Visual field in hysteria-reliability of visual field by Goldmann perimetry. Doc Ophthalmol 1989;71:61–7.

11. Slater E, Glithero E. A follow-up of patients diagnosed as suffering from hysteria. J Psychosom Res 1965;9:9–13.

12. Stone J, Smyth R, Carson A, et al. La belle indifference in conversion symptoms and hysteria: systematic review. Br J Psychiatry 2006;188:204–9.

13. Taich A, Crowe S, Kosmorsky GS, et al. Prevalence of psychosocial disturbances in children with nonorganic visual loss. J AAPOS. 2004;8(5):457–61.

14. Towle VL, Sutcliffe E, Sokol S. Diagnosing functional visual deficits with the P300 component of the visual-evoked potential. Arch Ophthalmol 1985;103(1):47–50.

20

DISORDERS OF HIGHER VISUAL FUNCTIONS, CORTICAL BLINDNESS, OTHER VISUAL DISORDERS AND AMBLYOPIA

AK Khurana, Rashmin A Gandhi, Ashwin Mohan

APPLIED ANATOMY OF VISUAL PATHWAYS
- Pre-cortical afferent visual system
- Cortical visual system
- Occipitofugal pathways—'what' and 'where' of vision

DISORDERS OF HIGHER VISUAL FUNCTIONS
- Area V1 disorders
- Area V2 and V3 (prestriate and peristriate cortex) disorders
- Area V5 disorders
- The dorsal occipitofugal pathway disorders

- The ventral occipitofugal pathway disorders

CORTICAL BLINDNESS

OTHER VISUAL DISORDERS
- Night blindness
- Day blindness
- Amaurosis

AMBLYOPIA
- Classification and terminology
- Pathogenesis and pathophysiology
- Clinical characteristics and laboratory findings
- Clinical evaluation and diagnosis
- Management of amblyopia

APPLIED ANATOMY OF VISUAL PATHWAYS

The retinal ganglion cells act as first order neurons projecting to the lateral geniculate (LGN) body. These first order neurons comprise the optic tracts. Second order neurons from here known as the optic radiations project to the calcarine cortex. Functional areas of the calcarine cortex and their pathology is what we will review in this chapter.

PRE-CORTICAL AFFERENT VISUAL SYSTEM

Three major types of retinal ganglion cells travel in the optic tracts, also referred to as the retinogeniculate pathway. This pathway, as the name implies travels from the ganglion cells in the retina to the LGN carrying the first order neurons. The midget ganglion cells project to areas 3–6 of the parvocellular LGN. Parasol ganglion cells project to areas 1–2 of the magnocellular LGN. Bistratified ganglion cells project to the koniocellular layers of the ganglion cells.

The parvocellular (P pathways) system is a static firing system concerned with wavelength selectivity that conveys low contrast high spatial resolution images. This pathway is concerned with fine resolution acuity, color and form of objects. The magnocellular (M pathways) system is a color blind system that conveys information that is of high contrast and low spatial resolution. This pathway is concerned with location and motion of objects. The koniocellular system (K pathway) conveys information concerning blue-yellow color opponency.

CORTICAL VISUAL SYSTEM

Pathways originate from V1 and travel through various association areas. V2 lying immediately adjacent to V1 receives feedforward connections from V1 going to V3, 4, 5 and 6 and receives feedback connections going back to V1.

The visual cortex is located in the calcarine ("spur" shaped) sulcus of the occipital lobe, hence also called the calcarine cortex. The calcarine visual cortex can be sub-divided into areas V1–V6 (based on experiments in the macaque monkeys). Area

Pathways originate from V1 and travel through various association areas. V2 lying immediately adjacent to V1 receives feedforward connections from V1 going to V3, 4, 5 and 6 and receives feedback connections going back to V1.

V1 is the primary visual cortex and corresponds to the striate cortex. It is also referred to as Brodmann area 17. Areas V2–V6 contain specialized maps of the visual field. Area V2 is also referred to as the parastriate cortex and Brodmann area 18. Area V3, Brodmann area 19 is also called the peristriate cortex. Area V4 located in the lateral occipital lobe is believed to involved in color processing. Area V5 or visual area MT (middle temporal) plays a major role in motion detection. Area V6 in the monkey is believed to be homologous to the visuospatial processing in the posterior parietal cortex.

The posterior parietal cortex is neither a purely sensory nor a purely motor area; rather, it combines characteristics of both. Thus, it serves as a junction between multimodal sensory input and motor output, linking the afferent and efferent arms of the visual pathways and providing the connection that encompasses the entire field of neuro-ophthalmology, from the eyes to the extraocular muscles.

OCCIPITOFUGAL PATHWAYS—"WHAT" AND "WHERE" OF VISION

The information processed by the striate cortex and visual associative areas is projected through two occipitofugal pathways: a ventral occipito-temporal pathway and a dorsal occipitoparietal pathway. The ventral occipitotemporal path-way, often called the "what" pathway, is involved in processing the physical attributes of a visual image that are important to the perception of color, shape, and pattern. This pathway from V1 travels through V2 to V4 (color perception) and the inferior temporal cortex. These, in turn, are crucial for object identification and object-based attention. It provides visual information to areas involved in visual identification, language processing, memory, and emotion. Thus, a lesion in this pathway may cause a variety of associative defects, including visual alexia and anomia, visual agnosia, visual amnesia, and visual hypoemotionality.

The dorsal occipitoparietal or "where" pathway is involved in visuospatial analysis, in the localization of objects in visual space, and in modulation of visual guidance of movements toward these objects. This pathway from V1 projects through V2, travels through V5/MT (motion detection) through to V6 (visuospatial processing). Thus, lesions of this pathway may cause a variety of visuospatial disorders, such as Bálint's syndrome and hemispatial neglect.

DISORDERS OF HIGHER VISUAL FUNCTIONS

The disorders of higher cortical function can be localized to lesions involving V1–V6 and the occipitofugal pathways. Table 20.1 is a short summary of the syndromes and their locations in the cortex.

Table 2.1 *Disorders of higher cortical function and their location in cortex*			
V1	*V2 and V3*	*V4*	*V5*
Anton syndrome	Quadrantic	Cerebral	Akinetopsia
Blindsight	Homonymous	Achromatopsia	Dyslexia
Riddoch	Hemianopsia		
Phenomenon			
Transient			
Achromatopsia			
Visual ataxia			
Dorsal Occipitofugal		**Ventral Occipitofugal**	
Bálint syndrome		Visual verbal (pure alexia, color and object anomia)	
Hemispatial neglect		Visual-visual (prosopagnosia, object agnosia)	
Visual allesthesia		Visual limbic (visual amnesia and hypoemotionality)	
Environmental rotation			

Information from these several pathways undergo complex combinations in the visual association areas of the brain, and an image of the world is created. Information based on position and category are separated and correlated with surrounding objects and sounds. A reference library is maintained for immediate recall. An understanding of these pathways can enable us to recognize characteristic syndromes.

AREA V1 DISORDERS

Anton syndrome

Denial of blindness, or Anton syndrome, is an uncommon form of anosagnosia that usually follows extensive damage to the striate cortex. Patients with Anton syndrome will deny they are blind and often confabulate to mask their visual loss. Geschwind noted that patients with this condition often had altered emotional reactivity, with a "coarse and shallow" affect similar to some patients with frontal lobe lesions. He attributed the denial of blindness to damage to higher cognitive centers.

Blindsight

Preserved higher levels of visual processing following an occipital stroke is referred to as blindsight. This entity encompasses a wide variety of visual processing mechanisms, all occurring without conscious awareness.

Riddoch phenomenon

In 1917, George Riddoch, a captain in the Royal Army Medical Corps, described 10 patients with wounds to the occipital area who were able to perceive movements within their blind hemifield. Riddoch phenomenon is the preservation of motion perception in an otherwise complete scotoma.

It has been suggested that patients who exhibit this phenomenon have preserved islands of function within the striate cortex. Clinically, the Riddoch phenomenon can be a useful prognostic indicator. For example, patients with the Riddoch phenomenon following an occipital stroke or in the setting of an occipital lobe tumor are more likely to recover function in the affected field, spontaneously in the first setting or after removal of the tumor in the second.

Cerebral achromatopsia is an acquired defect in color perception caused by damage to the ventromedial visual cortex. Affected patients describe a world that looks faded, gray, and washed out, or completely devoid of color, like a black-and-white photograph. This occurs in lesions of Area V4.

Transient achromatopsia

Transient achromatopsia resulting in some patients with vertebrobasilar insufficiency and visual ataxia are other presentations of lesions involving area V1.

Visual ataxia

Visual ataxia is a disorder of balance and results from a lesion in the occipital lobe. Patients with an homonymous hemianopia from an occipital lobe lesion may experience loss of balance associated with a sensation of falling toward the blind hemifield. Such patients have an intact vestibular system, and this "visual ataxia" is thought to be secondary to unopposed tonic input from the intact contralateral occipital lobe.

AREA V2 AND V3 (PRESTRIATE AND PERISTRIATE CORTEX) DISORDERS

Horton and Hoyt reported two patients with lesions thought to involve the superior parastriate and peristriate cortex. Both patients had homonymous quadrantic visual field defects that respected the horizontal and vertical meridians.

AREA V5 DISORDERS

Akinetopsia is the loss of perception of visual motion with preservation of the perception of other modalities of vision, such as form, texture, and color. This results from lesions involving Area V5.

Dyslexia is a broad term defining a learning disability that impairs a person's fluency or comprehension accuracy in being able to read, and spell. In a study using fMRI, Eden et al. found almost no activation of area V5 in dyslexic patients. The results of this study support previous psychophysiologic and anatomic data suggesting that patients with dyslexia have anomalous magnocellular responses.

THE DORSAL OCCIPITOFUGAL PATHWAY DISORDERS

This pathway originates in V1, traverses V2, V5/MT and continues to the posterior parietal cortex. This cortex contains various maps of the visual environment used in visually guided movement. These maps code the location of visual targets in a variety of coordinate systems tailored to the guidance of eye movements, head movements, and arm movements.

Bálint's syndrome

Bálint syndrome is classically defined as the combination of simultanagnosia, optic ataxia, and acquired oculomotor apraxia, also called psychic paralysis of gaze. The components of Bálint syndrome are not closely bound together and may occur in isolation or in association with other disorders of visuospatial perception. We will discuss each of these components separately.

Dorsal simultanagnosia: Patients with dorsal simultanagnosia can perceive whole shapes, but their perception of these shapes is limited to a single visual area because they are unable to shift visual attention.

Optic ataxia is a disorder of visual guidance of movements in which visual inputs are disconnected from the motor systems. Do not confuse this entity with visual ataxia which has been described earlier. Lesions of superior parietal cortex are more likely to damage areas involved with limb guidance, whereas inferior parietal lesions are more likely to affect visual attention and thus produce neglect syndromes.

Spasm of fixation is characterized by loss of voluntary eye movements with persistence of fixation on a target. However, in contrast to true ocular motor apraxia, saccades easily are made to peripheral targets in the absence of a fixation target.

There are other manifestations of injury to the where pathway. Hemifield neglect can be present on the contralateral side of the lesion. The subject fails to see objects in that hemifield with binocular stimulation, but sees objects in both the fields with uniocular testing. This is primarily because both the eyes and their visual pathways till the striate cortex are intact, but the processing after that is what is erroneous. Thus we may have a patient with homonymous hemianopia on binocular testing, but is normal with uniocular testing.

Classic visual allesthesia is a disorder of visuospatial perception in which the retinotopic visual field is rotated, flipped, or even inverted. If the environment is rotated instead it is termed environmental rotation. Here, the environment is rotated irrespective of head position, but in visual allesthesia, the vision changes with head position.

THE VENTRAL OCCIPITOFUGAL PATHWAY DISORDERS

Disorders of this pathway cause defects in recognition, identification and analysis of objects. The "Where" pathway mainly dealt with the relationship of the object in focus with the space around it. A few disorders worth mentioning are:

1. Agnosia—Failure in recognition of an object.
2. Anomia—Failure in naming the object.
3. Alexia—Difficulty in reading, although identification with other sensory modalities like tracing an alphabet may still be intact. These patients will be able to write. Hence, pure alexia is without agraphia—the inability to write.

Visual hallucinations

Hallucinations are internally generated perceptions. Activation of visual processing areas can result in internally generated visual stimuli that are perceived consciously.

This activation of visual processing areas can result from psychiatric disease states like schizophrenia, narcolepsy and mania, from neurological diseases like Alzheimer's disease and epilepsy, vascular conditions like stroke, metabolic derangements like alcohol withdrawal, and finally drug induced hallucinations.

Hallucinations can be simple or complex. Simple hallucinations consist of phosphenes, brief flashes of light, various shapes and textures. Complex hallucinations are specific objects like people, animals, plants or imaginary creatures.

Three main types of hallucinations are as under:

1. Release hallucinations or the Charles Bonnet syndrome
2. Visual migraine
3. Visual seizures

Charles Bonnet syndrome

Charles Bonnet, a Swiss naturalist, described complex formed hallucinations experienced by his 89-year-old grandfather, who, although cognitively intact, was blind from cataracts. These hallucinations were later described by Cogan as seen by blind or near blind people. It presumably occurs from deprivation of visual input, which results in a "Release" of previously perceived visual stimuli. These patients often tend to see images that they have previously seen when their vision was good.

As these hallucinations can occur during sensory deprivation, it can also occur with bilateral patching of the eyes, thus termed as black patch psychosis. Social deprivation and loneliness can also be an added risk factor. These patients are often aware that what they are seeing is unreal, and are afraid to mention it to their friends as they feel people will think they are crazy. This is in contrast to the hallucinations experienced by schizophrenics who believe what they see is real.

Thus vision loss—worse than 20/60 in the better eye and social isolation have been postulated as the main causative factors. Most patients are not disturbed by release hallucinations, and some patients may even enjoy them; however, identification of this syndrome is important to avoid unnecessary neuroimaging and psychiatric evaluations.

Treatment consists of removing the patient from social isolation and a few drugs like anticonvulsants, haloperidol and tiapride that have been tested with mixed success.

Visual migraine

The typical fortification spectra of visual migraines (migraine with visual aura or visual aura without headache) usually consist of a moving arc of either colored or black-and-white zigzag lines that expand toward the periphery with concurrent increase in the size of lines. These scintillations reflect the cytoarchitectural arrangement of the orientation columns as a wave of excitatory activity spreads across the striate cortex. The scotoma that trails behind fortification spectra represents an area of transient inactivation of cortical neurons. These phenomena usually last about 20 minutes and may or may not be followed by headache. A variety of atypical hallucinations also may occur during migraine attacks, including formed hallucinations, micropsia, macropsia, palinopsia, and visual allesthesia.

Visual seizures

Visual seizures involving the occipital or, occasionally, the temporal lobe may cause unformed hallucinations similar to those experienced during a classic migraine attack. Patients with visual seizures usually lack the typical history of migraines, have an atypical frequency and duration of hallucinations, and often exhibit other seizure phenomena such as eye deviation or rapid blinking. Temporal and even occipital lobe seizures may cause formed visual hallucinations, thus mimicking the Charles Bonnet syndrome. Although, a careful history usually will differentiate visual seizures from other visual hallucinations, the diagnosis in some cases can be made only by seizure monitoring.

Drug induced seizures

Drugs, both prescribed and illicit, can induce hallucinations. Some of the more common drugs associated with visual hallucinations are indomethacin, digoxin, bupropion, vincristine, cyclosporin, lithium, lidocaine, and dopamine. Visual hallucinations can also occur in patients given topical homatropine, scopolamine, atropine, or other topical agents. Withdrawal of certain medications, such as baclofen, may cause hallucinations. The most frequent types of visual hallucinations are release hallucinations, visual migraines, and visual seizures.

CORTICAL BLINDNESS

Cortical blindness (visual cortex disease) is produced by bilateral occipital lobe lesions. Unilateral occipital lobe lesions typically produce contralateral macular sparing congruous homonymous hemianopia.

Causes of cortical blindness include:

- *Vascular lesions* producing bilateral occipital infarction are the commonest cause of cortical blindness (e.g. embolization of posterior cerebral arteries).
- *Head injury* involving bilateral occipital lobes is the second common causes.
- *Tumors,* primary (e.g. falcotentorial meningiomas, bilateral gliomas) or metastatic are rare causes.
- *Other rare causes* of cortical blindness are migraine, hypoxic encephalopathy, Schilder's disease and other leukodystrophies.

Clinical features. Cortical blindness is characterized by:

- Bilateral loss of vision
- Normal papillary light reflexes
- Visual imagination and visual imagery in dream are preserved
- *Anton syndrome,* i.e. denial of blindness by the patients who obviously cannot see
- *Riddoch phenomenon,* i.e. ability to perceive kinetic but not static targets.

Management. A thorough neurological and cardiovascular investigative workup including MRI and MRI angiography should be carried out. Treatment depends upon the underlying cause. Partial or complete recovery may occur in patients with stroke progressing from cortical blindness through visual agnosia, and partially impaired perceptual function to recovery.

OTHER VISUAL DISORDERS

NIGHT BLINDNESS (NYCTALOPIA)

Night (scotopic) vision is a function of rods. Therefore, the conditions in which functioning of these nerve endings is deranged will result in night blindness. These include vitamin A deficiency, tapetoretinal degenerations (e.g.

retinitis pigmentosa), congenital high myopia, familial congenital night blindness and Oguchi's disease. It may also develop in conditions of the ocular media interfering with the light rays in dim light (i.e. with dilated pupils). These include paracentral lenticular and corneal opacities. In advanced cases of primary open angle glaucoma, dark adaptation may be so much delayed that patient gives history of night blindness.

DAY BLINDNESS (HEMERALOPIA)

It is a symptomatic disturbance of the vision, in which the patient is able to see better in dim light as compared to bright light of the day. Its causes are:

- Congenital deficiency of cones
- Central lenticular opacities (polar cataracts) and
- Central corneal opacities.

AMAUROSIS

It implies complete loss of sight in one or both eyes, in the absence of ophthalmoscopic or other marked objective signs.

1. Amaurosis fugax

It refers to a sudden, temporary and painless monocular visual loss occurring due to a transient failure of retinal circulation.

Common causes of amaurosis fugax are: carotid transient ischemic attacks (TIA), embolization of retinal circulation, papilledema, giant cell arteritis, Raynaud's disease, migraine, as a prodromal symptom of central retinal artery or carotid artery occlusion, hypertensive retinopathy, and venous stasis retinopathy. An attack of amaurosis fugax is typically described by the patients as a curtain that descends from above or ascends from below to occupy the upper or lower halves of their visual fields.

Clinical characteristics. The attack lasts for two to five minutes and resolves in the reverse pattern of progression, leaving no residual deficit. Due to brief duration of the attack, it is rarely possible to observe the fundus. When observed shortly after an attack, the fundus may either be normal or reveal signs of retinal ischemia such as retinal edema and small superficial hemorrhages. In some cases, retinal emboli in the form of white plugs (fibrin-platelet aggregates) may be seen.

2. Uremic amaurosis

It is a sudden, bilateral, complete loss of sight occurring probably due to the effect of certain toxic materials upon the cells of the visual center in patients suffering from acute nephritis, eclampsia of pregnancy and renal failure. The visual loss is associated with dilated pupils which generally react to light. The fundi are usually normal except for the coincidental findings of hypertensive retinopathy, when associated. Usually, the vision recovers in 12–48 hours.

AMBLYOPIA

Amblyopia by definition refers to a partial loss of sight in one or both eyes, caused by abnormal visual development secondary to abnormal visual stimulation in the absence of ophthalmoscopic or other marked objective signs. Literally speaking, amblyopia is a spectrum of visual loss, ranging from missing a few letters on the 20/20 lines to hand motion vision. However, for practical purposes, amblyopia is labelled, when there is at least two Snellen lines difference in the visual acuity between the eyes. Amblyopia occurring in a patient with strabismus is not a sensory adaptation per se, but the consequence of suppression which is a sensory adaptation.

CLASSIFICATION AND TERMINOLOGY

Despite the advanced electrophysiologic, psychophysical and histopathologic studies, the present knowledge of amblyopia is still inadequate, and therefore, no consensus has been reached regarding classification and terminology of amblyopia. Some of the older and newer concepts are as described as follows.

Functional versus organic amblyopia

Organic amblyopia, which is irreversible, refers to partial visual loss caused by undetectable organic lesions in the eye or in the visual pathway, e.g. toxic amblyopia. While *functional amblyopia* refers to obligatory psychical suppression of the retinal image. Functional amblyopia is reversible in large number of cases and depending on the cause, may be anisometropic, strabismic, meridional or stimulus deprivation.

Classification of amblyopia into organic and functional gives a broader view of the condition. However, some of the workers have suggested the term *developmental amblyopia* in place of functional amblyopia because of the following reasons:

- The term 'functional' in psychiatry and neurology means 'hysterical' or 'psychological' while the amblyopic condition under consideration is not such.
- Electrophysiological, psychophysical and histopathologic changes observed from the occipital cortex of experimental animals with such type of induced amblyopia constitute the ultimate refutation of the 'functional organic' dichotomy.

Amblyopia of arrest versus amblyopia of extinction

Chavasse divided the amblyopia that results from interference with the fixation reflex during period of visual immaturity (from birth to 6 years of age) into two types—amblyopia of arrest and amblyopia of extinction.

Amblyopia of arrest is a term used by Chavasse to define an amblyopia caused by a halt in visual development early in life. Since, it is now known that a 6/6 visual acuity in an infant is reached by 6 months of age, 'amblyopia of arrest' would be caused by an interference with the fixation reflex that begins before 6 months of age, i.e. during critical period of development.

Amblyopia of extinction was referred by Chavasse to denote an amblyopia resulting from the suppression of an already existing visual acuity. A related and more recent term *suppression amblyopia* is based on the idea that in order to avoid diplopia and confusion the deviating eye in strabismus becomes suppressed and that this suppression eventually takes on a permanent obligatory character. However, this is usually possible in children up to 6 years of age. In other words, it can be concluded that any strabismus or visual deprivation between the age of 6 months and 6 years would result in amblyopia of extinction or the so-called suppression amblyopia. Though, these terms are not in much use presently, they do help in understanding of the subject.

Congenital versus acquired amblyopia

The term *congenital amblyopia* had been used in the literature for the patients having low vision, nystagmus and poor color vision. Since these findings suggest a defective cone function, Goodman et al. have suggested that the term congenital amblyopia should be replaced by the term *cone deficiency syndrome.*

The term *congenital amblyopia* is also used for patients having reduced visual acuity in whom no obvious cause such as strabismus or ametropia, is present. These patients do not respond to treatment and it is assumed that they are caused by lesions somewhere along the visual pathway. Congenital amblyopia has been classified as one of the organic amblyopia.

Acquired amblyopia is a non-informative term which encompasses all other cases with amblyopia such as those due to strabismus, anisometropia, disuse, etc.

Present day terminologies for amblyopia

Many of the above described terminologies are not used in present day clinical practice. As already pointed out, no consensus has been reached regarding classification of amblyopia. The self-explanatory terms used for amblyopia in present day orthoptic practice are as follows:

1. Strabismic amblyopia

The term strabismic amblyopia is used for the amblyopia seen in those patients with unilateral constant squint who strongly favor one eye for fixation.

Strabismic amblyopia is a common form of amblyopia and typically shows following features that are uncommon in other forms of amblyopia:

- *Grating acuity* is often considerably less reduced than the Snellen's acuity. This is because forms seen by the affected eye are in a twisted or distorted manner that interfere more with letter recognition than with the simpler task of determining whether a grating is present or not.
- *Neutral density filter effect,* i.e. when illumination is decreased, the acuity of an eye with strabismic amblyopia does not decline further while it does so in organic amblyopia.
- *Laterality,* strabismic amblyopia is always unilateral and is caused by an active inhibition within the retinocortical pathways of visual input originating in the fovea of the deviating eye. Strabismic amblyopia follows through a stage of suppression, giving rise to the term suppression amblyopia.
- *Type of strabismus.* Strabismic amblyopia is seen far more often in esotropes than the exotropes. This might be related to the fact that in esotropia, the fovea of the deviating eye has to compete with the strong temporal hemifield of the fellow eye; while in exotropia, the fovea of the deviating eye has to compete with the weaker contralateral nasal hemifield.
- Strabismic amblyopia occurs very rarely in patients with hypertropia, as they usually manage to maintain fusion in some positions of gaze with an anomalous head posture.
- Patients with alternate strabismus do not have amblyopia but they do have abnormal binocular function.

2. Stimulus deprivation amblyopia or amblyopia of disuse (old term: Amblyopia ex anopsia)

The term amblyopia ex anopsia (amblyopia of disuse) has been used for years to label the amblyopia resulting in patients with strabismus (thinking that this eye is being disused). However, this term has been discarded in relation to strabismus. Since such an amblyopic eye is not prevented from use, von Noorden has suggested that the term amblyopia ex anopsia should be reserved for those conditions only wherein one eye is totally excluded from seeing early in life. Such conditions would include monocular congenital or traumatic cataract, complete ptosis, corneal opacity and prolonged patching of the normal eye for treatment of amblyopia (occlusion amblyopia). The literature of recent years reflects the tendency to accept the von Noorden's suggestion and the term *stimulus deprivation amblyopia* is preferred.

Deprivation amblyopia is characterized by following features:

- It is the least common but most damaging and difficult to treat form of amblyopia.
- Amblyopic visual loss resulting from unilateral deprivation is worse than that produced by bilateral deprivation of similar degree. This is because of the fact that in the unilateral deprivation, interocular effects add to the direct developmental impact of severe image degradation.

Note. Bilateral deprivational amblyopia may develop in small children with bilateral media opacities, e.g.:

- Bilateral congenital cataract
- Bilateral corneal opacities (Peter's anomaly)
- Bilateral vitreous haemorrhage

3. Anisometropic amblyopia

The term anisome tropic amblyopia refers to the amblyopia occurring in an eye having higher degree of refractive error than the fellow eye.

Anisohypermetropic versus anisomyopic amblyopia. It has been reported that amblyopia is more common and is of a higher degree in patients with anisohypermetropia than in those with anisomyopia. Even 1–2 dioptre hyperopic anisometropia may cause amblyopia while up to 3 dioptre myopic anisometropia usually does not cause amblyopia. However, unilateral high myopia (–6 D or more) often results in severe amblyopia. It has been presumed that both the forms, vision deprivation as well as the abnormal binocular interaction that is caused by unequal foveal images in the two eyes, might be playing role in the development of anisometropic amblyopia.

Strabismus is frequently associated with anisometropia. In such cases whether amblyopia occurs due to anisometropia or strabismus or both is very difficult to determine.

4. Meridional amblyopia

This refers to amblyopia occurring in patients with uncorrected astigmatic refractive error due to selective visual deprivation for visual stimuli of a certain spatial orientation. Thus, meridional amblyopia is a selective amblyopia for a specific visual meridian. Even small amount of unilateral astigmatism may cause amblyopia.

5. Isoametropic amblyopia

Isoametropic amblyopia is bilateral amblyopia occurring in children with bilateral uncorrected high refractive error. Hyperopia of more than +5.0 D and myopia in excess of –10.0 D have a risk of inducing bilateral amblyopia. Such amblyopia is usually of milder form. It is supposed to result from the effect of blurred retinal images alone (pattern vision deprivation). Bilateral meridional amblyopia is caused by bilateral astigmatism. Significant meridional amblyopia occurs with astigmatism greater than –2.5 D.

6. Amblyopia secondary to nystagmus

Bilateral amblyopia may occur secondary to nystagmus. But usually, it is very difficult to ascertain whether nystagmus is the cause or effect of reduced visual acuity. In some patients with bilateral amblyopia having apparently no amblyogenic factor, micro-nystagmus may be discovered while examining for fixation behavior with the visuscope or conventional direct ophthalmoscope containing a fixation target.

7. Idiopathic amblyopia

It refers to unilateral amblyopia occurring in apparently normal patients with a negative history for strabismus and in the absence of other usual amblyogenic factors. Clinically, such patients have foveal suppression and visual acuity improves after patching of the sound eye, but the amblyopia recurs, when treatment is suspended. von Noorden has postulated that perhaps it occurs due to some amblyogenic factors (such as transient anisometropia) which are present in infancy for a short period but disappear with advancing age.

PATHOGENESIS AND PATHOPHYSIOLOGY OF AMBLYOPIA

Despite an enormous research in this field, pathogenesis and pathophysiology of amblyopia is still not elucidated fully. However, the clinical features and laboratory findings in eyes with amblyopia permit certain conclusions for understanding the nature of the processes underlying amblyopia and its treatment. Psychophysical studies in human strabismic, anisometropic and visual deprivation amblyopia show differences between the function of the fovea versus the retinal periphery. Further, there are also differences in the severity and reversibility of the various types of amblyopia. However, the most pertinent factual knowledge about the changes occurring in amblyopia which has been obtained through experimental studies (electrophysiologic and histopathologic) in kittens suggests that the structural and functional involvement of the afferent visual pathway in different forms of amblyopia is the same as is the sensitive period during which amblyopia occurs, regardless of the etiology. Therefore, on the basis of this recent neurophysiologic reasearch, largely done in experimental animals, it has been postulated that the basic amblyogenic mechanisms are—light deprivation, foveal form vision deprivation, abnormal binocular interaction and active cortical inhibition.

Thus, the pathophysiology of amblyopia can be discussed under following headings:

• Amblyogenic factors
• Role of retina in the development of amblyopia
• Active cortical inhibition

A. AMBLYOGENIC FACTORS

The basic mechanisms responsible for amblyopia, which have been recognized on the basis of neurophysiologic research, largely done in experimental animals, are as follows:

• Deprivation of form vision
• Light deprivation
• Abnormal binocular interaction

1. Deprivation of form vision

• *Monocular deprivation of form vision* during the critical period of visual development results in amblyopia of the deprived eye. Since the deprived eye becomes dominated by the normal eye so a *competitive amblyopia* of profound intensity develops. Monocular visual deprivation works as an amblyogenic factor in strabismic, anisometropic, stimulus deprivation ambloypia.
• *Binocular deprivation of form vision* during the critical period of visual development results in bilateral deprivational amblyopia. Since in binocular deprivation, the binocular interaction is not disrupted so a competitive amblyopia is not superimposed; so the resultant amblyopia not so severe as in unilateral deprivation. Binocular deprivation plays the role of amblyogenic factor in children with bilateral cataract, ametropia and bilateral high refractive errors.

2. Light deprivation

Light deprivation works as an amblyogenic factor in children with unilateral as well as bilateral complete cataracts.

3. Abnormal binocular interaction

Abnormal binocular interaction is highly amblyogenic. It produces a profound amblyopia due to a competition amblyopia. Abnormal binocular interaction plays the role of amblyogenic factor in children with strabismic, anisometropic and unilateral stimulus deprivation amblyopia.

Thus, the amblyogenic factors for different types of amblyopia are same. However, their contribution to each may vary and so is the severity of amblyopia (Table 20.2).

Neurophysiological basis of role of amblyogenic factors

The above conclusions about the role of various amblyogenic mechanisms have been drawn from the various experimental studies done in cat, kitten and monkey. A few key studies to understand the neurophysiologic basis of normal binocular vision and amblyopia are described briefly here.

Neurophysiologic basis of normal binocular vision

Hubel and Wiesel are pioneers in the neurophysiologic studies of binocular vision. They have concluded that in normal cat or kitten:

• Approximately 80% neurons of striate cortex are derived from each eye, 10% from the contralateral eye and 10% from the ipsilateral eye only. The two receptive fields of binocularly driven cortical cells are found to have corresponding location in the two retinae.
• Of the binocularly driven cortical neurons, only 25% are stimulated equally well from each eye, while the remaining 75% show graded degree of influence from the right or left eye (disparity sensitive binocular cells).

Table 20.2 *Role of amblyogenic factors in different types of amblyopia*

Types of amblyopia	Amblyogenic factors			
	Light deprivation	*Deprivation of form vision*	*Abnormal binocular interaction*	*Severity of amblyopia*
• Stimulus deprivation amblyopia				
– Unilateral (e.g. cataract)	+	+	+	+ + +
– Bilateral (e.g. cataract)	+	+	–	+ +
• Strabismic amblyopia	–	+	+	+ +
• Anisometropic amblyopia	–	+	+	+ +
• Ametropic amblyopia	–	+	–	+

Stereopsis has been linked with horizontal disparity sensitive binocularly driven cortical neurons.

- It has been reported that at birth (i.e. without previous visual experience or training) the visual system of kittens gives responses which are in no way different from those obtained in adult cats. From this, the conclusion was drawn that the basis for visual recognition and binocular interaction is already fully developed at birth. The immaturity of visually dependent behavior in young animals, such as the lack of pursuit movements, therefore, cannot be explained by incomplete development but must be due to other factors, possibly lack of interpretation or of visuomotor cooperation.

- To understand the pathophysiologic mechanisms concerned with binocular vision and development of amblyopia, the visual pathway carrying visual sensations from the retina to visual cortex have been classified in X, Y and W-system (Fig. 20.1) as follows:

X-system. The fibers from the retinal ganglion cells carrying the sustained response to visual stimuli are found in the X cell system—the medium velocity system. The X-system is associated with central form vision, and therefore, central visual acuity. Cells of this system project only to the lateral geniculate nucleus.

Y-system. The fibers from the retinal ganglion cells carrying a transient response are in the Y cell, or fast system. The Y-system is associated with the peripheral retina and is concerned with the location of objects in space, which enables

fixation movements to be made. This system projects to both the lateral geniculate nuclei and superior colliculus.

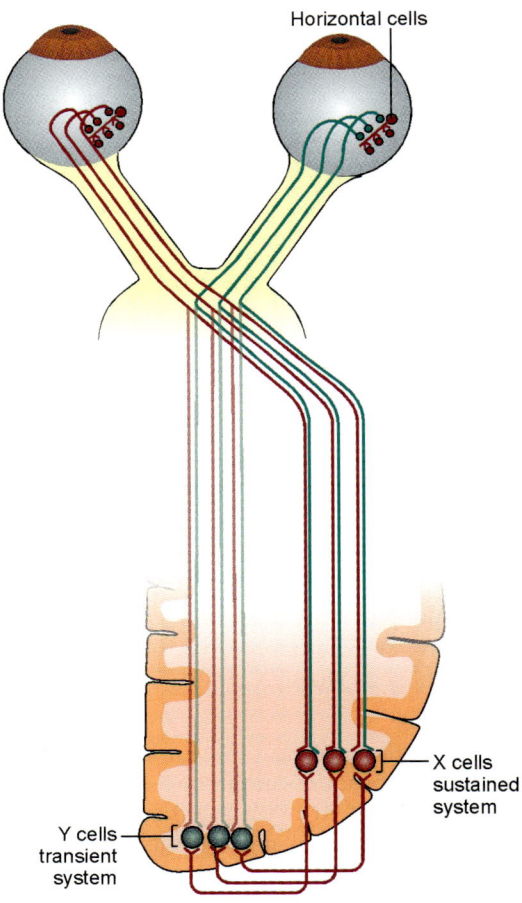

Fig. 20.1 *X, Y and W-system of cells in the visual cortex.*

W cell system (slow system). It is believed to be the pursuit system. It projects only to superior colliculus.

Neurophysiologic studies in experimental and clinical amblyopia

Neurophysiology of amblyopia is a complex mechanism and its understanding is far from complete. Some of the observations made from the study of experimental modification of visual experience in animals and laboratory testing of amblyopic human beings are given below.

Monocular deprivation studies

Methods

Monocular deprivation was produced in experimental animals (kitten and monkey) by suturing the eyelids of one eye during the critical period of development.

Observations

• Deprived eye developed amblyopia, probably because this eye was dominated by the normal eye due to the interruption in binocular co-operation.

• Changes observed in visual system neuron functions were as follows:

– In the lateral geniculate body, cells in those layers receiving input from the deprived eye showed a profound shrinkage. Larger cells shrank more than the smaller ones.

– Cells of primary visual cortex either lost their innate ability to respond to stimulation or showed significant functional deficiency.

It has been reported that there occurs a selective reduction in the number of cortical cells driven by Y-input from retina, suggesting that perhaps visual deprivation selectively involves the Y-system.

Note. Similar experiments in adult animals did not reveal such changes.

Conclusions

These studies indicate that uniocular visual deprivation produces amblyopia by changes in the visual system neurons. It has also been concluded that deprivation during the early part of critical period of development is more deleterious than at a later stage. This experimental work of uniocular deprivation closely resembles the clinical situation of unilateral cataract, severe congenital ptosis or corneal opacity producing profound amblyopia.

Binocular deprivation studies

Binocular visual deprivation was made by bilateral tarsorrhaphy in kittens and monkeys during sensitive period of development and also in visually mature animals and following observations were made:

• A mild bilateral amblyopia occurred in infant animals due to visual deprivation. Perhaps amblyopia was mild due to the fact that the competition amblyopia was not superimposed since the binocular interaction was not abnormal in binocular equal deprivation.

• Changes observed in visual system neuron functions were as follows:

– Cell shrinkage produced in lateral geniculate body was less than that produced in uniocular deprivation.

– There occurred a decrease in the specific responsiveness of cells and an increase in number of cells that respond sluggishly or abnormally. In addition, there were many cells that did not respond at all.

– The number of Y cells was reduced by 307%.

– It was postulated that in binocular deprivation, there may be a competition for synaptic space in the cortex between the X cells and the more disadvantaged Y cells.

Conclusions

The amblyopia produced by binocular deprivation was less severe than that produced by uniocular deprivation, owing to the fact that binocular interaction was not abnormal. This work closely resembles the clinical situations of bilateral amblyopia seen in children with bilateral cataract and also to some extent the ametropic amblyopia.

Experimentally produced strabismus studies

In monkeys made artificially strabismic, by disinserting lateral or medial rectus, only the binocular portion of the lateral geniculate body showed cell shrinkage, while in visually deprived monkeys, both the monocular and binocular portions of the lateral geniculate nucleus showed shrinkage. Thus, two different neural mechanisms appear to underlie the deprivational and strabismic amblyopia. However, it has been postulated that visual deprivation (since central fixation is not used in strabismus), abnormal binocular interaction and active cortical inhibition similar to that occurs, in suppression, all play a role in the amblyopia associated with strabismus. While this seems reasonable intuitively and laboratory findings suggest this, but definitive proof is still lacking.

B. ROLE OF RETINA IN DEVELOPMENT OF AMBLYOPIA

There is some evidence that the retina itself is abnormal in amblyopia. Whether retinal abnormality is the effect or cause of amblyopia is debatable. The views have differed, if retinal threshold and sensitivity have been affected in amblyopia. It is, however, widely believed and proved experimentally that there is a decreased sensitivity of foveal cones in amblyopia. Even flicker fusion threshold and differential thresholds are considerably affected. However, reduction of foveal cone and retinal sensitivity is much less than the reduction in visual acuity. Also electroretinography is found to be normal in amblyopic eyes. It, therefore, is improbable that a functional defect of foveal cones would be responsible for reduced visual acuity. However, amblyopic eye is not at its best under photopic condition than under mesopic conditions. In fact, it has been observed that there is a quicker dark adaptation in such eyes suggesting takeover of rod functions from decreased retinal foveal cones. It is, therefore, logical to believe that reduced inputs from the rods and cones in the affected eye cause certain neurophysiological changes, transmitted aberrantly to the CNS which triggers the onset of amblyopia. The vicious circle continues, till the process is reversed. It may become irreversible in later stages.

That retinal sensitivity is related to onset of amblyopia is further proved by the fact that eyes which had relatively poor sensitivity, responded to amblyopia treatment better than those which had better retinal thresholds. Perhaps a different mechanism is also responsible, i.e. a central suppression exists in amblyopia.

C. ACTIVE CORTICAL INHIBITION

The neurophysiologic research points out that visual deprivation and active cortical inhibition are the two fundamental mechanisms for the development of amblyopia. The role of active cortical inhibition is evidenced by following studies.

1. *Physiologic evidence.* In one study, in experimental animals, deprivation amblyopia was produced in one eye. After 5 months of deprivation, these animals, were divided into two groups. In group-I animals the normal eye was enucleated, while in group-II, the normal was retained and following observations were made:

In group-I animals (with normal eye enucleated), the amblyopic eye was found to drive 31% of the visual cortex cells. While in group-II animals, in which normal eye was retained, only 6% of the visual cortex cells were driven by the amblyopic eye. In other words, after removal of the normal eye, the deprived eye showed marked capacity for recovery indicating thereby that perhaps the normal eye may be responsible for an active cortical inhibition in unilateral amblyopia.

2. *Pharmacologic evidence.* It has been ascertained that under normal circumstances, most of the excitatory synapses in the visual cortex are cholinergic. Further, it has also been reported that the visual cortex is inhibited by the gamma aminobutyric acid (GABA)—an inhibitory neurotransmitter. The assumption that perhaps in amblyopia, active cortical inhibition might be mediated by GABA led the researchers to perform certain experiments.

Duffy et al. produced deprivation amblyopia in kittens and studied the effects of some anti-GABA agents. Following observations were made by them:

- *Intravenous injection of biculline* (an anti-GABA agent) led to stimulation of 60% visual cortex cells which were otherwise unresponsive due to deprivation amblyopia. However, convulsions were noted as a complication of this drug.
- *Intravenous injection of naloxone,* another anti-GABA agent, also restored binocular inputs in the visual cortex cells which were otherwise unresponsive due to deprivation amblyopia.

Kasamatsu and Pettigrew produced depletion of brain catecholamines by using 6-hydroxy-dopamine and norepinephrine and observed a failure of ocular dominance shift after mono-cular occlusion in kittens.

The above studies provide a pharmacologic evidence of the role of active cortical inhibition in the amblyopia. However, further studies will reveal as to where we stand in understanding the pathological basis of onset of amblyopia.

CLINICAL CHARACTERISTICS AND LABORATORY FINDINGS IN AMBLYOPIA

1. Visual acuity

Amblyopia, by definition, refers to a partial loss of sight in one or both eyes in the absence of ophthalmoscopic and other marked objective signs. It has been recommended that a difference of two lines on a visual acuity chart should be there to diagnose amblyopia. However, strictly speaking, any difference between the two eyes especially in strabismic amblyopia should be considered significant.

Certain clinical characteristics associated with visual acuity in patients with amblyopia are as follows:

i. Recognition acuity (Snellen's or similar charts) is more affected than the resolution acuity (Teller's chart or VER) and the detection acuity (Catford drum test or Bailey-Hall cereal test).

ii. Snellen's acuity and grating acuity are affected equally in anisometropic amblyopia whereas in strabismic amblyopia, the grating acuity is affected to half the extent of Snellen's acuity. Thus, strabismic amblyopia is under-estimated on grating test.

iii. Effect of neutral density filter. It has been reported that when visual acuity is tested with a neutral density filter placed in front of the affected eye, the visual acuity improves by one or two lines in patients with developmental amblyopia; while in patients with organic amblyopia, the visual acuity decreases by two to three lines. Therefore, the *neutral density filter test* has been recommended to differentiate between developmental amblyopia and organic amblyopia.

The neutral density filter test is based on the fact that under photopic conditions, visual acuity of amblyopic eye is less than that under scotopic conditions. Since the neutral density filter, when placed in front of an eye, produces a state of scotopic conditions, the vision of amblyopic eye improves.

iv. Crowding phenomenon. Crowding pheno-menon, also known as *separation difficulty*, refers to the inability of an amblyopic eye to distinguish letters (or other symbols) crowded together. Therefore, the vision in an amblyopic eye is better, when tested with isolated opto-types than when tested with line or Snellen's acuity charts having rows of letters. In other words, single optotype visual acuity is better than linear visual acuity. The larger the dis-crepancy between the linear and single letter acuity, the poorer the prognosis.

Crowding phenomenon is the result of contour-interaction between the neighbouring test targets because of decreased lateral inhibition in amblyopia.

2. Fixation pattern

Amblyopia may be associated with central fixation, eccentric viewing or eccentric fixation. In a normal eye, three characteristics of foveolar area, which appear to be responsible for maintaining the fixation reflex central, are:

a. Peak visual acuity in the foveolar region
b. A principal occulocentric direction of straight ahead
c. A retinomotor value of zero.

Amblyopia with central fixation. In amblyopia with foveolar fixation, the foveola has preserved the principal visual direction and its zero retinomotor value. Amblyopia is secondary to a central suppression scotoma.

Amblyopia with eccentric viewing. In amblyopia with eccentric viewing, patients prefer to view with an extrafoveal point bacause of the deep suppression scotoma, but the fovea has still not lost its principal visual direction. In eccentric viewing, patients look past the object they have been asked to fix. This can be demonstrated during visuscopic examination of a co-operative patient, who will tell the examiner that he/she is aware of the fact that he/she has to look over to one side to see the star clearly and when he/she looks straight ahead the fixation target appears blurred. The examiner can also observe that in eccentric viewing, patient will place the image of fixation target first on the fovea and then immediately from the fovea onto the paramacular retinal elements.

Amblyopia with eccentric fixation. In amblyopia with eccentric fixation, the fovea has lost its principal visual direction, its retinal motor value is no longer zero and an extrafoveal point is now the bearer of these properties. Patients report that they are looking straight at an object stimulating non-foveolar retinal area. If the image of an object is placed on the patient's fovea (by means of an instrument), this object is sensed as being in some other direction than straight ahead.

Types of eccentric fixation. Depending upon the retinal area with which the eyes appear to fixate, the eccentric fixation may be of following types (Fig. 20.2):

- *Parafoveolar*—just outside the foveal reflex.
- *Parafoveal*—outside but close to foveal wall.
- *Paramacular*—on or just outside the rim of the macula. Many workers have now abandoned the use of this term because of vague ophthalmoscopic definition of the macula.
- *Peripheral*—outside the macula, anywhere between the macula and extreme retinal periphery.

Steady versus wandering fixation. Central as well as eccentric fixation may be steady or wandering. Wandering fixation, which occurs only upon covering the sound eye, must be distinguished from the monocular, spontaneous, pendular and vertical oscillations that are occasionally found in deeply amblyopic eyes. This condition has been designated as the *Heimann-Bielschowsky phenomenon*. It is clinically similar to other forms of monocular nystagmus that may occur in connection with posterior fossa or brainstem disorders.

Paradoxical eccentric fixations. Ordinarily, there develop nasal eccentricity in esotropic and temporal eccentricity in exotropic patients. However, sometimes the eccentric fixation may be paradoxical, i.e. reverse of the expected situation. In other words, there may be nasal eccentricity in exotropic and temporal eccentricity in esotropic patients. Such a situation can occur under following circumstances:

- Following surgical overcorrection of the deviation.
- In patients with spontaneous reversal of the deviation.
- Following prolonged occlusion of the sound eye in amblyopia.
- With no obvious cause (rarely).

3. Absolute central scotoma

Monocular scotometry on visual field charting may plot an absolute central scotoma. Visual field charting for this purpose should never be done binocularly, otherwise, a facultative binocular suppression scotoma (present only with binocular viewing) may be mistaken as the absolute central scotoma. The scotometry may not be possible in amblyopic, patients with unsteady fixation.

4. Localization of an object of regard

Localization of an object of regard is normal in patients having amblyopia with central as well as eccentric fixation. However, in patients having amblyopia with eccentric viewing, localization of an object of regard is faulty.

5. Color vision

Color vision anomalies may occur in patients with amblyopia only if visual acuity is markedly reduced below 6/36. Anomalous

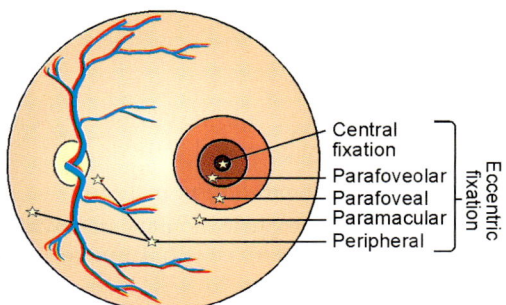

Central fixation
Parafoveolar
Parafoveal
Paramacular
Peripheral

Eccentric fixation

Fig. 20.2 *Types of fixation pattern.*

color vision in such cases has been related to peripheral eccentric fixation, i.e. a peripheral retinal area is being used for fixation rather than foveola.

6. Light perception

There occurs a dissociation of the form vision and light perception in amblyopia, since form vision is abnormal (especially under photopic condition) while absolute light threshold is found to be normal. However, differential threshold (i.e. how much brighter the test field must be than its surrounding so that a difference is perceived) is elevated in amblyopia.

7. Pupillary light reflexes

Generally speaking, pupillary light reflex is normal in amblyopes. However, rarely in patients with a deep amblyopia, an afferent pupillary defect may occur. It has been suggested that perhaps the afferent pupillary defect may result from synaptic inhibition in the retina, since this pathway does not reach the geniculate body.

8. Light and dark adaptation

Usually, dark adaptation is not abnormal in amblyopes, though a significant difference in adaptation between amblyopic and normal eyes has been found in the region of Kohlrausch's bend (the kink or bend in the adaptation curve normally produced by increased sensitivity of the rods).

9. Critical flicker frequency (CFF)

It has been reported that in amblyopia, central CFF tends to approach the CFF of peripheral retina or of rod mechanism. It has also been reported that CFF is significantly faster in amblyopic eyes that fixated eccentrically than in those with foveal fixation. Some workers have reported that examination of CFF with a simple apparatus is a useful tool to distinguish reduced visual acuity in maculopathies from amblyopia, since in the former the thresholds are below normal.

10. Electroretinography (ERG) and electro-oculography (EOG)

An enormous data is available on ERG studies in amblyopia, however, till date it has not been definitely answered whether ERG is normal or abnormal in amblyopia. Many studies report that ERG is essentially normal and EOG shows unsteadiness of fixation in amblyopia.

EVALUATION AND DIAGNOSIS

Diagnosis of amblyopia is made by a reduced best corrected visual acuity that cannot be entirely explained on the basis of physical ocular abnormalities. Clinical evaluation of a suspected case of amblyopia should include the following:

1. Evaluation of visual acuity
2. Neutral density filter test
3. Test for crowding phenomenon
4. Thorough ocular examination including fundus examination
5. Refraction
6. Evaluation for central versus eccentric fixation
7. Tests for other sensory anomalies.

MANAGEMENT OF AMBLYOPIA

Management of amblyopia includes:

• Prevention and early detection
• Treatment of amblyopia.

Prevention and early detection

Early detection as well as early intervention is most essential for the effective treatment of amblyopia. The best way for prevention and early diagnosis of amblyopia is adoption of some screening programme.

Treatment of amblyopia

Goal of amblyopia treatment is to maximize and potentially normalize visual acuity.

Strategies to treat amblyopia include:

• Elimination of the cause of visual deprivation and provision of clear retinal image in the amblyopic eye
• Correction of ocular dominance
• Perceptual training.

BIBLIOGRAPHY

1. Andersen RA, Zipser D. The role of the posterior parietal cortex in coordinate transformations for visual-motor integration. Can J Physiol Pharmacol 1988;66:488–501.

2. Andersen RA. Multimodal integration for the representation of space in the posterior parietal cortex. Philos Trans R Soc Lond B Biol Sci 1997;352:1421–8.

3. Anton G. Über Herderkrankungren der Gehirns, welche vom Patienten selbst nicht wahrgenommmen werden. Wiener Klinsche Wochenshrift 1989;33:227–9.

4. Argenta PA, Morgan MA. Cortical blindness and Anton syndrome in a patient with obstetric hemorrhage. Obstet Gynecol 1998;91:810–2.

5. Balint R. Seelenlähmung des Schauens, optische Ataxie, räumliche Strörung der Aufmerksamkeit. Monatsschr Psychiat Neurol 1909;25:51–81.

6. Bonnet C. Essai Analytique Sur Les Facultes de L'Ame. Copenhagen, Philber 1769;2.

7. Cogan DG. Visual hallucinations as release phenomena. Al- brecht von Graefes: Arch Klin Exp Ophthalmol 1973;188:139–50.

8. Colby CL, Duhamel JR. Spatial representations for action in parietal cortex. Brain Res Cogn Brain Res 1996;5:105–15.

9. Dacey DM, Lee BB. The blue-on opponent pathway in primate retina originates from a distinct bistratified ganglion cell type. Nature 1994;367:731–5.

10. Dacey DM. Circuitry for color coding in the primate retina. Proc Natl Acad Sci USA 1996;93:582–8.

11. Eden GF, VanMeter JW, Rumsey JM, et al. Abnormal processing of visual motion in dyslexia revealed by functional brain imaging (see comments). Nature 1996;382:66–9.

12. Essen DC, Zeki SM. The topographic organization of rhesus monkey prestriate cortex. J Physiol (Lond) 1978;277:193-226.

13. Farah MJ. Visual Agnosia Disorders of Object Recognition and What they Tell us about Normal Vision. Cambridge, MIT Press, 1990.

14. Friedrich FJ, Egly R, Rafal RD, et al. Spatial attention deficits in humans: a comparison of superior parietal and temporal-parietal junction lesions. Neuropsychology 1998;12:193–207.

15. Girkin C, Miller NR. Central Disorders of Vision in Humans. Surv Ophthalmol, 2001.

16. Goldberg ME, Segraves MA. Visuospatial and motor attention in the monkey. Neuropsychologia 1987;25:107–18.

17. Haxby JV, Grady CL, Horwitz B, et al. Dissociation of object and spatial visual processing pathways in human extrastriate cortex. Proc Natl Acad Sci USA 1991;88:1621–5.

18. Horton JC, Hoyt WF. Quadrantic visual field defects. A hallmark of lesions in extrastriate (V2/V3) cortex. Brain 1991;114:1703–18.

19. Hupp SL, Kline LB, Corbett JJ. Visual disturbances of migraine. Surv Ophthalmol 1989;33:221–36.

20. Kolmel HW. Colored patterns in hemianopic fields. Brain 1984;107:155–67.

21. Lapresle J, Metreau R, Annabi A. Transient achromatopsia in vertebrobasilar insufficiency. J Neurol 1977;215:155–8.

22. Lessel S. Higher disorders of visual function: negative phenomena, in Glaser J, Smith J (Eds): Neuro-ophthalmology, St. Louis, Mosby 1975;8:3–4.

23. Livingstone MS, Hubel DH. Psychophysical evidence for separate channels for the perception of form, color, movement, and depth. J Neurosci 1987;7:3416–68.

24. Livingstone MS, Rosen GD, Drislane FW, et al. Physiological and anatomical evidence for a magnocellular defect in developmental dyslexia [published erratum appears in Proc Natl Acad Sci USA 1993 Mar 15;90(6):2556]. Proc Natl Acad Sci USA 1991;88:7943–7.

25. McKeefry DJ, Zeki S. The position and topography of the human color center as revealed by functional magnetic resonance imaging. Brain 1997;120:2229–42.

26. Ogren MP, Mateer CA, Wyler AR. Alterations in visually related eye movements following left pulvinar damage in man. Neuropsychologia 1984;22:187–96.

27. Perenin MT, Vighetto A. Optic ataxia: a specific disruption in visuomotor mechanisms. I. Different aspects of the deficit in reaching for objects. Brain 1988;111:643–74.

28. Riddoch G. Dissociation of visual perceptions due to occiptial injuries, with especial reference to appreciation of movement. Brain 1917;15–7.

29. Rondot P, Odier F, Valade D. Postural disturbances due to homonymous hemianopic visual ataxia. Brain 1992;1(115):179–88.

30. Shipp S, Zeki S. Segregation of pathways leading from area V2 to areas V4 and V5 of macaque monkey visual cortex. Nature 1985;315:322–5.

31. Sokolski KN, Cummings JL, Abrams BI, et al. Effects of substance abuse on hallucination rates and treatment responses in chronic psychiatric patients. J Clin Psychiatry 1994;55:380–7.

32. Stoerig P, Cowey A. Blindsight in man and monkey. Brain 1997;120:535–59.

33. Sveinbjornsdottir S, Duncan JS. Parietal and occipital lobe epilepsy: a review (published erratum appears in Epilepsia Mar-Apr 1994; 35(2):467). Epilepsia 1993;34:493–521.

34. Teunisse RJ, Cruysberg JR, Hoefnagels WH, et al. Visual hallucinations in psychologically normal people: Charles Bonnets syndrome (see comments). Lancet 1996;347:794–7.

35. Troost BT, Newton TH. Occipital lobe arteriovenous malformations. Clinical and radiologic features in 26 cases with comments on differentiation from migraine. Arch Ophthalmol 1975; 93:250–6.

36. Ungerleider LG, Mishkin M. Two cortical visual systems, in I. DJ, G. MA and M. RJW (Eds): Analysis of Visual Behaviour. Cambridge, MIT Press 1982;549–86.

37. von Noorden GK, Middleditch PR. Histology of the monkey lateral geniculate nucleus after unilateral lid closure and experimental strabismus: further observations. Invest Ophthalmol 1975; 14:674–83.

38. Williamson PD, Thadani VM, Darcey TM, et al. Occipital lobe epilepsy: clinical characteristics, seizure spread patterns, and results of surgery. Ann Neurol 1992;31:3–13.

39. Zeki S. Color coding in the cerebral cortex: the reaction of cells in monkey visual cortex to wavelengths and colors. Neuroscience 1983;9: 741–65.

Section

VI

Ocular Manifestations of Diseases of Central Nervous System

21

OCULAR MANIFESTATIONS OF INTRACRANIAL INFECTIONS

AK Khurana, Ankita Phogat, Aruj K Khurana, Bhawna Khurana

INTRODUCTION
- Applied anatomical considerations
- General considerations

PRESENTING OCULAR FEATURES AND CLINICAL EVALUATION

Presenting Ocular Feature

Clinical Evaluation
- History
- Examination
- Investigations

COMMON INTRACRANIAL INFECTIONS
- Bacterial infections

- Viral infections
- Fungal infections
- Parasitic infections
- Prion diseases

CLINICAL PRESENTATIONS OF INTRA-CRANIAL INFECTIONS
- Epidural (extradural) abscess, subdural empyema/abscess and brain abscess
- Meningitis
- Encephalitis
- Cavernous sinus thrombosis

INTRODUCTION

APPLIED ANATOMICAL CONSIDERATIONS

- Ocular signs of intracranial involvement can be readily explained by anatomy of that particular part of nervous system
- Brain is protected by thick bony skull which inturn is covered by scalp. The meninges covering the brain are: innermost being the pia mater, followed by arachnoid mater and outermost lining being the dura mater.
- Inside the meninges lies the brain parenchyma.
- Blood vessels run in the subarachnoid space.
- Optic nerve is the direct continuation of the brain bringing with it the meninges. So, any infection involving the meninges can spread to optic nerve.
- Raised intracranial pressure hampers venous drainage of eye presenting as papilledema.
- The 3rd, 4th, and 6th cranial nerves supplying the eye arise from different brainstem nuclei and their involvement (easily seen on ocular examination) may point towards intracranial pathology.

- The venous drainage of eye into the cavernous sinus is an important link as this sinus also receives drainage from the brain.
- The path traveled by optic nerve in brain as tract and radiation can be affected by various pathologies presenting as visual field defects.
- The horizontal and vertical gazes of eye being controlled by pons and midbrain respectively, their paralysis points to the area of pathology. Also, the supranuclear control of gazes by frontal lobe can direct us to any localized abscess in the lobes if gaze area is involved.

GENERAL CONSIDERATIONS

Eyes can be considered as the mirror for intracranial pathologies. When carefully looked for, many ocular signs can point to involvement of the brain. Infact, many a times such patients with intracranial pathologies first report to an ophthalmologist either with a cranial nerve palsy or a visual field defect. This chapter deals with various ophthalmic manifestations which can point towards intracranial infections and might help in diagnosis of specific etiology.

Intracranial infections are not uncommon. Their incidence has increased in this era of acquired immunodeficiency syndrome (AIDS) and other forms of immunosuppression.

Common intracranial infections include:

- Meningitis
- Encephalitis
- Brain abscess, and
- Neurosyphilis

PRESENTING OCULAR FEATURES AND CLINICAL EVALUATION

PRESENTING OCULAR FEATURES

Ocular signs which are cardinal of most intracranial infections include:

- *Ptosis* (3rd cranial nerve involvement)
- *Strabismus*/ocular movement dysfunction (3rd, 4th, and 6th cranial nerve involvement)
- *Corneal anesthesia* (5th cranial nerve)
- Pupillary abnormalities
  - Argyll Robertson pupil (neurosyphilis).
  - Adie's pupil (viral encephalitis)
  - Horner's syndrome (viral encephalitis, posterior fossa lesions)
- *Visual field defects*, e.g. bitemporal hemianopia in pituitary adenoma.
- *Parkinson's sign* (intracavernous 6th cranial nerve palsy with post-ganglionic Horner's syndrome as here 6th nerve is joined by sympathetic branches from paracarotid plexus)
- *Accommodation paralysis*
- *Nystagmus* and nystagmoid movements (viral encephalitis)
- *Gaze palsies*
  - Horizontal (internuclear ophthalmoplegia in encephalitis)
  - Vertical (perinaud dorsal mid brain syndrome in meningitis)
- *Papillitis*
  - Infectious optic neuritis
  - Parainfectious optic neuritis
- *Neuro-retinitis*
- *Papilledema*
- *Choroiditis/retinitis*
- *Retinal hemorrhages* and cotton wool spots.

CLINICAL EVALUATION OF PATIENT

History

Following history should be taken from all patients suspected of having intracranial infection:

- *Fever:* Onset, duration, diurnal variation (evening rise of temperature), if associated with chills or rigors, grade.
- *Headache:* Onset, duration, site, recent change in character, aggravating factors like bending, diurnal variation, associated with nausea or vomiting
- *Neck stiffness*
- *Alteration* in mental status
- *Nausea and projectile vomiting* due to raised intracranial tension
- *Seizures:* Focal (due to focal arterial ischemia or infarction or edema), generalized (due to fever, hyponatremia or cerebral anoxia, antimicrobial toxicity)
- *Skin rash* or petechiae (meningococcal meningitis)
- *Focal neurological deficits.*

Examination

Findings on examination of patient which suggest intracranial infection are:

- *Fever*
- *Signs of raised intracranial tension* like papilledema, focal neurological deficits
- *Signs of meningeal irritation,* i.e. nuchal rigidity tested by Kernig and Brudzinski's maneuvers which stretch the inflamed spinal structures leading to pain and reflex extension of the neck and flexion of hips and knees.
- *Focal neurological signs* due to abscess or edema like hemiplegia or paresis, cranial nerve palsies, paresthesias.
- *Ocular signs* as mentioned above.

Investigations

Following investigations should be ordered whenever an intracranial infection is suspected:

- Blood culture
- Cerebrospinal fluid examination (increased intracranial pressure, raised WBC and cloudy appearance, raised protein and low sugar with identification of microorganism on culture or gram stain).
- Cranial MRI or CT scan (MRI preferred over CT)
- Biopsy of petechial skin lesions

COMMON INTRACRANIAL INFECTIONS

BACTERIAL INFECTIONS

Common bacteria causing intracranial infections are:
- *Streptococcus pneumoniae*
- *Neisseria meningitidis*
- *Haemophilus influenzae*

Others lesser common bacteria include:
- Group B streptococci (in neonates), and
- *Listeria monocytogenes* or *Enterobacteriaceae* species (in elderly or immunocompromised).
- Even in HIV+ patients, *S. pneumoniae* is most common, but non-typhi *Salmonella* species can cause acute meningitis.

MENINGITIS

Meningitis, i.e. infection and inflammation of the meanings surrounding the brain, is basically of two types:
- Suppurative bacterial meningitis, and
- Tubercular meningitis

Suppurative bacterial meningitis

Acute meningitis is usually severe with complications like death, seizures, learning disorders and hearing loss.

Clinical features

Pathogenesis involves inflammation and accumulation of pus in subarachnoid space
   Interference with CSF flow may result in obstructive hydrocephalus

Systemic features meningococci present with characteristic skin rash or petechial lesions with dermal seeding of organism revealed on biopsy.

Ophthalmic signs and symptoms are as described earlier for intracranial infections. Ophthalmic signs are non-specific and may include any of the above described depending upon the area of brain involved but most commonly seen are:
- Papilledema
- Papillitis
- Cranial nerve involvement.

Treatment

Includes appropriate intravenous antibiotics, maintenance of adequate fluid and electrolyte balance.

VIRAL INFECTIONS

Common viruses responsible for intracranial infections are:
- Enterovirus (polio virus)
- Arbovirus like Japanese encephalitis virus
- HIV
- HSV-2

Less common viruses include:
- HSV-1
- Lymphocytic choriomeningitis virus (LCMV)
- Mumps virus.

Rare viruses causing intracranial infections are:
- Adenoviruses
- Cytomegalovirus (CMV)
- Epstein-Barr virus (EBV)
- Measles; influenza A, B; parainflenza; rubella; varicella zoster virus (VZV)

Note. Herpes simplex and herpes zoster can cause infection in patients with immuno-suppression like AIDS.

VIRAL LESIONS

Encephalitis and aseptic meningitis

- More common compared to bacterial meningitis.
- Infection is mild and self-limiting which recovers in 2–3 weeks. Complications can occur but less frequently than in bacterial meningitis.
- Nuchal rigidity is minimal and Kernig's and Brudzinski's sign are not elicitable.
- Focal neurological deficits and cranial nerve palsies usually do not occur in uncomplicated viral meningitis.
- *Headache* is usually retro-orbital and frontal with associated photophobia.
- Rabies virus spreads centripetally to brain. It causes hydrophobia, behavioral disturbances and other signs and symptoms seen in rabies.
- VZV should be suspected in the presence of concurrent chickenpox or shingles.
- *Ophthalmic findings* include panuveitis, vitritis, retinal arteritis, papillitis, and necrotizing retinitis initially sparing the posterior pole.

- *Acute retinal necrosis* produces photophobia, ocular pain, floaters and decreased visual acuity.

Treatment in usual case is symptomatic and hospitalization is not required. Exceptions include immunosuppression, neonates, severe infection or possibility of bacterial or other non-viral cause.

- *Oral or intravenous acyclovir* in HSV, VZV and EBV meningitis.
- *Vaccination* for preventing meningitis due to polio, measles and mumps.

FUNGAL INFECTIONS

Common fungi associated with intracranial infections include:

- Aspergillosis
- Fungi zygomycetes causing mucormycosis
- Cryptococcosis
- Fungi causing intracranial infections like meningitis is rare
- Typically limited to people who have had surgical procedures or have impaired immune systems due to cancer and other diseases affecting immune function.

ASPERGILLOSIS

Clinical profile

Invasive aspergillosis typically occurs in immunocompromised individuals and CNS infection occurs secondarily by either direct or hematogenous spread of organisms. Mortality is very high.

Aspergilloma or fungal ball may involve brain or orbit. Extension to optic canal, cavernous sinus, optic nerves, and optic chiasm produces neuro-ophthalmic findings.

Ophthalmic manifestations include:

- Acute retrobulbar optic neuropathy
- Endophthalmitis
- Orbital apex syndrome
- Cavernous sinus syndrome

Cerebral infarction or hemorrhage may occur due to vascular invasion.

Treatment

- *Medical treatment* comprising systemic steroids and anti-fungal agents like amphotericin B.

- *Surgical treatment* is required in invasive aspergillosis and aspergillomas.

MUCORMYCOSIS

- Fungus is of low virulence and inhabit decaying matter
- It has predilection for blood vessels. Therefore, hemorrhages, thrombosis and ischemic necrosis are hallmarks.

Ophthalmic involvement occurs in two types of mucormycosis:

- Rhinocerebral mucormycosis, and
- CNS mucormycosis

Rhinocerebral mucormycosis

Rhinocerebral mucormycosis occurs in diabetics, those on steroids or neutropenic patients taking antibiotics.

Spreads from facial skin, nasal mucosa, paranasal sinuses or hard palate to nearby vessels and then to orbital vessels, carotid arteries, cavernous sinuses or jugular veins with high mortality.

Neurologic signs include:

- Hemiparesis
- Aphasia
- Seizures
- Altered mental status.

Ocular manifestations include:

- Orbital swelling, conjunctival chemosis, ophthalmoplegia and visual loss.
- Retinal infarction, ophthalmic artery occlusion and optic nerve infiltration
- Painful diplopia, cranial neuropathy
- Orbital apex, cavernous sinus or chiasmal syndrome.

Central nervous system mucormycosis

Central nervous system mucormycosis is rare. Spreads to brain from nose or paranasal sinuses. But no orbital, nasal or paranasal disease detectable when neurological manifestations appear.

Presents as meningitis, cranial nerve involvement, abscess and seizures.

Diagnosis is madle when CT scan shows bone destruction, soft tissue alteration in paranasal sinuses and orbit, air-fluid levels in sinuses.

Definitive test is biopsy.

Treatment includes aggressive surgical debridement and systemic amphotericin B administration.

CRYPTOCOCCOSIS

- Most commonly caused by *Cryptococcus neoformans* found in pigeon droppings and contaminated soil.
- Most common life-threatening mycosis in patients with AIDS.
- Adhesive arachnoiditis is one of its manifestations.
- Insidious onset with waxing and waning course

Systemic manifestations include headache, nausea, vomiting, dizziness and mental status changes most commonly seen

Ophthalmic manifestations are as follows:
- Papilledema from meningitis is most common
- Unilateral or bilateral 6th nerve palsy, other cranial neuropathies
- Photophobia, blurred vision and retrobulbar pain
- Homonymous visual field defects or nystagmus.
- Retrobulbar neuritis
- Retinochoroiditis and cotton wool spots.

Diagnosis by demonstrating *C. neoformans* capsular antigen or yeast in CSF. Serum antigen titres are helpful.

Treatment includes antifungal agents like amphotericin B and flucytosine.

PARASITIC INFECTIONS

Common parasitic infections are caused by:
- Protozoal organisms (toxoplasmosis), and
- Helminthic organisms (cysticercosis, echinococcosis)

TOXOPLASMOSIS

- Caused by *Toxoplasma gondii* which is an obligate intracellular protozoan.
- Cats act as definitive host and humans as intermediate hosts.
- Organisms exist in three forms: sporozoites, bradyzoites and tachyzoites.

Sporozoites:
- Contained in oocyst (sporocyst)
- Result from sexual reproduction in intestinal mucosa of cats
- Excreted in faeces

Bradyzoites
- They are present in tissue cysts
- Most commonly develop in brain, eye, heart, skeletal muscles and lymph nodes.
- Lie dormant for many years without any inflammatory reaction

Tachyzoites (trophozoites)
- They are the active forms
- They are responsible for destruction and inflammation after rupture of cyst wall containing bradyzoites.

Humans are infected by
- Ingestion of undercooked meat (pork, beaf, lamb)
- Ingestion of sporocysts due to contaminated hands or ingestion of dirt (pica, especially in children)
- Transplacental spread when pregnant women are infected

Types
Toxoplasmosis is mainly of two types:
- Congenital toxoplasmosis, and
- Acquired toxoplasmosis

Congenital toxoplasmosis

- Severity of disease in fetus depends on duration of gestation at the time of infection in mother. Early is the gestation, more severe is the disease.
- Most cases are subclinical and detected later in life on observing bilateral healed chorioretinal scars.
- Intracranial calcification may be detected on CT scan.
- Infection occurring at end of 2nd trimester may result in macular scar detected at birth.
- When infection occurs later in 3rd trimester, child may be normal at birth but later develops uveitis or neurological disease.

Acquired toxoplasmosis

Immunocompetent individuals may present with any of the following:
- *Subclinical presentation* is the most common.
- *Lymphadenopathic syndrome* which consists of fever, malaise, pharyngitis and cervical lymphadenopathy.
- *Meningoencephalitis,* where patient presents with altered consciousness and convulsions.

- *Exanthematous presentation* where patient presents with skin lesions and resembles rickettsial infection.

Immunocompromised individuals, e.g. patients with AIDS usually present with life-threatening disease.
- Most common manifestation is a space occupying lesion resembling an abscess on MRI.
- CNS toxoplasmosis produces multifocal lesions with predilection for basal ganglia and the frontal, parietal and occipital lobes leading to headaches, focal neurological deficits, seizures.
- Life long antitoxoplasmosis treatment is necessary to prevent recurrence.

Ocular features
- Toxoplasmosis is the most frequent cause of infectious retinitis in immunocompetent individuals
- Most cases are acquired postnatally but few can result from reactivation of prenatal disease.
- Retinal lesions are usually found adjacent to blood vessels
- Neuroretinitis may occur
- Optic neuritis is rare
- Neuro-ophthalmic findings include: homonymous hemianopia and quadrantopia, ocular motor palsies, and gaze palsies.

ECCHINOCOCCOSIS

Ecchinococcosis is caused by *Echinococcus granulosis* and cysticercosis by *Cysticercus cellulosae*, the larval form of *Taenia solium.*
- Cysts may form in lungs, muscles and brain
- Patient may present with headache, seizures and focal neurological deficits due to cyst in brain (neurocysticercosis).
- *Ocular disease* usually manifests as cysticercous cysts in retina or vitreous.
- Neuroimaging detects the calcified cyst with scolex.

PRION DISEASES

- These are caused by transmission of infectious proteins called prions.
- Example includes Creutzfeldt-Jakob disease (CJD), Kuru, Bovine spongiform encepahalo-pathy, fatal familial insomnia.

- Only some are known to occur in humans.
- Transmission occurs by:
  - Ingestion of infected meat
  - Iatrogenic spread by dura mater grafts and contaminated human growth hormone.
- Patient presents with non-specific features like malaise, loss of weight, headache and insomnia.
- Seizures, cerebellar ataxia, extra-pyramidal dysfunction resembling parkinsonism and progressive dementia can occur.
- *Ocular features* include:
  - Visual impairment due to optic atrophy, and
  - Supranuclear gaze palsies.
- Any patient dying of non-specific neurological disease is suspected of having prions infection
- No specific treatment is available.
- Prevention is achieved by complete inactivation of prions by sterilization using autoclaving at 132°C for 5 hours.

CLINICAL PRESENTATIONS OF INTRACRANIAL INFECTIONS

EPIDURAL (EXTRADURAL) ABSCESS, SUBDURAL EMPYEMA/ABSCESS AND BRAIN ABSCESS

Causal organism (polymicrobial)
- *Streptococcus pyogenes*
- Microaerophilic/anaerobic streptococci
- *Staphylococcus aureus*
- Enteric gram –ve bacilli
- Pneumococci and meningococci (rare)

Epidural abscess is collection of pus in the potential space between cranium and dura mater.

Subdural abscess is the collection of pus in the potential space between the dura mater and the arachnoid mater.

Brain abscess. Collection of pus in the brain parenchyma with necrosis causes formation of brain abscess.

Clinically present as space occupying lesions with focal neurological deficits depending on the location of the abscess.

Ocular findings depend on the location of abscess. Papilledema can be present due to raised intracranial tension.

Neuroimaging CT scan is more sensitive and preferred over MRI for diagnosis.

Treatment is by neurosurgical drainage under cover of antibiotics.

MENINGITIS

Meningitis is the term used to define infection involving the covering of brain mainly pia-arachnoid resulting in accumulation of pus (inflammatory exudate) in the subarachnoid space and cerebrospinal fluid.

Clinical types

Clinically it can be:

- Fulminant acute meningitis progressing over hours.
- Sudacute meningitis progressing over days
- Chronic meningitis persisting for more than 4 weeks.

Bacterial meningitis

Community acquired acute bacterial meningitis is caused by:

- *Streptococcus pneumoniae* which is most common
- *Neisseria meningitidis* is the next common
- Group B streptococci and *Listeria monocytogenes*

Hospital acquired meningitis is mostly caused by *Staphylococcus aureus* and coagulase-negative staphylococci.

Chronic meningitis is mostly due to partially treated suppurative meningitis, *Mycobacterium tuberculosis*, Lyme disease, syphilis.

Tuberculous meningitis

Ocular manifestations include:

- Bilateral papillitis
- Miliary tubercles in choroid mostly seen near the disc in miliary TB
- 6th and 3rd nerve paresis (bilateral 3rd nerve palsy rare or unknown, differential diagnosis from syphilitic basal meningitis where its present)
- Kinetic conjugate deviation of eyes and head to one side
- Intracranial tuberculomas produce ocular signs as in brain tumors.
  Treatment involves administration of anti-tubercular drugs.

Ocular manifestations

Acute meningococcal (epidemic) meningitis

- Papillitis due to descending infective peri-neuritis
- Papilledema rarely
- Kinetic strabismus or conjugate lateral deviation of eyes in early stages
- Widely open palpebral aperture with infrequent blinking: *characteristic sign*
- 6th and/or 3rd nerve paralysis
- Pupils are miotic in early stages and later when coma sets in, pupils get dilated, loss of reaction to light is rare
- Metastatic endophthalmitis

Acute basal meningitis

- *Complete amaurosis* with normal pupillary reactions and fundi due to actions of toxins on higher visual centers.
- *Blindness persists* for several weeks even when other symptoms subside

Chronic basal meningitis

- Same feature as in acute
- Optic neuritis and post-neuritic atrophy due to secondary hydrocephalus and pressure of distended 3rd ventricle on chiasma.

Meningitis of middle ear origin

- Papillitis or papilledema due to sinus thrombosis or cerebral abscess
- 6th or rarely 3rd nerve paralysis
- Lagophthalmos due to facial nerve paralysis
- Conjugate deviation of eyes.

Chronic chiasmal arachnoiditis

It is defined as localized infection of meninges around chiasma and optic nerve.

Etiology

- Idiopathic (unknown)
- Sepsis of nasal sinuses
- Sarcoidosis

Ocular lesions include bilateral optic atrophy with central scotoma and irregular contraction of visual fields.

Differential diagnosis from pituitary tumor:

- Negative radiological evidence
- Deformation of chiasmal cistern on CT cisternography.

ENCEPHALITIS

- It is defined as the infection predominantly affecting the brain parenchyma.
- Mainly caused by viruses as already described in viral infections

Encephalitis lethargica or von Economo disease is an atypical form of encephalitis.
- Also known as "sleepy sickness"
- Patient appears to be in a state of coma, motionless and speechless

Ocular manifestations
- *Ocular palsies* are common
- *Ptosis* is the commonest feature due to 3rd nerve palsy
- *Diplopia* and nystagmus
- *Papilledema* rarely seen and pupils are usually normal.
- *Spasmodic conjugate* deviation of eyes (*oculogyric crises*) in later stages. Oculogyric crises sometimes result from phenothiazine idiosyncrasy. Relieved by Benzedrine
- Acute polioencephalitis can result in *paralytic squint*. 6th cranial nerve is most commonly involved.

CAVERNOUS SINUS THROMBOSIS

- Usually results from suppurative infection in the "dangerous area" of face or orbit.
- Patient presents with fever, retro-orbital and frontal pain and hypesthesia of face along ophthalmic and maxillary divisions of trigeminal nerve.

Ocular manifestations include:
- Conjunctival chemosis
- Restriction of extraocular movements
- 6th nerve palsy is the most consistent early neurological sign
- Proptosis, ptosis and absent corneal sensations
- Tortuous dilated retinal veins, papilledema
- Loss of vision from exposure keratopathy
- Optic nerve involvement due to raised intraorbital pressure or secondary to septic vasculitis and ischemia.

BIBLIOGRAPHY

1. Ahlm C, Lindén C, Linderholm M, et al. Central nervous system and ophthalmic involvement in nephropathia-epidemica, Journal of Infection, March 1998;36(2):A2-32;137–248.

2. Berglöff J, Gasser R and Feigl B. Ophthalmic Manifestations in Lyme Borreliosis: A Review, Journal of Neuro-ophthalmology, March 1994, Vol 14, Issue 1:61–65.

3. Edward F. Gonyea, Kenneth M. Heilma: Neuro-ophthalmic Aspects of Central Nervous System Cryptococcosis: Internuclear and Supranuclear Ophthalmoplegia, Arch Ophthalmol 1972; 87(2):164–68.

4. Emmett T Cunningham (Jr), Jane E Koehler. Ocular bartonellosis, American Journal of Ophthalmology Sept 2000;130(3):340–49.

5. Garg S, Jampol LM. Systemic and intraocular manifestations of West Nile virus infection, Survey of Ophthalmology Jan-Feb 2005;50(1): 3–13.

6. Ormerod, L. David Keith A Skolnick, Matthew M Menosky, et al. Retinal and choroidal manifestations of cat-scratch disease. Ophthalmology, June 1998;105(6):1024–31.

7. Leah Levi, Matthew R Jones, Robert Bhisitkul, et al. Optic disk edema associated with peripapillary serous retinal detachment: an early sign of systemic Bartonella henselae infection, American Journal of Ophthalmology Sep 2000;130(3):327–34.

8. Lesser RL. Ocular manifestations of Lyme disease, The American Journal of Medicine, Supplement 1,1995;98(4):60–62.

9. Ostler HB, Thygeson P. The ocular manifestations of herpes zoster, varicella, infectious mononucleosis, and cytomegalovirus disease. Survey of ophthalmology 1976;2(2):148–59.

10. William V. Anninger, Mark D. Lomeo, Jack Dingle, et al. Epstein and Martin Lubow: West nile virus-associated optic neuritis and chorioretinitis, American Journal of Ophthalmology Dec. 2003;136(6):1183–5.

22 INTRACRANIAL ANEURYSMS AND CAROTID-CAVERNOUS FISTULAE

Devendra V Venkatramani

INTRACRANIAL ANEURYSMS
- Applied anatomy
- Clinical features
- Investigations
  — MRI versus CT scan
  — Conventional angiography
- Management
  — Clipping
  — Coiling

CAROTID-CAVERNOUS FISTULAE
- Applied anatomy
- Classification
- Etiology and epidemiology
- Pathophysiology
- Clinical features
- Investigations
- Management

INTRACRANIAL ANEURYSMS

INTRODUCTION

Aneurysms are localized out-pouchings of the vessel wall. In the intracranial circulation they could be an isolated finding, or could be associated with systemic hypertension, connective tissue disorders (Ehlers-Danlos syndrome, Marfan syndrome) polycystic kidney disease, or coarctation of the aorta.

About 3.6 to 6 per cent of the adult population harbor unruptured intracranial aneurysms.

Aneurysm rupture is often a catastrophic event that results in death in more than half of victims who reach the hospital alive. Unruptured aneurysms are much less dangerous, however the annual risk of rupture for an aneurysm 10 mm or more in diameter is approximately 1 per cent.

APPLIED ANATOMY

Sacular ('berry') aneurysms are located at the bifurcations of large to medium-sized arteries;

85–90 per cent of these are found in the circle of Willis, an anastomotic septagon located at the base of the brain (Fig. 22.1). Around one-fifth of patients have more than one aneurysm, often at a bilaterally symmetric site.

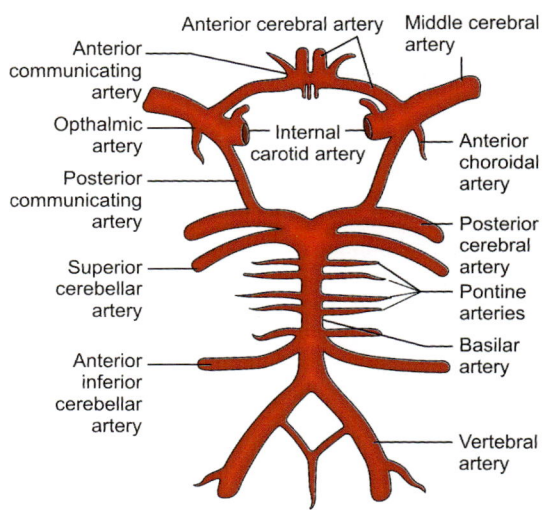

Fig. 22.1 *Circle of Willis.*

233

It is important to note the close relation of structures of neuro-ophthalmic significance to sites of aneurysmal dilatation. The oculomotor and trochlear nerves travel in the sub-arachnoid space, passing between the posterior cerebral and superior cerebellar arteries. They then travel parallel (and lateral) to the posterior communicating artery before they pierce the dura to enter the cavernous sinus. Here they are located in the lateral wall of the sinus (Fig. 22.2), and gain access to the orbit through the superior orbital fissure.

The abducent nerve comes in contact with vascular structures chiefly in the cavernous sinus, as it passes through the substance of the sinus is close association with the internal carotid artery.

CLINICAL FEATURES

Intracranial aneurysms can produce symptoms due to mass effect on surrounding structures (Table 22.1), or due to subarachnoid haemorrhage as a result of rupture.

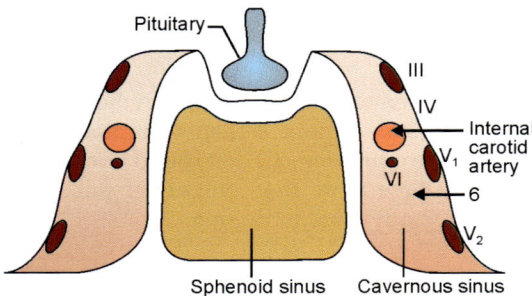

Fig. 22.2 *Course of the oculomotor nerve in the subarachnoid space.*

For all practical purposes, compressive lesions of the oculomotor nerve (including aneurysmal compression) result in ipsilateral ophthalmoparesis with a mid-dilated, non-reactive pupil—a 'pupil-involving' palsy. Nerve fibres supplying the sphincter pupillae are located more peripherally in the nerve substance, and draw their nutrition from the delicate surrounding pial vessels. These vessels are readily occluded by extrinsic compression, resulting in pupilloplegia. Thus it is a clinical maxim that pupil-involving third nerve palsy is an indication for urgent neuro-imaging to detect compressive lesions. It is important to remember, however, that pupil-involvement may develop a few days after ophthalmoparesis. Therefore all patients with acute third nerve palsy presenting without pupil involvement must be followed closely in the early stages to detect pupilloplegia.

Another important feature of aneurysmal compression is pain. This probably arises from stretching of pain sensitive structures in the dura mater, or from compression of the trigeminal nerve branches in the cavernous sinus. The latter produces referred pain to the ipsilateral half of the face. However, pain may also be a feature of ischaemic (pupil-sparing) third nerve palsy. Additionally, pain may be absent in unruptured aneurysms.

"The worst headache of my life" is the descriptive term used by a patient with a subarachnoid haemorrhage. Other features are nausea, vomiting and neck stiffness. Abducent palsy (unilateral or bilateral) and papilloedema may occur due to raised intracranial pressure.

Table 22.1 *Compressive effects of intracranial aneurysms*	
Clinical scenario	*Remarks*
Isolated oculomotor nerve palsy	Classically pupil-involving
Aberrant regeneration of oculomotor nerve	Primary, i.e. without antecedent paresis
Isolated trochlear nerve palsy	10% of acquired palsies
Painful ophthalmoplegia (multiple cranial nerves)	Compression of other ocular motor nerves, especially by intracavernous aneurysms
Atypical migraine	Especially suspect in ophthalmoplegic migraine
Carotid-cavernous fistula	Direct fistula due to rupture of intracavernous aneurysm. 3rd, 4th, 6th cranial nerve palsies, facial pain, Horner syndrome constitute the cavernous syndrome.
Visual pathway compression	Optic nerve, chiasma, less commonly optic tract

In some patients, vitreous, prehyaloid and/or intraretinal haemorrhages may be seen, an association known as Terson syndrome. Some patients may provide history of recent severe headaches, suggestive of 'sentinel bleeds' due to small ruptures and leaks. Sub-arachnoid haemorrhage is a neurosurgical emergency.

Aneurysms may also compress the visual pathway, presenting with a variety of visual field defects including monocular hemianopia, bitemporal hemianopia, homonymous hemianopia, and junctional scotoma.

INVESTIGATIONS

Intracranial aneurysms can present to the ophthalmologist in a variety of ways. A third nerve palsy is one situation which requires careful handling. Any patient presenting with an acute, pupil-involving third nerve palsy requires urgent neuroimaging. Risk-stratification schemes exist, based on the likelihood of aneurysm as the cause for third nerve palsy. Essentially, these weigh the degree of internal and external ophthalmoplegia, and other risk factors such as vasculopathic diseases.

MRI versus CT scan

The initial investigation of choice is a magnetic resonance imaging (MRI) scan, coupled with magnetic resonance angiography (MRA), a non-invasive, gadolinium contrast-based technique that allows excellent delineation of vascular structures. Additionally, as MRI is better than computerised tomography (CT) scanning in the evaluation of non-aneurysm causes of third nerve palsy, it is often the preferred modality.

CT scanning is preferred in the evaluation of acute intracranial haemorrhage, if an emergent scan is needed, or in patients in whom MRI is otherwise contraindicated. Like MRA, CT angiography (CTA) is also non-invasive and has comparable sensitivity in detecting intracranial aneurysms (LEE, HAYMAN, BRAZIS et al.). It utilizes iodine-based contrast which may be more nephrotoxic than gadolinium, but scanning and processing times are shorter than MRA.

Conventional angiography

The gold-standard for aneurysm detection, however, remains conventional catheter angiography. The risks of this technique (especially stroke) need to be weighed against the likelihood of an aneurysm. Broad guidelines for its use include worsening of ophthalmoparesis or pupilloparesis beyond 14 days, no recovery of function within three months, or signs of aberrant regeneration.

MANAGEMENT

Aneurysmal rupture and resultant sub-arachnoid haemorrhage is a neurosurgical emergency. The role of an ophthalmologist is mainly limited to the diagnosis and prompt referral of unruptured aneurysms to a neurosurgeon. *Unruptured aneurysms* can be repaired through an open (craniotomy) approach, or by endovascular interventions.

A large, multicentre study found a relatively low risk of rupture in small aneurysms (<10 mm in diameter) without history of subarachnoid haemorrhage, and also noted that morbidity and mortality rates associated with surgical intervention exceeded the risk of rupture in these patients.

Two techniques exist for treating unruptured aneursyms—clipping and coiling:

- *Clipping* involves placing a surgical clip across the neck of the aneurysm, thereby pinching it off from (and simultaneously preserving) the parent artery.
- *Coiling* involves the endovascular placement of detachable platinum coils (for example, the Guglielmi detachable coil system) within the aneurysm. The coils mechanically occlude the aneurysm, and promote thrombosis which ultimately obliterates the aneurysm. Potential complications common to treatments include cerebral ischaemia, haemorrhage, vessel wall rupture, migration of the implant, and distal thromboembolism.

CAROTID-CAVERNOUS FISTULAE

APPLIED ANATOMY

A fistula is an anomalous connection between two cavities or spaces, or between a cavity and the external environment. A carotid-cavernous fistula connects the carotid arterial system with the cavernous sinus.

The cavernous sinus is a large blood filled space, which in cadaver sections resembles cavernous tissue. In reality, it may be more accurately described as a plexus, which extends from the superior orbital fissure to the apex of the petrous temporal bone longitudinally, with a length of 2 cm and a width of 1 cm as shown in Fig. 22.3. The internal carotid artery (and a surrounding sympathetic plexus) travels forwards within the sinus, along with the more inferotemporally placed abducent nerve. The oculomotor, trochlear, and first and second branches of the trigeminal nerve run forwards in the lateral wall, but do project into the sinus. Additionally, the sphenoid sinus and the pituiutary gland are located medially. Because of its intimate relation to these structures, the sinus is of great neuro-ophthalmic significance.

The internal carotid artery enters the petrous temporal bone through the carotid canal and runs anteriorly over the foramen lacerum. It gives off the cavernous, hypohyseal, and meningeal branches within the cavernous sinus. The ophthalmic, anterior cerebral, middle cerebral, posterior communicating, and anterior choroidal arteries are branches of its cerebral segment.

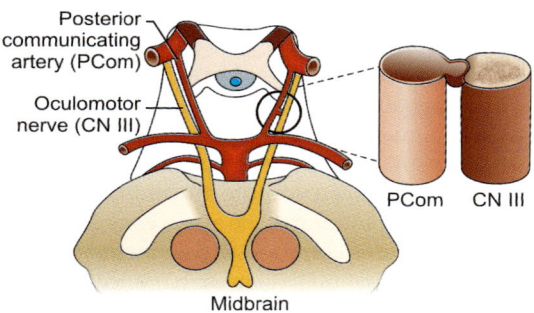

Posterior communicating artery (PCom)

Oculomotor nerve (CN III)

PCom   CN III

Midbrain

Fig. 22.3 *Diagram showing the cavernous sinuses and their relations.*

The external carotid artery's larger terminal branch, the maxillary artery, produces the middle meningeal artery which is responsible for supplying large areas of the dura and cranium.

CLASSIFICATION

Fistulae can be grouped into 'direct' and 'indirect' types. This grouping has clinical as well as therapeutic significance, as outlined later. A direct fistula is a communication involving the intracavernous internal carotid artery, whereas an indirect one involves smaller arterial branches but not the main trunk.

The most clinically relevant classification is still the one given by Barrow, in which there are 4 types of fistulae (Table 22.2):
- *Type A* refers to a direct fistulous communication.
- *Types B–D* imply an indirect communication with the cavernous sinus; via a branch of the internal carotid artery (Type B), a branch of the external carotid artery (Type C), or via branches of both the internal and external carotid arteries (Type D).

A clinical classification groups fistulae into high-flow or low-flow types, depending on the severity of the clinical features.

ETIOLOGY AND EPIDEMIOLOGY

A fistula is the result of rupture or a breach in the arterial wall. This breach can occur spontaneously, as a consequence of trauma, or in an area of already weakened arterial wall. Spontaneous fistulae (without a history of preceding trauma) may occur in subjects with connective tissue disorders, especially Ehlers-Danlos syndrome type IV.

Traumatic fistulae are seen at a young age. These are more likely to produce high-flow, direct (Type A) communications. Likely mechanisms include vascular injury from fractures

Type	Pathogenesis	Arterial supply	Haemodynamics
A	Head trauma/aneurysm rupture	Internal carotid	High flow
B	Spontaneous	Internal carotid—dural branches	Low flow
C	Spontaneous	External carotid—dural branches	Low flow
D	Spontaneous	Internal and external carotid—dural branches	Low flow

Table 22.2 *Barrow classification of carotid-cavernous fistulae*

(especially those involving the skull base), torsional or stretching forces on the carotid siphon, and acceleration-deceleration injuries. Iatrogenic fistulae have also been reported following rhinoplasty, trans-sphenoidal surgery, and carotid angioplasty and stenting.

Fistulae may occur in the setting of a weakened arterial wall. High-flow lesions may occur due to rupture of an intracavernous aneurysm. Low-flow lesions are more likely to be seen in elderly patients with atherosclerotic disease.

PATHOPHYSIOLOGY

A communication between an artery (high pressure) and a vein (low pressure) results in shunting of blood into the venous system. This results in an increase in venous pressure chiefly in the superior ophthalmic vein and its tributaries, and a reduction in arterial pressure and perfusion.

Venous hypertension produces swelling of extraocular muscles and soft tissues. Venous pressure is also conducted to the episcleral vessels, interfering with aqueous humour outflow. Ocular perfusion may also be compromised.

CLINICAL FEATURES

The classic clinical triad of carotid-cavernous fistula is proptosis, chemosis and orbital bruit. However, the clinical pictures varies greatly depending upon the type of fistula. In direct fistulae, there is often a history of preceding head trauma, following which ocular signs and symptoms develop. Tinnitus is often of a pulsatile nature; many patients hear a 'whooshing' sound that coincides with the pulse. Headache may be quite severe. If associated with contralateral neurodeficit it indicates retrograde interference with cortical venous drainage, which may result in fatal intracerebral haemorrhage.

Proptosis is usually axial, progressive, and can be seen in up to 80 per cent of patients. It can occasionally be severe enough to result in lagophthalmos and exposure keratopathy. Conjunctival prolapse may also interfere with lid functions. Visual loss may occur due to compression of the optic nerve at the orbital apex.

Eye movements may be limited due to the engorgement of extraocular muscles, or due to compressive effects on ocular motor nerves, either in the cavernous sinus itself or in the orbit. The abducent nerve is most commonly involved due to its vulnerable location within the substance of the cavernous sinus. Involvement of the first two divisions of the trigeminal nerve localizes the lesion to the cavernous sinus, stressing the importance of cranial nerve examination in these patients.

In patients with indirect fistulae, the clinical picture is subtler. These patients may present with unilateral conjunctival congestion, and are often misdiagnosed as chronic blepharo-conjunctivitis. Careful slit lamp examination reveals the presence of 'cork-screw' capillaries due to arterialization of the conjunctival and episcleral vessels.

Anterior segment ischaemia can be seen in up to 20 per cent of subjects, and may produce corneal oedema, anterior chamber flare, iris atrophy or rubeosis, and cataract.

Elevated intraocular pressure secondary to raised episcleral venous pressure has been noted in up to 65 per cent of patients. Posterior segment findings include venous stasis retinopathy, and optic neuropathy that can be glaucomatous, ischaemic, or compressive in nature.

Differential diagnoses for carotid-cavernous fistula are cavernous sinus thrombosis, orbital cellulitis, thyroid orbitopathy, idiopathic orbital inflammatory disease (orbital pseudotumour), and neoplastic infiltration of the orbit.

INVESTIGATIONS

In the setting of acute trauma and intracranial haemorrhage, a non-contrast computerized tomography (CT) scan is the preliminary investigation to be performed. While a contrast-enhanced CT scan may demonstrate a fistula, the investigation of choice to delineate the fistula is magnetic resonance imaging (MRI). A dilated superior ophthalmic vein (SOV) is highly suggestive of carotid-cavernous fistula, but may also been seen in other orbital conditions. The cavernous sinus and extraocular muscles also appear enlarged. T1-weighted scanning with fat-suppression enhances visualization of the SOV. Magnetic resonance angiography (MRA) is also an excellent non-invasive tool. CT angiography helps to define the lesion and has been noted to be more sensitive than MRA.

The gold standard however is (invasive) catheter digital subtraction angiography (DSA). This may be reserved for patients with ambiguous MRA or CTA findings, or those in whom intervention is planned in the same sitting.

MANAGEMENT

Direct fistulae seldom close spontaneously, due to the high flow-rate and volume of blood passing through them. On the other hand, the rate of closure of indirect fistulae can be as high as 75 per cent even without invasive intervention.

Conservative management

Conservative management is thus indicated in patients with indirect fistulae, with minimal symptoms, and without signs of visual system compromise.

- *Carotid self-compression* involves intermittent manual application of pressure on the external carotid artery for up to 10 seconds. This manoeuvre has been shown to induce closure in 30 per cent of patients with indirect fistulae. It is to be avoided in patients with hypertensive carotid sinus syndrome, atherosclerotic stenosis, and in those with a history of cerebral ischaemia or stroke.
- *Other general measures* include cessation of anti-platelet therapy unless medically necessary.

Surgical management

Direct fistulae often need surgical intervention, especially when complicated by glaucoma, diplopia, intolerable headache or bruit, or severe proptosis. Cerebral ischaemia also warrants intervention. The goal of therapy is to ensure complete fistula closure, but also to maintain patency of the feeding artery. Internal carotid artery ligation is today performed only in patients in whom endovascular intervention fails.

The endovascular approach is possible through either transarterial (internal carotid artery) or transvenous (superior ophthalmic vein or inferior petrosal sinus) routes. Detachable balloon occlusion is typically performed transarterially. This technique has a high success rate of 88–99 per cent in direct fistulae, but may be complicated by cerebral infarction in up to 4 per cent of patients. Use of n-butyl cyanoacrylate (n-BCA) and other polymers like Onyx (ethylene vinyl alcohol copolymer in dimethyl sulfoxide solvent) has also been described.

Detachable coils can be placed either by transarterial or transvenous routes. The transvenous route is preferred in dural fistulae, where the artery may be too small to cannulate. Venous access can be gained through tributaries of the facial vein, inferior petrosal sinus, or through an enlarged superior ophthalmic vein, the latter either after surgical exposure or percutaneously. *Complications of treatment* include cerebral ischaemia, damage and rupture of vascular structures (especially in patients with Ehlers-Danlos syndrome type IV), cranial nerve paresis due to the mass effect of coils, and incomplete occlusion. Venus occlusion can lead to severe ocular hypertension, intraocular haemorrhage, and vision loss.

Management of secondary ocular effects

Secondary ocular effects such as diplopia, exposure keratopathy, glaucoma, neovascularization, and vascular occlusions need to be managed accordingly.

BIBLIOGRAPHY

1. Barrow DL, Spector RH, Braun IF, et al. Classification and treatment of spontaneous carotid-cavernous sinus fistulas. J Neurosurg 1985; 62:248–56.
2. Biousse V, Mendicino ME, Simon DJ, et al. The ophthalmology of intracranial vascular abnormalities. Am J Ophthalmol 1998;125:527–44.
3. Brisman JL, Song JK, Newell DW. Cerebral aneurysms. N Engl J Med 2006;355(9):928–39.
4. Chen CC, Chang PC, Shy CG, et al. CT angiography and MR angiography in the evaluation of carotid-cavernous sinus fistula prior to embolization: a comparison of techniques. AJNR Am J Neuroradiol 2005;26:2349–56.
5. Farley MK, Clark RD, Fallor MK, et al. Spontaneous carotid-cavernous fistula and the Ehlers-Danlos syndromes. Ophthalmology 1983; 90:1337–42.

6. Goldberg RA, Goldey SH, Duckwiler G, et al. Management of cavernous sinus-dural fistulas. Indications and techniques for primary embolization via the superior ophthalmic vein. Arch Ophthalmol 1996;114:707–14.

7. Gupta N, Kikkawa DO, Levi L, et al. Severe vision loss and neovascular glaucoma complicating superior ophthalmic vein approach to carotid-cavernous sinus fistula. Am J Ophthalmol 1997; 124:853–5.

8. Higashida RT, Halbach VV, Tsai FY, et al. Interventional neurovascular treatment of carotid-cavernous fistula with detachable balloons. AJR Am J Roentgenol 1989;153:577–82.

9. Higashida RT, Hieshima GB, Halbach VV, et al. Closure of carotid-cavernous sinus fistulae by external compression of the carotid artery and jugular vein. Acta Radiol Suppl 1986; 369:580–83.

10. Ishijima K, Kashiwagi K, Nakano K, et al. Ocular manifestations and prognosis of secondary glaucoma in patients with carotid-cavernous fistula. Jpn J Ophthalmol 2003;47:603–08.

11. Kupersmith MJ, Berenstein A, Choi IS, et al. Management of nontraumatic vascular shunts involving the cavernous sinus. Ophthalmology. 1988;95:121–30.

12. Kupersmith MJ, Berenstein A, Choi IS, et al. Management of nontraumatic vascular shunts involving the cavernous sinus. Ophthalmology. 1988;95:121–30.

13. Lee AG, Hayman LA, Brazis PW. The evaluation of isolated third nerve palsy revisited: an update on the evolving role of magnetic resonance, computed tomography, and catheter angiography. Surv Ophthalmol 2002;47:137–57.

14. Lee AG, Johnson MC, Policeni BA, et al. Imaging for neuro-ophthalmic and orbital disease-a review. Clinical and Experimental Ophthalmology 2009;37:30–53.

15. Lewis AI, Tomsick TA, Tew JM (Jr). Management of 100 consecutive direct carotidcavernous fistulas: results of treatment with detachable balloons. Neurosurgery 1995;36:239–44; discussion 244-235.

16. Lewis AI, Tomsick TA, Tew JM (Jr). Management of 100 consecutive direct carotid-cavernous fistulas: results of treatment with detachable balloons. Neurosurgery 1995;36:239–44; discussion 244–235.

17. Liang W, Xiaofeng Y, Weiguo L, et al. Traumatic carotid-cavernous fistula accompanying basilar skull fracture: a study on the incidence of traumatic carotid cavernous fistula in the patients with basilar skull fracture and the prognostic analysis about traumatic carotid cavernous fistula. J Trauma, 2007; 63:1014–20; discussion 1020.

18. Liu HM, Wang YH, Chen YF, et al. Long-term clinical outcome of spontaneous carotid-cavernous sinus fistulae supplied by dural branches of the internal carotid artery. Neuroradiology 2001;43:1007–14.

19. Miller N, Newman Nancy J, Biousse V, et al. (Eds). Walsh & Hoyt's Clinical Neuro-ophthalmology. 6th Ed. Lippincott Williams & Wilkins; 2004:

20. Monsein LH, Debrun GM, Miller NR, et al. Treatment of dural carotid-cavernous fistulas via the superior ophthalmic vein. AJNR Am J Neuroradiol 1991;12:435–9.

21. Park YS, Jung JY, Ahn JY, et al. Emergency endovascular stent graft and coil placement for internal carotid artery injury during trans sphenoidal surgery. Surg Neurol. Dec 2009; 72(6):741–6. Epub 2009, Jul 14.

22. Rinkel GJ, Djibuti M, Algra A, et al. Prevalence and risk of rupture of intracranial aneurysms: a systematic review. Stroke 1998;29:251–6.

23. Song IC, Bromberg BE. Carotid-cavernous sinus fistula occurring after a rhinoplasty. Case report. Plast Reconstr Surg Jan 1975;55(1):92–6.

24. Subramanian PS, Williams ZR. Arteriovenous malformations and carotid-cavernous fistulae. International Ophthalmology Clinics 2009; 49(3): 81–102.

25. Suzuki S, Lee DW, Jahan R, et al. Transvenous treatment of spontaneous dural carotid-cavernous fistulas using a combination of detachable coils and Onyx. AJNR Am J Neuroradiol 2006;27:1346–9.

26. Theron J, Guimaraens L, Coskun O, et al. Complications of carotid angioplasty and stenting. Neurosurg Focus Dec 15, 1998 ;5(6):e4.

27. Unruptured intracranial aneurysms-risk of rupture and risks of surgical intervention. International Study of Unruptured Intracranial Aneurysms Investigators. N Engl J Med 1998; 339:1725–33.

28. Wardlaw JM, White PM. The detection and management of unruptured intracranial aneurysms. Brain 2000;123(2):205–21.

29. Yu SC, Cheng HK, Wong GK, et al. Transvenous embolization of dural carotid-cavernous fistulae with transfacial catheterization through the superior ophthalmic vein. Neurosurgery 2007; 60:1032–7; discussion 1037–8.

23 INTRACRANIAL TUMOURS OF OPHTHALMIC SIGNIFICANCE

Devendra V Venkatramani

INTRODUCTION

CLINICAL APPROACH
- Clinical presentation
- Examination of pupils
- Ophthalmoscopy
- Perimetry
- Diplopia and squint
- Nystagmus and nystagmoid movements

SPECIFIC INTRACRANIAL TUMOURS AND THEIR NEURO-OPHTHALMIC SIGNIFICANCE
- Pituitary adenomas
- Craniopharyngiomas
- Meningiomas
- Gliomas

CONCLUSIONS

INTRODUCTION

Intracranial tumors can be either primary or metastatic. Brain and vertebral metastases are more prevalent than primary tumors; about 15 percent of patients who die of cancer in the United States have symptomatic brain metastases.

Primary tumors arise from various cells of origin within the central nervous system and are classified accordingly into tumors of neuro-epithelial origin, of mesodermal origin, of ectodermal origin, and developmental malformations (craniopharyngiomas and germinomas, Table 23.1).

CLINICAL APPROACH

Clinical presentation

Half of all patients with a brain tumor have ophthalmic signs and/or symptoms. These can be attributed to either the visual pathway or the

Table 23.1 *Intracranial tumors and their origin*

Germ-line of origin	Tumors
Neuroepithelium	Glioblastoma
	Oligodendroglioma
	Astrocytoma
	Ependymoma
	Medulloblastoma
	Choroid plexus papilloma
	Pinealoma
Mesodermal	Meningioma
Ectodermal	Pituitary adenoma
Developmental	Craniopharyngioma
malformations	Germinoma

ocular motor system. Patients may also present with non-specific complaints like headache.

Syndromic presentations of brain tumors are depicted in Fig. 23.1.

The likelihood of a particular tumor being present varies with the age of the patient. In childhood, the commoner tumors are medullo-blastomas, ganglioneuromas and gliomas. A

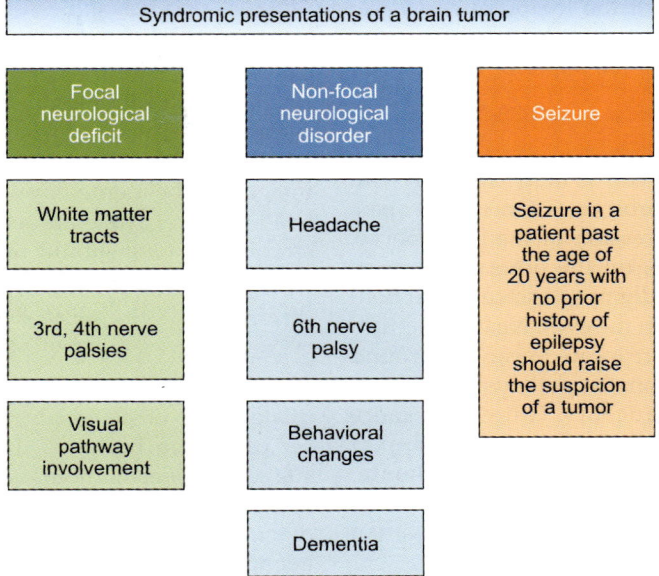

Fig. 23.1 *Syndromic presentations of a brain tumor (asterisks indicate features that may cause the patient to present first to an ophthalmologist).*

chiasmal syndrome in a child should raise suspicion of a glioma or craniopharyngioma rather than a pituitary tumor. In adults, astrocytomas, meningiomas and pituitary tumors are more likely. In elderly patients, lymphomas and metastases should be suspected.

Headache could be a result of localized irritation of pain-sensitive structures (especially dura mater), or due to raised intracranial pressure. Headaches suggestive of raised intracranial pressure include a frequency of more than once a day, worsening with recumbent posture, associated vomiting, and precipitation by sneezing, coughing or straining.

Other systemic signs and symptoms are discussed later, along with specific tumors.

Examination of pupils

Examination of the pupillary light reflexes may reveal a relative afferent pupillary defect (RAPD) in patients with unequal affection of the anterior visual pathways. In most cases the lesion is ipsilateral to the eye with the RAPD; optic tract lesions, however, can produce a small *contralateral* RAPD, due to the fact that nasal fibers crossing at the optic chiasm outnumber

the temporal fibers from the same eye that do not cross.

Optic nerve function tests that should be performed (in each eye, separately) include color vision, red color desaturation test, and brightness comparison.

Ophthalmoscopy

Optic disc evaluation by ophthalmoscopy is essential in each case. Bilateral disc oedema may be due to raised intracranial pressure (papilledema), and warrants urgent neuroimaging and referral to a neurologist. Bilateral disc involvement can also occur with chiasmal compression. Unilateral disc oedema or optic atrophy indicates affection of the optic nerve prior to the chiasm, either within the orbit, the optic canal, or within the cranium. A notable clinical entity is optic disc edema on one side, with optic atrophy on the other (Foster-Kennedy syndrome), which may be seen with frontal lobe tumors. The tumor compresses the ipsilateral optic nerve producing atrophy, while raised intracranial pressure causes disc edema in the other eye. 'Bow-tie' or band atrophy may be seen with contralateral optic tract lesions, due to atrophy of the crossed nasal fibers. Pallor of the temporal and nasal quadrants of the optic disc produces a central band of pallor, while the superior and inferior poles appear pink.

Perimetry

Decrease in visual acuity is more common with tumors within the orbit or at the orbital apex, due to direct compression of the optic nerve. Intracranial tumors, on the other hand, may present with gradually progressive visual field defects in one or both the eyes. Nearly one-fifth of all brain tumors are located near and around the chiasma. Occasionally, patients are misdiagnosed to have glaucoma. Clues to a more sinister etiology include field defects that respect the vertical midline, junctional scotomata, bitemporal defects, and progressive field loss despite of normal intraocular pressure (apparent normal-tension glaucoma).

Junctional scotomas are the product of injury to the anterior chiasm at its junction with the optic nerve. These are characterized by a central scotoma or blind eye on one side, with a superotemporal defect directed towards fixation in the other eye. This defect in the other eye has been thought to be due to damage to inferonasal retinal fibers that cross in the chiasm and pass anteriorly for approximately 4 millimeters into the contralateral optic nerve (von Willebrand's knee), before continuing into the optic tract. The existence of von Willebrand's knee has been called into question. It does, however, help to explain this specific field defect.

Bitemporal hemianopias may be denser superiorly (due chiasmal compression from below, e.g. a pituitary adenoma) or denser inferiorly (due to compression from above, e.g. by a craniopharyngioma). A more important determinant may be the chiasmal fixation pattern, as explained later.

Retrochiasmal pregeniculate lesions produce homonymous hemianopia involving the contralateral hemifield.

Confrontation visual field examination has been shown to have a high sensitivity when multiple techniques are combined, and can serve as useful bedside tests which can be performed in patients unable to sit for automated perimetry.

Diplopia and squint

In patients presenting with diplopia or squint due to ocular motor nerve palsies, a detailed history and examination of ocular motility is required. Diplopia appears suddenly, may produce a sensation of nausea, and often the two images can be merged by adopting a particular head posture. These are features of incomitant strabismus. One should measure the angle of strabismus with prisms and document motility limitations with 9-gaze photographs in each case.

A third nerve palsy associated with an ipsilateral dilated, non- or sluggishly reacting pupil should set off alarm bells, as this entity is highly suggestive of oculomotor nerve compression by a mass lesion. In cases without pupillary involvement, the patient may be observed closely if his/her age is over 40 years *and* if there are vasculopathic risk factors. Subsequent appearance of pupilloplegia, signs of aberrant regeneration, and failure of the squint to improve and resolve by 3 months are indications for neuroimaging and referral.

The trochlear nerve has the longest intracranial course and may be affected by intracranial tumors, producing a vertical diplopia with a torsional component. While the commonest cause of acquired fourth nerve palsy is probably ischemia, onset following trivial head trauma points towards an intracranial space-occupying lesion that may have tethered the nerve, making it more vulnerable to injury.

The sixth nerve has a long and 'dangerous' intracranial course. Raised intracranial pressure may lead to downward displacement of the brainstem and stretching of the nerve between its exit at the pons and entry into Dorello's petroclinoid canal. This has earned the sixth nerve the moniker of 'barometer of the cranium'. Sixth nerve palsy due to elevated intracranial pressure is thus a false localizing sign, as it wrongly suggests that a lesion lies along the course of the abducent nerve. Isolated sixth nerve palsy in an adult over 40 years of age is likely to be ischaemic. One may closely observe such patients if they have vasculopathic risk factors and if they show signs of improvement.

In children, however, the likelihood of intracranial tumor is much higher, with some studies showing a risk as high as 39 per cent.

Nystagmus and nystagmoid movements

Specific forms of nystagmus and nystagmoid movements have been described in conjunction with intracranial tumors.

Acquired monocular nystagmus in a child should raise suspicion of an anterior visual pathway tumor, commonly a glioma. Neuro-imaging is a must prior to making a diagnosis of spasmus nutans, a relatively benign self-limiting entity characterised by abnormal head posture, head nodding, and nystagmus (which may be monocular or highly asymmetric between the two eyes).

See-saw nystagmus of Maddox is a pendular nystagmus in which one eye elevates and intorts while the other depresses and extorts. It is associated with suprasellar mass lesions, especially craniopharyngioma.

Brun's nystagmus may be seen in patients with cerebellopontine angle tumors which compress the eighth cranial nerve as well as the brainstem. On ipsilateral gaze the patient has large amplitude, low frequency horizontal nystagmus, which becomes reduces in amplitude and increases in frequency on contralateral gaze.

Convergence-retraction nystagmus, along with other features of Parinaud's dorsal midbrain syndrome (light-near dissociation of pupils, lid retraction, vertical gaze palsy, skew deviation) may be seen in children with pinealomas. Nystagmus occurs on attempted convergence and is associated with retraction of the eyeballs due to extraocular muscle co-contraction.

Other forms of nystagmus that may be associated with intracranial tumors include vertical nystagmus (down-beat or up-beat) and gaze-evoked nystagmus. Ocular bobbing, characterised by a fast downward movement followed by a slow upward drift to primary position, occurs in patients with large pontine tumors.

SPECIFIC INTRACRANIAL TUMORS AND THEIR NEURO-OPHTHALMIC SIGNIFICANCE

PITUITARY ADENOMAS

Adenomas are benign tumors arising from glandular tissue. Pituitary tumors can be secretory (two-thirds) or non-secretory in nature. The most common type is the prolactinoma, which accounts for nearly one-third of all pituitary adenomas.

Pituitary adenomas are relatively common, accounting for roughly 10 percent of all intracranial tumors. Middle-aged adults are most affected and there is no gender predilection. Occasionally, tumors may have systemic associations such as multiple endocrine neoplasia (MEN) 1 and McCune-Albright syndrome.

Classification

Pituitary tumors can be classified based upon their size-microadenomas are smaller than, and macroadenomas are larger than 10 millimeters in size. In general, tumors larger than 3 mm can be detected radiologically.

Clinical features

Clinically, these tumors present in one of two ways.

Secretory tumors tend to be smaller at the time of diagnosis (microadenomas) and come to light due to their distant endocrine effects (Table 23.2).

Table 23.2 *Secretory pituitary adenomas and their relative frequency*

Pituitary hormone	Relative frequency
Prolactin	30%
Growth hormone (somatotropin)	15%
Luteinizing hormone (LH), follicle-stimulating hormone (FSH)	10%
Adrenocorticotropin (ACTH)	5%
Thyroid-stimulating hormone (TSH), more than one hormone	Rare

Non-secretory tumors are generally larger macroadenomas which present with features of local compression.

- *Bitemporal hemianopia* is the most common ophthalmic presentation. The gland is located in the bony sella turcica, the dorsal roof of which presents the least resistance to expansion. Depending on the positional relationship between the chiasm and the pituitary gland, visual field defects in the early stages vary. Patients with a post-fixed chiasm develop highly asymmetric field loss, whereas those with a pre-fixed chiasm develop homonymous defects due to optic tract compression (Fig. 23.2).
- *Diplopia.* Less commonly, patients may present with diplopia due to compression of the third, fourth and/or sixth cranial nerves within the cavernous sinus.
- *Reduced facial sensations.* Compression of the first two divisions of the trigeminal nerve can lead to reduced facial sensation.
- *Pituitary apoplexy* is an endocrine emergency caused by sudden hemorrhage within the pituitary gland; it may occur in patients with a pre-existing adenoma, in the postpartum state (Sheehan syndrome), or in association with vasculopathic diseases like hypertension and diabetes. Massive enlargement of the gland leads to compression of surrounding sellar structures and necrosis of viable gland tissue. Patients present with headache, meningeal irritation, visual field defects and ophthalmoplegia. Severe cases may develop hypoglycemia, hypotension and shock. Up to 10 percent of pituitary adenomas may present in this manner.

Treatment

Treatment of pituitary adenomas depends on their size and level of hormonal activity.

- *Medical management* may be sufficient for patients with secretory microadenomas. For prolactinomas, dopamine agonists (bromocriptine, cabergoline) are the treatment of choice.
- *Surgical management.* Larger tumors, ACTH-secreting tumors (which lack effective medical treatment) and non-secretory macroadenomas require surgical debulking, most commonly performed via a trans-sphenoidal approach. Stabilization of hormonal levels is a must prior to contemplating any surgical procedure, and there is a risk of postoperative hypopituitarism.
- *Radiation therapy* may be used as an adjunct to medical or surgical therapy, stereotactic radiosurgery being a recent modality.

CRANIOPHARYNGIOMAS

These relatively uncommon tumors arise from Rathke's pouch near the pituitary stalk, and are therefore suprasellar in location. A biphasic age distribution has been noted, with most patients under the age of 30 years with a second peak at 60 years.

Clinical features

Craniopharyngiomas are large, often cystic and partially calcified. Cystic spaces contain a viscous fluid likened in appearance to motor oil—sterile meningitis produced by rupture of these cysts has been termed 'acute craniopharyngioma'. Craniopharyngiomas commonly present with features of raised intracranial pressure, such as headache, vomiting and papilledema. Visual field defects occur in two-thirds and reflect the posterior-dorsal compression of the chiasm. Hypopituitarism due to pituitary gland compression, and hydrocephalus are often present at the time of diagnosis.

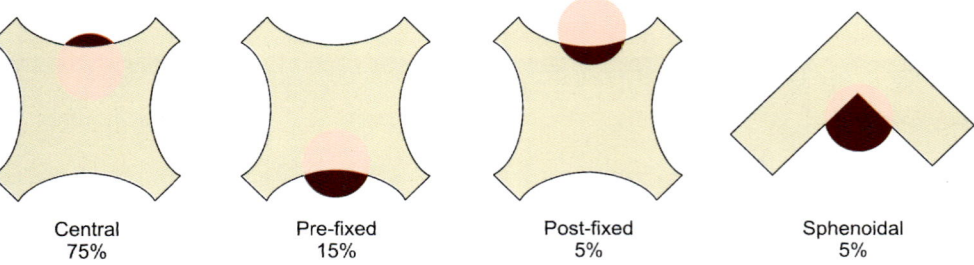

| Central | Pre-fixed | Post-fixed | Sphenoidal |
| 75% | 15% | 5% | 5% |

Fig. 23.2 *Patterns of chiasmal fixation in relation to the pituitary gland.*

Treatment

Treatment is mainly limited to surgical resection by either transcranial or trans-sphenoidal routes, followed by directed radiotherapy. Most patients require pituitary hormone replacement.

MENINGIOMAS

Meningiomas comprise up to one-fifth of all intracranial tumors. There is an association with neurofibromatosis types 1 and 2. These tumors have a predilection for females between the ages of 40 and 60 years, and grow rapidly during pregnancy.

Clinical features

Meningiomas can arise from nearly any location within the cranium, as well as the optic nerve sheaths, but nearly 40 percent arise from the basal dura mater. Those arising from the tuberculum sellae, anterior clinoid process, and sphenoidal wing meningiomas can present first to an ophthalmologist.

Meningiomas of the tuberculum sellae usually grow asymmetrically, initially compressing the optic nerve on that side and subsequently affecting the anterior chiasm. This produces a junctional scotoma (central scotoma in one eye with a superotemporal defect in the other).

Tumors arising from the clinoid process and the sphenoid together constitute a quarter of all meningiomas. Hyperostotic reaction leads to exophthalmos (which can also be a result of orbital extension via the superior orbital fissure) and fullness of the temporal fossa visible externally. Visual field defects could be unilateral or bilateral, the latter due to optic tract involvement.

Neuroimaging. Meningiomas are often calcified and can be picked up on computerized tomographic (CT) scanning, which also reveals the extent of hyperostosis. On magnetic resonance imaging (MRI) they enhance brilliantly with contrast.

Treatment

Treatment is chiefly surgical, however this is seldom more than a debulking due to proximity to neural tissue and blood vessels. Stereotactic radiotherapy appears to be an attractive adjunct or alternative to surgery.

GLIOMAS

Clinical profile

- Gliomas are tumors arising from glial cells and include astrocytomas (the most common type), ependymomas, and oligodendrogliomas. Based upon location, they can be supratentorial, which constitute the majority in adults, or infratentorial, which are mostly found in children.
- The optic nerve is a rare location, except in children with neurofibromatosis type 1. Optic nerve gliomas may extend along the nerve to reach the chiasm and the intracranial space. Those located more anteriorly in the orbit may present with proptosis and/or strabismus with relatively good vision. On the other hand, those nearer the orbital apex usually present later, with very poor vision.
- Gliomas may also involve the hypothalamus and the third ventricle, producing hydrocephalus.
- Secondary effects due to compression of nearby structures include diabetes insipidus, delayed sexual maturation, and behavioral changes.

Neuroimaging

Imaging reveals a fusiform tumor along the optic nerve with expansion of the optic canal in cases of intracranial extension. The limits of intracranial extension are best delineated by MRI.

Treatment

Treatment is controversial. In eyes with very poor vision and disfiguring proptosis, surgical excision is recommended.

- Patients with good vision and fair cosmesis may be observed for evidence of tumor growth.
- Tumors with intracranial extension and/or hydrocephalus need surgical removal.
- For hypothalamic tumors radiotherapy is a useful modality. These tumors may also be observed if stability of size is documented.
- Chemotherapy is preferred in children under the age of 5 years with chiasmal hypothalamic tumors because of the associated morbidity with radiotherapy.

CONCLUSIONS

Patients with life-threatening intracranial neoplasia may first present to the ophthalmologist. Careful history and examination can help in the diagnosis, and to differentiate them from commoner ophthalmological 'mimics'. The ophthalmologist also plays an important role in the follow-up of patients known to have brain tumors. Documentation of visual acuity, optic disc findings and visual field examinations allow for serial comparison and may detect early recurrence.

BIBLIOGRAPHY

1. Kerr NM, Chew SSL, Eady EK, et al. Diagnostic accuracy of confrontation visual field tests. Neurology 2010;74(15):1184–90.

2. Leo-Kottler B. Brain Tumors Relevant to Clinical Neuro-ophthalmology. In: Schiefer U, Wilhelm H, Hart W (Eds). Clinical Neuro-ophthalmology—A Practical Guide. 1st edn. Heidelberg: Springer-Verlag 2007;171–83.

3. Melmed S, Jameson JL. Disorders of the Anterior Pituitary and Hypothalamus. In: Kasper DL, Braunwald E, Fauci AS, et al. (Eds). Harrison's Principles of Internal Medicine. 16th edn. The McGraw-Hill Companies, Inc: New York 2005;2076–98.

4. Robertson DM, Hines JD, Rucker CW. Acquired sixth nerve paresis in children. Arch Ophthalmol 1970;83:574–9.

5. Reddy SSK, Hamrahian AH. Pituitary Disorders and Multiple Endocrine Neoplasia Syndromes. In: Mandell, Brian F. Stoller, James K et al. (Eds). The Cleveland Clinic Foundation intensive review of internal medicine, 5th edn. Hagerstwon, MD: Lippincott Williams and Wilkins 2009;526.

24 DEMYELINATING DISORDERS AND GUILLAIN-BARRÉ SYNDROME

Devendra V Venkatramani

DEMYELINATING DISORDERS

INTRODUCTION

Myelin was discovered by the 'Father of modern pathology', Rudolf Virchow, in 1854. It is composed of water, glycolipid (galactocerebroside), and proteins (including myelin basic protein—MBP, and myelin oligodendrocyte glycoprotein—MOG).

The myelin sheath (Fig. 24.1) is an investing structure that wraps around neuronal axons, and is formed by Schwann cells in the peripheral nervous system and by oligodendrocytes in the central nervous system (CNS).

Myelin is an insulator, that is, it does not allow the passage of ions. Conduction of the nerve impulse (action potential) can thus occur only at areas along the axon which lack myelin. Such areas are present at regular intervals and are called nodes of Ranvier. The electric impulse 'jumps' from one node to the next, appearing to skip the myelinated segment in between. This

Saltatory conduction

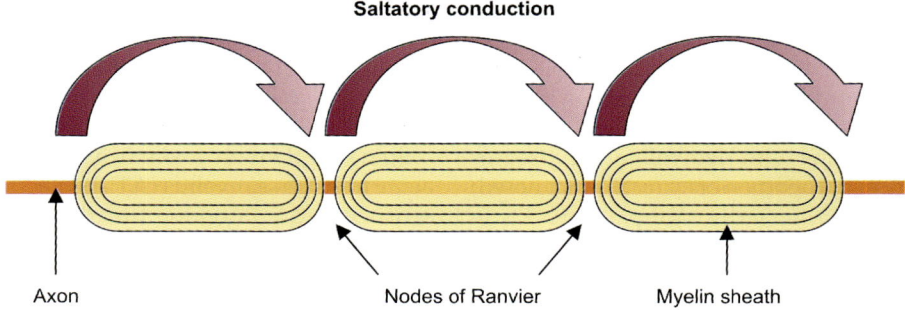

Axon   Nodes of Ranvier   Myelin sheath

Fig. 24.1 *The myelin sheath and saltatory conduction.*

'jumping' has been called saltatory conduction (Fig. 24.1) and is the secret behind the high speed with which signals can be carried by myelinated nerve fibers. Myelinated fibers carry impulses at a speed of approximately 70 meters per second, in comparison to the slower 1 metre per second velocities of non-myelinated fibers.

Demyelinating disorders are characterized by inflammatory destruction of the myelin sheath. These disorders chiefly affect the myelinated axons of the CNS, sparing the peripheral nervous system.

Demyelinating disorders include:
- Neuromyelitis optica
- Multiple sclerosis
- Diffuse sclerosis

NEUROMYELITIS OPTICA

Nuromyelitis optica (NMO) (Devic's disease or Devic's syndrome) is an autoimmune demyelinating disease with a predilection for the spinal cord and optic nerves. In 1894, Eugene Devic and Fernand Gault, his PhD student, described 16 cases of unilateral or bilateral vision loss associated with features of acute spinal cord involvement. NMO was long thought to be a subtype of multiple sclerosis, but has notable differences in its pathophysiology and clinical course.

Epidemiology

Neuromyelitis optica can occur at any age, but has been noted to occur at a later mean age of 40–50 years compared to multiple sclerosis. This may be true for the relapsing form of the disease. NMO is much more common in females than MS, with some studies suggesting a ratio of 8 : 1. This again may be more applicable to relapsing disease.

NMO is thought to be uncommon among Caucasians compared with Asians and Africans. Studies in Asians with demyelinating diseases reveal a higher proportion of (clinically diagnosed) NMO, up to 6% in India, compared to 1% in Causcasians. These findings may be biased by the clinical overlap between MS and NMO, and may change with the more widespread use of antibody assays.

Pathophysiology

NMO is now thought to be an autoimmune channelopathy, due to the presence of IgG antibodies against the *aquaporin-4* water channel. Aquaporin-4 is part of the dystroglycan protein complex present in the foot processes of astrocytes, which contribute to the blood–brain barrier. Humoral mechanisms are thought to be responsible for the spinal cord (and possibly optic nerve) lesions, which are characterized by extensive demyelination, cavitation and necrosis. Immunopathological studies show large numbers of perivascular eosinophils, a high degree of complement activation, and loss of oligodendrocytes. Glial scarring is much less compared to MS.

The antibody IgG-NMO has been reported to have a very high sensitivity and specificity for neuromyelitis optica (91 and 100% respectively, according to some studies).

Clinical features

Presentation

Patients can present with either optic neuritis or transverse myelitis, both scenarios occurring with similar frequencies. Less commonly, optic neuritis and myelitis occur simultaneously. The interval between myelitis and optic neuritis is usually 3 months, although intervals of up to 2 years have been described.

A 'viral' prodrome can precede the onset of symptoms in one-third of all patients, consisting of fever, headache, myalgia, respiratory and/or gastrointestinal symptoms. This points towards an infectious trigger.

Optic neuritis in NMO is acute and classically bilateral, although patients with unilateral optic neuritis have an identical disease course. It is usually severe, some patients experiencing an inability to perceive light in that eye. Visual field defects described include central scotomata, altitudinal, and even chiasmal defects.

Spinal cord involvement in NMO is classically acute transverse myelitis (ATM) affecting motor, sensory and autonomic functions bilaterally. Weakness may progress to paraplegia or quadriplegia (depending on the level of the lesion). Sensory system involvement manifests as paresthesias, complete sensory loss caudal to the lesion, and deep, radicular pain. Other features include loss of deep tendon reflexed and incontinence of urine.

Disease course and prognosis

Patients may have monophasic or a relapsing course, the latter occurring in 70–90% of patients. Patients with the relapsing form are more to have onset at a later age (late thirties), a history of autoimmune disease, and a presentation with either optic neuritis or myelitis only (non-synchronous). Other predictive factors are mentioned in Box 24.1.

Relapses in NMO occur at extremely variable intervals, and can involve either the spinal cord or the optic nerves. Visual recovery may take several weeks to months, and is often incomplete. While the initial event is often more severe in monophasic NMO, the effect of multiple recurrences lends a poorer outcome in relapsing NMO as a result of cumulative damage.

Visual recovery is generally poorer than in optic neuritis associated with MS. Subsequent relapses also tend to occur earlier in patients with NMO. A small sub-group of patients may have a progressive form of disease (as in MS), wherein neurological function deteriorates rapidly on attempting to taper or stop steroids.

Patients with relapsing NMO have a higher 5-year mortality rate, the highest difference reported as 32% as opposed to 10% in the monophasic form. Cause of death is most commonly respiratory failure secondary to severe cervical myelitis.

Investigations and diagnosis

The clinical diagnosis of NMO is made by the presence of bilateral optic neuritis with myelitis, without clinical evidence of cerebral white matter demyelination. Certain investigations, however, help to establish a level of diagnostic certainty.
- *Magnetic resonance imaging* (MRI) of the brain and spinal cord is useful in distinguishing NMO from MS. Patients with MS have characteristic enhancing periventricular and white matter lesions (demyelinating 'plaques'), whereas these are conspicuous by their absence in patients with NMO. The latter may have a few punctate, nonspecific cerebral lesions. Spinal cord MRI in patients with NMO reveals the presence of gadolinium-enhancing, cavitatory lesions that are relatively extensive and contiguous. Extension over three or more vertebral segments differentiates them from the shorter lesions seen in patients with MS.

- *Cerebrospinal fluid (CSF) analysis* shows oligoclonal banding of IgG antibodies in as many as 97% of patients with MS. In those with NMO however, their prevalence is as low as 27% and is transient. CSF in NMO shows pleocytosis of more than 50 white blood cells/mm^3 at the time to myelitis, a finding not seen in typical MS.

- *Anti-NMO antibodies* (against the aquaporin-4 channel) have a very high sensitivity and specificity for NMO. A subset of MS, the opticospinal (Japanese) form, also shows a high level of seropositivity, suggesting that this disorder may represent a form of NMO.

- *Various diagnostic criteria* have been proposed for NMO. The Mayo Clinic revised diagnostic criteria for NMO (2006) require both absolute criteria to be fulfilled along with at least two supportive criteria (Box 24.2). Using this combination yields 99% sensitivity and 90% specificity for NMO. CNS involvement beyond the optic nerves and spinal cord is compatible with NMO.

Box 24.1 *Risk factors for relapsing NMO (Wingerchuk and Weinshenker, 2003)*

A longer first inter-attack interval (more than several weeks)
Female gender
Better motor recovery after the first myelitis event

Box 24.2 *Diagnostic criteria for neuromyelitis optica (Mayo Clinic, revised 2006)*

Absolute criteria
1. Optic neuritis
2. Myelitis

Supportive criteria
1. MRI evidence of a contiguous spinal cord lesion 3 or more segments in length
2. Onset brain MRI non-diagnostic for multiple sclerosis
3. NMO-IgG seropositivity

Differential diagnosis of NMO

Table 24.1 depict the differentiating features between multiple sclerozni and neuromyelitis optica.

Management

Treatment of acute presentation. In patients with acute relapses, corticosteroids are the drug of choice. Intravenous methylprednisolone in a dose of 1 gram per day is given for 5 days, followed by a tapering course of oral prednisolone.

Prevention of relapses forms an important part of patient management. An immunosuppressant is preferred, either alone or in combination with a corticosteroid in reduced doses. Azathioprine-prednisolone combination has been shown to reduce the frequency of relapses in relapsing NMO, and allowed improvement in neurological function. Azathioprine is used at a relatively high dose of 2.5 to 3 mg/kg/day. Blood cell counts (leukocyte and platelets) and liver function tests need to be monitored during therapy.

- *Mycophenolate mofetil* can be used in patients who do not tolerate azathioprine, as it does not affect leukopoiesis and has fewer gastrointestinal effects.
- *Rituximab*, a monoclonal antibody against CD-20 present on B-lymphocytes, has potential benefit. A small case series showed disease stability and fewer relapses after administration, with a moderate improvement in neurological function. Rituximab is given as two intravenous injections separated by a period of 2 weeks. Adverse effects include reactivation of latent infections such as hepatitis and tuberculosis, and infusion reactions such as fever, chills, flushing and bronchospasm.

- *Interferon beta-1b* has been used in MS, especially the relapsing-remitting form, but clinical experience with NMO does not support its use. A randomized controlled trial, however, did find a reduction in relapse rates in patients with opticospinal MS as well (which may be the same disease as NMO).
- *Intravenous immunoglobulin (IVIg)* may be effective in NMO, as it is an antibody-mediated immune disorder. While anecdotal evidence exists showing its efficacy in preventing relapses, further studies are needed.
- *Plasmapheresis* can be used in patients with severe exacerbations. A marked functional improvement was noted in the majority of patients with NMO, which was rapid and sustained. However, plasma exchange is unsuitable as a routine preventive measure.

Conclusions

Neuromyelitis optica is a debilitating and in some cases, fatal demyelinating disease. Epidemiological data suggests that it may be a fairly common cause of demyelinating optic neuritis in India and other parts of Asia. Distinguishing it from multiple sclerosis appears to be important for reasons of management and prognostication (Table 24.1).

Table 24.1 *Differentiating features between multiple sclerosis and neuromyelitis optica*

	Multiple sclerosis	*Neuromyelitis optica*
Age	20–40 years	Late thirties to forties
Race	Caucasians, temperate climates	Asians, Africans > Caucasians
Gender predilection	F : M = 2 : 1	F : M >> 2 : 1, may be as high as 8 : 1
Optic neuritis	Unilateral, bilateral (non-synchronous)	Unilateral, bilateral (synchronous, non-synchronous) more likely
Visual loss	Less severe	More severe
Cerebral, brainstem involvement	Present	Absent
Immune markers	Oligoclonal IgG banding in cerebrospinal fluid	Antibodies to aquaporin-4 water channel
Magnetic resonance imaging (MRI)	Cerebral (periventricular or white matter) demyelinating plaques	Spinal cord lesions—enhancing, cavitatory, extending over three or more vertebral segments
Visual prognosis	Better	Poor

MULTIPLE SCLEROSIS

Etiology. Multiple sclerosis (MS) is a demyelinating disorders of unknown etiology, affecting women more often than men, usually in the 15–50 year age group.

Pathologically, the condition is characterized by a patchy destruction of the myelin sheaths throughout the central nervous system.

Clinical course of the condition is marked by remissions and relapses.

Ocular lesions include:
- *Optic neuritis* which is usually unilateral (for details see page 142–147).
- *Other ocular lesions* include internuclear ophthalmoplegia and nystagmus (vestibular or cerebellar).

Systemic lesions include:
- Muscular weaknesses
- Gait abnormalities, and
- Seizures

Magnetic resonance imaging (MRI) is the neuroimaging technique of choice for suspected cases of demyelinating disorder.

DIFFUSE SCLEROSIS (SCHILDER'S DISEASE)

Features. It typically affects children and adolescents and is characterized by progressive demyelination of the entire white matter of the cerebral hemispheres.

Ocular lesions include: optic neuritis (papillitis or retrobulbar neuritis), cortical blindness (due to destruction of the visual centers and optic radiations), ophthalmoplegia and nystagmus.

GUILLAIN-BARRÉ SYNDROME

Guillain-Barré syndrome (GBS) is an acute, autoimmune polyradiculoneuropathy, characterized clinically by areflexia, ascending motor paralysis, and variable sensory involvement. GBS has an acute, sometimes fulminant course with a mortality rate of up to 5 percent, chiefly due to pulmonary complications. The vast majority, however, experience near-complete neurological recovery, often over several months to a year.

ETIOLOGY

Evidence suggests that GBS is an autoimmune disease, triggered by infection with *Campylobacter* *jejuni*, cytomegalovirus, or Epstein-Barr virus, or recent immunization (older 'neural' rabies vaccines). The mechanism of 'molecular mimicry', wherein non-self antigens bear an epitopal resemblance to self antigens which subsequently become targets to the immune response, has been implicated in GBS. The self antigens are neural gangliosides; these are located on the plasma membrane of neurons and are particularly abundant at nodes of Ranvier.

CLINICAL PROFILE

GBS is a clinical entity comprising various subtypes. These include:
- Acute inflammatory demyelinating polyneuropathy (AIDP, the most common subtype), acute motor axonal neuropathy (AMAN),
- Acute motor sensory axonal neuropathy (AMSAN), and
- Miller Fisher syndrome (MFS).

Note. Of these, AIDP and MFS are demyelinating in nature, while AMAN and AMSAN demonstrate axonal damage on electrodiagnostic testing.

Miller Fisher Syndrome

Clinical features

The Miller Fisher syndrome presents clinically as a triad of ataxia, areflexia of limbs, and ophthalmoplegia. Onset is with diplopia, myalgia and paresthesias, vertigo, and ataxia. A respiratory prodrome has been reported to be the most common antecedent event.

Ophthalmoplegia is commonly bilateral and asymmetric. Unilateral paresis has been reported but is distinctly uncommon. Approximately 50 percent of patients show pupilloparesis. Pupillary involvement has been described as a presenting feature of MFS. Light-near dissociation has also been noted.

Involvement of other cranial nerves has been described in more than half of patients, with the 7th nerve, followed by the 9th and 10th, being the most common.

Visual impairment has been noted, suggesting central nervous system involvement, unlike other form of GBS.

Pathophysiology

GQ1b is a ganglioside (Fig. 24.2) found in high concentration in the oculomotor, trochlear and

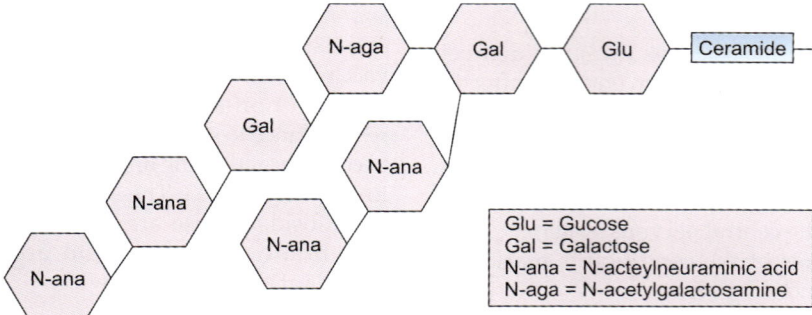

Fig. 24.2 *Structure of ganglioside GQ1b.*

abducens nerves. Antibodies to this ganglioside have been found in over 90 percent of patients with MFS, pointing towards a causative role.

Differential diagnosis

Wernicke's encephalopathy closely mimics MFS, and presents with ophthalmoplegia, ataxia, and global confusion. It is also often precipitated by infection, commonly in a person with severe nutritional deficiency. Other possibilities include botulism, stroke, and myasthenia gravis.

Clinically and immunologically, MFS, GBS with ophthalmoplegia, acute opthalmoparesis without ataxia, and Bickerstaff's brainstem encephalitis (BBE) may form a spectrum of disease linked by the presence of anti-GQ1b antibody.

Management and outcome

The natural course of the disease is favorable, with recovery in the majority of cases with or without treatment. Plasmapheresis has been tried with contradictory results. Intravenous immunoglobulin (IVIg) may reduce the duration between onset of ophthalmoplegia and ataxia and the onset of recovery.

BIBLIOGRAPHY

1. Bae JS, Kim JK, Kim SH, et al. Bilateral internal ophthalmoplegia as an initial sole manifestation of Miller Fisher syndrome. Journal of Clinical Neuroscience 2009;16(7):963–4.

2. Beck GM. A case of diffuse myelitis associated with optic neuritis. Brain 1927;50:687–703.

3. Berlit P, Rakicky J. The Miller Fisher syndrome. Review of the literature. J Clin Neuro-ophthalmol 1992;12(1):57–63.

4. Colding-Jørgensen E, Vissing J. Visual impairment in anti-GQ1b positive Miller Fisher syndrome. Acta Neurol Scand 2001;103(4):259–60.

5. Cree BA, Lamb S, Morgan K, Chen A, Waubant E, Genain C. An open label study of the effects of rituximab in neuromyelitis optica. Neurology 2005;64(7):1270–2.

6. Fisher M. An unusual variant of acute immune polyneuritis (syndrome of ophthalmoplegia, ataxia, and areflexia). N Engl J Med 1956;255: 57–65.

7. Hogancamp WE, Rodriguez M, Weinshenker BG. The epidemiology of multiple sclerosis. Mayo Clin Proc 1997;72(9):871–8.

8. Keegan M, Pineda AA, McClelland RL, et al. Plasma exchange for severe attacks of CNS demyelination: predictors of response. Neurology 2002;58(1):143–6.

9. Lucchinetti CF, Mandler RN, McGavern D, et al. A role for humoral mechanisms in the pathogenesis of Devic's neuromyelitis optica. Brain 2002;125(7):1450–61.

10. Mandler RN, Ahmed W, Dencoff JE. Devic's neuromyelitis optica: a prospective study of seven patients treated with prednisolone and azathioprine. Neurology 1998;51(4):1219–20.

11. Mori M, Kuwabara S, Fukutake T, et al. Clinical features and prognosis of Miller Fisher syndrome. Neurology 2001;56:1104–06.

12. Mori M, Kuwabara S, Fukutake T, Hattori T. Intravenous immunoglobulin therapy for Miller Fisher syndrome. Neurology 2007;68(14): 1144–6.

13. Nitta T, Kase M, Shinmei Y, et al. Mydriasis with light-near dissociation in Fisher's syndrome. Jpn J Ophthalmol 2007;51(3):224–7.

14. Odaka M, Yuki N, Hirata K. Anti-GQ1b IgG antibody syndrome: clinical and immunological range. J Neurol Neurosurg Psychiatry 2001; 70(1):50–5.

15. Saida T, Tashiro K, Itoyama Y, et al. Interferon Beta-1b Multiple Sclerosis Study Group of Japan. Interferon beta-1b is effective in Japanese RRMS patients: a randomized, multicenter study. Neurology 2005;64(4):621–30.

16. Shibasaki H, McDonald WI, Kuroiwa Y. Racial modification of clinical picture of multiple sclerosis: comparison between British and Japanese patients. J Neurol Sci 1981;49:253–71.

17. Singhal BS. Multiple sclerosis-Indian experience. Annals of the Academy of Medicine, Singapore 1985;14:32–6.

18. Smith J, Clarke L, Severn P, et al. Unilateral external ophthalmoplegia in Miller Fisher syndrome: case report. BMC Ophthalmology 2007;7:7.

19. Takahashi T, Fujihara K, Nakashima I, et al. Antiaquaporin-4 antibody is involved in the pathogenesis of NMO: a study on antibody titre. Brain 2007;130:1235–43.

20. Tourtellotte WW, Staugaitis SM, Walsh MJ, et al. The basis of intra-blood-brain barrier IgG synthesis. Ann Neurol 1985;17:21–7.

21. VA, Kryzer TJ, Pittock SJ, Verkman AS, Hinson SR. IgG marker of optic-spinal multiple sclerosis binds to the aquaporin-4 water channel. Journal of Experimental Medicine 2005;202(4):473–7.

22. Wingerchuk DM, Hogancamp WF, O'Brien PC, et al. The clinical course of neuro-myelitis optica (Devic's syndrome). Neurology 1999;53:1107–14.

23. Wingerchuk DM, Lennon VA, Pittock SJ, et al. Revised diagnostic criteria for neuromyelitis optica. Neurology 2006 66(10):1485–9.

24. Wingerchuk DM, Weinshenker BG. Neuromyelitis optica: clinical predictors of a relapsing course and survival. Neurology 2003;60(5):848–53.

25. Yuan C-L, Wang Y-J, Tsai C-P. Miller Fisher syndrome: a hospital-based retrospective study. European Neurology 2000;44(2):79–85.

25 OPHTHALMIC MANIFESTATIONS OF HEAD INJURY

Devendra V Venkatramani

GENERAL CONSIDERATIONS
Introduction
Clinical Examination
• History
• External examination
• Pupillary examination
OPHTHALMIC MANIFESTATIONS
OF HEAD INJURY
Pupillary Signs

Optic Nerve Dysfunctions
Ocular Motility Disturbances
• 3rd, 4th, and 6th cranial nerves
• Nystagmus, other ocular movements
Retinopathies
• Purtscher retinopathy
• Terson syndrome

GENERAL CONSIDERATIONS

INTRODUCTION

Head injury is a common cause of morbidity and mortality in an urban industrialized environment. It may arise in the setting of road-traffic accidents, as a consequence of workplace injuries, domestic accidents, or assault. Young males appear to be at particular risk, but infants and the elderly also are commonly affected. Special scenarios include the shaken-baby syndrome and seemingly innocuous trauma in the elderly.

The role of the ophthalmologist in management of head injury is manifold. He or she may be the first health care provider to come in contact with the patient, as in the instance of shaken-baby syndrome. Ophthalmic referral may be sought for interpreting abnormal extraocular motility, pupillary reflexes, or in the setting of vision loss due to traumatic optic neuropathy (the latter is discussed elsewhere).

Clinical findings need to be interpreted considering the level of patient awareness, which may be objectively documented using the Glasgow Coma Scale (GCS) (Table 25.1).

Table 25.1 *Glasgow Coma Scale (GCS)*			
Score	*Eye opening*	*Speech*	*Motor function*
6			Obeys
5		Oriented	Localizes
4	Spontaneous	Confused at times	Withdraws
3	To voice	Inappropriate words	Abnormal flexion
2	To pain	Incomprehensible	Abnormal extension
1	None	None	None

Traditionally, a score of 13–15 indicates mild injury, a score of 9–12 indicates moderate injury, and a score of 8 or less indicates severe injury.

CLINICAL EXAMINATION

Patients with head injury will be variably arousable and aware of their surroundings. This complicates the examination, and one thus primarily relies on testing of reflexes that do not require the patient's active participation.

History

Certain points in the patient's history need to be elicited either from the patient himself, or from by-standers.
- A history of loss of consciousness points towards significant neurological injury.
- Remote or current use of alcohol or recreational drug abuse can alter examination findings.
- It is useful if history of visual function prior to the injury is available, as well as any prior ocular surgery.

External examination

On external examination the ophthalmologist should note the presence and extent of periorbital ecchymosis.
- *Bilateral ecchymosis* ('raccoon eyes') may result from hemorrhage in the scalp which tracks down into the eyelids, but also indicates a fracture of the base of the skull.
- *Bony orbital crepitus and discontinuity* of the orbital rim are evidence for orbital wall fractures.
- *Apparent telecanthus* (increase in the distance between the two medial canthii) is seen in fractures of the nasal bones, and when coupled with rounding of the medial canthus suggests a dinsertion or avulsion of the medial canthal tendon.
- *Globe hypotropia* may be seen in cases of orbital floor blow-out.

These findings are important when interpreting the results of pupillary examination and ocular motility, as they can be local confounding factors.

Pupillary examination

Pupillary examination as described below is most important and reveals the different happenings.

OPHTHALMIC MANIFESTATIONS OF HEAD INJURY

Ophthalmic manifestations of head injury include:
- Pupillary signs
- Optic nerve dysfunctions
- Ocular motility disturbances, and
- Retinopathies

PUPILLARY SIGNS

Just as the pupils are the 'windows to the eyes', so too can they be windows to the central nervous system. Pupillary evaluation should be interpreted after considering factors like prior ocular surgery (evidenced by the presence of an intraocular lens, limbal scar, etc.), and concurrent ocular or orbital injury.

Points to be considered are pupil size, shape, reaction to light (direct, consensual, and the presence of relative afferent pupillary defect or RAPD), and reaction to accommodation in specific cases.

Abnormalities of pupil size could be bilaterally symmetrical or asymmetrical (anisocoria) (Fig. 25.1). For anisocoria to be considered significant, an inter-eye difference of 2 millimeters or more is required.

Bilaterally constricted pupils are an ominous sign as they are associated with pontine hemorrhage, which generally has a poor prognosis.

A fixed and dilated pupil (FDP) may be the result of direct 3rd nerve (oculomotor) injury, or due to the mass effect of a remote intracranial hemorrhage producing transtentorial herniation of the nerve.

Hutchinson's pupil demonstrates the stages of increasing intracranial hemorrhage. Initially, compression of the oculomotor nerve (by an ipsilateral hematoma) stimulates it, causing ipsilateral pupillary contriction. Further compression and herniation paralyse the nerve, producing ipsilateral dilation. Ultimately the contralateral 3rd nerve may also get compressed leading to bilaterally fixed and dilated pupils.

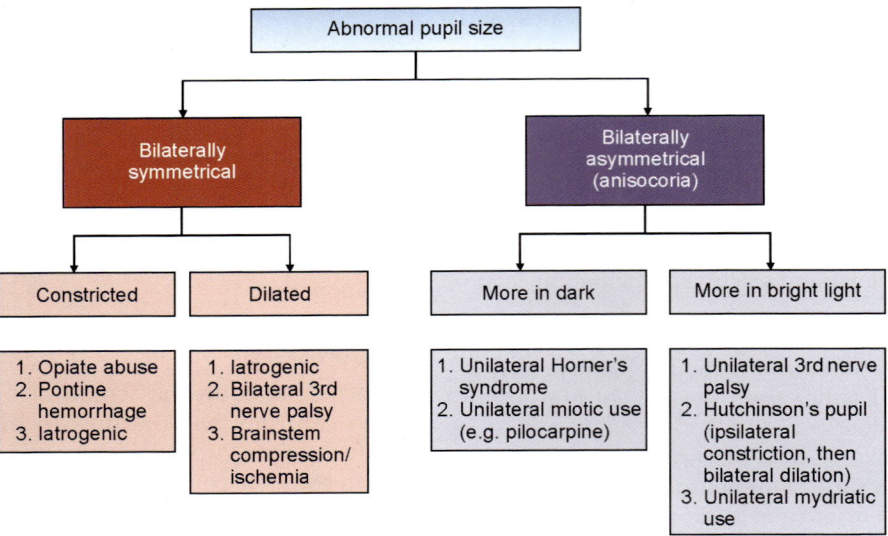

Fig. 25.1 *Evaluation of a patient with head injury and abnormal pupil size.*

A FDP is more likely to be due to 3rd nerve injury, whereas bilateral FDPs are thought to be associated with hypoperfusion and ischemic damage to the brainstem. Bilateral fixed and dilated pupils are associated with high mortality and need urgent neurosurgical intervention.

Horner's syndrome following head injury could be central in origin, or preganglionic due to associated neck trauma. The classic signs of acquired Horner's syndrome are miosis, ptosis, apparent enophthalmos and anhidrosis.

OPTIC NERVE DYSFUNCTION

Optic nerve lesions

Optic nerve involvement may be in the form of:

- Papilledema
- Traumatic optic neuropathy
- Optic nerve avulsion

Clinical examination

Visual acuity It is often not possible to objectively test visual acuity in patients with acute head injury. Bedside examination involves finger counting at various distances and a subjective comparison of vision between the two eyes. *Confrontation visual field estimation* is a subjective but fairly accurate test in cooperative patients, and should be a part of routine examination.

Ophthalmoscopy in the acute setting generally shows a normal optic nerve head.

- *Papilledema* (bilateral optic nerve head swelling secondary to raised intracranial pressure) may take a few hours to develop.

- *Optic disc pallor* may set in after weeks; optic atrophy may be secondary to chronic papilledema (secondary optic atrophy with gliotic disc changes and absence of cupping), or due to traumatic optic neuropathy (primary optic atrophy).

- *Optic nerve avulsion* may be appreciated before it is obscured by hemorrhage.

Electrophysiologic testing, namely the visual-evoked potential (VEP), will objectively demonstrate visual pathway damage anywhere from the eye to the occipital cortex. This test, therefore, has poor localizing value, but has utility in suspected traumatic optic neuropathy or suspected functional visual loss.

OCULAR MOTILITY DISTURBANCES

Limitations of ocular motility may arise due to neurological injury in the brainstem, along the intracranial course of the ocular motor nerves, as secondary effects of elevated intracranial pressure, or due to restrictive orbital pathology. *Supranuclear causes of ocular motility abnormalities* after head injury include Parinaud's dorsal midbrain syndrome and internuclear ophthalmoplegia (INO).

Cranial neuropathy most commonly affects the abducens (6th) cranial nerve. This nerve is particularly vulnerable to the downward displacement of the brainstem due to raised (supratentorial) intracranial pressure, as it is tethered between its exit from the brainstem and Dorello's canal. Palsy may be bilateral and is a non-localizing sign. Fractures of the base of the skull may extend to the apex of the petrous temporal bone and damage the 6th nerve there. This may be associated with Battle's sign (retroauricular ecchymosis) and leakage of cerebrospinal fluid from the ear.

The trochlear (4th) nerve may be damaged in the midbrain resulting in a nuclear injury producing contralateral superior oblique palsy and often associated with contralateral Horner's syndrome. Bilateral 4th nerve palsies can occur due to a contrecoup type of injury wherein the nerves are damaged against the free tentorial edge. Acquired trochlear nerve palsy is most often due to trauma.

Oculomotor or 3rd cranial nerve injury can occur as it passes over the tentorial edge, where it is related superiorly to the uncal portion of the temporal lobe. Raised intracranial pressure compresses the nerve against the tentorium and produces the sequence of pupillary changes known as Hutchinson's pupil (described above).

Oculomotor nerve palsy is thus pupil involving or of the 'surgical' type, with variable ptosis and limitation of ocular motility. Oculomotor palsy following seemingly trivial head trauma should arouse suspicion of a compressive lesion along the course of the third cranial nerve.

Nystagmus may develop following head injury. Various types described include down-beat nystagmus, vestibular nystagmus (both peripheral following vestibulocochlear nerve injury, and central forms), and ocular bobbing in patients with pontine hemorrhage.

RETINOPATHIES
Purtscher retinopathy

It may occur after head injury, as well as due to severe chest compression, fractures of long bones, and liver injury.

Symptoms and signs are usually bilateral although sometimes asymmetrical. The chief complaints is of painless vision loss, within a few hours after the trauma. Vision typically ranges between 20/200 and counting fingers close to the face.

Ophthalmoscopy characteristically shows superficial retinal hemorrhages, dilated and tortuous vessels, confluent soft exudates (cotton wool spots) in a peripapillary location, optic disc swelling, and occasionally serous macular detachment.

Fluorescein angiography shows blocked choroidal fluorescence in the early phases. Hypofluorescence may also be due to focal areas of arteriolar obstruction and capillary non-perfusion. There may be late leakage of dye from posterior pole vessels including arterioles, venules and capillaries, and late vascular staining.

Treatment. There is no specific treatment and the retinal hemorrhages resolve spontaneously over a period of weeks. Variable degrees of retinal pigment epithelial migration can occur. Visual recovery may be very good, but can be limited by pigment alterations and optic atrophy, and non-specific visual field changes may also persist.

Terson's syndrome

It is defined as concomitant vitreous hemorrhage with any form of acute intracranial hemorrhage, including subarachnoid (the most common form), subdural, or extradural. Intraocular bleeding may occur at other sites in up to one-fifth of eyes.

Fundus examination shows vitreous hemorrhage along with multiple preretinal, intraretinal, and subretinal hemorrhages. Terson's syndrome is thus a differential diagnosis for intraocular hemorrhage at multiple levels, especially if bilateral. Studies have directly correlated the presence of intraocular hemorrhage to increased morbidity and mortality in patients with ruptured intracranial aneurysms. Vitrectomy may be required in select cases, as in amblyopia-susceptible children, or in eyes with associated retinal detachment.

BIBLIOGRAPHY

1. Clusmann H, Schaller C, Schramm J. Fixed and dilated pupils after trauma, stroke, and previous intracranial surgery: management and outcome. J Neurol Neurosurg Psychiatry 2001;71:175–81.

2. Frizzel R, Kuhn F, Morris R, et al. Screening for ocular hemorrhages in patients with ruptured cerebral aneurysms: a prospective study on 99 patients. Neurosurgery 1997;41: 529–34.

3. Garfinkle AM, Danys IR, Nicolle DA, et al. Terson's syndrome: a reversible cause of blindness following subarachnoid hemorrhage. J Neurosurg 1992;76:766–71.

4. Ropper AH. The opposite pupil in herniation. Neurology 1990;40:1707–9.

section

VII

Ocular Motor System

ANATOMY AND LESIONS OF OCULOMOTOR, TROCHLEAR AND ABDUCENT NERVES

AK Khurana, Indu Khurana, Aruj K Khurana, Bhawna Khurana

OCULOMOTOR NERVE

The oculomotor (third cranial) nerve is entirely motor in function. It supplies all the extraocular muscles except lateral rectus and superior oblique. It also supplies the intraocular muscles namely sphincter pupillae and ciliary muscle.

FUNCTIONAL COMPONENTS

1. *Somatic efferent component* is concerned with the movements of the eyeball.
2. *General visceral efferent* (parasympathetic) component of the nerve is meant for accommodation and contraction of the pupil.
3. *General somatic afferent* component of the nerve is associated with proprioceptive impulses from the extraocular muscles supplied by the somatic efferent component of this nerve.

OCULOMOTOR NUCLEAR COMPLEX

The nuclear complex of the oculomotor nerve is situated in the midbrain at the level of superior colliculus, in the ventromedial part of the central grey matter that surrounds the cerebral aqueduct (Fig. 26.1).

It is a longitudinal column of about 10 mm length. It extends above to the level of floor of third ventricle and below it is related to nucleus of the trochlear nerve (Fig. 26.2). The oculomotor nucleus complex has two motor nuclei:
- The *main motor nucleus* of large multipolar neurons
- The *accessory parasympathetic nucleus* (Edinger-Westphal nucleus) of small multipolar neurons.

Main motor nucleus

The main motor nucleus is composed of the subnuclei (Figs 26.3A and B) supplying individual extraocular muscles as follows:

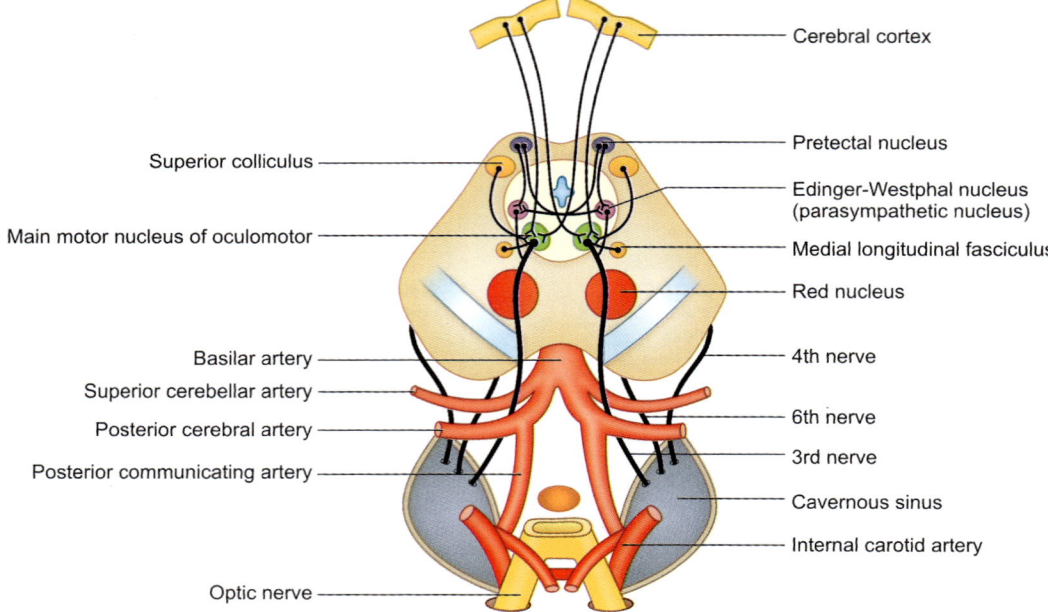

Fig. 26.1 *Oculomotor nerve nuclei, their central connections and course of fascicular part and basilar part of the nerve.*

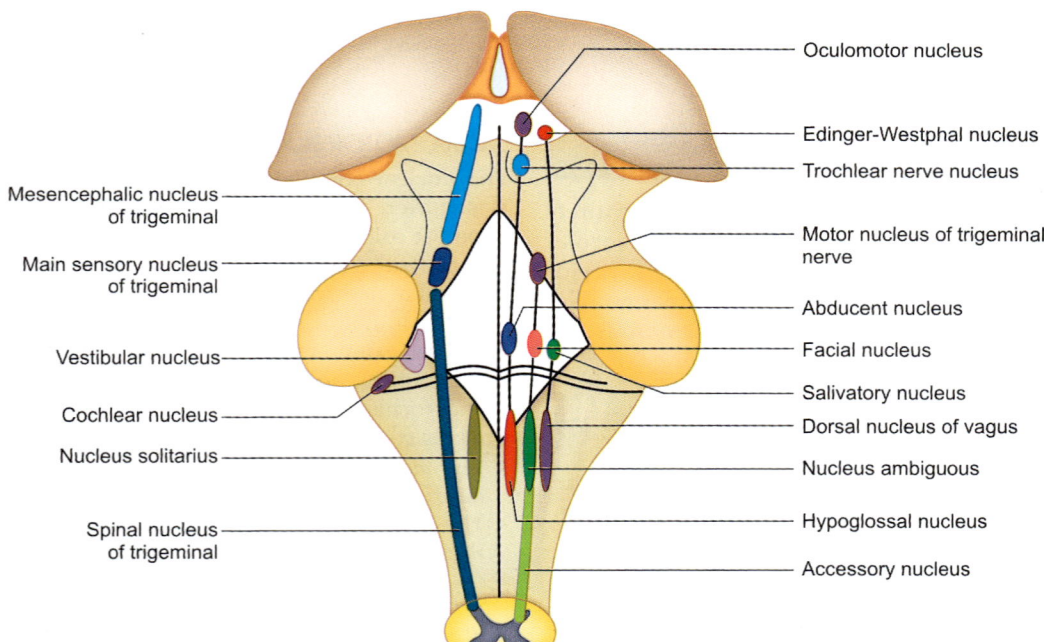

Fig. 26.2 *The cranial nerve nuclei as projected onto the posterior surface of the brainstem.*

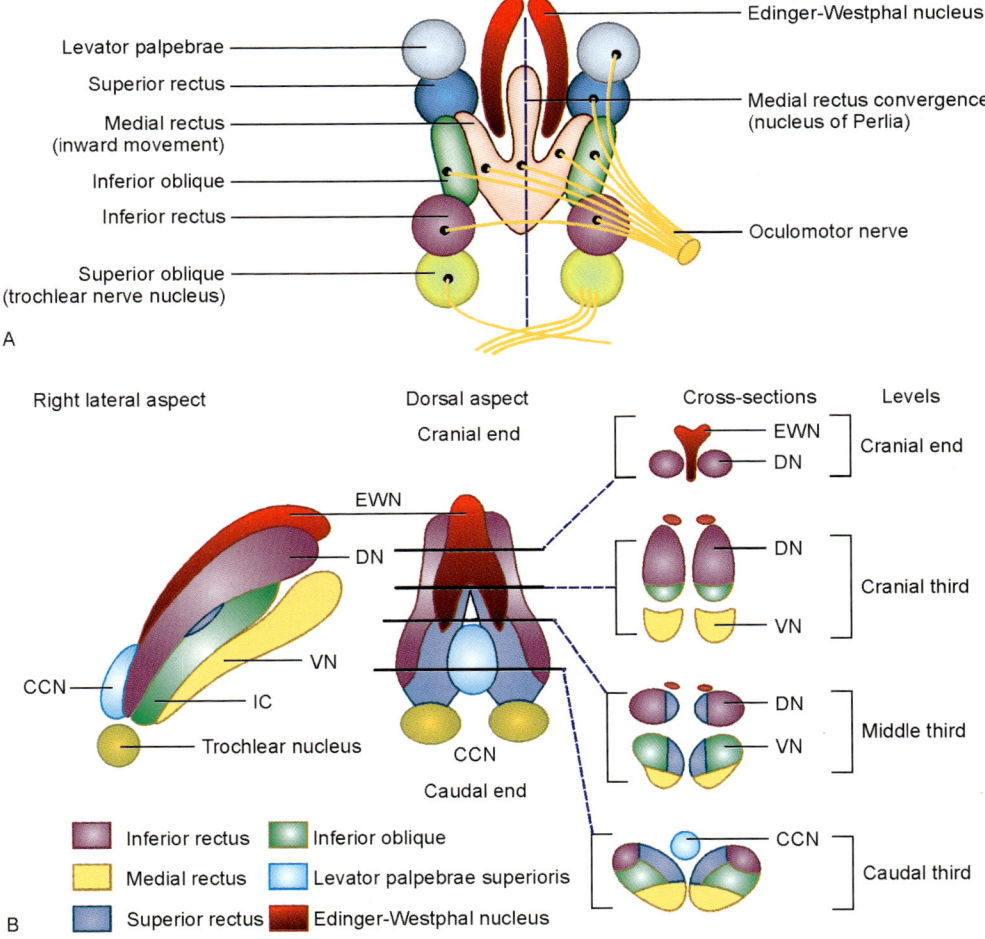

Fig. 26.3 *Components of oculomotor nucleus complex: (A) Old outdated concept; (B) Modern concept.*

1. *Dorsolateral nucleus:* Ipsilateral inferior rectus.
2. *Intermedial nucleus:* Ipsilateral inferior oblique.
3. *Ventromedial nucleus:* Ipsilateral medial rectus.
4. *Paramedial (scattered) nucleus:* Contralateral superior rectus.
5. *Caudal central nucleus:* Bilateral levator palpebrae superioris.

• *Accessory motor muscles.* The accessory motor nucleus (Edinger-Westphal nucleus). It is situated posterior to the main oculomotor nucleus mass. It sends preganglionic parasympathetic fibers along the other oculomotor fibers. It consists of a median and two lateral components. Perhaps the cranial half of the nucleus is concerned with light reflexes and the caudal half with accommodation. The median part is fork-shaped (nucleus of Perlia) and its role in convergence is questionable.

Connections of the nucleus

The oculomotor nucleus is connected with the following:

1. *Cerebral cortex*
   • *Motor cortex* (precentral gyrus) of both sides through the corticonuclear tracts.
   • *Visual cortex* through the superior colliculus and the tactobulbar tract.
   • *Frontal eye field* (FEF).
2. *Nuclei of 4th, 6th and 8th cranial nerves* through the medial longitudinal bundle.

3. *Pretectal nucleus* of both sides (for light reflex).
4. *Vertical and torsional gaze centers* through the medial longitudinal bundle.
5. *Cerebellum* through the vestibular nuclei.

COURSE AND DISTRIBUTION

For the purpose of description, the course of the oculomotor nerve can be divided into: fascicular, basilar, intracavernous and intra-orbital parts.

The fascicular part

The fasciculus consists of efferent fibers which pass from the third nerve nucleus through the red nucleus and the medial aspect of the cerebral peduncle. They then emerge from the midbrain and pass into the interpeduncular space (Fig. 26.1).

The basilar part

The basilar part starts as a series of 15 to 20 rootlets in the interpeduncular fossa. These coalesce to form a large medial and a small lateral root, which unite to form a flattened nerve, which gets twisted bringing the inferior fibers superiorly and superior fibers inferiorly; and thus the nerve becomes a rounded cord. The nerve then passes between the posterior cerebral artery and the superior cerebellar artery and runs forwards in the interpeduncular cistern (running lateral to and parallel with the posterior communicating artery) to reach the cavernous sinus (Figs 26.1 and 26.4).

The intracavernous part

The nerve enters the cavernous sinus by piercing the posterior part of its roof on the lateral side of the posterior clinoid process (Fig. 26.5). It then descends to the lateral wall of the sinus, where it lies above the trochlear nerve (Fig. 26.6). In the anterior part of the cavernous sinus, the nerve divides into superior and inferior divisions which enter the orbit through the middle part of the superior orbital fissure within the annulus of Zinn (Fig. 26.7). In the fissure, the nasociliary nerve lies in between the two divisions, while the abducent nerve lies inferolateral to them.

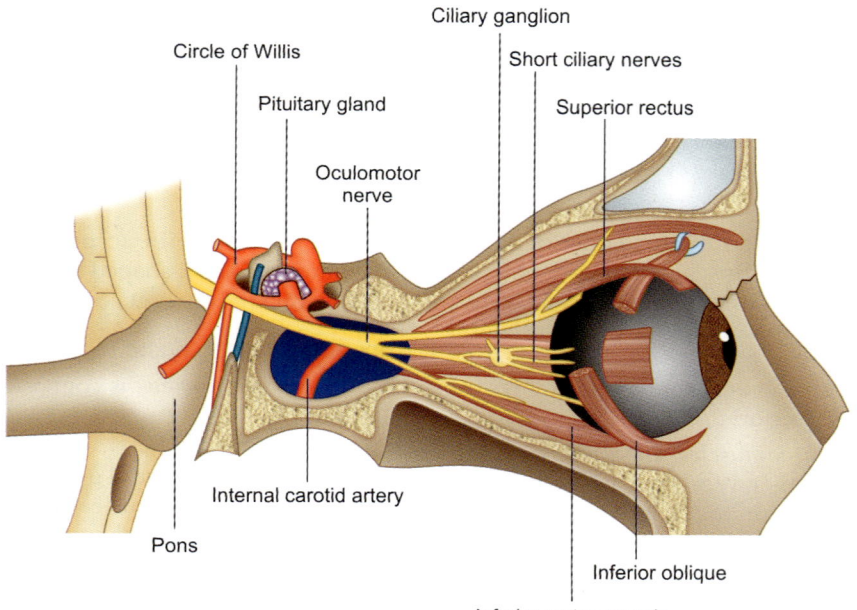

Ciliary ganglion
Circle of Willis
Short ciliary nerves
Pituitary gland
Superior rectus
Oculomotor nerve
Internal carotid artery
Pons
Inferior oblique
Inferior rectus muscle

Fig. 26.4 *Course of oculomotor nerve.*

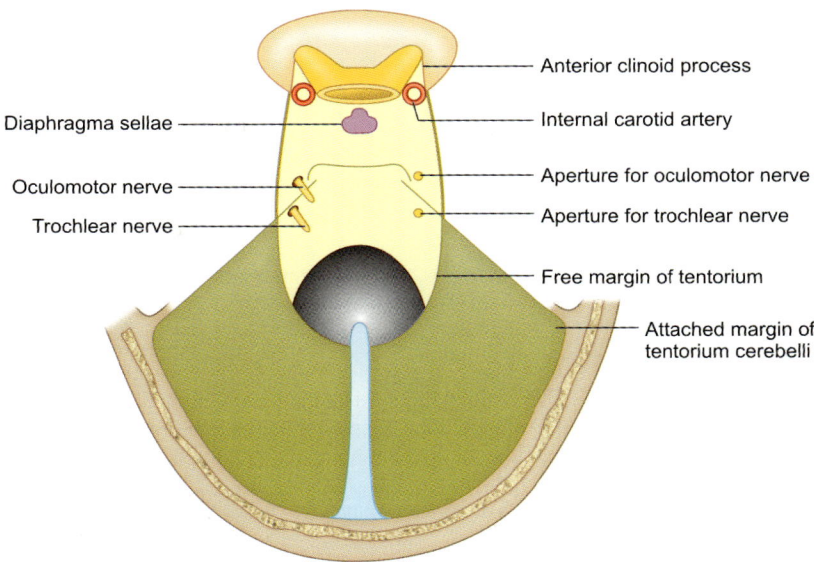

Fig. 26.5 *Entry of oculomotor nerve and trochlear nerve into the cavernous sinus from its root.*

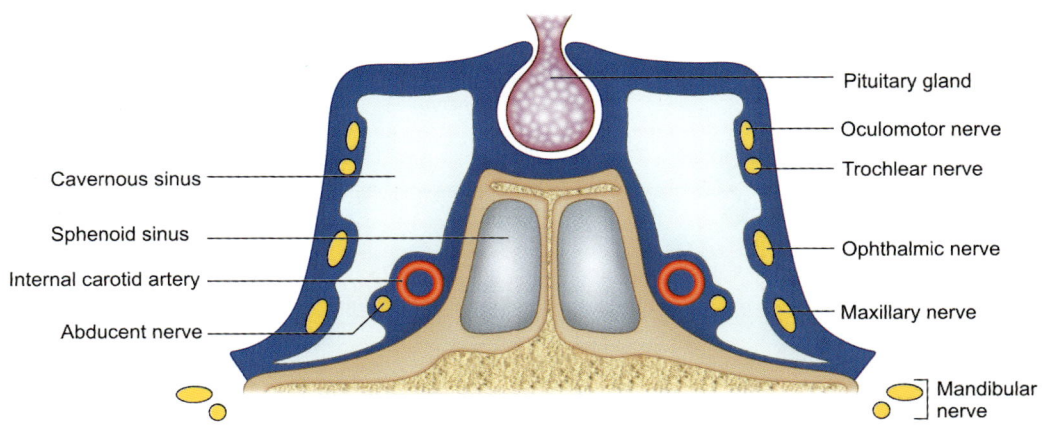

Fig. 26.6 *Coronal section through the middle cranial fossa showing the relations of cranial nerves (3rd, 4th, three divisions of 5th and 6th) with each other in the lateral wall of the cavernous sinus.*

The intraorbital part

In the orbit, the smaller *superior division* ascends on the lateral side of optic nerve and supplies the superior rectus and the levator palpebrae superioris (Fig. 26.4). The larger, *inferior division* divides into three branches:

1. *Nerve to the medial rectus* passes inferior to the optic nerve

2. *Nerve to inferior* rectus passes downward and enters the muscle on its upper aspect

3. *Nerve to inferior oblique* (longest of the three branches) passes in between the inferior rectus and lateral rectus and supplies the inferior oblique from its posterior border. It gives off the motor root to the ciliary ganglion (Fig. 26.8).

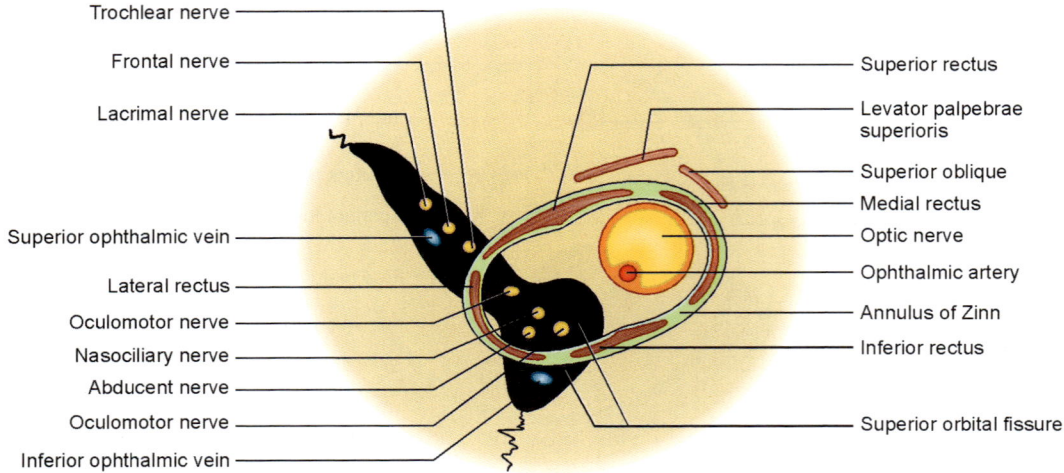

Fig. 26.7 *Apical part of the orbit showing the origin of extraocular muscles, the common tendinous ring and the structures passing through the superior orbital fissure.*

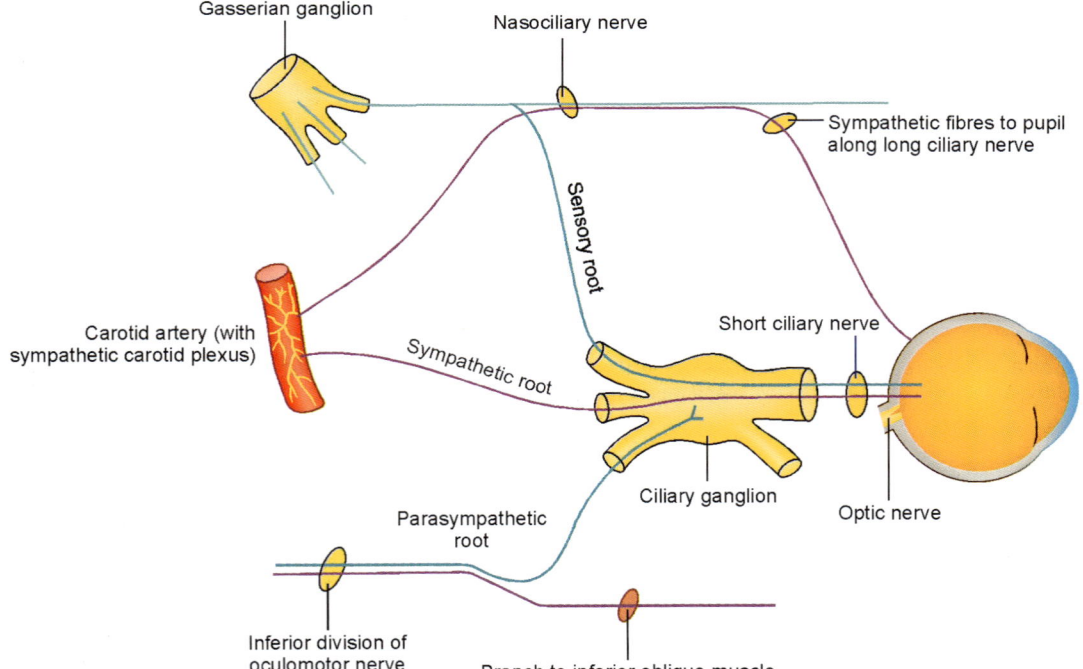

Fig. 26.8 *Ciliary ganglion and its roots and branches.*

Ciliary ganglion

This is a peripheral parasympathetic ganglion placed in the course of oculomotor nerve. It lies near the apex of the orbit between the optic nerve and the tendon of the lateral rectus muscle (Fig. 26.8).

Roots of ciliary ganglion

1. *Sensory root* comes from nasociliary nerve. It contains sensory fibers from the eyeball. These fibers do not relay in the ganglion.
2. *Parasympathetic root* arises from the nerve to inferior oblique muscle. It contains preganglionic fibers that begin in the Edinger-Westphal nucleus. These fibers relay in the ganglion. Postganglionic fibers arising in the ganglion pass through the short ciliary nerves and supply the sphincter pupillae and the ciliary muscle.
3. *Sympathetic root* is a branch from the internal carotid plexus. It contains postganglionic fibers arising in the superior cervical ganglion. These fibers do not relay in the ciliary ganglion. They pass out of the ganglion in the short ciliary nerves and supply the blood vessels of the eyeball. They may also supply dilator pupillae muscle when it is not supplied by the usual course via the nasociliary nerve.

Branches of ciliary ganglion

The ganglion gives 8 to 10 branches which divide into 15 to 20 short ciliary nerves, which pierce the sclera around the entrance of the optic nerve. These contain fibers from all the three roots of the ganglion.

CLINICALLY APPLIED ASPECTS

ANATOMICAL BASIS OF CLINICAL FEATURES OF THIRD NERVE PALSY

A complete and total third nerve palsy is of common occurrence. It may be congenital or acquired. Clinical features of complete third nerve palsy (Fig. 26.9) include the following:

1. *Ptosis* due to paralysis of the LPS muscle.
2. *Deviation.* Eyeball is turned down, out and slightly intorted due to unopposed action of the lateral rectus and superior oblique muscles.
3. *Ocular movements* are restricted due to paralysis of the muscles as follows:

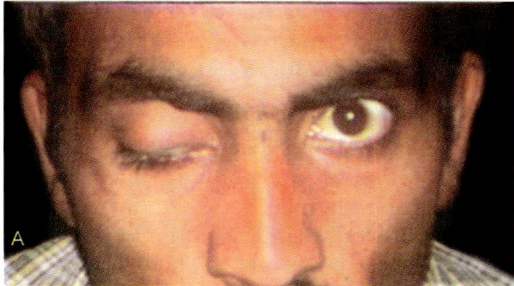
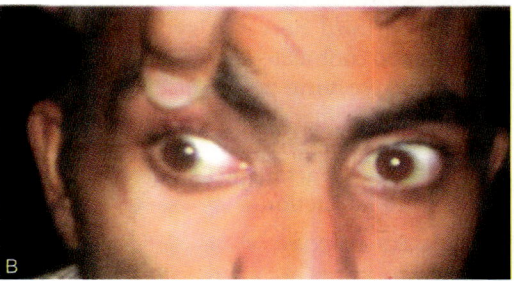

Fig. 26.9 *A patients with third cranial nerve paralysis showing (A) ptosis; (B) divergent squint.*

- Adduction—due to medial rectus
- Elevation—due to superior rectus and inferior oblique
- Depression—due to inferior rectus
- Extorsion— due to inferior rectus and inferior oblique.

4. *Pupil is fixed and dilated* due to paralysis of the sphincter pupillae muscle.
5. *Accommodation* is completely lost due to paralysis of the ciliary muscle.
6. *Crossed diplopia,* elicited on manually raising the eyelid, occurs due to paralytic divergent squint.
7. *Head posture.* If the pupillary area is uncovered, head takes a posture consistent with the directions of actions of the paralysed muscles, i.e. head is turned on the opposite side, tilted towards the same side and chin is slightly raised.

FEATURES AND CAUSES OF THIRD NERVE LESIONS AT VARIOUS LEVELS

1. Supranuclear lesions

Lesions of cerebral cortex and supranuclear pathway (supranuclear paralysis of third nerve) produce *conjugate paresis* which affect both eyes equally. In supranuclear lesions although position and movements of the eyes are abnormal, they maintain their relative coordination and produce no diplopia.

2. Nuclear lesions

- Lesions involving purely the third nerve nucleus complex are relatively uncommon.
- *Common causes* include: Vascular diseases, demyelination, primary tumors and metastasis.
- Lesions involving *entire nucleus* cause an ipsilateral third nerve palsy with ipsilateral sparing and contralateral-weakness of elevation.
- Lesions involving *paired medial rectus* subnuclei (ventromedial nucleus) cause a wall-eyed bilateral internuclear ophthalmoplegia (WEBINO), characterized by defective convergence and adduction.

3. Fascicular lesions

- *Causes* are similar to nuclear lesions.
- *Benedikt's syndrome* characterized by ipsilateral third nerve palsy associated with tremors and jerky movements of the contralateral side, occurs due to lesions at the intermediate level of the midbrain. Third nerve paralysis occurs due to involvement of fasciculus as it passes through the red nucleus.

- *Weber's syndrome.* In it fascicular part of the nerve is involved, while passing through the cerebral peduncle. The syndrome is characterized by ipsilateral third nerve palsy, contralateral hemiplegia and facial palsy of upper motor neuron type.

4. Lesions involving basilar part of the nerve

As the nerve runs in the subarachnoid space at the base of skull unaccompanied by any other cranial nerve, *isolated third nerve palsies are frequently basilar.*

Causes

1. *Aneurysms* at the posterior communicating artery cause isolated third nerve palsy with involvement of pupil.

2. *Extradural hematoma* which may cause tentorial pressure cone with downward herniation of the temporal lobe. This compresses the third nerve as it passes over the tentorial edge (Fig. 26.10). Initially, there occurs fixed dilated pupil, which is followed by a total third nerve palsy.

3. *Diabetes* causes isolated third nerve palsy with sparing of the pupillary reflexes.

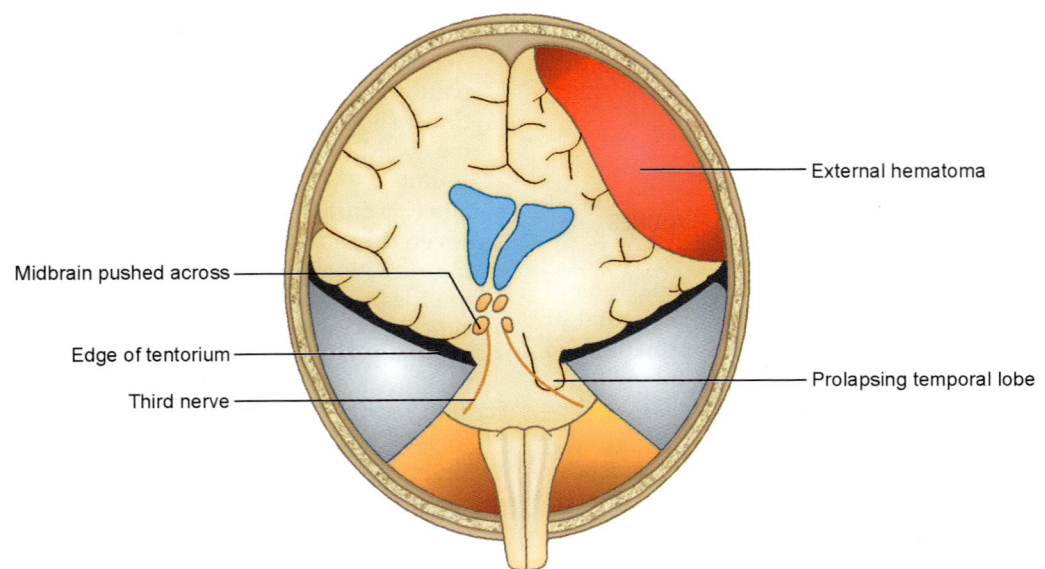

Fig. 26.10 *Mechanism of third nerve palsy in extradural hematoma.*

5. Lesions involving intracavernous part of the nerve

- Because of its close proximity to other cranial nerves, intracavernous third nerve palsies are usually associated with involvement of the fourth and sixth nerves, and the first division of the trigeminal nerve.
- In intracavernous third nerve palsy, pupil is spared. Sometimes, pupil may be constricted owing to involvement of sympathetics.

Causes

1. *Diabetes* may cause vascular palsy
2. *Pituitary apoplexy* may cause a third nerve palsy as a result of hemorrhagic infarction of a pituitary adenoma (e.g. after childbirth), with lateral extension into the cavernous sinus.
3. *Intracavernous lesions* which may cause a third nerve palsy include aneurysms, meningiomas, carotid cavernous fistulae and Tolosa-Hunt syndrome (granulomatous inflammation).

6. Lesions of the intraorbital part of the nerve

- May cause isolated extraocular muscle palsies or may involve either superior division or inferior division or both divisions.

Causes

Orbital tumors, pseudotumors, trauma, and vascular diseases.

7. Lesions of pupillomotor fibers

- Between the brainstem and the cavernous sinus pupillomotor fibers are located superficially in the superior median quadrant of the nerve. They derive their blood supply from the pial blood vessels, whereas the main trunk of the third nerve is supplied by vasa nervorum (Fig. 26.11).

- *Surgical lesions* such as aneurysms, trauma and uncal herniation characteristically involve the pupil by compressing the pial blood vessels and the superficially located pupillary fibers (Fig. 26.11).

- *Medical lesions* such as diabetes and hypertension usually spare the pupil. This is because the microangiopathy associated with these diseases involves the vasa nervorum, causing infarction of the main trunk, but sparing the superficial pupillary fibers.

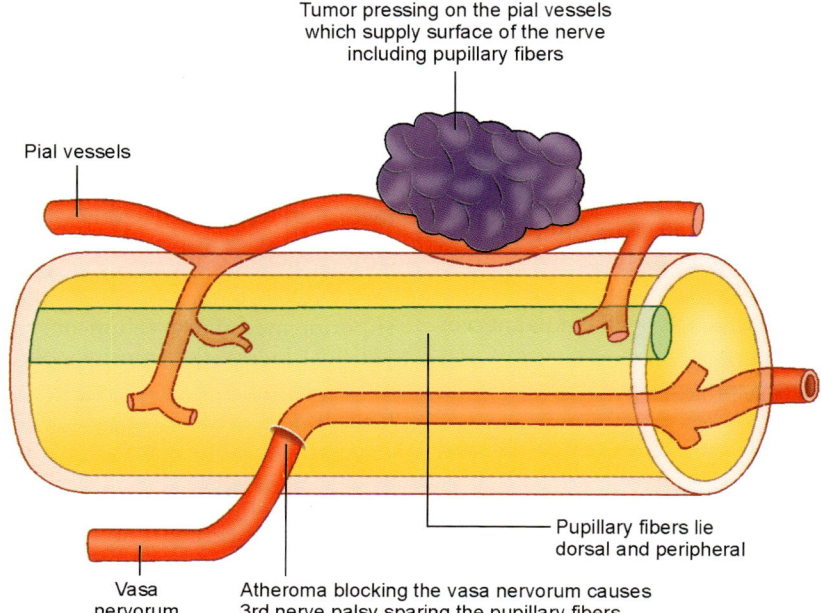

Tumor pressing on the pial vessels
which supply surface of the nerve
including pupillary fibers

Pial vessels

Pupillary fibers lie
dorsal and peripheral

Vasa
nervorum

Atheroma blocking the vasa nervorum causes
3rd nerve palsy sparing the pupillary fibers

Fig. 26.11 *The location of pupillomotor fibers within third nerve trunk and their involvement by surgical lesions.*

Isolated third nerve palsy

Causes of isolated third nerve palsy are as below:

1. *Idiopathic.* In about 25 percent cases, cause is not known.
2. *Vascular diseases.* Diabetes and hypertension are the common medical causes of pupil sparing isolated third nerve palsy.
3. *Trauma* is also an important cause of isolated third nerve paralysis. Mechanism of third nerve involvement by an extradural hematoma is shown in Fig. 26.10.
4. *Aneurysms* at the junction of the posterior communicating artery with the internal carotid artery is an important cause of isolated, painful third nerve palsy with involvement of the pupil. Other causes of painful third nerve palsy are migraine, Tolosa-Hunt syndrome and diabetes.
5. *Miscellaneous.* Other rare causes include tumors, vasculitis associated with collagen disorders, syphilis and tuberculosis.

TROCHLEAR NERVE

The trochlear (fourth cranial) nerve is entirely motor in function and supplies only the superior oblique muscle of the eyeball. It differs from other cranial nerves in being:

1. The only cranial nerve to arise from the dorsal aspect of the brain (midbrain).
2. The only cranial nerve to cross completely on the other side (i.e. the trochlear nerve arises from the contralateral nucleus).
3. The longest and thinnest of all cranial nerves.

FUNCTIONAL COMPONENTS

1. *Somatic efferent* component of the nerve is concerned with the movement of the eyeball through the superior oblique muscle.

2. *General somatic afferent* component carries proprioceptive impulses from the superior oblique muscle. These impulses are relayed to the mesencephalic nucleus of the trigeminal nerve.

NUCLEUS

The trochlear nucleus is situated in the ventromedial part of the central grey matter of the midbrain at the level of inferior colliculus (Fig. 26.12). It is caudal to and continuous with the third nerve nucleus complex (Fig. 26.2). It belongs to somatic efferent column of nuclei and is closely related to the medial longitudinal bundle (Fig. 26.12).

Connections of the nucleus

1. *Cerebral cortex*
   - *Motor cortex* (precentral gyrus) of both sides through the corticonuclear tracts.
   - *Visual cortex* through the superior colliculus and the tactobulbar tract.
   - *Frontal eye fields.*
2. *Nuclei of 3rd, 6th and 8th cranial nerves* through the medial longitudinal bundle.
3. *Superior colliculi* through the descending pre-dorsal bundle.
4. *Vertical and torsional gaze centers*
5. *Cerebellum* through the vestibular nuclei.

COURSE AND DISTRIBUTION

For the purpose of description, the course of the trochlear nerve can be divided into fascicular, precancerous, intracavernous and intraorbital.

The fascicular part

The fasciculus consists of efferent fibers which after leaving the nucleus, pass posteriorly around the aqueduct in the central grey matter and decussate completely in the anterior medullary velum (Fig. 26.12).

Pre-cavernous part

The trochlear nerve trunk emerges from the superior medullary velum near the frenulum veli just below the inferior colliculus, on the dorsal aspect of midbrain. It then winds round the superior cerebellar peduncle and the cerebral peduncle just above the pons (Figs 26.12 and 26.13). It runs beneath the free edge of the tentorium, and like third nerve passes between the posterior cerebral and superior cerebellar arteries to appear ventrally lateral to cerebral peduncle. It then pierces the dura on the posterior corner of the roof of the cavernous sinus to enter into it (Fig. 26.5).

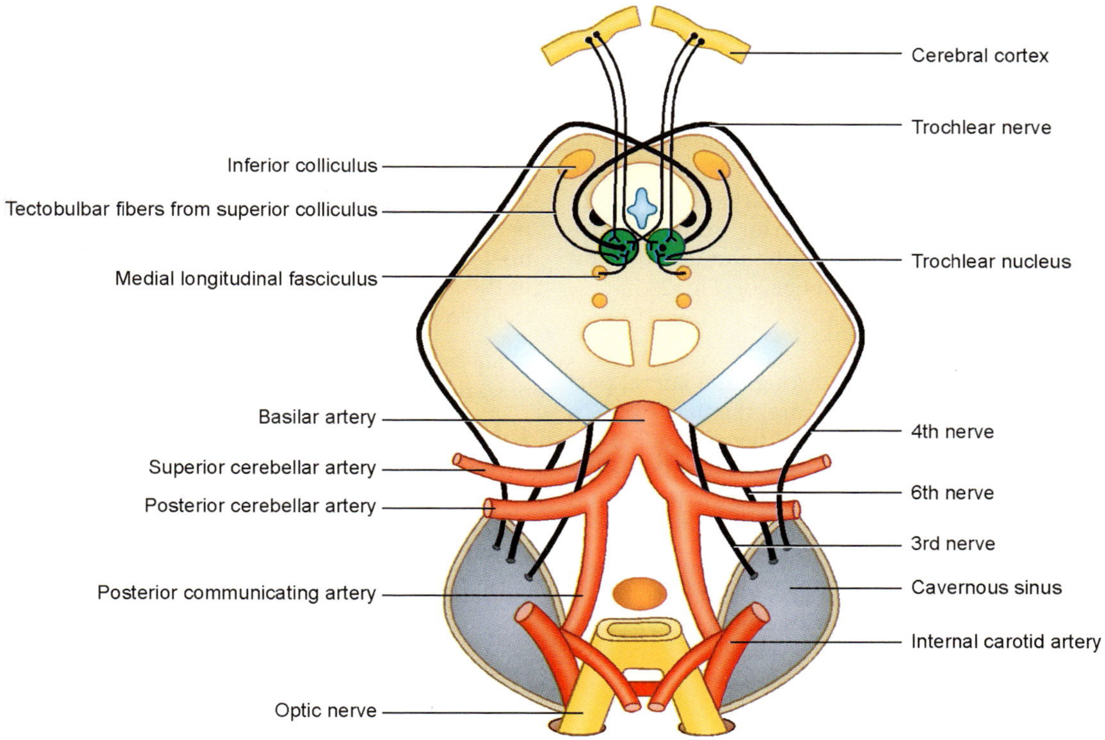

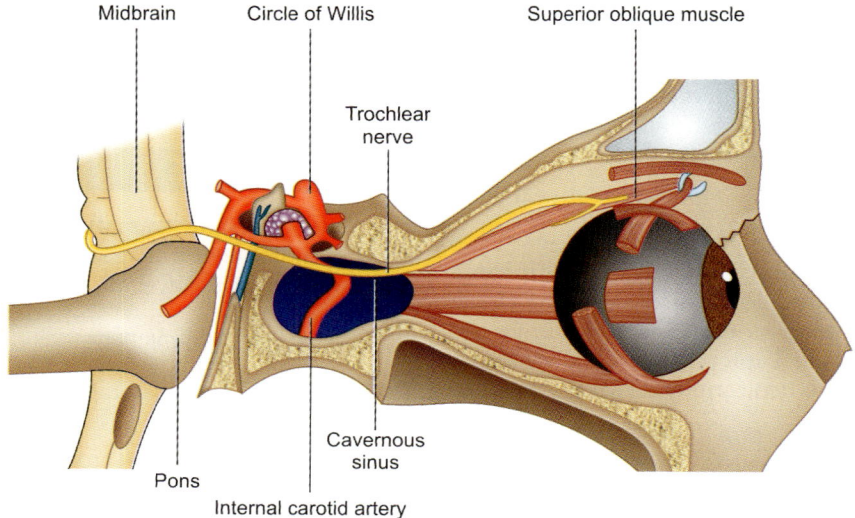

Fig. 26.12 *Trochlear nerve nucleus, its central connections and course of fascicular and basilar part of the nerve.*

Fig. 26.13 *The course of trochlear nerve.*

Intracavernous part

In the cavernous sinus, the nerve runs forwards in its lateral wall lying below the oculomotor nerve and above the first division of the fifth cranial nerve (Fig. 26.6). In the anterior part of the cavernous sinus, it rises, crosses over the third nerve and leaves the sinus to pass through the lateral part of the superior orbital fissure (where it lies superolateral to annulus of Zinn and medial to the frontal nerve) (Fig. 26.7).

Intraorbital part

After entering the orbit through the lateral part of the superior orbital fissure, the nerve passes medially above the origin of levator palpebrae superioris (Fig. 26.13) and ends by supplying the superior oblique muscle through its orbital surface.

The number of fibers in the intraorbital part of the trochlear nerve are greater than its intracranial part. These extra fibers carrying the proprioceptive impulses from the superior oblique muscle leave the trochlear nerve to join the ophthalmic division of the fifth nerve, in the cavernous sinus. Ultimately, these fibers relay in the mesencephalic nucleus of the fifth cranial nerve.

CLINICALLY APPLIED ASPECTS

FEATURES OF FOURTH NERVE PALSY

1. *Hyperdeviation.* The involved eye is higher as a result of the weakness of the superior oblique muscle. This becomes more obvious when the head is tilted towards ipsilateral shoulder (Bielschowsky's head tilt test).

2. *Ocular movements.* Depression is limited in adduction. Extorsion is also limited.

3. *Diplopia.* Homonymous vertical diplopia occurs on looking downwards. Usually, vision is single so long as the eyes look above the horizontal plane. Diplopia is especially noticed by the patient when coming down the stairs.

4. *Abnormal head posture.* To avoid diplopia head takes a posture towards the action of superior oblique muscle, i.e. face is slightly turned to the opposite side, chin is depressed and head is tilted towards the opposite shoulder.

CAUSES OF FOURTH NERVE PARALYSIS

In order of frequency, following are the causes of fourth nerve paralysis:

1. *Congenital paralysis* is quite frequent (about 40% cases).

2. *Trauma* is another important cause of fourth nerve paralysis (about 34%). It frequently causes bilateral trochlear nerve palsy due to an impact in the area of anterior medullary velum, where the two nerves decussate.

3. *Idiopathic.* In about 20 percent cases, cause is not known.

4. *Vascular and neurologic* causes account for about 3 to 5 percent. Aneurysms and tumors are rare causes. Ocular *myasthenia gravis* may present as an isolated unilateral superior oblique paralysis with an insidious courses.

Comparative incidence of fourth nerve palsy

It has been reported that superior oblique paralysis is the most common form of paralytic squint.

Supranuclear lesions

Supranuclear lesions cause loss of conjugate movements of the eyeball.

Nuclear lesions

When the lesions involve the nucleus and the fibers of the nerve within the midbrain before their decussation, there occurs paralysis of the contralateral superior oblique muscle.

ABDUCENT NERVE

The abducent (sixth cranial) nerve is a small, entirely motor nerve that supplies the lateral rectus muscle of the eyeball.

FUNCTIONAL COMPONENTS

1. *Somatic efferent,* for lateral movement of the eye.

2. *General somatic afferent,* for proprioceptive impulses from the lateral rectus muscle. These impulses ultimately reach the mesencephalic nucleus of the trigeminal nerve.

NUCLEUS

The abducent nucleus is situated in the lower part of pons, close to the midline, beneath the floor of the fourth ventricle. It is closely related to the fasciculus of the facial nerve (Fig. 26.14). It consists of two types of multipolar cells—large and small. The large multipolar cells give rise to fibers of the abducent nerve, while the fibers of the small multipolar cells relay in the oculomotor nucleus via the medial longitudinal fasciculus. The small multipolar cells are believed to form the para-abducent nucleus. Since the abducent nucleus belongs to the group of somatic efferent nuclei, it lies in line with nuclei of fourth and third nerves above and with the nucleus of hypoglossal nerve below (Fig. 26.2).

Connections of the nucleus

1. *Cerebral cortex*
   - *Motor cortex* (precentral gyrus) through the afferent corticonuclear fibers from both cerebral hemispheres (principally contra-lateral).
   - *Visual cortex*, through the superior colliculus and tactobulbar tract.
   - *Frontal cortex* (frontal eye fields).
2. *Nuclei of 3rd, 4th and 8th* cranial nerves through the medial longitudinal bundle.

3. *Pretectal nucleus* of both sides through the tectobulbar tract.
4. *Horizontal gaze center* (paramedian pontine reticular formation—PPRF) through the medial longitudinal bundle.
5. *Cerebellum* through vestibular nuclei.

COURSE AND DISTRIBUTION

For the purpose of description, the course of the abducent nerve can be divided into fascicular, basilar, intracavernous and intraorbital parts.

The fascicular part

The fasciculus consists of efferent fibers which start from the nucleus, pass forward traversing the medial leminiscus and pyramidal tract. These then emerge prominence (of medulla). The rootlets join to form one nerve, at varying distance from the origin (Fig. 26.14).

The basilar part

The nerve then runs forwards, upwards and slightly laterally through the cisterna pontis between the pons and the occipital bone. The nerve runs upwards on the back of the petrous temporal bone near its apex. At the sharp upper border of the petrous bone, the nerve bends forward at right angle under petrosphenoidal ligament and enters the cavernous sinus by

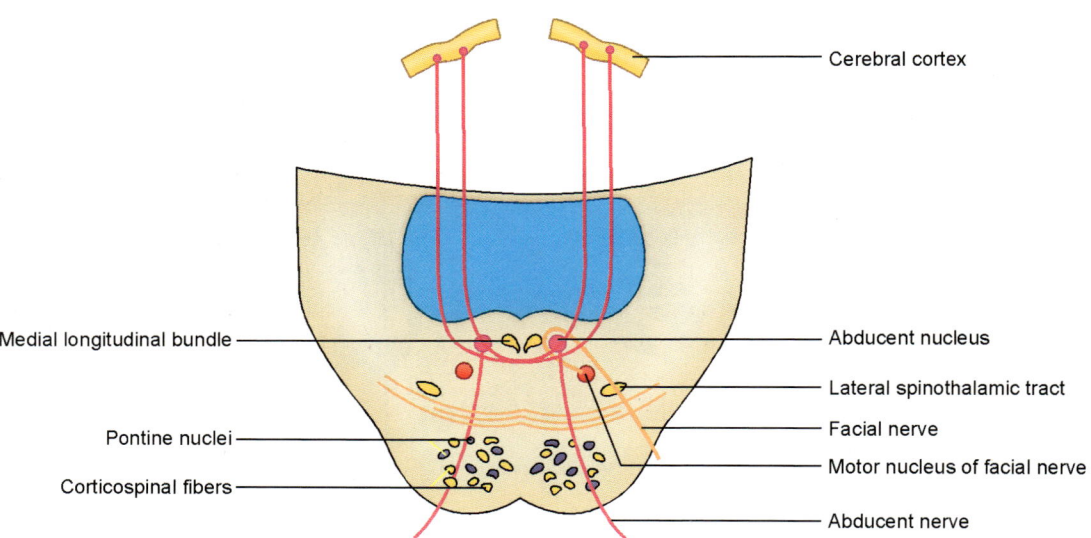

Fig. 26.14 *Abducent nerve nucleus and its central connections.*

Labels: Cerebral cortex; Medial longitudinal bundle; Pontine nuclei; Corticospinal fibers; Abducent nucleus; Lateral spinothalamic tract; Facial nerve; Motor nucleus of facial nerve; Abducent nerve.

piercing its posterior wall at a point lateral to the dorsum sellae and superior to the apex of petrous temporal bone (Fig. 26.15).

The intracavernous part

In the cavernous sinus, the nerve runs almost horizontally forward, occupying a position below and lateral to the internal carotid artery (Fig. 26.6). The internal carotid artery is surrounded by sympathetic plexus. The nerve then leaves the cavernous sinus to enter the orbit through the middle part of the superior orbital fissure within the annulus of Zinn (Fig. 26.7). In the superior orbital fissure, the abducent nerve lies inferolateral to the oculomotor and naso-ciliary nerves.

The intraorbital part

In the orbit, the nerve runs forwards and enters the ocular surface of the lateral rectus muscle just behind its middle portion after dividing into three or four branches (Fig. 26.15).

CLINICALLY APPLIED ASPECTS

CLINICAL FEATURES OF SIXTH NERVE PALSY

1. *Deviation.* In primary position, eyeball is converged due to unopposed action of the medial rectus muscle.
2. *Ocular movements.* Abduction is limited due to weakness of the lateral rectus muscle.

3. *Diplopia.* Uncrossed horizontal diplopia occurs, which becomes worse toward the action of paralysed muscle.
4. *Head posture.* The face is turned towards the action of paralysed muscle to minimize diplopia.

FEATURES AND CAUSES OF SIXTH NERVE LESIONS AT VARIOUS LEVELS

1. Supranuclear lesions

Supranuclear lesions cause loss of conjugate movements of eyeball.

2. Nuclear lesions

Nuclear lesions never cause isolated sixth nerve palsy. A lesion in and around the sixth nerve nucleus causes the following:
  i. Ipsilateral sixth nerve palsy.
 ii. Ipsilateral seventh nerve palsy of upper motor neuron type due to concomitant involvement of facial fasciculus.
iii. Loss of conjugate movements to the same side. resulting from involvement of horizontal gaze center in the pontine paramedian reticular formation (PPRF).

3. Fascicular lesions

Foville's syndrome results due to lesions of dorsal pons involving sixth nerve fasciculus as it passes through PPRF and is characterized by the following:

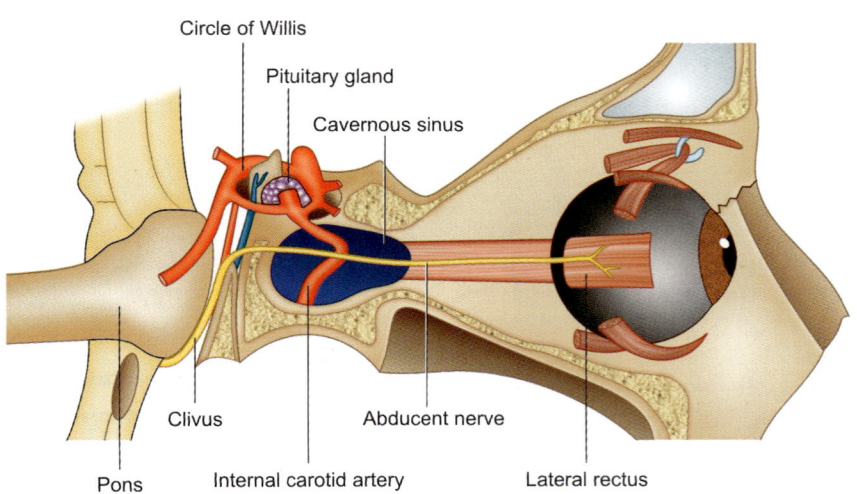

Circle of Willis

Pituitary gland

Cavernous sinus

Clivus

Abducent nerve

Pons

Internal carotid artery

Lateral rectus

Fig. 26.15 *Courses of sixth cranial nerve.*

- Ipsilateral sixth nerve palsy
- Loss of conjugate movements to the same side
- Ipsilateral facial nerve palsy
- Facial analgesia from involvement of the sensory portion of the fifth nerve
- Deafness

Millard-Gubler syndrome results due to lesions of the ventral pons involving fasciculus as it passes through pyramidal tracts and is characterized by the following:

- Ipsilateral sixth nerve palsy
- Contralateral hemiplegia
- Variable number of signs of dorsal pontine lesions.

4. Lesions of the basilar part of sixth nerve

The important causes which may damage the basilar part of the sixth nerve include acoustic neuroma, nasopharyngeal tumors and fracture base of the skull. It should be emphasized that the first symptom of acoustic neuroma is hearing loss and the first sign is diminished corneal sensations. Therefore, hearing and corneal sensations should be tested in all patients with sixth nerve palsy.

Gradenigo syndrome the involvement of petrous bone from otitis media. It is characterized by the following:

- Ipsilateral sixth nerve palsy
- Deafness
- Neuralgia in the distribution of first division of trigeminal nerve
- Facial weakness

Involvement in raised intracranial pressure

Sixth nerve paralysis is one of the commonest *false localizing sign* in cases with raised intracranial pressure. Its susceptibility to such damage is due to its long course in the cisterna pontis, to its sharp bend over the superior border of the petrous temporal bone and the downward shift of the brainstem (towards the foramen magnum) produced by raised intracranial pressure (Fig. 26.16).

5. Lesions of the intracavernous part of sixth nerve

- Since the sixth nerve runs through the middle of the cavernous sinus, it is most prone to damage than the other nerves from the

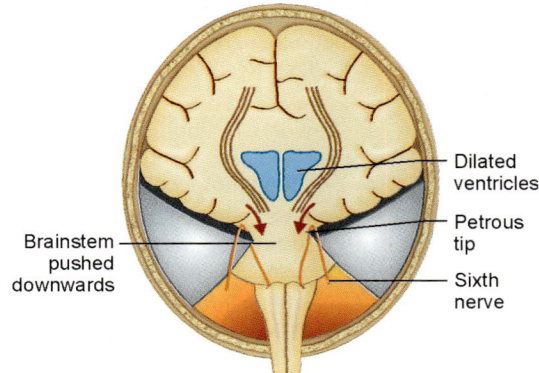

Fig. 26.16 *Mechanism of bilateral sixth nerve palsy resulting from raised intracranial pressure.*

intracavernous lesions such as aneurysms, meningioma, carotid cavernous fistulae and Tolosa-Hunt syndrome (granulomatous inflammation). In contrast to third nerve, aneurysms rarely cause a sixth nerve palsy. *Vascular causes* such as diabetes and hypertension are, however, common causes of sixth nerve palsy.

- Since, in its intracavernous part, the sixth nerve is joined by the sympathetic branch from paracarotid plexus, so occasionally sixth nerve palsy may be accompanied by Horner's syndrome.

6. Lesions of the intraorbital part of sixth nerve

Isolated sixth nerve palsy due to intraorbital lesions is not so common. However, it is involved in the lesions producing

- *Orbital apex syndrome,* and
- *Superior orbital fissure syndrome*

BIBLIOGRAPHY

1. Barr D, Kupersmith M, Turbin R, et al. Synkinesis following diabetic third nerve palsy. Arch Ophthalmol 2000;118:132–4
2. Bhatti MT, Eisenschenk S, Roper SN, et al. Superior divisional third cranial nerve paresis: clinical and anatomical observations of 2 unique cases. Arch Neurol 2006;63:771–6.
3. Carrasco JR, Savino PJ, Bilyk JR. Primary aberrant oculomotor nerve regeneration from a posterior communicating artery aneurysm. Arch Ophthalmol 2002;120:663–4.

4. Custer PL. Lagophthalmos: an unusual manifestation of oculomotor nerve aberrant regeneration. Ophthal Plast Reconstr Surg 2000;16: 50–51.

5. Donahue SP, Taylor RJ. Pupil-sparing third nerve palsy associated with sildenafil citrate (Viagra). Am J Ophthalmol 1998;126:476–7.

6. Foroozan R, Slamovits TL, Ksiazek SM, et al. Spontaneous resolution of aneurysmal third nerve palsy. J Neuro-ophthalmol 2002; 22:211–4.

7. Galetta SL, Smith JL. Chronic isolated sixth nerve palsies. Arch Neurol 1989;46:79–82.

8. Hoya K, Kirino T. Traumatic trochlear nerve palsy following minor occipital impact-four case reports. Neurol Med Chir (Tokyo) 2000; 40: 358–60.

9. Ksiazek S, Behar R, Savino PJ, et al. Isolated acquired fourth nerve palsies. Neurology 1988; 38(suppl 1):246.

10. Lee AG, Brazis PW. Clinical Pathways in Neuro-Ophthalmology: An Evidence-based Approach. 2nd edn. New York: Thieme Medical Publishing; 2003.

11. Moster ML, Savino PJ, Sergott RC, et al. Isolated sixth nerve palsies in younger adults. Arch Ophthalmol 1984;102:1328–330.

12. Umapathi T, Koon SW, Mukkan RP, et al. Insights into the three-dimensional structure of the oculomotor nuclear complex and fascicles. J Neuro-ophthalmol 2000;20:138–44.

13. von Noorden GK, Murray E, Wong SY. Superior oblique paralysis. A review of 270 cases. Arch Ophthalmol 1986;104:1771–6.

27 SUPRANUCLEAR CONTROL AND DISORDERS OF OCULAR MOTILITY

AK Khurana, Indu Khurana, Aruj K Khurana, Bhawna Khurana

SUPRANUCLEAR CONTROL OF EYE MOVEMENTS

There exists a highly accurate, still not fully elucidated, supranuclear control of eye movements which keeps the two eyes yoked together so that the image of the object of interest is simultaneously held on both foveas despite the movements of the perceived object or the observer's head and/or body. For the purpose of understanding, the neural control of eye movements can be discussed under two parts: (1) supranuclear ocular motor neural pathway and (2) supranuclear eye movement systems.

SUPRANUCLEAR OCULAR MOTOR NEURAL PATHWAY

The supranuclear pathway concerned with the control of various ocular movements include (Fig. 27.1):

- Cortical control centers
- Subcortical control centers.

CORTICAL CONTROL CENTERS

The cortical control centers include:
- Frontal ocular motor area
- Parieto-occipito-temporal (POT) junction.

I. Frontal ocular motor area

The frontal ocular motor area is primarily involved in the saccadic eye movement system. It is thought to control voluntary rapid conjugate gaze, both vertically and horizontally. Recently, four main cortical areas involved in the generation of saccades have been recognized. These include: (1) frontal eye field (FEF), (2) supplementary eye field (SEF), (3) dorsolateral prefrontal cortex (DLPFC), and (4) posterior eye field (PEF).

The frontal eye fields (FEFs) are located at Brodman's area 8, the posterior end of the second frontal convolution.

Role of FEFs is as below:
- *Horizontal gaze movements* result, when the extraocular muscles receive signals from one hemisphere (contralateral) only. Stimulation

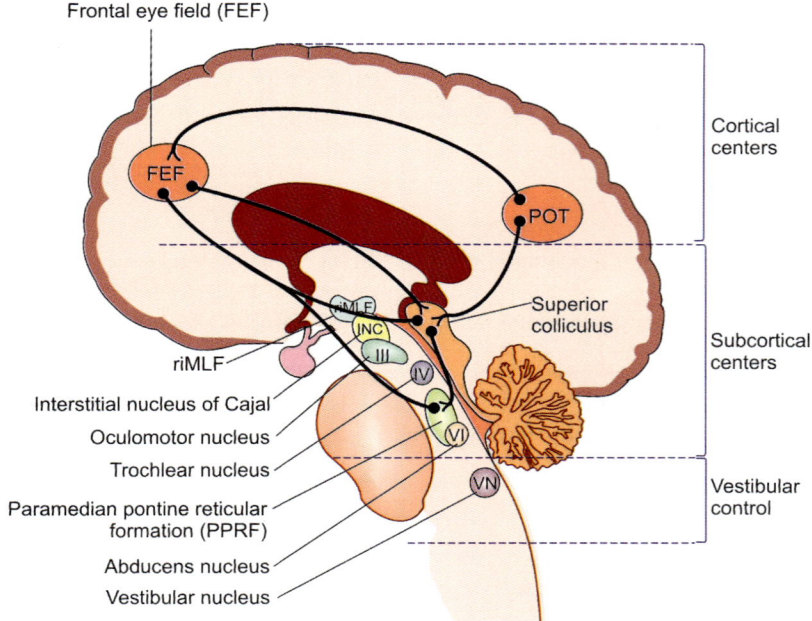

Fig. 27.1 *Supranuclear connections of ocular motor neural pathway.*

of the frontal lobe area, on the right, for instance, leads to conjugate movements of both eyes to the left (Fig. 27.2).

- *Voluntary vertical conjugate gaze movements* occur, when equal signals are transmitted simultaneously from both the frontal ocular motor areas (Figs 27.3 and 27.4).

II. Parieto-occipito-temporal (POT) junction

The ipsilateral parieto-occipital ocular motor area is primarily concerned with the fixation and pursuit movements. Recently, following cortical areas have been identified in relation with the pursuit movements:

- Middle temporal (MT) visual area
- Medial superior temporal (MST) visual area.

i. *Middle temporal (MT) visual area.* The cerebral cortex in the region of the POT junction is important in the control of smooth pursuit eye movements and object tracking in space. This area is known as the middle temporal (MT) area in non-human primates. The area of the human brain that is the equivalent of the MT cortex of the non-human primate is Flechsig's area 10. The MT receives visual information from the striate

and prestriate cortex. It projects to the brainstem, cerebellum, superior colliculi, and the FEF. The latter projections modulate visually directed saccadic eye movements. The POT junction cortex plays the key supranuclear role in the visual ocular reflex by way of projections to the PPRF and riMLF. This reflex keeps a moving image projecting on the fovea. There are specific efferent fibers for horizontal, vertical, and torsional movements.

Damage to only one side of the MT cortex slows ipsilateral slow pursuit, requiring catch-up saccades. Such lesions also temporarily impair pursuit responses to fast targets in moving in either direction.

ii. *Medial superior temporal (MST) visual area:* In human, it is considered to lie superior and a little anterior to MT area within the inferior parietal lobe.

SUBCORTICAL CONTROL CENTERS

The brainstem control centers include:
- Paramedian pontine reticular formation (PPRF)
- Rostral interstitial nucleus of medial longitudinal fasciculus (riMLF)

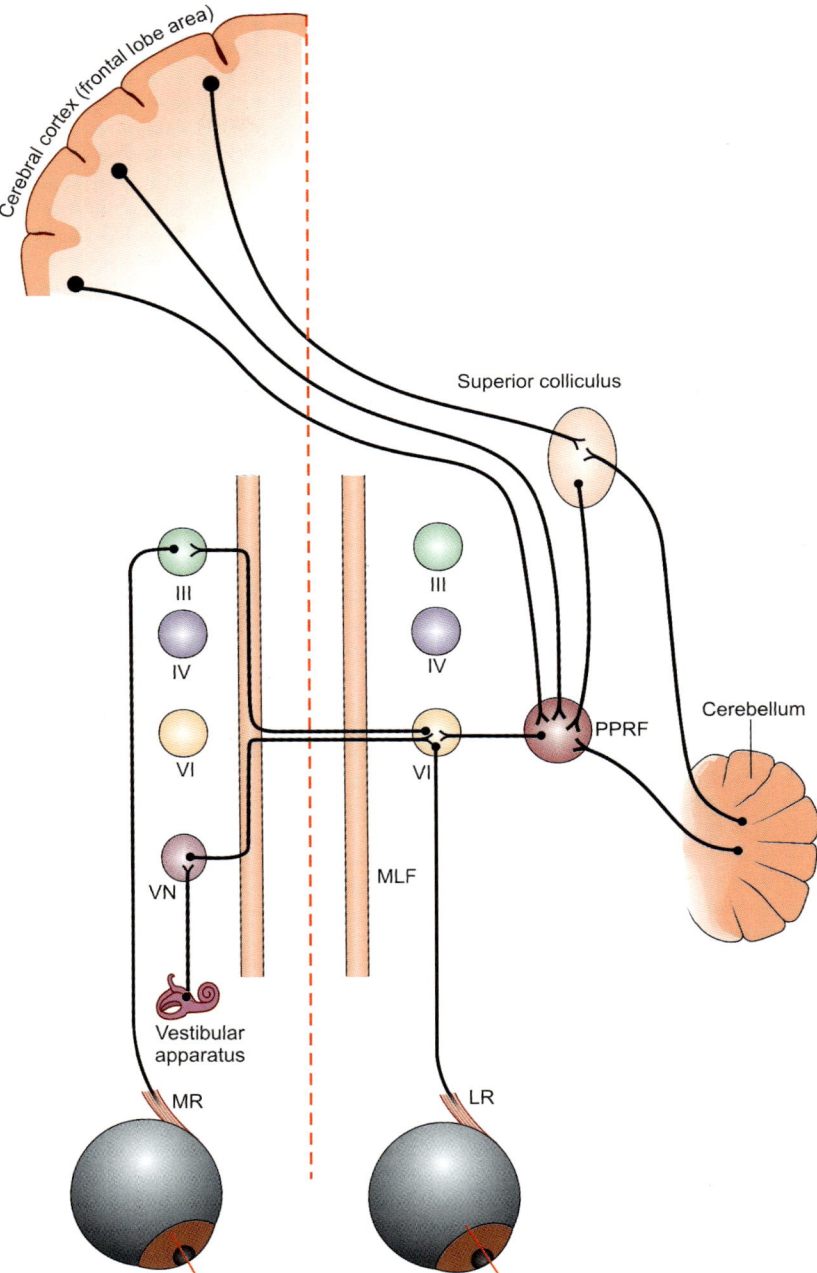

Fig. 27.2 *Pathway for horizontal gaze saccadic eye movements. The horizontal gaze center (present in PPRF) is connected with ipsilateral lateral rectus (LR) muscle and with abducens internuclear neurons whose axons cross the midline and travel in the medial longitudinal fasciculus (MLF) of the opposite side to that part of the nucleus of IIIrd nerve which innervates the medial rectus (MR) muscle.*

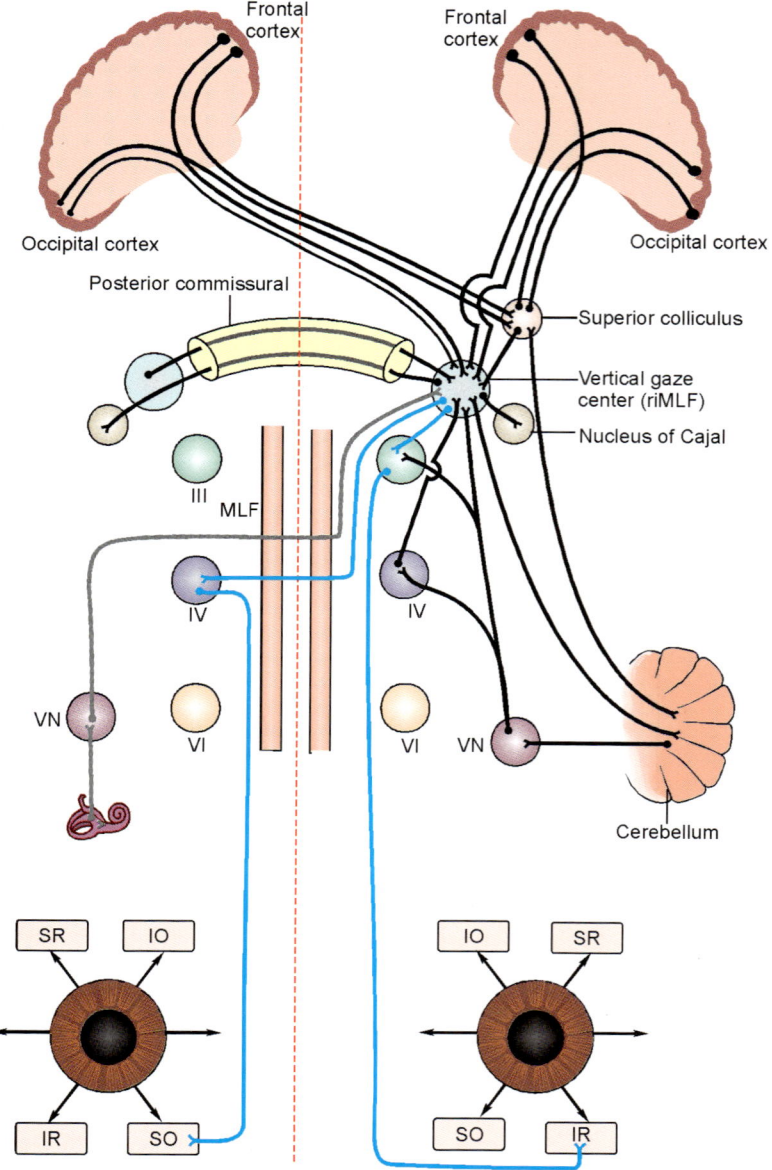

Fig. 27.3 *Pathway for vertical gaze (downgaze) saccadic eye movements.*

- Convergence and divergence center
- Posterior commissure
- Superior colliculus
- Vestibular apparatus
- Cerebellum
- Medial longitudinal fasciculus.

1. Paramedian pontine reticular formation

Horizontal gaze center. The paramedian pontine reticular formation (PPRF) is the primary center responsible for generating horizontal conjugate gaze. The PPRF is positioned ventral to the medial longitudinal fasciculus (MLF). It extends

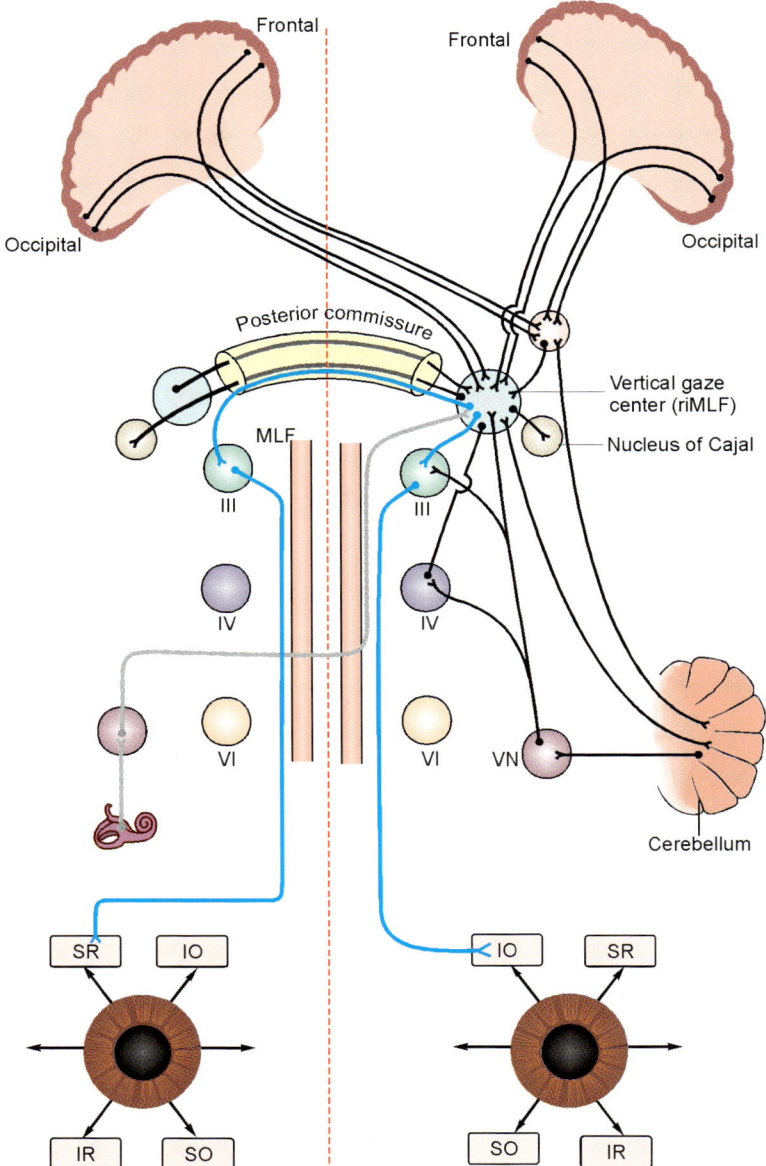

Fig. 27.4 *Pathway for vertical gaze (upgaze) saccadic eye movements.*

from the level of the trochlear nerve nucleus to the abducens nerve nucleus (Fig. 27.1).

• *Afferent connections.* Most afferent connections to the PPRF are through the vestibular nucleus. It receives signals from both the frontal cortical areas concerned with generation of saccades and

ipsilateral occipitoparietal cortical area concerned with generation of pursuits directly (for voluntary movements) and through the superior colliculus (for involuntary movements). Vestibular input for horizontal eye movements comes from the contralateral vestibular apparatus by way of the vestibular nuclei. An axon from the vestibular nucleus crosses to the opposite abducens nucleus, where it innervates a motor neuron and an internuclear neuron for horizontal gaze in the opposite direction (Fig. 27.2).

• *Efferent connections.* The center for horizontal gaze movements in turn is connected with the homolateral abducent nucleus present next to it. The axons of the internuclear neurons of the abducent cross the midline and travel through the medial longitudinal fasciculus (MLF) of the opposite side to that part of nucleus of the oculomotor nerve which innervates the medial rectus muscle (Figs 27.2 and 27.5). Therefore, impulses from this center produce contraction

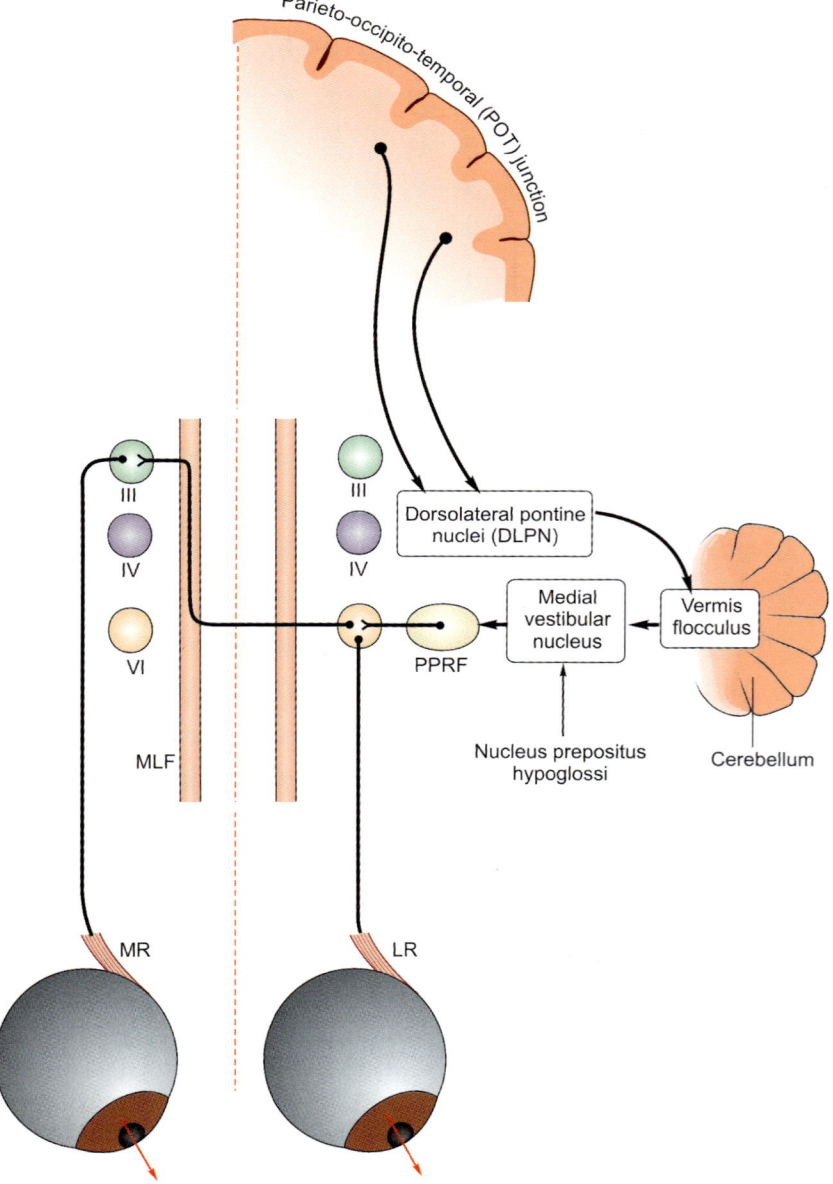

Fig. 27.5 *Neural pathway of horizontal pursuit eye movements.*

of the homolateral lateral rectus muscle and the opposite medial rectus, hence binocular gaze movements to the side of the stimulated center.

2. Rostral interstitial nucleus of medial longitudinal fasciculus

Vertical gaze center. The vertical gaze center is the rostral interstitial nucleus of the medial longitudinal fasciculus (riMLF) located at the level of upper pole of the red nucleus. Slightly caudal to the riMLF and directly connected to it lies the interstitial nucleus of Cajal (INC). This nucleus contains neurons which appear to be involved in vertical gaze holding and vertical pursuit.

- *Afferent connections.* The vertical gaze center (riMLF) receives impulses from both the frontal and occipital cortical ocular motor centers as well as from the superior colliculus.
- *Efferent connections.* The riMLF nucleus projects through the posterior commissure to its equivalent on the other side of the mesencephalon as well as directly to the nuclei of III and IV cranial nerves supplying the extraocular muscles concerned with the vertical movements (Figs 27.3, 27.4 and 27.6).

3. Posterior commissure

Dorsal and rostral to the riMLF is the posterior commissure, a fiber tract that contains some scattered neuronal cell bodies. Lesions in this region produce abnormalities of upward gaze. It is likely that the fibers for upward gaze leave the riMLF and pass through this region before reaching the oculomotor and trochlear nuclei. Involvement of the posterior commissure may be part of the dorsal midbrain syndrome (Parinaud syndrome). In this syndrome, there is impairment of upwardly directed saccades or, in extreme cases, loss of all vertical movement. Other signs include pupillary mydriasis and light-near pupillary dissociation, corectopia, and convergence-retraction nystagmus.

4. Convergence and divergence center

At present, nothing is known about the location of a subcortical divergence center. In fact, there is no evidence that such a center exists at all. Similarly, a subcortical center for convergence also may not exist at all and convergence as well

as divergence may be purely cortical functions. However, clinical evidence points that the pretectal area is probable site for the subcortical convergence center; since lesions in this area abolish convergence. The impulses to the so-called convergence center come from the frontal and the occipital ocular motor centers. Convergence occurs only upon simultaneous bilateral stimulation of either the frontal or the occipital motor centers. These impulses are relayed to the nuclei of both third nerves which innervate the medial recti muscles (Fig. 27.8).

5. Superior colliculus

These structures in the dorsal midbrain play a role in both ocular motor and sensory function. The superior colliculus receives visual input directly from branches of retinal ganglion cell axons. Visual input also comes indirectly from the visual cortex, the parietal and frontal lobes, and the substantia nigra. There are efferent projections to the brainstem premotor areas. The superior colliculus can generate visually directed saccades independently and may play a role in the control of pursuit eye movements. In primates, ablation of both FEFs and both superior colliculi is necessary to produce permanent saccadic defects.

6. Vestibular apparatus

Reflex eye movements that compensate for changes in the position of head or body originate from the vestibulum. They are called statokinetic reflexes. If, for instance, the head is turned to the left, the eyes perform an involuntary compensatory movement to the right which allows continuous fixation of the object. These reflexes are innate and unconditioned, occurring even in blind. The vestibular apparatus is a receptor specialized to sense changes of equilibrium and position. It is part of the inner ear and is comprised three semicircular canals, the sacculus and the utriculus, all of which belong to the membranous labyrinth. The apparatus derives its name from the vestibulum, which is the bony cavity housing the utriculus and the sacculus.

Semicircular canals

The semicircular canals contain receptor organs called cristae that sense movements of the head.

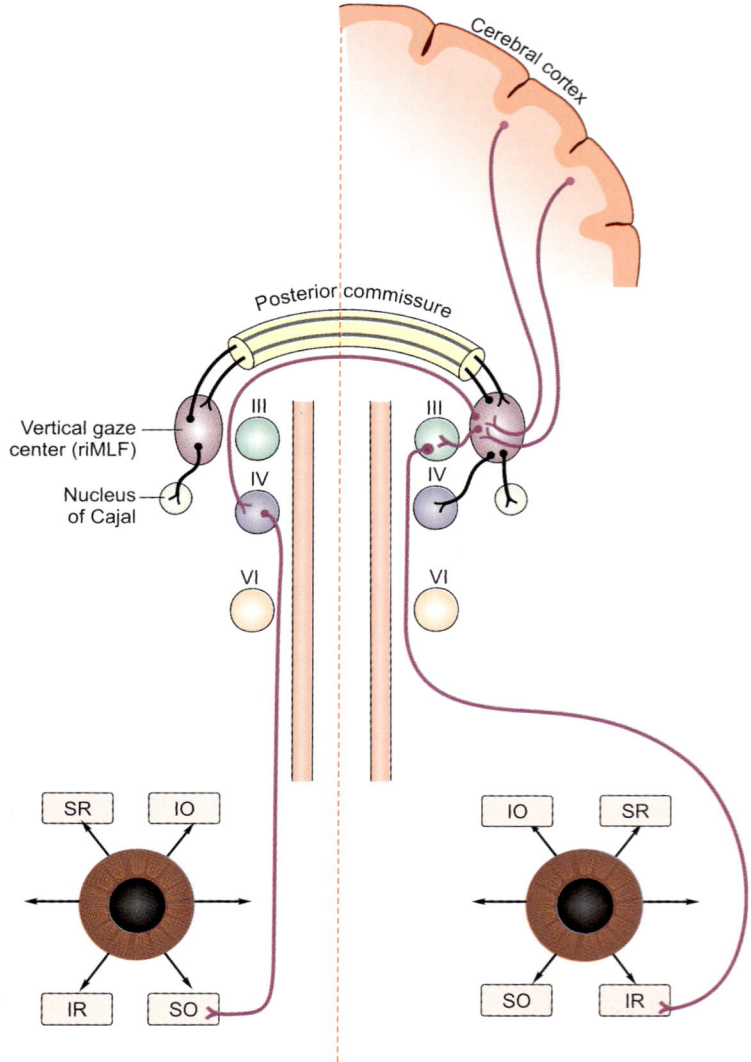

Fig. 27.6 *Neural pathway of vertical pursuit (downgaze) eye movements.*

Each of the canals is oriented perpendicular to the other two so that a three-dimensional structure is formed roughly coinciding with the horizontal, vertical, and frontal planes. The canals are filled with a watery fluid, the endolymph. When the head moves, the endolymph is subjected to inertia and exerts a certain pull on the sensory hair of the cristae. This stimulus excites the receptor cells and elicits a nerve impulse that is transmitted through the vestibular nerve (part of nerve VIII) to the vestibular nuclei in the brainstem.

Sacculus and utriculus

The sacculus and the utriculus each contains a macula that functions in a manner similar to that of the cristae of the semicircular canals. Whereas, the cristae respond to head movements (statokinetic reaction), the macula of the utricle responds to gravity (static reaction). On top of each macula rests a gelatinous plate into which protrudes hair from the surface of the macula. The plates, which contain mineral crystals, follow the force of gravity and slide to whichever side is dependent, thereby pulling on the hair. This leads to stimulation of the terminal branches of the vestibular nerve that supply the maculae. The function of the sacculus is not known.

Vestibular nerve

The vestibular nerve (part of nerve VIII) enters the brainstem at the level of the lower end of the pons and terminates in the vestibular nuclei. The vestibular nuclei, in turn, are connected directly to the abducens nuclei and to the nuclei of the ocular motor nerves through the medial longitudinal fasciculi (Figs 27.3 to 27.7). Stimulation of a labyrinth or of a vestibular nerve causes conjugate deviation of the eyes to the opposite side. Depending on the nature of the stimulus, the eyes may remain in the deviate position or a nystagmus may result. A

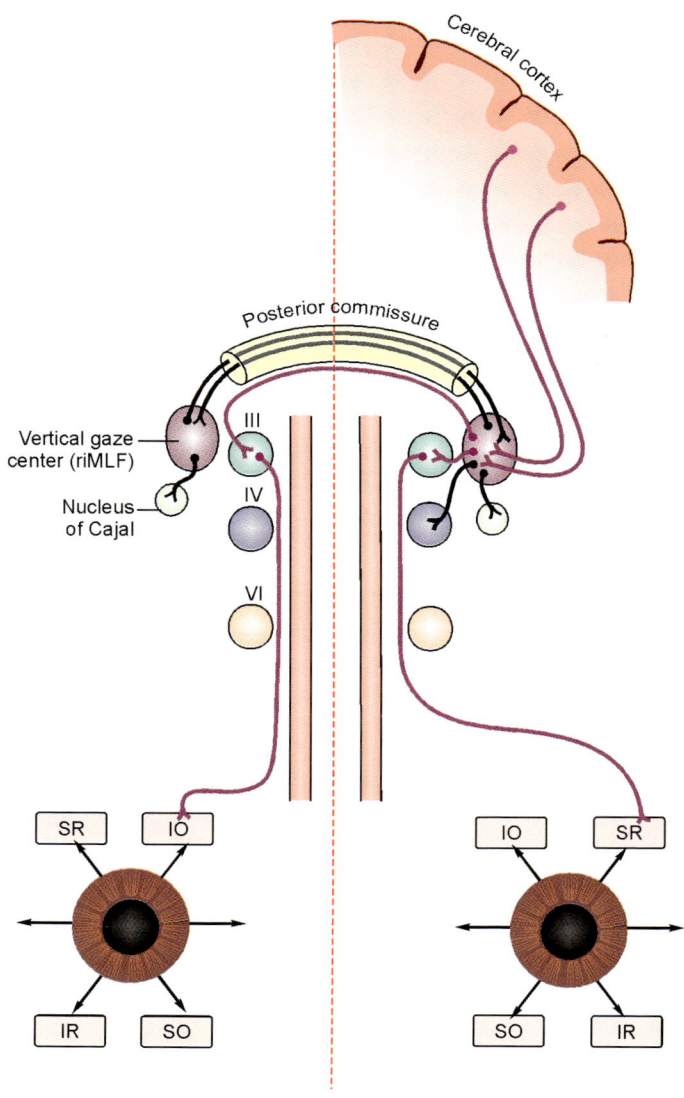

Fig. 27.7 *Neural pathway of vertical pursuit (upgaze) eye movements.*

nystagmus is an oscillatory movement of the two eyes. Both eyes turn in the same direction and are suddenly pulled back into the primary position by a fast, jerky movement, where upon the cycle begins again with conjugate deviation. Usually, the first phase of nystagmus, the conjugate deviation, is distinctly slower than the second phase in which the corrective movement takes place. Diagnostically, vestibular nystagmus can be produced to test the integrity of the vestibular reflex mechanism. For this, the patient is either submitted to rotation on a revolving chair (rotatory vestibular nystagmus) or his/her external auditory canals are irrigated nystagmus).

7. Medial longitudinal fasciculus

The medial longitudinal fasciculus (MLF) is a fiber tract that extends from the spinal cord to the oculomotor nerve nucleus. It contains primarily ascending fibers, the majority of which arise in the superior and medial vestibular nuclei. The MLF is in close proximity to the ocular motor nuclei and influences both ipsilateral and contralateral nuclei.

Functions of MLF. The medial longitudinal fasciculus plays an important role in the pathway of ocular movements. Its main functions can be summarized as follows (Fig. 27.9):

- It connects the ocularmotor nuclei with one another.
- It transmits signals from the subcortical–horizontal gaze center for the horizontal versions to the opposite medial rectus muscle.
- It transmits impulses originating from the vestibular nucleus (in response to statokinetic stimulation) to the ocular motor nuclei as well as to nucleus innervating muscles of head and neck.
- It relays signals from the proprioceptors of the head and neck muscles to the ocular motor nuclei.

Lesions of MLF. An abnormality of the MLF causes problems with horizontal and vertical gaze co-ordination of the two eyes. The clinically most important connection passing through the

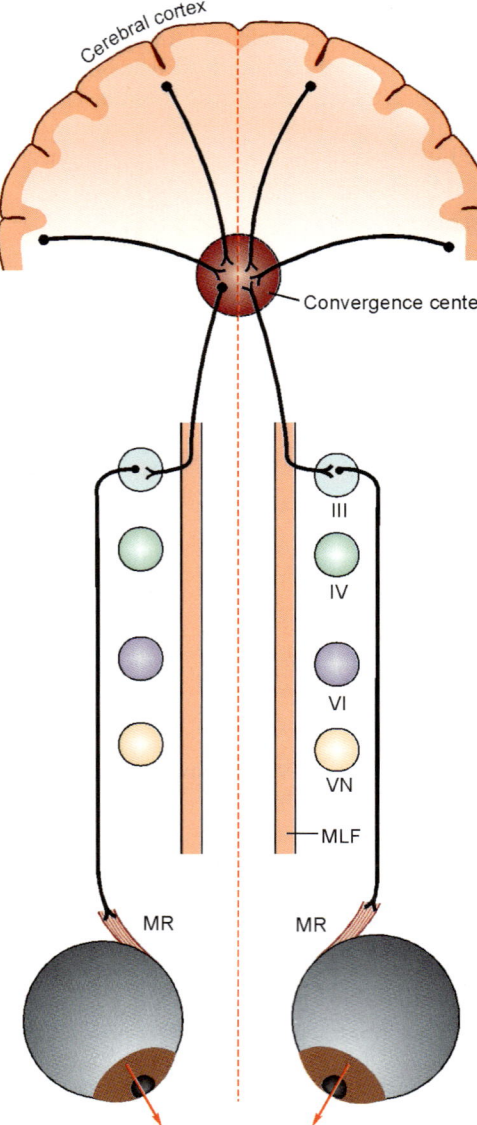

Fig. 27.8 *Presumptive pathway of convergence.*

MLF links, the contralateral abducens nucleus with the ipsilateral medial rectus subnucleus. Abnormalities of this tract produce an internuclear ophthalmoplegia. Such a lesion produces slowed or complete loss of adduction of the ipsilateral eye and abducting nystagmus of the fellow eye.

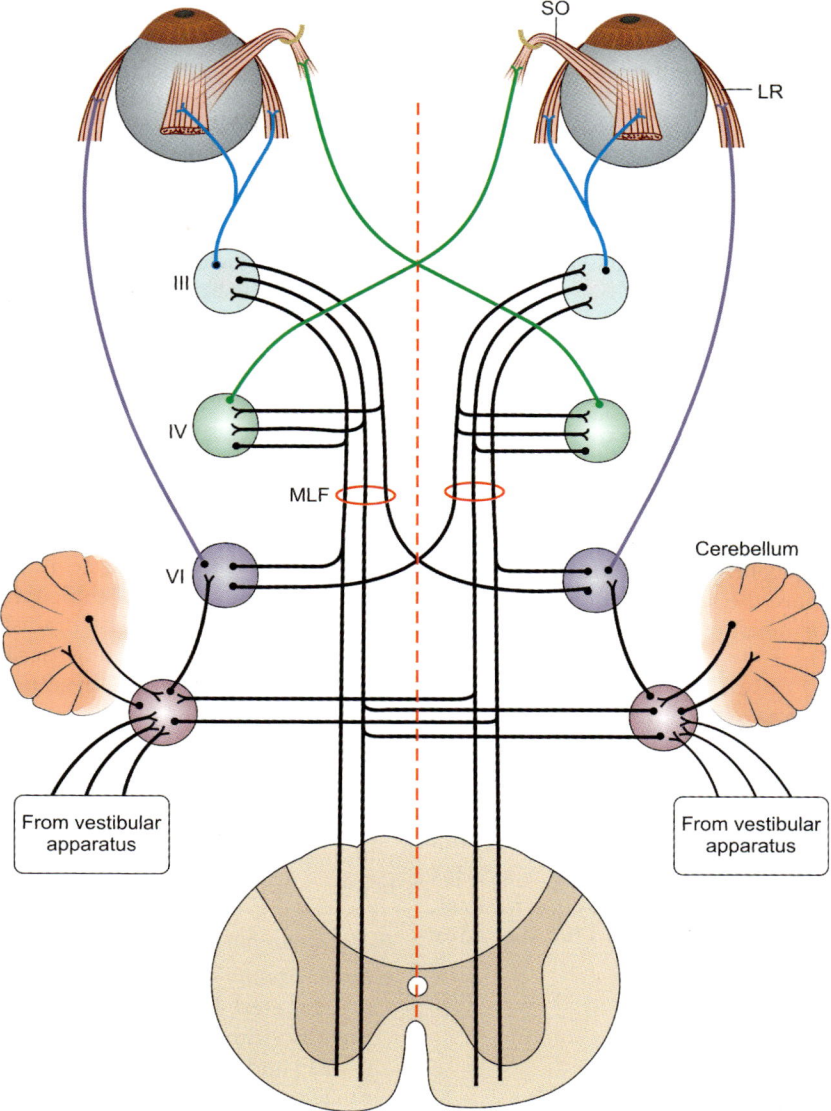

Fig. 27.9 *Connections of medial longitudinal fasciculus (MLF).*

8. Cerebellum

The cerebellum appears to be involved in the immediate modulation of ongoing eye movements, as well as in the long-term adaptive processes that compensate for ocular motor dysmetria. The cerebellum controls and adjusts the size of saccades. The latter ability is essential for maintaining accurate ocular motor performance during growth and aging, during and after ocular motor disease, or even while using spectacles. For instance, the use of aniso-metropic spectacles produces a varying anisophoria in different directions of gaze, which must be compensated in each direction of gaze.

Hemicerebellectomy produces ipsilateral saccadic and contralateral pursuit defects, while total cerebellectomy creates persistent saccadic dysmetria and abolishes smooth pursuit. The cerebellum has numerous connections to nuclear and supranuclear ocular motor centers.

SUPRANUCLEAR EYE MOVEMENT SYSTEMS

Following supranuclear eye movement systems have been recognized:

- Saccadic system
- Smooth pursuit system
- Vergence system
- Vestibular system
- Optokinetic system
- Position maintenance system

All these systems perform specific functions and each one is controlled by a different neural system but share the same final common path, i.e. the motor neurons that supply the extraocular muscles.

SACCADIC SYSTEM

Saccades are sudden, jerky conjugate eye movements that occur as the gaze shifts from one object to another. Thus they are performed to bring the image of an object quickly on the fovea. Though normally voluntary, saccades may be involuntary aroused by peripheral, visual or auditory stimuli. The saccades include:

- Horizontal saccades
- Vertical saccades.

Neural pathway

Cortical areas

The pathway originates in the premotor cortex of the frontal motor area. From there, the fibers for voluntary saccades pass directly and for involuntary saccades through the superior colliculus to the contralateral horizontal gaze center in PPRF (Fig. 27.2).

Pathways involved in the cortical generation of saccades

It appears that there are three pathways involved in the cortical generation of saccades:

i. ***Ventral pathway.*** The ventral pathway projects by way of the posterior portion of the anterior limb of the internal capsule and the medial part of cerebral peduncle to reach the pons, where there is a partial decussation and termination in the PPRF.

ii. ***The dorsal pathway*** passes from the FEF through the thalamus, the pulvinar, the pretectal nuclei, and the superior colliculus to reach the brainstem.

iii. ***The intermediate pathway*** extends from the FEF to the rostral ocular motor nuclei and the interstitial nucleus of Cajal.

Brainstem pathway

Recent evidence suggests that the saccades (horizontal as well as vertical) are generated by groups of neurons located in the brainstem and are controlled by higher frontal system (for voluntary saccades) and collicular system (for involuntary saccades). The brainstem neurons concerned with generation of saccades form the final premotor circuits. These neurons are of three types:

1. Excitatory burst neurons (EBN)
2. Inhibitory burst neurons (IBN)
3. Pause neurons (PN).

Brainstem pathway for saccades is described below.

Pathway for horizontal saccades

- *For horizontal saccades,* the excitatory neurons are located in horizontal gaze center in paramedian pontine reticular formation (PPRF) and project to the ipsilateral abducens nucleus. The axons from these cells synapse in the abducens nucleus on motor neurons that innervate the ipsilateral lateral rectus and on the interneurons that innervate contralateral medial rectus subnucleus by way of the contralateral MLF (Fig. 27.2).

Pathway for vertical saccades

For the vertical saccades, the excitatory neurons are located in the vertical gaze center formed by rostral interstitial nucleus of medial longitudinal fasciculus (riMLF) and other neurons in the region of posterior commissure.

- *For downward saccades* (Fig. 27.3), the activated neurons in the riMLF send impulse directly through the fibers that synapse upon the inferior rectus subnucleus of the ipsilateral IIIrd nerve and contralateral IVth nerve nucleus for superior oblique muscles. riMLF nuclei of both sides are connected by a commissure which projects into the interstitial nucleus of Cajal (INC) and to the ipsilateral IIIrd nerve nucleus.

- *For upward saccades* (Fig. 27.4), the activated neurons in the riMLF send impulse through the fibers that synapse upon the inferior oblique subnucleus of the ipsilateral IIIrd nerve; and through the fibers which pass via posterior commissure and synapse upon the superior rectus subnucleus of the contra-lateral IIIrd nerve.

Activities of brainstem involved in generation of saccades neurons

As mentioned above, three types of neurons are involved in generation of saccades: Excitatory burst neurons (EBN), inhibitory burst neurons (IBN) and pause neurons (PN). These neurons generate saccades by a 'pulse-step' innervation system (Fig. 27.10). The 'pulse' is created by sudden firing of the neurons to the extraocular muscles. After the eyeball is moved to the new position; to keep it in the same position, sustained contraction of the muscle is required. This is called a step and is affected by tonic contraction of muscles due to continuous discharge from neurons.

Excitatory burst neurons

The excitatory burst neurons (EBNs) discharge at high frequencies just prior to and during the saccades and provide the eye velocity commands known as the pulse (Fig. 27.10). Burst cells discharge, only when there is need for a fast eye movement and do not discharge during fixation, pursuit or vergence eye movements.

The EBNs send impulses to the neurons of cranial nerve nuclei supplying to yoke muscles for the gaze movements.

Inhibitory burst neurons (IBNs)

The inhibitory burst neurons (IBNs) send impulses through the medullary reticular formation to the neurons of cranial nerve nuclei supplying to the

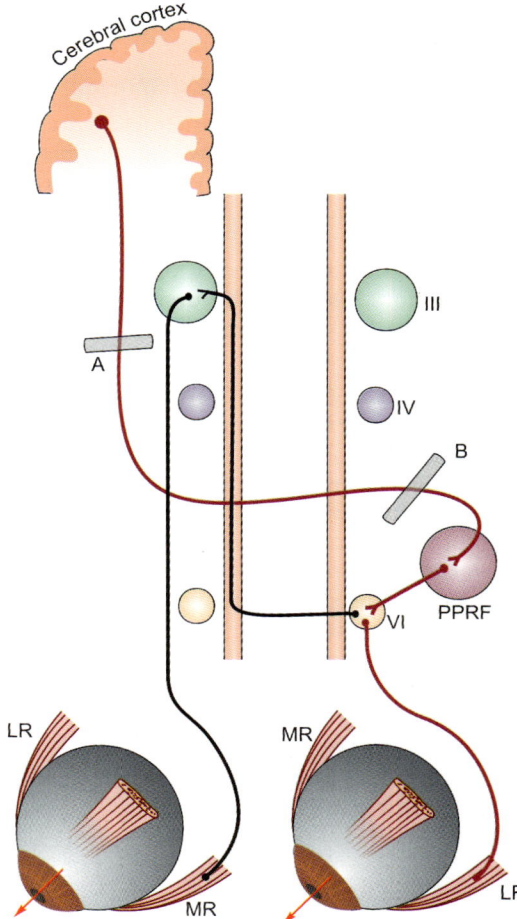

Fig. 27.10 *Relation between the three sets of neurons (excitatory burst neurons, pause neurons and inhibitory burst neurons) concerned with generation of saccades.*

antagonist muscles of the yoke muscles for the concerned gaze movement and thus inhibit these muscles and allow the gaze movement to occur.

Their firing rate is inversely proportional to the excitatory burst cells.

Pause neurons

These neurons discharge tonically, except just before and during saccades, when they pause. They appear to exert an inhibitory influence on the burst neurons preventing extraneous saccades occurring during fixation. These cells inhibit the burst cells within the ipsilateral PPRF. These cells are important during fixation and smooth pursuit. Abnormalities of these cells lead to opsoclonus and ocular flutter.

SMOOTH PURSUIT EYE MOVEMENT SYSTEM

Smooth pursuit movements are tracking movements of the eye as they follow moving objects. These occur voluntarily, when the eyes track moving objects but take place involuntarily, if a repetitive visual pattern is displayed continuously. When the velocity of the moving object is more, the smooth pursuit movement is replaced by small saccades (catch-up saccades).

Neural pathway for pursuit movements originates in the cortex of the perieto-occipito-temporal (POT) junction. The fibers then descend and terminate in the ipsilateral PPRF for horizontal pursuits (Fig. 27.5) and the ipsilateral mesencephalic reticular formation for the vertical pursuits (Figs 27.6 and 27.7); and then possibly directly to the ocular motor nuclei. The right occipital lobe, therefore, controls pursuits to the right and the left occipital lobe those to the left. The cerebellum is closely associated with normal pursuit movements. The FEF and the superior colliculi play a modulating role in the production of pursuit eye movements by POT junction. Lesions in the POT area produce ipsilateral pursuit defects.

VERGENCE MOVEMENT SYSTEMS

Vergence movements allow focussing of an object which moves away from or towards the observer or when visual fixation shifts from one object to another at a different distance. Vergence movements are very slow (about 20°/sec) disjugate movements. They have a latency of about 160 msec.

Neural pathway. The exact neuroanatomical substrate is not known. Stimulation of parieto-occipital region (area 19 or 22) provokes vergence movements in monkeys. Premotor signals are thought to originate in the mesenchephalic reticular formation with separate population of cells for convergence and divergence. The fibers travel then to the relevant cranial nuclei (Fig. 27.8). This link seems to course outside the MLF, since the MLF lesions usually spare convergence.

VESTIBULAR EYE MOVEMENT SYSTEM

Vestibular movements are usually effective in compensating for the effects of head movements in disturbing visual fixation (vestibulo-ocular reflex—VOR). These movements operate through the vestibular system (*see* page 283). Most rotations of the head do not involve angular rotations as fast as 300°/sec and the vestibular system can compensate for these. However, when the body is rotated at great speeds around a vertical axis (e.g. a skater performing a spin), eye movements show the so-called oculovestibular nystagmus, with a slow motion of the eyes in the opposite direction to that of rotation—this is initiated by the vestibular mechanism—followed by a quick jerky binocular 'return' movement in the direction of rotation. This sequence is repeated as long as the angular acceleration lasts. It is likely that the fast component of nystagmus is mediated by mechanisms similar to those responsible for saccades.

OPTOKINETIC SYSTEM

This system helps to hold the images of the seen world steady on the retinae during sustained head rotation. This system becomes operative, when the vestibular reflex gets fatigued after 30 seconds. The optokinetic response is evoked by rotation of the visual field before the eyes. It consists of a movement following the moving scene, succeeded by a rapid saccade in the opposite direction. In fact, the transient head rotation stimulates both the vestibulo-ocular reflex with a latency of only 10 ms and the optokinetic reflex with a latency of 70 ms. However, during sustained rotation with eyes open, the vestibulo-ocular reflex ceases while the optokinetic system maintains a steady discharge from the vestibular nuclei to sustain the compensatory optokinetic nystagmus.

POSITION MAINTENANCE SYSTEM

This system helps to maintain a specific gaze position by means of rapid micromovements called 'flicks' and slow micromovements called 'drifts'. This system coordinates with other systems.

Neural pathway for this system is believed to be the same as for saccades and smooth pursuits.

SUPRANUCLEAR DISORDERS OF EYE MOVEMENTS

INTRODUCTION

Anatomic background and site of lesions

As described above, the supranuclear pathways connect the frontal lobe, occipital lobe and cerebellum with the mesencephalon, i.e. midbrain and pons (containing the nuclei controlling the extraocular muscles and the centers for horizontal and vertical conjugate gazes). The pathway transmitting impulses from the frontal lobe centers to the mesencephalon may be referred to as *frontomesencephalic pathway* and that connecting occipital lobe centers with mesencephalon as *occipitoparietomesencephalic pathway*.

Supranuclear disorders thus result from the lesions involving the cortical centers or the lesions interrupting the frontomesencephalic pathway, occipitoparietomesencephalic pathway, cerebellar pathways, centers for horizontal and vertical conjugate gazes and medial longitudinal fasciculus.

Characteristic of supranuclear disorders

The basic characteristic of supranuclear lesions (other than those interrupting vergence mechanism and the medial longitudinal fasciculus) is that both eyes are affected equally and that the disturbance is one of deficient or defective conjugate eye movements. They usually do not produce diplopia because both eyes are equally involved.

List of common supranuclear disorders

Some of the common supranuclear disorders are as follows:

- Horizontal conjugate gaze paralysis
- Internuclear ophthalmoplegia
- One-and-a-half syndrome
- Vertical conjugate gaze paralysis
- Skew deviation
- Cogwheeling
- Ocular dysmetria, ocular flutter and opsoclonus
- Oculomotor apraxia
- Double elevator paralysis
- Nystagmus
- Comitant squint. (It is considered the most common supranuclear disorder. It is being presumed that the comitant squint represents primarily a deficiency in the vergence movement mechanism.)

HORIZONTAL CONJUGATE GAZE PARALYSIS

Horizontal conjugate gaze paralysis refers to equal paralysis of same sided horizontal movement in both eyes, i.e. either levoversion or dextroversion is deficient or defective.

Site of lesion

As described earlier, the frontal lobe is connected with the mesencephalon through the frontomesencephalic pathway. This pathway descends into the internal capsule and is thought to cross completely at the level of fourth nerve nucleus (Figs 27.2 to 27.4). It is primarily involved in the saccadic eye movement system.

A destructive lesion in the cortical center or frontomesencephalic pathway above decussation (Fig. 27.11A) produces defects in conjugate gaze to the opposite side. Lesions below the decussation (Fig. 27.11B) produce defects in conjugate gaze to the same side as the lesion. Lesions involving 6th nerve nucleus (1 in Fig. 27.14) and PPRF (2 in Fig. 27.14) can also produce horizontal gaze palsy on the same side. It is important to note that since the area of the frontal lobe concerned with horizontal eye movements is so large, small lesions of the frontal lobe rarely affect conjugate horizontal gaze.

Efferent fibers from the occipital lobe connecting the mesencephalon from the occipitoparietomesencephalic pathway. This pathway also crosses to the opposite side at the level of 4th nerve nucleus. Lesions involving this pathway will also produce conjugate movements to the opposite side or same side depending upon the site of lesions similar to frontal lobe lesions. However, the conjugate paralysis caused by lesions of occipitoparietal pathway is of lesser magnitude than that caused by lesions involving the frontal voluntary system.

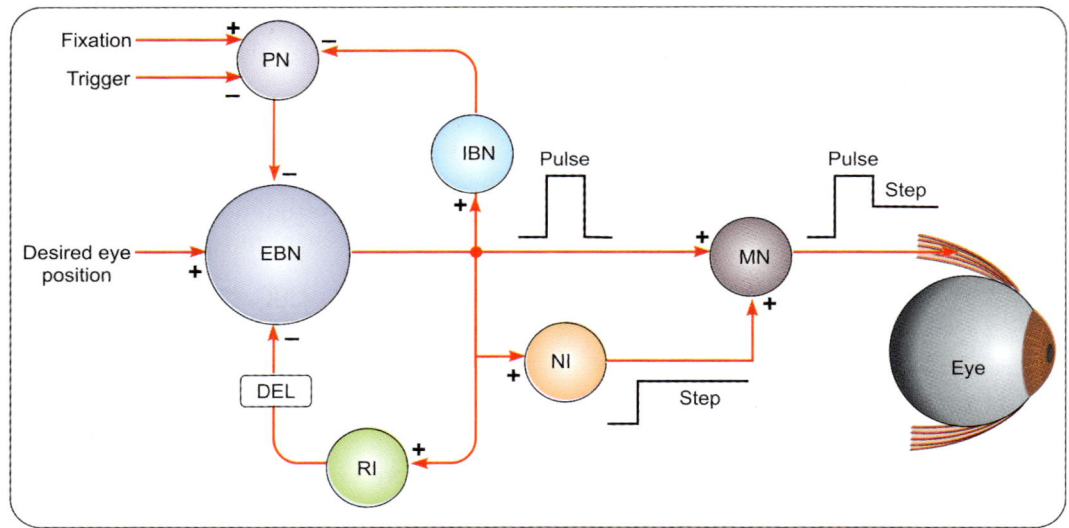

Fig. 27.11 *Site of lesions producing conjugate paralysis to the opposite side* (A) *and the same side* (B).

Causes of conjugate paralysis

1. Vascular lesions producing infarctions or haemorrhages
2. Inflammatory lesions
3. Tumors

Clinical features

As described above, when the frontomesencephalic tract is interrupted by a lesion above the crossing, there is a deficit of rapid eye movements to the opposite side; thus the right-sided lesion will affect:

1. Saccades to the left.
2. The fast phase of the optokinetic nystagmus, when it is to the left.
3. The fast phase of caloric or vestibular nystagmus when it is to the left.
4. On looking to the left, there may be a gaze paretic nystagmus with the fast phase to the left with varying amplitude and rhythm.
5. Gaze paralysis and conjugate deviations caused by hemispheric lesions are usually transient, probably due to compensation from the contralateral uninvolved hemisphere. While, paralysis resulting from lesions in the brainstem are less marked but last as long as the lesion exists since no compensation of function occurs.

6. Lesions causing gaze paralysis (e.g. infarction, haemorrhages and tumors) also produce severe neurologic signs such as hemiplegia and thus the eye signs are usually over-shadowed.

INTERNUCLEAR OPHTHALMOPLEGIA

Internuclear ophthalmoplegia (INO) results from a lesion of the medial longitudinal fasciculus (MLF) that interrupts fibers passing from the subcortical center for horizontal gaze of one side to the nucleus of the third nerve on the other side (Fig. 27.12A). It is the only supranuclear defect that does not result in a gaze paralysis.

Etiology

- *Disseminated sclerosis* is the most common cause of bilateral INO.
- *Cerebrovascular accident and brain tumor* can also cause bilateral INO.
- *Infarct of small branch of the basilar artery* is usually associated with unilateral INO.

Clinical features

Unilateral INO. As is clear from the Fig. 27.11, patient with unilateral INO on version movements will exhibit:
- Tropia in the involved side.
- *Limitation of adduction* on the involved side (Fig. 27.13A), and

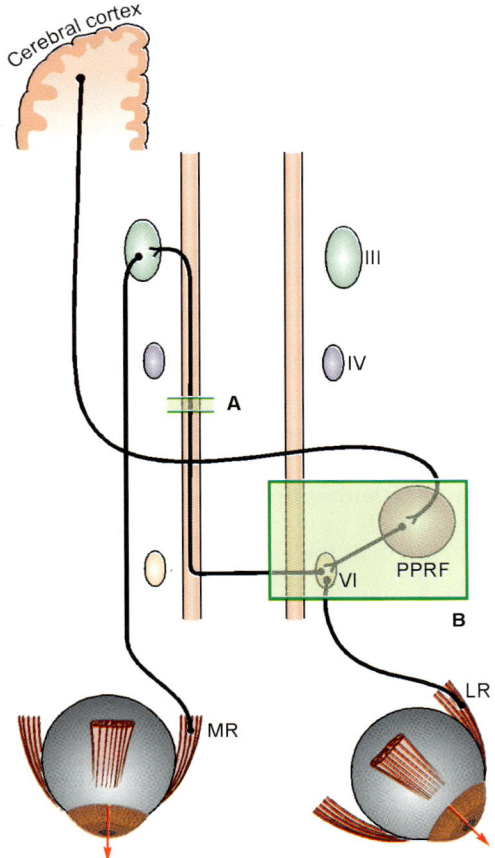

Fig. 27.12 *Site of lesion: Producing internuclear ophthalmoplegia (A), and one- and A-half syndrome (B).*

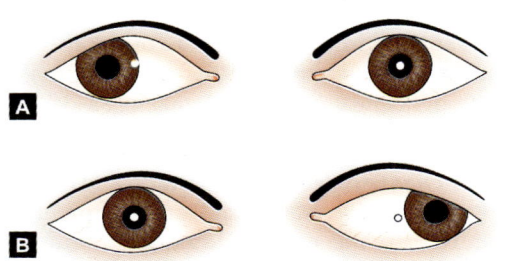

Fig. 27.13 *Diagrammatic depiction of right internuclear ophthalmoplegia. Note right exotropia in primary position (A) and limitation of adduction in the right eye with normal abduction in the left eye (B).*

- *Normal abduction* of the opposite eye (Fig. 27.13B).
- *Nystagmus* is associated with abduction of the opposite side. Nystagmus in INO is a secondary response to the weakness of adduction and not caused directly by the central defect.
- *Convergence* is normal in many patients and thus both eyes adduct normally to fixate a near object.
- *Skew deviation* of some degree may be noted with the eye ipsilateral to the lesion slightly higher than the other.

Bilateral INO is more frequent than unilateral INO. Depending upon the site of lesion, other cranial nuclei and convergence mechanism may also be involved.

Differential diagnosis

1. *Isolated medial rectus palsy* needs to be differentiated from the INO.

2. *Pseudointernuclear ophthalmoplegia* should be distinguished from the true INO. Pseudo-INO, i.e. a condition characterised by limitation of adduction and nystagmus of the abducting eye caused by lesions other than lesions of MLF, such as:

- That occurring due to myasthenia gravis
- That following recession and retroequatorial posterior fixation of both medial rectus muscles.

Treatment

Unfortunately, still there is no effective treatment for INO.

ONE-AND-A-HALF SYNDROME

One-and-a-half syndrome (paralytic pontine exotropia) consists of a unilateral internuclear ophthalmoplegia and a contralateral-horizontal gaze palsy.

Etiology

An extensive caudal lesion in the pons can affect the horizontal gaze center and the adjacent MLF, resulting in a palsy of both medial rectus muscles and one lateral rectus (i.e. gaze palsy plus INO) (Fig. 27.12B and 4 in Fig. 27.14). Causes include demyelination, vascular, tumor and inflammation.

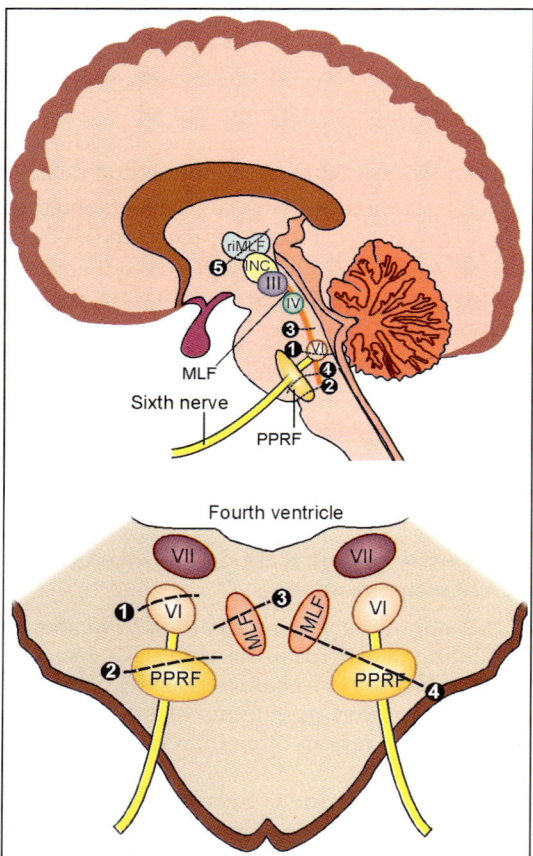

Fig. 27.14 *Site of lesions producing supranuclear disorders. Horizontal gaze palsy may result from a lesion involving 6th nerve nucleus (1) and PPRF (2); Internuclear ophthalmoplegia may result from a lesion of medial longitudinal fasciculus (3), one-and-a-half syndrome results from a lesion involving both the MLF and PPRF (4); and vertical gaze palsy may result from a lesion involving riMLF (5).*

Features

The main clinical and diagnostic features are as follows: The only remaining horizontal movement is abduction by the unaffected lateral rectus, which is associated with the typical abducting nystagmus. When the patient attempts to fixate with this eye in the primary position, the nystagmus will reduce or cease. There is, therefore, a palsy of conjugate gaze on one side and an INO on looking to the other side. A marked compensatory head posture may be adopted to achieve fixation with the preferred

eye. Although complete 'one-and-a-half' syndromes are rare, partial or incomplete syndromes are more common. They can be diagnosed on clinical assessment. A Hess chart is useful in monitoring the condition. However, care must be taken in its interpretation, as synergist muscles are affected in patients with lesions involving the horizontal gaze center as well as the MLF (partial one-and-a-half syndrome). Since the basis of the Hess chart is a comparison of action of synergistic muscles, the test is comparing abnormal with abnormal and, if viewed in isolation, the gaze palsy element may be missed.

VERTICAL CONJUGATE GAZE PARALYSIS

Vertical conjugate gaze paralysis refers to paralysis of either upward gaze or downward gaze or both upward and downward gazes equally in both the eyes.

Site of lesion, causes and clinical features

As mentioned earlier (page 283), the vertical gaze centers (riMLF) are located at the level of upper pole of red nucleus and that a vertical version occurs only upon simultaneous stimulation from both the hemispheres. Therefore, vertical gaze paralysis will occur, if there is a lesion of similar extent in each hemisphere involving riMLF (5 in Fig. 27.14). Further, the fact that paresis of upward gaze may occur while the downward gaze is unaffected and *vice versa*, indicates that there must be some separation of the two centers anatomically.

The upgaze palsy is typically caused by lesions involving the posterior commissure and characteristically occurs in Parinaud's dorsal midbrain syndrome. The most common cause of a Parinaud's syndrome is a pinealoma in which deficiency of upward gaze is associated with pupillary abnormalities.

The downgaze palsy is less common and occurs, when both sides of the midbrain tegmentum posterior to the red nucleus are damaged. Downgaze palsy is frequently associated with convergence paresis and thus it can be assumed that perhaps the convergence center and the pathway mediating convergence are in close approximation to the center for downgaze.

SKEW DEVIATION

Skew deviation is a vertical strabismus resulting from a disruption of input into the oculomotor and trochlear nuclei. Cyclotorsion is often a feature and other symptoms and signs of central nervous system disease are usually present.

Etiology

Skew deviation arises from a peripheral or central imbalance of otolith inputs to the oculomotor and trochlear nuclei.

Structures involved in the pathogenesis of skew deviation include: The middle ear and the vestibular nerve; the vestibular nuclei in the brainstem; the cerebellum; the medial longitudinal fasciculus; the interstitial nucleus of Cajal in the midbrain.

Features

The features of skew deviation are: A vertical strabismus, which can be transient or permanent. Transient deviations are common in unilateral internuclear ophthalmoplegia. A deviation, which may be concomitant or incomitant. Incomitant skew deviation must be differentiated from a cyclovertical muscle palsy, and typically resembles a unilateral or bilateral inferior rectus muscle or a unilateral superior rectus underaction. Incyclotorsion of the hypertropic eye. This is similar to one-half cycle of see-saw nystagmus and reflects the common occurrence of both disorders with lesions involving the interstitial nucleus of Cajal. Other signs of central nervous system disease, usually, involving the brainstem and cerebellum. The strabismus can be monitored using a Hess chart.

COGWHEELING

Defects in slow pursuit tracking to the opposite side may be produced by lesions affecting one occipital lobe. These pursuit movements may be interrupted by saccadic movements; this sign is known as cogwheeling. A lesion interrupting the occipitoparietomesencephalic pathway above the decussation in the midbrain will cause a breakdown in tracking or following objects to the opposite field. When the lesion is below the crossing of fibers, the defect is to the same side.

OCULAR DYSMETRIA, OCULAR FLUTTERS AND OPSOCLONUS

Ocular dysmetria. It is a defect in the saccadic eye movement mechanism believed to be caused by lesions of the cerebellum and cerebello-mesencephalic pathway. Normally, when a patient is asked to make saccadic movement from one target to another, there is a small undershoot and a precise end point is reached. In ocular dysmetria, there is tendency of both eyes to overshoot the object of regard, and small oscillations occur until a stable endpoint is reached.

Ocular flutter. It refers to rapid horizontal oscillations of the eyes in primary position. It is thought to be related to fixation difficulties.

Opsoclonus. It refers to a sequence of saccadic eye movements that may be in either direction but are predominantly horizontal. These movements are spontaneous and may show a rhythm to their amplitude and frequency.

OCULOMOTOR APRAXIA

A total loss of voluntary conjugate gaze in all directions is known as oculomotor apraxia. In order to bring their eyes into the desired gaze position, patients with oculomotor apraxia characteristically have a head thrusting movement. Oculomotor apraxia can be congenital or acquired.

Congenital oculomotor apraxia

Etiopathogenesis

It is a rare disorder of unknown etiopathogenesis. It is more common in males than females and may be familial.

- Agenesis of the corpus callosum and hydrocephalus have been reported to be associated with some cases.
- Mass lesions of cerebellum compressing the rostral part of the brainstem have been reported in many infants presenting with oculomotor apraxes.

Clinical features

Clinical features include:

- An inability to generate normal, voluntary horizontal saccades.

- Changes in horizontal fixation are made by a head thrust that overshoots the target followed by a rotation of the head back in the opposite direction once fixation is established.
- Vertical saccades and random eye movements are intact.
- Vestibular and optokinetic nystagmus are impaired.
- Reading can be difficult with this condition.
- Developmental delay, especially motoric, may be present.

Acquired oculomotor apraxia

Bilateral lesions of the frontoparietal cortex have been reported to be associated with the acquired oculomotor apraxia. It needs to be differentiated from the conditions that affect the generation of voluntary saccades, including metabolic and degenerative diseases such as Huntington's chorea.

BIBLIOGRAPHY

1. Bender MB. The oculomotor decussation. Am J Ophthalmol 1962;54:591.
2. Bizzi E. Discharge of frontal eye field neurons during eye movements in unanesthetized monkey. Science 1967;157:1588.
3. Bizzi E. Discharge of frontal eye fields neurons during saccadic and following eye movements in unanesthetized monkey. Exp Brain Res 1968;6:69.
4. Daroff RB. Control of ocular movement. Br J Ophthalmol 1974;58:217.
5. Daroff RB. Physiologic, anatomic and pathophysiologic considerations of eye movements. Trans Ophthalmol Soc UK 1970;90:410.
6. Gay AJ, Newman NM, Keltner JL, Stroud MH. Eye Movement Disorders. St Louis. CV Mosby Co., 1974.
7. Weber R. Daroff RB. The metrics of horizontal saccadic eye movements in normal humans. Vision Res 1971;2:921.

28 | NYSTAGMUS AND RELATED OSCILLATIONS

AK Khurana, Aruj K Khurana, Bhawna Khurana

NYSTAGMUS

DEFINITION AND FEATURES

Definition

Nystagmus comes from the Greek word *nystagmos* (to nod) and may be defined as repetitive, to and fro involuntary movement of one or both eyes that is initiated by a slow phase (drift). The movements which are not regular and rhythmic are called *nystagmoid movements*.

Features of nystagmus movements

1. *Type of waveform.* Nystagmus may be pendular or jerk type.
- *Pendular nystagmus* is characterized by the movements which are of equal velocity in each direction (Fig. 28.1A). It may be horizontal, vertical, oblique, rotatory or mixed.

- *Jerk nystagmus* is characterized by the movements which have a slow component in one direction and a fast component in the other direction; the latter being a recovery phenomenon aimed at refixation. The direction of jerk nystagmus is defined by the direction of fast component (phase). For instance, if the fast phase beat to the right, this is called *right beating* nystagmus. Likewise the jerk nystagmus may be left, up, down or rotatory.

Waveform can further be characterized and documented by the nature of the slow phase as shown in Figs 28.1B to E.

297

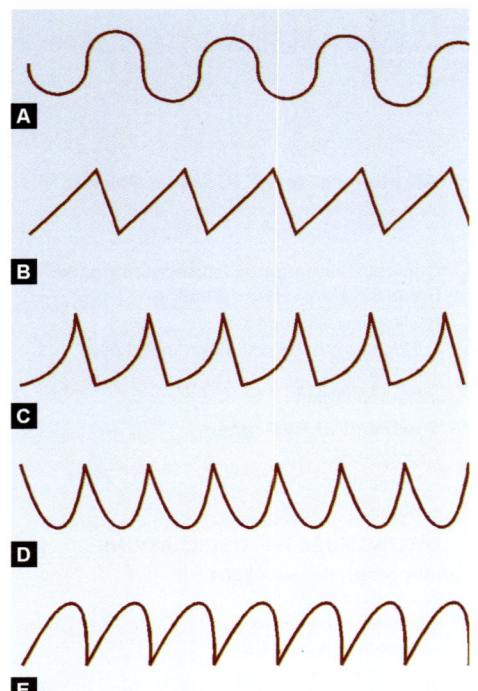

Fig. 28.1 *Waveform characteristics of: pendular nystagmus (A) and, jerk nystagmus (B to E), B, Jerk nystagmus with slow components of constant velocity; C, Jerk nystagmus with slow components of exponentially increasing velocity; D, Jerk nystagmus with slow components of exponentially increasing velocity with extended foveation periods that follow slow movements; E, Jerk nystagmus with slow components of exponentially decreasing velocity.*

2. **Direction.** Direction or plane of nystagmus can be horizontal, vertical, oblique, torsional or mixed. For a jerk nystagmus, the direction is described according to the fast phase. For simplicity of recording the direction of nystagmus in case notes, the following method may be used:

a. *Pendular nystagmus*

• Horizontal
• Vertical
• Rotatory
• Oblique

b. *Jerk nystagmus with quick phase*

• To the right
• To the left
• Up

• Down
• Right rotatory (anticlockwise)
• Left rotatory (clockwise)
• Oblique up to right   or left
• Oblique down to right   or left

3. **Conjugacy.** Nystagmus may be of conjugate, disconjugate or dissociative type.

• *Conjugate nystagmus.* Binocular nystagmus with symmetric direction, amplitude and rate in both eyes.
• *Disconjugate nystagmus.* Monocular or binocular with different directions and frequencies in two eyes.
• *Dissociative nystagmus refers to* unidirectional but asymmetrical nystagmus in two eyes. Such type of nystagmus is seen in internuclear ophthalmoplegia.

4. **Amplitude.** The amplitude is measured in degrees and represents the extent of movement between the start of drift away from fixation and the start of corrective movement in the opposite direction. The amount of movement should be approximately equal. In majority of cases, the amplitude increases, when the patient looks in the direction of the fast phase (*Alexander's law*). When the patient looks in the opposite direction, the amplitude reduces, the oscillation ceases or the direction of the nystagmus may reverse. There are very few exceptions to this rule, but in some cases of vertical nystagmus, the amplitude increases on looking in the direction of the slow phase.

Grading of amplitude. The amplitude is graded as small, medium or large as below:
• *Fine (small)*— excursions less than 3°
• *Medium*— excursions between 5° and 15°
• *Coarse (large)*— excursions more than 15°

A dissociated nystagmus has different amplitudes in both eyes. Subtle forms of nystagmus, due to low amplitude or inconsistent presence, require prolonged observation over 2–3 minutes. Low amplitude nystagmus may be detected only by viewing the patient's retina with an ophthalmoscope. In case records amplitude is recorded by the thickness of arrows or increasing lines in arrows, e.g.:

- Small ⟩—→ or ——→
- Medium ⟫—→ or ——→→
- Large ⟫—→ or ——→→→

5. Frequency. Frequency of nystagmus refers to number of beats, i.e. to and fro movements per second.
Grading and recording of frequency. It is done into low (slow), moderate and high (fast):
- Low (Lo): 1–2 Hz
- Moderate (M): 3–4 Hz
- High (H): > 5 Hz

6. Intensity. Intensity of nystagmus is the product of amplitude and frequency.
Grading of intensity. Nystagmus of each type may be seen in the primary position or it may be made apparent, only when the visual axes are deviated. On these grounds, nystagmus may be graded as to its intensity into:
Recording of frequency
- *First degree nystagmus.* In it, the movements occur only in that direction of the gaze in which the quick phase occurs.
- *Second degree nystagmus.* In it, the movements are also present in the primary position.
- *Third degree nystagmus.* In it, movements are also present in the direction of the gaze to the side opposite to that of the quick phase.

7. Foveation period. It is the period in the waveform where eye velocity is at minimum and thus visual acuity is maximum (Fig. 28.2). The foveation period is maximum in the null position of gaze and increases with the decrease in intensity of nystagmus.

8. Null zone and neutral zone
- *Null zone* refers to the position of eyes where a zerk nystagmus is absent. Some patients may assume a head posture to bring the eyes in the null zone.
- *Neutral zone* is the point from where fast component of nystagmus changes its direction. It may be different than the null zone or may be the same.

9. Trajectories of nystagmus
Not infrequently patients with nystagmus show a waveform that has vertical, horizontal and rotary components. When a horizontal and a vertical component coexist and are superimposed on each other, three characteristic nystagmus trajectories can be observed (Fig. 28.3):

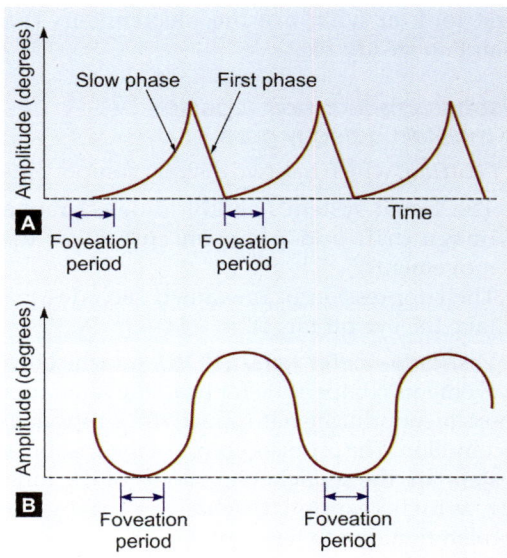

Fig. 28.2 *Foveation period in:* (A) *Jerk nystagmus;* (B) *Pendular nystagmus.*

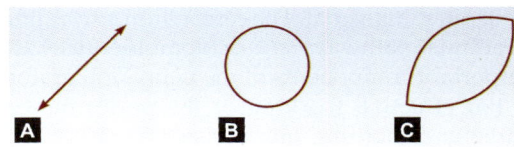

Fig. 28.3 *Trajectories of nystagmus:* (A) *Oblique;* (B) *Circular;* (C) *Elliptical.*

a. *Oblique trajectory* occurs when vertical and horizontal components are of equal frequency and amplitude and in phase with each other.
b. *Circular trajectory* occurs when vertical and horizontal components are of equal frequency and amplitude and are 90°, out of phase with each other.
c. *Elliptical trajectory* occurs when vertical and horizontal components are of equal frequency but unequal amplitudes and are 90° out of phase with each other.

PATHOPHYSIOLOGY OF NYSTAGMUS

Nystagmus and other related conditions in essence disrupt steady fixation and thereby degrade vision. To understand the pathophysiology of nystagmus, we must, therefore, first look at what are the mechanisms that maintain steady fixation.

Mechanisms that work together to maintain a steady gaze

1. *Fixation*, which has two distinct components:

a. The visual system's ability to detect retinal image drift and program corrective eye movements.

b. The suppression of unwanted saccades that take the eye off target.

2. *Vestibulo-ocular reflex (VOR)*, by which eye movements compensate for head movements at short latency during natural activities, especially locomotion. The proprioceptors of the vestibular system are the semicircular canals of the inner ear, which respond to changes in angular acceleration due to head rotation.

3. *Neural integrator*, ability of the brain to hold the eye at an eccentric position in the orbit against the elastic pull of the suspensory ligaments and extraocular muscles. A gaze-holding network called the neural integrator generates this signal. The cerebellum, ascending vestibular pathways, and oculomotor nuclei are important components of the neural integrator.

For effective working of the performance, three gaze-holding mechanisms are tuned by adaptive mechanisms (recalibration) that monitor the visual consequences of eye movements. A nystagmus is caused by defect in any of these mechanisms or their adaptive tuning. In other words, nystagmus occurs due to disturbances in the sensory or motor systems responsible for neuromuscular coordination of the extraocular muscles, which in turn provides a steady fixation under normal circumstances. The retina, the vestibular system and the proprioceptive endorgans of the cervical musculature constitute the essential sensory system; the motor system being the extrinsic ocular muscles innervated by the oculomotor cranial nerves. The cerebellum controls the muscle tone and facilitates the smooth operation of the reflex responses involved.

CLASSIFICATION

Many classifications have been proposed for the nystagmus, and so, the reader will find different classifications in different books. It is important to note here that the terms motor and sensory nystagmus are no longer being considered. National Eye Institute Workshop has developed a new classification in 2001 called the classification of eye movement abnormalities and strabismus (CEMAS). In this volume, a simple classification has been adopted by slightly modifying CEMAS as below:

A. *Physiological nystagmus*
1. Optokinetic nystagmus
2. Endpoint nystagmus
3. Physiological vestibular nystagmus

B. *Pathological nystagmus*

I. *Nystagmus occurring in infancy*

1. Infantile nystagmus syndrome (includes old names such as 'congenital', 'motor', 'sensory', idiopathic and nystagmus blockage)
2. Fusion maldevelopment nystagmus syndrome (old names "latent, manifest latent," nystagmus blockage)
3. Spasmus nutans syndrome
   - Without optic pathway glioma
   - With optic pathway glioma

II. *Acquired nystagmus.* This group includes various forms of nystagmus acquired after infancy, which can be further classified as follows:

1. *Nystagmus due to disorders of visual fixations.* (vision loss nystagmus)
   - Prechiasmal
   - Chiasmal
   - Postchiasmal

2. *Nystagmus caused by vestibular imbalance*
   i. Peripheral vestibular imbalance, e.g. Menière and drug toxicity nystagmus
   ii. Central vestibular imbalance
       - Downbeat
       - Upbeat
       - Torsional
       - Horizontal
   iii. Instability of vestibular mechanisms periodic alternating nystagmus

3. *Nystagmus due to disorders of gaze holding*
   - Gaze-evoked nystagmus

- Dissociated nystagmus (ataxic nystagmus)
- Bruns' nystagmus
- Convergence-retraction nystagmus
- Centripetal and rebound nystagmus

4. *Acquired pendular nystagmus*
  - Central myelin
  - Oculopalatal
  - Whipple
  - Drug toxicity

Note. Only a very brief account of the various types of nystagmus is given here just as a passing reference. For detailed accounts, the readers should consult certain standard textbooks on neuro-ophthalmology.

PHYSIOLOGICAL NYSTAGMUS

1. **Optokinetic nystagmus.** It is a physiological jerk nystagmus induced by presenting to gaze the objects moving serially in one direction; such as strips of a spinning optokinetic drum. The eyes will follow a fixed strip momentarily and then jerk back to reposition centrally to fix up a new strip. Similar condition occurs while looking at outside things from a moving train.

2. **Endpoint nystagmus.** It is a fine jerk horizontal nystagmus seen in normal persons on extreme right or left gaze.

3. **Physiological vestibular nystagmus.** It is a jerk nystagmus which can be elicited by stimulating the tympanic membrane with hot or cold water. It forms the basis of caloric test. If cold water is poured into right ear, the patient develops left jerk nystagmus (rapid phase towards left) while the reverse happens with warm water, i.e. patient develops right jerk nystagmus. It can be remembered by the mnemonic COWS (Cold Opposite, Warm-Same).

PATHOLOGICAL NYSTAGMUS

I. NYSTAGMUS OCCURRING IN INFANCY

The three most common forms of nystagmus seen in childhood begin in infancy and are, therefore, not congenital. These include:
1. Infantile nystagmus syndrome
2. Fusion maldevelopment nystagmus syndrome
3. Spasmus nutans syndrome

1. Infantile nystagmus syndrome

Infantile nystagmus syndrome (INS) is the new name given in the CEMAS system for the old 'congenital nystagmus, motor and sensory nystagmus'.

Etiology. It may be: (I) *idiopathic* or (II) *associated with sensory deprivation* due to any of the following causes:

- *Ocular albinism*, characterized by iris transillumination defects and foveal hypoplasia.
- *Aniridia,* i.e. bilateral near total congenital iris absence.
- *Leber's congenital amaurosis*, characterized by markedly abnormal or flat electroretinogram.
- *Other causes* include, bilateral congenital cataract, achromatopsia, congenital stationary night blindness, bilateral optic nerve hypoplasia, bilateral congenital toxoplasmosis and bilateral macular hypoplasia.

Characteristic features. It is characterized by erratic waveform with or without roving eye movement associated with reduced visual acuity due to above mentioned conditions.

CEMAS criteria for INS is summarized below:
- Infantile onset
- Ocular motor recordings show diagnostic (accelerating) slow phases
- Waveforms may change in early infancy
- Head posture usually evident by 4 years of age
- Vision prognosis dependent on integrity of sensory system.

Symbolic recording of an idiopathic case of INS is shown in Fig. 28.4.

Common associated findings
- Conjugate, horizontal-torsional, increases with fixation attempt
- Progression from pendular to jerk
- Family history often positive
- With or without associated sensory system deficits (e.g. albinism, achromatopsia) associated strabismus or refractive error
- Null and neutral zones present
- Associated head posture or head shaking may exhibit a "latent" component, "reversal" with OKN stimulus or periodicity to the oscillation.
- May decrease with induced convergence, increased fusion, extraocular muscle surgery, contact lenses, and sedation.

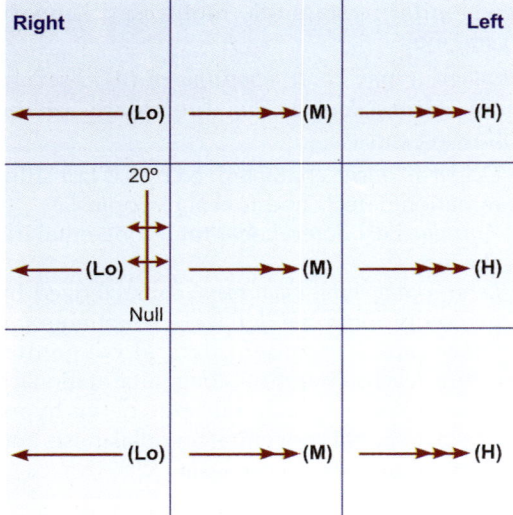

Fig. 28.4 *Symbolic recording of a case of idiopathic infantile nystagmus syndrome (INS) depicting left beating horizontal jerk nystagmus of medium amplitude and moderate frequency in primary position. Intensity of nystagmus increases in left gaze and decreases in right gaze. There is null zone in right gaze with pendular waveform.*

2. Fusion maldevelopment nystagmus syndrome

Fusion maldevelopment nystagmus syndrome (FMNS) is the new name for the old term-latent/latent manifest nystagmus as described in CEMAS.

Characteristic features

CEMAS criteria for FMNS are summarized below:

- Infantile onset
- Associated strabismus
- Ocular motor recordings show two types of slow phases (linear and decelerating) plus high-frequency
- Low-amplitude pendular nystagmus (dual-jerk waveform), jerk in direction of fixing eye
- Intensity decreases with age
- Nystagmus is not present, when both eyes are open. It appears when one eye is covered. It is a jerk nystagmus with rapid phase towards the uncovered eye
- While testing visual acuity in such patients, one eye should be fogged (by adding plus lenses in front) rather than occluding to minimize induction of latent nystagmus.
- May be associated with congenital esotropia and dissociated vertical deviation (DVD).
- Becomes manifest under monocular viewing conditions, i.e. in the presence of decreased vision in one eye as in anisometropic amblyopia, strabismic amblyopia, etc.

Symbolic recording of a case of FMNS is shown in Fig. 28.5.

Common associated findings

Conjugate, horizontal, uniplanar; usually no associated sensory system deficits (e.g. albinism, achromatopsia), may change with exaggerated convergence ("blockage"), head posture associated with fixing eye in adduction, no head shaking, may exhibit "reversal" with OKN stimulus, no periodicity to the oscillation. Dissociated strabismus may be present. Decreases with increased fusion (binocular function).

3. Spasmus nutans syndrome

Spasmus nutans syndrome (SNS) is the 3rd most common nystagmus seen in infancy.

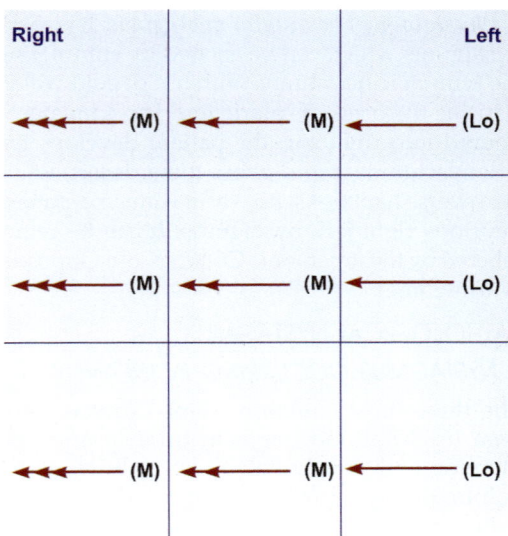

Fig. 28.5 *Symbolic recording of a case of fusion maldevelopment nystagmus syndrome (FMNS) depicting right beating horizontal jerk nystagmus of medium amplitude and moderate frequency. Intensity of the nystagmus increases in the right gaze and decreases in left gaze.*

Characteristic features

CEMAS criteria for SNS are as follows:

- Infantile onset
- Variable conjugacy, small-frequency, low-amplitude oscillation
- Abnormal head posture and head oscillation, improves (disappears) during childhood
- Normal MRI/CT scan of visual pathways
- Ocular motility recordings—high-frequency (>10 Hz), asymmetric, variable conjugacy, pendular oscillations
- Usually, spontaneously remits clinically in 2 to 8 years, remains present with eye movement recordings.

Common associated findings

Dysconjugate, asymmetric, multiplanar, family history of strabismus, may be greater in one (abducting) eye, constant, head posture/oscillation (horizontal or vertical), usually no associated sensory system deficits may have associated strabismus and amblyopia, may increase with convergence, head bobbing, head posture may be compensatory; normal fundus exam; decreases with increased fusion (binocular function).

II. ACQUIRED NYSTAGMUS

Nystagmus associated with diseases of the visual system

As mentioned in pathogenesis, fixation disorders can lead to nystagmus. The smooth visual fixation mechanism stops the eyes from drifting away from a stationary object of regard. This fixation mechanism depends upon the motion detection (magnocellular) portion of the visual system which is inherently slow, with a response time of about 100 milliseconds that encumbers all visually mediated eye movements, including fixation, smooth pursuit, and optokinetic responses. If the response time is delayed further by disease of the visual system, then the attempts by the brain to correct eye drifts leads to ocular oscillations.

Vision is also needed for recalibrating and optimizing all types of eye movements. These functions depend on visual projections to the cerebellum. Thus, signals go from secondary visual areas concerned with motion-vision project via the pontine nuclei and middle cerebellar peduncle to the cerebellum. For calibration of the ocular motor system, visual signals are compared with eye movement commands. At present, it is not certain how or where this function is performed. A group of cells in the paramedian tracts (PMT) in the lower pons have been suggested as a probable center.

Diseases affecting any part of the visual system, from retina to cortical visual areas, or interrupting visual projections to pons and cerebellum, may be associated with nystagmus.

Clinical features of nystagmus with lesions affecting the visual pathways

Disease of the retina

Congenital or acquired retinal disorders causing blindness, such as Leber's congenital amaurosis, lead to continuous jerk nystagmus with components in all three planes, which changes direction over the course of seconds or minutes. This is due to inability to calibrate the ocular motor system. This nystagmus often shows the increasing-velocity waveform earlier thought to be specific for congenital nystagmus.

Disease affecting the optic nerves

Optic nerve disease is associated with pendular nystagmus. With unilateral disease of the optic nerve, nystagmus affects the abnormal eye. The nystagmus has vertical, low-frequency, bidirectional drifts (pendular), unidirectional horizontal drifts with corrective quick-phases (jerk) are less common. When disease affects both optic nerves, the amplitude of nystagmus is greater in the eye with poorer vision (Heimann-Biels-Chowsky phenomenon). In infants, a monocular, vertical pendular nystagmus could be due to optic nerve tumor and thus, neuroimaging studies should be performed.

Disease affecting the optic chiasma

Parasellar lesions such as pituitary tumors that affect the chiasma are associated with see-saw nystagmus. See-saw nystagmus has two types—pendular and jerk. Pendular see-saw is seen in lesions of optic chiasma. It is because of the fact that, crossed visual inputs are important for optimizing vertical-torsional eye movements and if interrupted, lead to see-saw oscillations.

Disease affecting the postchiasmal visual system

Horizontal nystagmus is seen in patients with unilateral disease of the cerebral hemispheres. This nystagmus has constant-velocity slow phases toward the intact hemisphere and quick phases directed toward the side of the lesion, which are low amplitude. There is also asymmetry of horizontal smooth pursuit, with decreased response towards the side of the lesion.

Acquired pendular nystagmus

Acquired pendular nystagmus is one of the most common forms of nystagmus associated with disease affecting the visual system or its brainstem-cerebellar projections and is associated with distressing visual symptoms. Its pathogenesis is not entirely clear with more than one mechanism responsible.

Features: Acquired pendular nystagmus has horizontal, vertical, and torsional components with the same frequency, although one component may predominate. (In congenital pendular nystagmus, the oscillation usually is predominantly horizontal.) Depending on the phase difference between various directions, a pendular nystagmus may be oblique if the horizontal and vertical oscillatory components are in phase), elliptical. (If the horizontal and vertical oscillatory components are out of phase) or circular (phase difference of 90° and equal amplitude of the horizontal and vertical components.) Further, the nystagmus may be conjugate, or may appear convergent-divergent.

The frequency of oscillations ranges from 1 to 8 Hz, with an average value of 3.5 Hz and remains constant for a given patient. Acquired pendular nystagmus may be suppressed or brought out by eyelid closure or evoked by convergence.

Symbolic recording of a case of acquired pendular nystagmus is shown in Fig. 28.6.

Conditions associated with acquired pendular nystagmus are:

• Visual loss (including unilateral disease of the optic nerve)
• Disorders of central myelin, such as:
 – Multiple sclerosis
 – Pelizaeus-Merzbacher disease

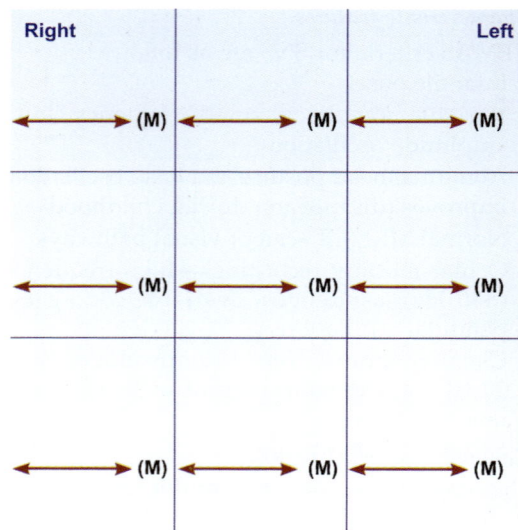

Fig. 28.6 *Symbolic recording of a case of horizontal acquired pendular nystagmus of a low amplitude and moderate frequency.*

 – Peroxisomal assembly disorders
 – Cockayne's syndrome
 – Toluene abuse
• Oculopalatal myoclonus
• Acute brainstem stroke
• Whipple's disease
• Spinocerebellar degenerations
• Congenital nystagmus

Nystagmus caused by vestibular imbalance

Nystagmus related to imbalance in the vestibular pathway can be caused by damage to peripheral or central structures.

Nystagmus caused by peripheral vestibular imbalance

Disease affecting the peripheral vestibular pathway (i.e. the labyrinth, vestibular nerve, and its root entry zone) causes nystagmus with linear slow phases, which reflect an imbalance in the level of tonic neural activity in the vestibular nuclei. The slow phase of the lesion is towards the side of the lesion. Gaze in the direction of the fast component increases the nystagmus intensity, and gaze in the direction of the slow component decreases the intensity (Alexander's law). An imbalance of vestibular tone also causes vertigo and a tendency to fall towards the side of the lesion. The nystagmus is suppressed by visual fixation and sometimes may only become apparent, when visual fixation is prevented. This is because in presence of normal visual functions, the calibration mechanisms discussed above prevent the drifting of eyes.

Vestibular nystagmus is categorized as follows:
- *First degree*— if it is present only on looking in the direction of the quick phases.
- *Second degree*— if it is also present in the central position.
- *Third degree*— if it is present on looking in all directions of gaze.

Pure vertical or pure torsional nystagmus. almost never occur with peripheral vestibular disease.

Diagnosis of specific types of peripheral vestibular nystagmus can be aided by observing the effect of head position on nystagmus as below:
- Complete unilateral labyrinthine destruction leads to a mixed horizontal-torsional nystagmus
- In benign paroxysmal positional vertigo (BPPV), a mixed upbeat-torsional nystagmus reflecting posterior semicircular canal stimulation is seen.
- Patients with dehiscence of the superior semicircular canal develop vestibular symptoms and nystagmus, when exposed to certain sounds (Tullio's phenomenon).

Peripheral vestibular nystagmus induced by caloric or galvanic stimulation
During caloric stimulation, a temperature gradient across the temporal bone induces a convection current in the endolymph of a semicircular canal, if it is orientated vertical to the earth:
- The subject is placed supine and the neck is flexed at 30°.
- A cold stimulus (30°C) induces horizontal slow phase components directed towards the stimulated ear (quick phases in the opposite direction).
- A warm stimulus (44°C) and the same head orientation, quick phases are towards the stimulated ear (mnemonic, COWS: Cold-Opposite, Warm-Same).

Symbolic recording of a case of peripheral vestibular nystagmus is depicted in Fig. 28.7.

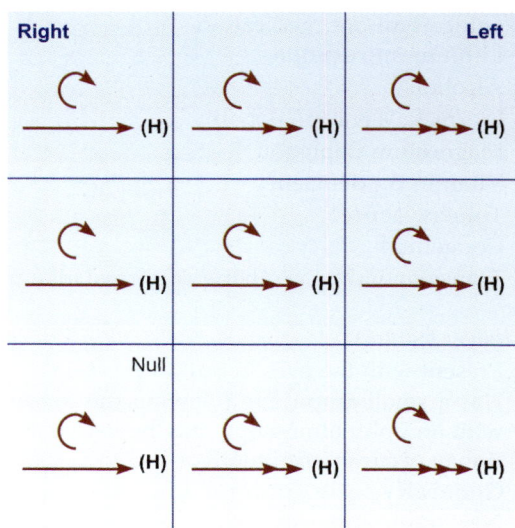

Fig. 28.7 *Symbolic recording of a case of peripheral vertibular nystagmus depicting left beating mixed horizontal jerk and rotary waveform caused by a right-sided lesion. Intensity of the nystagmus increases to the left (i.e. away from the site of lesion) and decreases to the right (i.e. towards the site of lesion).*

Nystagmus caused by central vestibular imbalance

Imbalance of central vestibular connections commonly leads to downbeat, upbeat, and torsional nystagmus.

Downbeat nystagmus

Causes

- Downbeat nystagmus is usually associated with lesions that effect the excitatory projections from posterior semicircular canals, sites include vestibulocerebellum, flocculus, paraflocculus, nodulus and uvula and the underlying medulla
- Cerebellar degeneration, including familial episodic ataxia, and paraneoplastic degeneration.
- Craniocervical anomalies, including Arnold-Chiari malformation
- Infarction of brainstem or cerebellum
- Dolichoectasia of the vertebrobasilar artery
- Multiple sclerosis
- Cerebellar tumor
- Syringobulbia
- Head trauma

- Anticonvulsant medication
- Lithium intoxication
- Alcohol
- Wernicke's encephalopathy
- Magnesium depletion
- Vitamin B$_{12}$ deficiency
- Toluene abuse
- Congenital
- Transient finding in otherwise normal infants.

Clinical features

- Present with the eyes in central position.
- Has a small amplitude (viewing the fundus with an ophthalmoscope may be necessary). It may occur intermittently.
- Generally, Alexander's law is obeyed: Nystagmus intensity is greatest in downgaze and least in upgaze.
- The waveform is linear, but it may be increasing in velocity.
- Downbeat nystagmus may be evoked by placing the patient in a head-hanging position.
- Convergence may influence the amplitude and frequency of the nystagmus or convert it to upbeat nystagmus.
- Other ocular motor abnormalities accompany downbeat nystagmus and reflect coincident cerebellar involvement.
- Vertical smooth pursuit and the vertical VOR are abnormal because of impaired ability to generate smooth downward eye movements.
- Impairment of eccentric horizontal gaze-holding, smooth pursuit, and combined eye-head tracking.
- The visual consequences of downbeat nystagmus are oscillopsia and postural instability.

Symbolic recording of a case of downbeat nystagmus is shown in Fig. 28.8.

Upbeat nystagmus

Causes

- Upbeat nystagmus is most commonly seen in patients with lesions affecting excitatory connections from the anterior semicircular canals. These include:
  - The perihypoglossal nuclei and adjacent medial vestibular nucleus (structures important for gaze-holding).

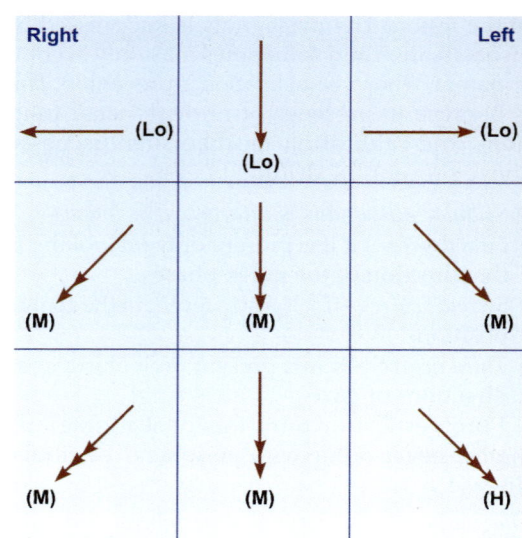

Fig. 28.8 *Symbolic recording of a case of downbeat nystagmus in primary position with a superimposed horizontal gaze-evoked nystagmus. Intensity of downbeat nystagmus increases in downgaze and laterally. Oblique trajectory shown in lateral gaze is due to superimposed horizontal gaze-evolved nystagmus.*

  - Ventral tegmentum (containing projections from the vestibular nuclei that receive inputs from the anterior semicircular canals)
  - Caudal medulla
  - Anterior vermis of the cerebellum
  - Brachium conjunctivum and midbrain
- Cerebellar degenerations, including familial episodic ataxia
- Leber's congenital amaurosis or other congenital disorder of the anterior visual pathways
- Infarction of medulla, midbrain, or cerebellum
- Tumors of the medulla, midbrain, or cerebellum
- Wernicke's encephalopathy
- Brainstem encephalitis
- Behçet's syndrome
- Meningitis
- Multiple sclerosis
- Thalamic arteriovenous malformation
- Organophosphate poisoning
- Tobacco
- Associated with middle ear disease
- Congenital
- Transient finding in otherwise normal infants

Clinical features

- It is present with the eyes close to central position.
- Nystagmus intensity is usually greatest in upgaze.
- It does not increase on right or left gaze.
- Removal of visual fixation has little influence on slow-phase velocity.
- Convergence can enhance, suppress, or convert upbeat nystagmus to downbeat.
- Placing the patient in a head-hanging position increases the nystagmus in some individuals.
- There are asymmetries of vertical vestibular and smooth pursuit eye movements, as well as associated cerebellar eye movement findings.

Torsional nystagmus

Causes

- Syringobulbia
- Brainstem stroke (Wallenberg's syndrome) or arteriovenous malformation
- Brainstem tumor
- Multiple sclerosis
- Oculopalatal myoclonus
- Head trauma
- Congenital
- Associated with the ocular tilt reaction

Clinical features

- Least common form of central vestibular nystagmus.
- It is difficult to detect and requires careful observation of conjunctival vessels or noting the direction of retinal movement on either side of the fovea.
- Modulation by head rotations is similar to upbeat and downbeat nystagmus.
- There are variable slow-phase waveforms
- Convergence suppresses the nystagmus.

Periodic alternating nystagmus

Causes

Periodic alternating nystagmus (PAN) does not fall in a single pathological category. It occurs in lesions affecting the cerebellum most notably nodulus and uvula. These areas determine the eye velocity of nystagmus seen after rotation (both VOR and OKN). Their destruction leads to un-inhibited, prolonged vestibular impulses which leads to nystagmus.

Clinical features

- Spontaneous horizontal nystagmus, present in central gaze.
- Reverses direction approximately every 90–120 seconds.
- Acquired PAN has the same characteristics in light or in darkness.
- Smooth pursuit and optokinetic nystagmus are usually impaired.

See-saw and hemi-see-saw nystagmus

Causes

Jerk see-saw nystagmus (hemi-see-saw nystagmus) occurs in patients with lesions in the region of the interstitial nucleus of Cajal (INC). The associated ocular tilt reaction is due to an imbalance of central otolithic projections from vestibular nuclei to the INC.

Clinical features

- One-half-cycle consists of elevation and intorsion of one eye and synchronous depression and extorsion of the other eye. In the next half-cycle, the vertical and torsional movements reverse (Fig. 28.9).
- The waveform may be pendular or jerk. Some authorities label the pendular form as see-saw and jerk form as hemi-see-saw.
- See-saw nystagmus may be congenital, or acquired.
- Patients often have a contralateral ocular tilt reaction.
- With a right-sided lesion, the reaction consists of a left head tilt, a skew deviation with a right hypertropia, tonic intorsion of the right eye and extorsion of the left eye, and misperception that earth—vertical is tilted to the left.

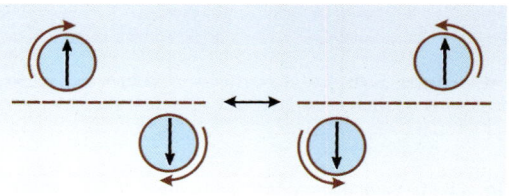

Fig. 28.9 *Symbolic recording of a case of see-saw nystagmus (for explanation see text).*

Nystagmus due to abnormalities of the mechanism for holding eccentric gaze

Gaze-evoked nystagmus

Nystagmus that is induced by turning the eye to an eccentric position in the orbit is called gaze-evoked nystagmus. It is the most common form of nystagmus encountered in clinical practice. Gaze-evoked nystagmus is a general term that includes both physiologic and pathologic nystagmus. When the nystagmus is physiologic, the term endpoint nystagmus should be used. When the nystagmus is associated with a paresis of gaze, e.g. ocular motor nerve palsies or weakness of the extraocular muscles, the term gaze-paretic nystagmus is appropriate.

- Gaze-evoked nystagmus usually occurs on lateral (Fig. 28.10) or upward gaze, seldom on looking down.
- Waveform is dependent on effect of fixation.
- If fixation is impaired the slow phases consist of exponentially decaying waveform.
- If visual fixation is possible, however, the slow phase has a linear profile.

To hold gaze at an eccentric position, the elastic force of the fascia and ligaments has to be overcome. This is achieved by a tonic contraction of the extraocular muscles. The neural signal involved in this contraction has been termed 'step', that is generated by the gaze-holding network, also called the neural integrator. This network includes the vestibulo-cerebellum, the medial vestibular nucleus and adjacent nucleus prepositus hypoglossy in the medulla, and the interstitial nucleus of Cajal (INC) in the midbrain.

Etiology. Gaze-evoked nystagmus is caused by a deficient step, so that the eyes cannot be maintained at an eccentric orbital position and are pulled back toward central position by the elastic forces of the orbital fascia. Corrective quick phases then move the eyes back towards the desired position in the orbit.

Additionally, lesions that produce gaze-evoked nystagmus also impair visual fixation and smooth pursuit.

Causes of gaze-evoked nystagmus include:
- Medications, including alcohol, anticonvulsants and sedatives.
- Structural lesions that damage the gaze-holding neural network.
- Nucleus prepositus hypoglossi/medial vestibular nucleus region.
- Interstitial nucleus of Cajal.
- Rarely, cerebellar lesions.
- Familial episodic ataxia type 2 (EA 2), which also has attack of ataxia and vertigo.

Endpoint nystagmus is a gaze-evoked nystagmus encountered in normal subjects. It typically occurs on looking far laterally and is poorly sustained. The nystagmus is primarily horizontal. It is usually symmetric. Differentiating features from a pathological nystagmus are that this nystagmus has lower intensity (i.e. slower drift) and is not accompanied by other ocular motor abnormalities.

Dissociated nystagmus (ataxic nystagmus): It is a special type of pathologic gaze-evoked nystagmus, most commonly associated with an internuclear ophthalmoplegia (INO). Dissociated nystagmus includes a series of saccades followed by postsaccadic drift that occurs, when the patient attempts to look laterally away from the side of the lesion. Since the saccades initiate the oscillations, this is not a true nystagmus. It

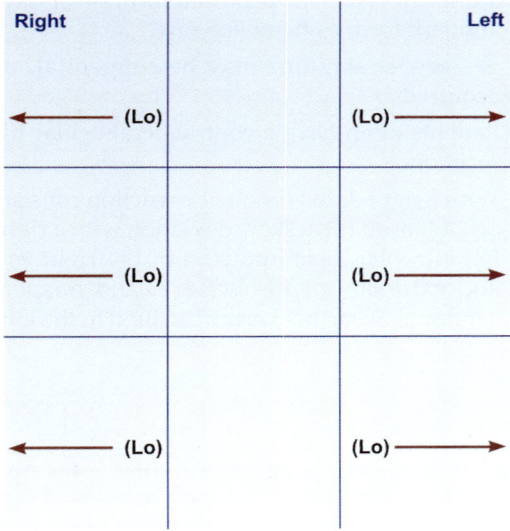

Fig. 28.10 *Symbolic recording of a case of bilateral gaze-evoked nystagmus. Note horizontal jerk nystagmus of small amplitude and low-frequency with fast phase in the direction of gaze.*

represents an attempt by the brain to adaptively correct hypometric saccades due to the weak medial rectus muscle, which because of Hering's law of equal innervation leads increase in the innervation to the normal, abducting eye, thereby resulting in overshooting saccades and postsaccadic drift of the normal eye if the patient attempts to fixate with the diseased eye. Thus, whenever a patient habitually prefers to fixate with a paretic eye, the normal eye, will show a dissociated nystagmus while looking in the direction of action of the paretic muscle, regardless of the pathogenesis of the weakness.

Other causes of dissociated nystagmus are:
- Previous extraocular muscle surgery
- Myasthenia gravis
- Miller Fisher syndrome

Bruns' nystagmus

Tumors in the cerebellopontine angle, produce a low-frequency, large-amplitude nystagmus, when the patient looks toward the side of the lesion, and a high-frequency, small-amplitude nystagmus, when the patient looks toward the side opposite the lesion. The nystagmus that occurs on gaze towards the side of the lesion is gaze-evoked nystagmus caused by defective gaze holding, whereas the nystagmus that occurs during gaze towards the side opposite the lesion is caused by vestibular imbalance. This is called Bruns' nystagmus (Fig. 28.11).

Convergence-retraction nystagmus

It is characterized by quick phases that converge or retract the eyes on attempts to look up. Affected patients usually have impaired or absent upward gaze for both pursuit and saccadic eye movements. It is a saccadic disorder rather than nystagmus because the primary adductive movements are asynchronous saccades. Causes include:
- Lesions of the mesencephalon that damage the posterior commissure, e.g. pineal tumors
- Chiari malformation
- Epileptic seizures

Centripetal and rebound nystagmus

If a patient with gaze-evoked nystagmus attempts to look eccentrically for a sustained period, the nystagmus begins to decrease in

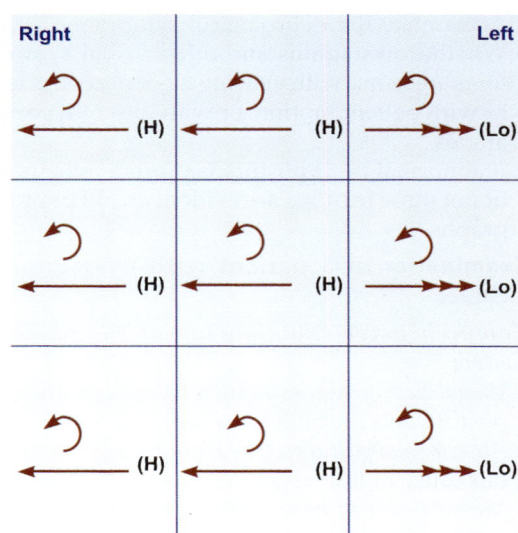

Fig. 28.11 *Symbolic recording of a case of Bruns' nystagmus depicting a high frequency, small amplitude, right beating horizontal and rotary waveform.*

amplitude and may even reverse direction, this is called centripetal nystagmus. If the eyes are then returned to the central position, a short-lived nystagmus with slow drifts in the direction of the prior eccentric gaze occurs. This is called rebound nystagmus. Both centripetal and rebound nystagmus reflect an attempt by brainstem or cerebellar mechanisms to correct for the drift of gaze-evoked nystagmus. Rebound nystagmus occurs in patients with:
- Cerebellar disease
- In normal subjects with typical gaze-evoked nystagmus
- Lateral medullary infarction
- Tumor confined to the flocculus.

CLINICAL EVALUATION, ELECTRO-PHYSIOLOGICAL RECORDING AND NEUROIMAGING

A. CLINICAL EVALUATION

It is often possible to diagnose the cause of nystagmus through careful history and systematic examination of the patient.

History should include:
- Duration of nystagmus
- Whether it interferes with vision and causes oscillopsia

- Accompanying neurological symptoms
- Whether nystagmus and other visual symptoms are worse with viewing far or near objects, or with patient motion, or with different gaze angles.
- If abnormal head posture is present, whether or not these features are evident on old photographs.

Examination of a patient with nystagmus include:

Comprehensive examination of the visual system

- *Visual acuity* assessment with and without posture and for both near and distance
- *Anterior and posture segment examination* to rule out cause of low vision. Especially look for
- *Measurement of head posture.* All the components of head posture, i.e. face turn, chin elevation or depression and head tilt should be noted. Face turn can be measured using the Goniometer (Fig. 28.12) or by simply using a scale and a protractor.

Systematic examination of each functional class of eye movements (vestibular, optokinetic, smooth-pursuit, saccades, vergence) and their effect on nystagmus.

Examination of nystagmus in a systematic manner. It is essential to have a mental checklist during clinical examination. **ABCDEF** is a suggested pneumonic for systematic examination of nystagmus where:

    A is amplitude
    B is basic shape or waveform
    C is conjugacy
    D is direction
    E is effect of gaze position and fixation. For example:

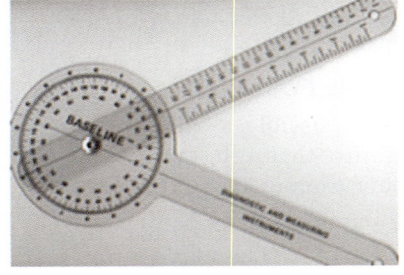

Fig. 28.12 *Goniometer: An orthopaedic instrument which can be used to measure face turn.*

- The stability of fixation (with the eyes close to primary position) viewing near and far targets, and at eccentric gaze angles.
- In patients with head turn or tilt, the eye should be observed in various directions of gaze, when the head is in that position as well as when the head is held straight.
- During fixation, occlude each eye in turn to check for latent nystagmus.
- The effect of removal of fixation (with Frenzelor high-plus spherical lenses).

F is frequency.

Note. Details of the features of nystagmus and method of their clinical documentation has been described earlier (page 297–299).

B. *ELECTROPHYSIOLOGICAL RECORDING OF EYE MOVEMENTS*

Electrophysiological recording of ocular motility has provided a new basis for eye movement abnormality classification, etiology and treatment. Only salient features of some of the techniques available for ocular motility recordings are mentioned here.

1. Electro-oculography

Electro-oculography (EOG) is based on the measurement of resting potential of the eye which exists between the cornea (+ve) and back of the retina (–ve).

Technique of recording is shown in Figs 28.13 A and B. Electrodes are placed over the orbital margin near the medial and lateral canthi serve as *active electrodes* (E1–E4 in Fig. 28.13A). A forehead electrode serves as a *ground electrode* or indifferent electrodes (E5 in Fig. 28.13A).

Salient features

- Horizontal range of measurement of 1 to 40° with a resolution of 1°.
- Useful for horizontal and some vertical movements.
- A bitnoisy–1°.
- Best clinical all-rounder with good electrodes.

2. Electronystagmography

Electronystagmography (ENG) is an adaption of electro-oculography (EOG). For ENG like EOG (Fig. 28.13) a ground electrode is attached to the forehead and three recording electrodes

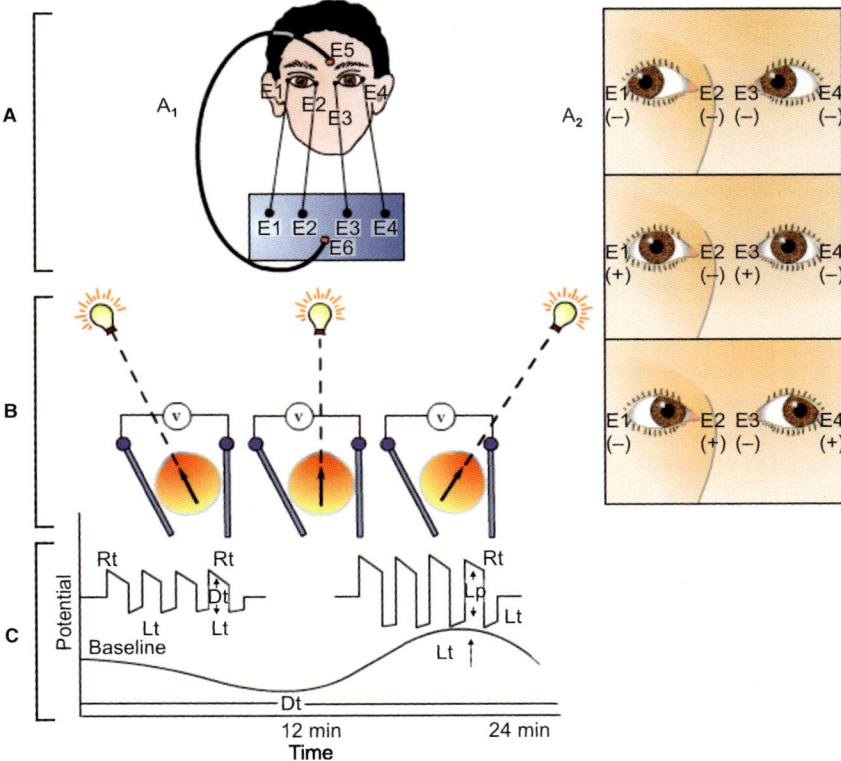

Fig. 28.13 *Technique of recording electro-oculogram:* (A) *Position of electrodes;* (B) *Ocular movements during recording.*

are placed one each to the side, above and below each eye which measure the eye movement.

Tests performed with ENG include:

- *Oculomotor tests*. ENG is used to record nystagmus during oculomotor tests such as saccades, pursuit and gaze testing and optokinetics. Abnormal oculomotor test results may indicate either systemic or central pathology as opposed to peripheral (vestibular) pathology.

- *Positional testing* is performed to see the effect of head or body movements on the eye movements.

- *Caloric test* is performed to assess the vestibular system.

3. Binocular infrared reflectance oculography (BIRO)

- Useful for horizontal and some vertical movements.

- Has a restricted range.
- Noise–0.1°

4. Electromagnetic scleral search coil method

- Useful for horizontal, vertical and torsional movements.
- Good resolution and frequency response.
- Requires mind bending mathematical analysis.
- Eye has to be anesthetized and a thick silicone lens is needed.
- Expensive.

5. Videonystagmography

Videonystagmography (VNG) is a sophisticated technique in which nystagmus is recorded with the help of the infrared video camera which is incorporated in the specially designed infrared camera goggles (worm by the patient during the recording technique (Fig. 28.14). A very sensi-

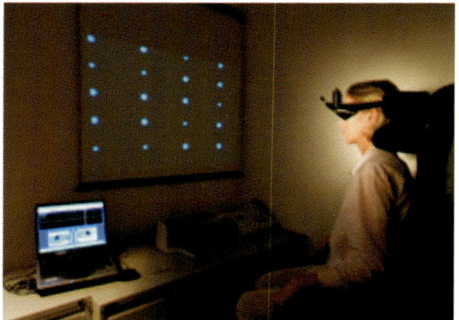

Fig. 28.14 *Technique of videonystagmography with infrared goggles worn by the patient.*

tive head movement sensors are also incorporated in it.

Tests performed with VNG. Similar to ENG, there are three parts of VNG testing:

- Ocular and optokinetic testing
- Positional nystagmus testing, and
- Caloric testing

Advantages of VNG over ENG

- *Less combursome* and less time-consuming as electrodes are not required.
- *Direct observation* of video images of eye movements available.
- *Simultaneous comparison* of waveform can be performed.
- *Computerized record* allows storage, processing and analysis.
- *Provides more information than ENG.* In addition to information about amplitude, frequency and intensity obtained from ENG; the VNG also provides information about slow phase velocity and foveation window with the help of intrinsic software.

Clinical uses of eye movement recording

Important clinical uses of eye movement recording are as follows:

- Identifies much congenital type nystagmus on the basis of waveform.
- Allows classification of acquired nystagmus with greater certainty.
- Measures slowness of saccades which can be diagnostic, e.g. internuclear ophthalmoplegia.
- Allows observation of motility in darkness (vestibular nystagmus).

- Allows temporal resolution of very fast eye movements such as flutter, opsoclonus, convergence nystagmus, dysmetria which are difficult to evaluate with the naked eye.
- Trains one to interpret what is 'seen'.

C. NEUROIMAGING

Neuroimaging is indicated to find out associated CNS abnormalities especially in patients with acquired nystagmus, periodic alternating nystagmus, see-saw nystagmus, spasmus nutans syndrome and infantile nystagmus syndrome with pallor disc and poor vision.

TREATMENT OF NYSTAGMUS
Aims of treatment

- To improve *visual acuity* by stabilizing the eyes
- To shift the *null zone*, if any, in the primary position, i.e. to reduce abnormal head posture.
- To correct the associated *strabismus*.
- To decrease any *oscillopsia* wherever possible.

Treatment modalities

Treatment modalities for nystagmus include:

- Optical
- Medical
- Surgical

I. OPTICAL TREATMENT

1. *Correction of refractive error* may sometimes significantly decrease nystagmus, especially in patients with bilateral aphakia. Although refraction is difficult in the presence of nystagmus but every effort should be made to correct any significant refractive error. Retinoscopy may be performed in null zone, whenever, it is present. Further, contact lenses are more useful than the spectacles (especially in high myopes), since these move with the movement of eye and so the visual axes always coincide with their optical axes. In addition to optical advantage, a tactile feedback from the contact lenses have also been reported to decrease the nystagmus.

2. *Stimulating accommodative convergence* by over correcting minus lenses may improve visual acuity at distance fixation by dampening the nystagmus.

3. *Prismotherapy* in nystagmus may be useful as follows:

i. *Base-out prisms* may stimulate fusional convergence (especially in patients with congenital motor nystagmus) and thus improve the visual acuity by dampening the nystagmus.

ii. *Prisms with base opposite to preferred* direction of gaze may be helpful in correcting the head posture. For example, in a patient with head turn to the left, the null zone is in dextro-version and a prism base-in before the right eye and base-out before the left eye will be helpful in correcting the abnormal head posture (Fig. 28.15).

Similarly, the appropriate prisms can also be used to correct the vertical and oblique head turns. Because of optical disadvantages, the long-term use of prisms incorrecting the head posture is discouraged. However, on the basis of patient's response to prismotherapy, the results of surgery for head turn can be predicted.

4. *Galilean arrangement of contact lenses and glasses* (optical device by Rushton and Cox) can be used to stabilize the retinal images in patients with acquired nystagmus and oscillopsia.

II. MEDICAL TREATMENT

1. *Cyclopentolate* used as 1% eye-drops twice a day has been reported to reduce the amplitude, velocity and frequency of latent nystagmus in about 60% of patients.

2. *Botulinum toxin* injected into the retrobulbar space (dose 10–25 U in 0.1–1 ml) every 3–4 months has been reported to dampen nystagmus and improve visual acuity in patients with acquired nystagmus and oscillopsia.

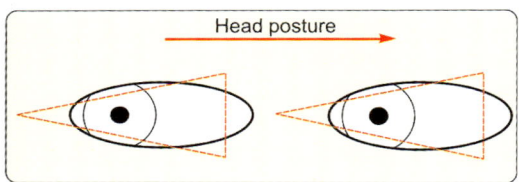

Fig. 28.15 *Use of prism to correct head posture (for explanation see text).*

3. *Baclofen* has been observed to suppress the acquired periodic alternating nystagmus. The initial recommended dose is 5 mg TDS, which in case of no response can be increased stepwise every 3 days to a maximum of 80 mg/day.

4. *Clonazepam* may be useful in patients with downbeat nystagmus.

5. *Carbamazepine* is useful in superior oblique myokymia.

6. *Propranolol* is reported to be effective for opsoclonus.

III. SURGICAL TREATMENT

Indications

1. To eliminate abnormal head posture by shifting the null point.

2. To decrease the intensity of nystagmus in patients having no abnormal head posture.

3. Both of the above.

Important points to be considered while planning surgery for nystagmus are as follows:

1. Surgical intervention is useful in patients with congenital motor nystagmus and nystagmus blockage syndrome.

2. Surgery should be performed, only if the abnormal head posture causes a significant cosmetic disturbance, i.e. when head turn—or tilts more than 15°.

3. Surgery should always be performed after the age of 5–6 years; since spontaneous improvement in abnormal head posture can occur in some cases up to this age.

General principles of surgery

1. The null point needs to be shifted in primary position. For this, the eyes should always be moved in the same direction as the abnormal head posture.

2. In the presence of strabismus and an abnormal head posture due to nystagmus, the head position can be corrected only by operating on the fixing eye.

3. Surgical therapy should be based on the greatest amount of abnormal head position that is measured at distance.

NYSTAGMUS LIKE OCULAR MOTOR OSCILLATIONS

Nystagmus like oscillations can be described as below:

- Inappropriate saccades
- Voluntary saccadic oscillation 'nystagmus'
- Roving eye movements

Inappropriate Saccades

Involuntary inappropriate saccades include:

Saccadic Intrusion's

These are basically transient breaks in fixation. These may occurs as:

- *Square wave jerks.* These are small amplitude conjugate saccades (<5°) which moves the eye away from fixation and back again (Fig. 28.16A).
- *Square wave pulse* also known as *macro-square wave jerk* have a large ampitude (>5°) and a shorter intersaccadic latency (100–150 ms) (Fig. 28.16B). They are usually and indication of neurological malfunction.

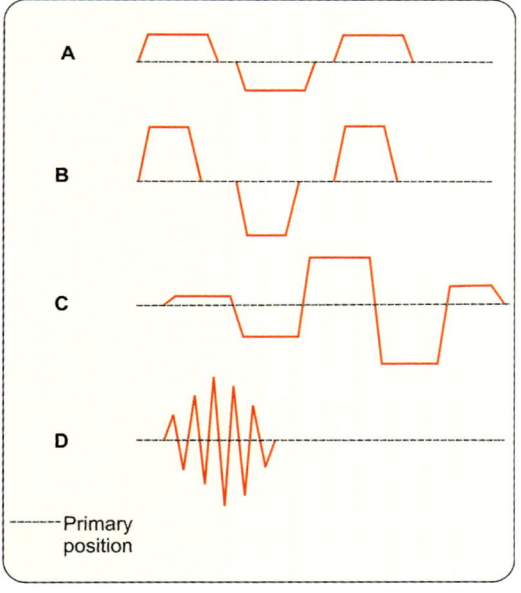

Fig. 28.16 *Inappropriate saccades:* A, *Square wave jerk;* B, *Macro-square wave jerks;* C, *Macro-saccadic oscillations;* and D, *Ocular flutter.*

Saccadic Oscillation

These movments oscillate across fixation and usually have amplitude large than 5°. Saccadic oscillations are of following types:

- *Macro-saccadic oscillation.* They have a similar intersaccadic latency to square wave jerk (Fig. 28.16C). They can reliably distinguished from ocular flutter only by eye movement recording.
- *Ocular flutter* occurs due to interruption of cerebellar connection to brainstem. It is characterized by horizontal oscillation and inability to fixate after change of gaze. Ocular flutter represent back to back horizontal scaddes without any interscaddic latency (Fig. 28.16D)
- *Opsoclonus* refers to combined horizontal, vertical and/or torsional oscillations associated with myoclonic movement of face, arms and legs. It is seen in patient with encephalitis. Opsoclonus has a similar waveform to ocular flutter but is multidirection and associated with ossilopsia.
- *Superior oblique myokymia* is characterized by monocular, rapid, intermittent, torsional vertical movements (which are best seen on slit-lamp examination).
- *Ocular bobbing* refers to rapid downward deviation of the eyes with slow updrift. It occurs due to pontine dysfunctions.

Voluntary Saccadic Oscillations 'Nystagmus'

Voluntary saccadic oscillations 'nystagmus' refers to the voluntary, poorly sustained conjugate oscillation of the eyes consisting of rapidly alternating small-amplitude saccades.

Characteristic features. The oscillations are conjugate, usually horizontal and symmetrical, and consist of back-to-back saccades. The oscillations can be sustained only for a matter of seconds; convergence is usually associated with either the initiation or the maintenance of the oscillation. The amplitude of the movement is small and the frequency high. There may be a familial basis for the ability to initiate voluntary 'nystagmus' or it may be learned. Voluntary 'nystagmus' can be readily differentiated from acquired nystagmus and does not require further investigation.

Roving eye movements

Roving eye movements refers to conjugate large amplitude low-frequency horizontal pendular-like movements. The movements are apparent soon after birth and are generally associated with severe anterior visual pathway disease such as Leber's congenital amaurosis and severe forms of bilateral optic nerve hypoplasia. With time the amplitude becomes smaller and a congenital nystagmus waveform may become superimposed on the roving pattern or may replace it.

BIBLIOGRAPHY

1. Abadi RV, Scallan CJ. Ocular oscillation on eccentric gaze. Vis Res 2001;41(22):2895–907.

2. Boman DK, Hotson JR. Smooth pursuit training and disruption: directional differences and nystagmus. Neuro-ophthal 1987;7(4):185–94.

3. Boman DK, Hotson JR. Smooth pursuit training and disruption: directional differences and nystagmus. Neuro-ophthal 1987;7(4):185–94.

4. Cesarelli M, Bifulco P, Loffredo L, et al. Relationship between visual acuity and eye posi-tion variability during foveation in congenital nystagmus. Doc Ophthalmol 2000;101(1):59–72.

5. Dell' Osso LF, Jacobs JB. An expanded nystagmus acuity function: intra- and intersubject prediction of best-corrected visual acuity. Doc Ophthalmol 2002;104(3):249–76.

6. Ettinger U, Kumari V, Crawford TJ, Davis RE, Sharma T, Corr PJ. Reliability of smooth pursuit, fixation, and saccadic eye movements. Psychophysiology 2003;40:620–8.

7. Krauzlis RJ. Recasting the smooth pursuit eye movement system. J Neurophysiol 2004;91:592–603.

29 | ANATOMY AND LESIONS OF FACIAL NERVE

AK Khurana, Indu Khurana, Aruj K Khurana,
Bhawna Khurana

ANATOMY OF FACIAL NERVE

The facial (seventh cranial) nerve is both a motor and sensory nerve.

FUNCTIONAL COMPONENTS

1. *Branchial efferent* for facial expression and elevation of hyoid bone.
2. *General visceral efferent component* is concerned with parasympathetic supply of the lacrimal gland, submandibular and sublingual salivary glands and the nasal, palatine and pharyngeal glands.
3. *Special visceral afferent* for taste sensations from the presulcal area of the tongue and the palate.
4. *General somatic afferent* for sensations from the concha of the auricle.

NUCLEI

The facial nerve has three types of nuclei:

1. Main motor nucleus
2. The parasympathetic nuclei
3. The sensory nucleus.

Main motor nucleus

This lies deep in the reticular formation of the lower part of the pons (Fig. 29.1); in the column of other branchial efferent nuclei (Fig. 29.2). The part of the nucleus that supplies the muscles of the upper part of the face receives corticonuclear fibers from both cerebral hemispheres. The part of the nucleus that supplies the muscles of the lower part of the face receives corticonuclear fibers from the opposite cerebral hemisphere only (Fig. 29.3).

These pathways explain the voluntary control of facial muscles. However, another involuntary pathway exists, which is separate and controls mimetic or *emotional changes in facial expression*. The origin and course of this upper motor neuron pathway is unknown.

Parasympathetic nuclei

These include the superior salivatory and lacrimatory nuclei. These are situated posterolateral to the main motor nucleus in the column of general visceral efferent nuclei (Fig. 29.2).

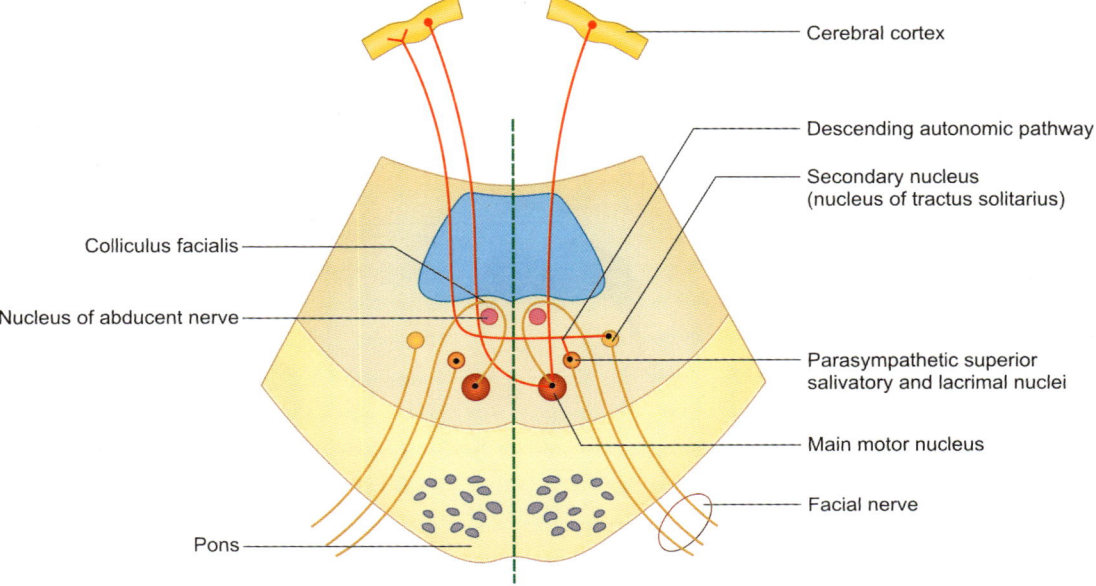

Cerebral cortex

Descending autonomic pathway

Secondary nucleus
(nucleus of tractus solitarius)

Colliculus facialis

Nucleus of abducent nerve

Parasympathetic superior
salivatory and lacrimal nuclei

Main motor nucleus

Facial nerve

Pons

Fig. 29.1 *Cranial nerve nuclei as projected onto the posterior surface of the brainstem.*

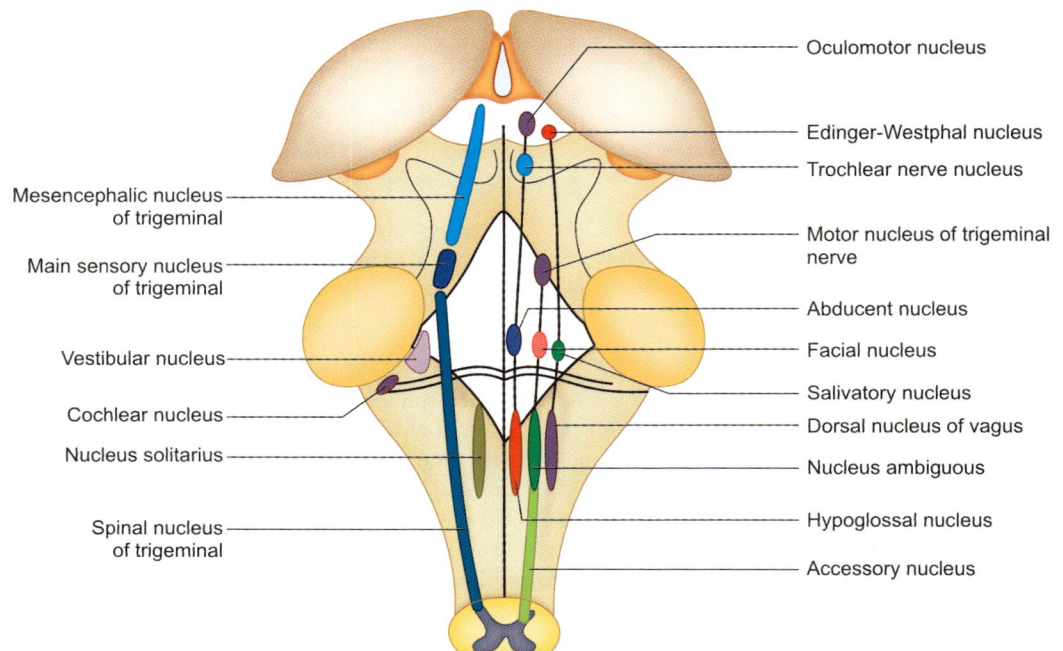

Oculomotor nucleus

Edinger-Westphal nucleus

Trochlear nerve nucleus

Mesencephalic nucleus
of trigeminal

Main sensory nucleus
of trigeminal

Motor nucleus of trigeminal
nerve

Abducent nucleus

Vestibular nucleus

Facial nucleus

Salivatory nucleus

Cochlear nucleus

Dorsal nucleus of vagus

Nucleus solitarius

Nucleus ambiguous

Spinal nucleus
of trigeminal

Hypoglossal nucleus

Accessory nucleus

Fig. 29.2 *Facial nerve nuclei and their central connections.*

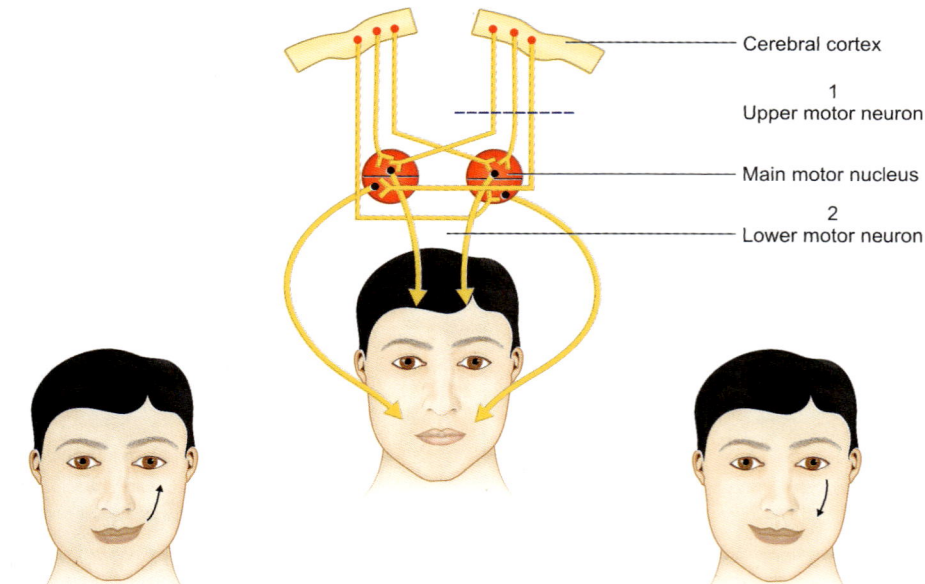

Cerebral cortex

1
Upper motor neuron

Main motor nucleus

2
Lower motor neuron

1. Upper motor neuron lesion

2. Lower motor neuron lesion

Fig. 29.3 *Facial nerve nucleus connections vis-à-vis supply to upper and lower parts of the face; and facial expression defects associated with lesions of (1) upper motor neurons, and (2) lower motor neurons.*

The *superior salivatory nucleus* receives afferent fibers from the hypothalamus through the descending autonomic pathway. Information concerning taste also is received from the nucleus of the solitary tract from the mouth cavity. It sends preganglionic fibers which innervate the submaxillary and sublingual salivary glands.

The *lacrimatory nucleus* receives afferent fibers from the hypothalamus for emotional responses and from the sensory nuclei of the trigeminal nerve for reflex lacrimation secondary to irritation of the cornea or conjunctiva. It sends preganglionic fibers for innervation of the lacrimal gland.

Sensory nucleus

The upper part of the *nucleus tractus solitarius* constitutes the sensory nucleus of the facial nerve. It belongs to the group of special visceral afferent nuclei. It is situated in the upper part of the medulla oblongata in line with the other nuclei of its group (Fig. 29.2). It receives afferent fibers (central processes of neurons of the geniculate ganglion of the facial nerve) carrying the sensations of taste and also afferents from the concha of the auricle. The *efferent* fibers from the

nucleus tractus solitarius cross the median plane and ascend to the ventral posterior medial nucleus of the opposite thalamus and also a number of hypothalamic nuclei. From the thalamus, the axons of the thalamic cells pass through the internal capsule and corona radiata to end in the taste area of the cortex in the lower part of the postcentral gyrus (Fig. 29.1).

COURSE AND DISTRIBUTION OF THE FACIAL NERVE

INTRACRANIAL COURSE

The facial nerve consists of a motor and a sensory root. Fibers of the *motor root*, after arising from the motor nucleus, first travel posteriorly from the medial side of the abducent nucleus (Fig. 29.1) and then pass around this nucleus beneath facial colliculus, in the floor of the fourth ventricle and finally pass anteriorly to emerge from the brainstem.

The *sensory root (nervous intermedius)* consists of central processes of the unipolar cells of geniculate ganglion. It also contains the preganglionic parasympathetic fibers from the parasympathetic nuclei.

The two roots of the facial nerve emerge from the junction of pons and medulla just medial to the 8th cranial nerve. Then the two roots run laterally and forwards (with the 8th nerve) to reach the internal acoustic meatus. *In the meatus*, the motor root lies in a groove on the 8th nerve, with the sensory root intervening. Here the 7th and 8th nerves are accompanied by the labyrinthine vessels. At the bottom (fundus) of the meatus, the two roots (sensory and motor) fuse to form a single trunk, which lies in the petrous temporal bone.

Within the canal, in the petrous part of temporal bone, the course of the nerve can be divided into three parts by two bends (Fig. 29.4). The first part is directed laterally above the vestibule; the second part runs backwards in relation to the medial wall of the middle ear above the promontory; the third part is directed vertically downwards behind the promontory. The first bend (at the junction of the first and second parts) is sharp. It lies over the anterosuperior part of the promontory, and is also called the *genu*. The geniculate ganglion of the nerve is so-called because it lies on the genu. The second bend is gradual, and lies between the promontory and the *aditus* to the mastoid antrum.

The facial nerve leaves the skull by passing through the stylomastoid foramen.

EXTRACRANIAL COURSE

In its extracranial course, the facial nerve crosses the lateral side of the base of the styloid process. It enters the posteromedial surface of the parotid gland, runs forward through the gland crossing the retromandibular vein and the external carotid artery. Behind the neck of the mandible, it divides into its five terminal branches which emerge along the anterior border of the parotid gland (Fig. 29.5).

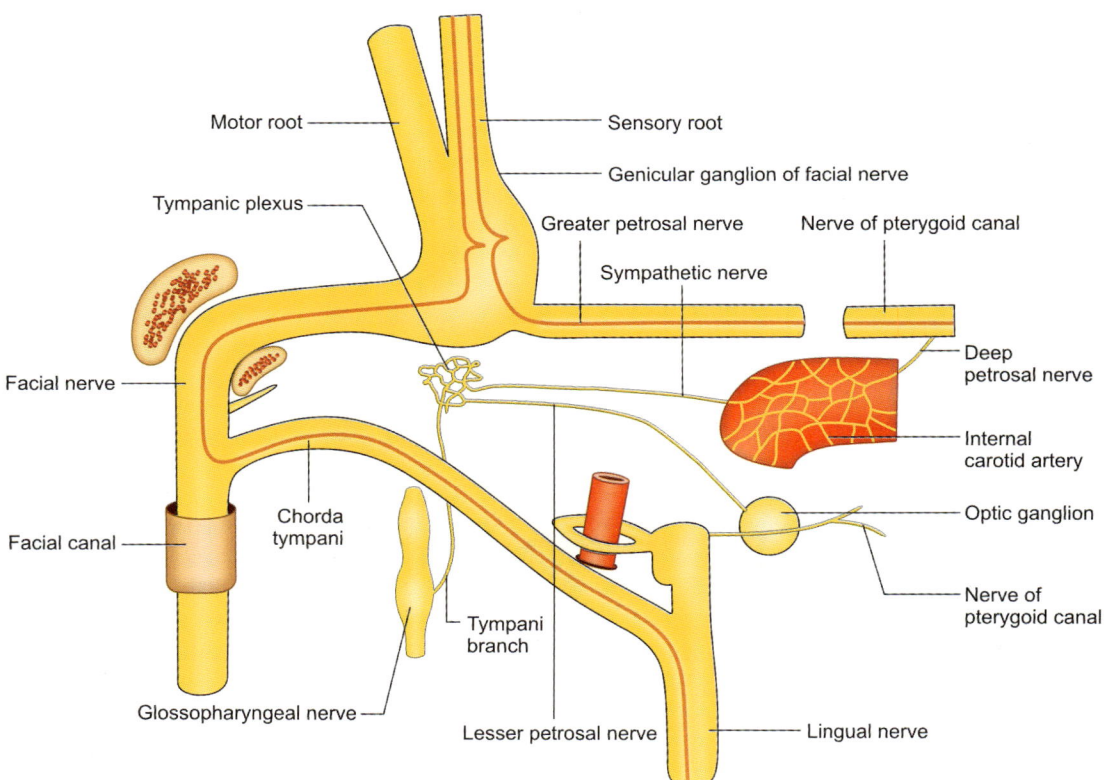

Fig. 29.4 *Course of the facial nerve within petrous part of temporal bone.*

BRANCHES

A. Branches within the facial canal

1. **Greater petrosal nerve.** This starts from the geniculate ganglion and contains mainly taste fibers from the palatal mucosa and also preganglionic parasympathetic fibers travelling to the pterygopalatine ganglion and said to be relayed through the zygomatic and lacrimal nerves to the lacrimal gland and through the nasal and palatine nerves to the nasal and palatine mucosal glands. It receives a ramus from the tympanic plexus, traverses the hiatus on the anterior surface of the petrous temporal bone and enters a groove on it, passing under the trigeminal ganglion to the foramen lacerum. Here it is joined by the *deep petrosal nerve* from the internal carotid sympathetic plexus to become the vidian nerve or *nerve of the pterygoid canal* which traverses the pterygoid canal to end in the pterygopalatine ganglion. Gustatory fibers pass without interruption through or over the pterygopalatine ganglion into its palatine branches.

2. The *nerve to the stapedius arises* opposite the pyramid of the middle ear and supplies the stapedius muscle. The muscle dampens excessive vibrations of the stapes caused by high-pitched sounds. In paralysis of the muscle, even normal sounds appear too loud (hyperacusis).

3. The *chorda tympani arises* in the vertical part of facial canal about 6 mm above the stylomastoid foramen. It runs upwards and forwards in a bony canal. It enters the middle ear and runs forwards in close relation to the tympanic membrane. It leaves the middle ear by passing through the petrotympanic fissure. It then passes medial to the spine of the sphenoid and enters the infratemporal fossa. Here it joins the lingual nerve through which it is distributed. It carries (a) preganglionic secretomotor fibers to the submandibular ganglion for supply of the submandibular and sublingual salivary glands; and (b) taste fibers from the anterior two-thirds of the tongue.

B. Branches at its exit from the stylomastoid foramen (Fig. 29.5)

1. The *posterior auricular nerve* arises just below the stylomastoid foramen. It ascends between the mastoid process and the external acoustic meatus and supplies:

a. The auricularis posterior

b. The occipitalis

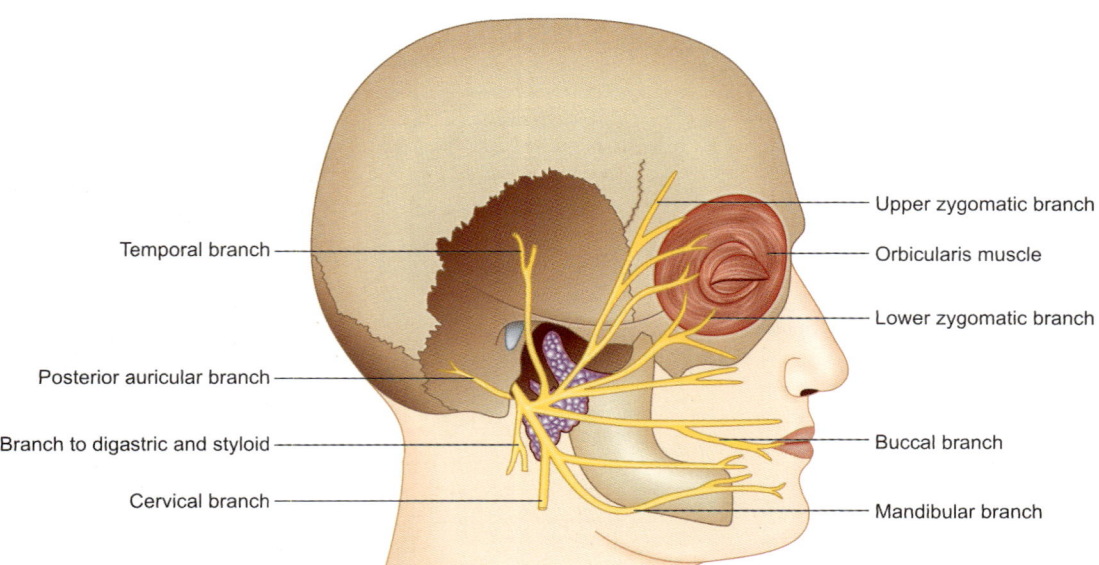

Temporal branch

Posterior auricular branch

Branch to digastric and styloid

Cervical branch

Upper zygomatic branch

Orbicularis muscle

Lower zygomatic branch

Buccal branch

Mandibular branch

Fig. 29.5 *Branches of facial nerve after emerging from the stylomastoid foramen.*

c. The intrinsic muscles on the back of the auricle.

2. The *digastric branch* arises close to the previous nerve. It is short and supplies the posterior belly of the digastric.

3. The *stylohyoid branch, which* may arise with the digastric branch, is long and supplies the stylohyoid muscle.

C. Terminal branches within the parotid gland

1. The *temporal branches* cross the zygomatic arch and supply (a) the auricularis anterior, (b) the auricularis superior, (c) the intrinsic muscles on the lateral side of the ear, (d) the frontalis, (e) the orbicularis oculi, and (f) the corrugator supercilii.

2. The *zygomatic branches* run across the zygomatic bone and supply the orbicularis oculi.

3. The *buccal branches* are two in number. The upper buccal branch runs above the parotid duct and the lower buccal branch below the duct. They supply muscles in that vicinity.

4. The *mandibular branch* (marginal mandibular) runs below the angle of the mandible deep to the platysma. It crosses the body of the mandible and supplies muscles of the lower lip and chin.

5. The *cervical branch* emerges from the apex of the parotid gland and runs downwards and forwards in the neck to supply the platysma.

D. Communicating branches

For effective coordination between the movements of the muscles of the first, second and third branchial arches, the motor nerves of the three arches communicate with each other. The facial nerve also communicates with the sensory nerves distributed over its motor territory.

GANGLIA

The ganglia associated with the facial nerve are as follows:

1. *The geniculate ganglion* is located on the first bend of the facial nerve, in relation to the medial wall of the middle ear. It is a *sensory ganglion*. The taste fibers present in the nerve are peripheral processes of pseudounipolar neurons present in the geniculate ganglion.

2. The submandibular ganglion

It is a *parasympathetic ganglion* for relay of secreto-motor fibers to the submandibular and sublingual glands.

3. Pterygopalatine ganglion or Sphenopalatine ganglion

This is the largest parasympathetic peripheral ganglion. It serves as a relay station for secreto-motor fibers to the lacrimal gland and to the mucous glands of the nose, the paranasal sinuses, the palate and the pharynx. Topographically, it is related to the maxillary nerve, but functionally, it is connected to the facial nerve (through its greater petrosal branch). The flattened ganglion lies in the pterygopalatine fossa just below the maxillary nerve, in front of the pterygoid canal and close to the sphenopalatine foramen.

Connections of sphenopalatine ganglion

1. **The *motor or parasympathetic root*** of the ganglion is formed by the nerve of the pterygoid canal. It carries preganglionic fibers that arise from neurons of lacrimatory nucleus, and pass through the nervus intermedius, the facial nerve, the geniculate ganglion, the greater petrosal nerve and the nerve of the pterygoid canal to reach the ganglion. The fibers relay in the ganglion. Post-ganglionic fibers arising in the ganglion supply secretomotor nerves to the lacrimal gland and to the mucous glands of the nose, the paranasal sinuses, the palate and the nasopharynx.

2. **The *sympathetic root*** is also derived from the nerve of pterygoid canal. It contains postganglionic fibers arising in the superior cervical sympathetic ganglion which pass through the internal carotid plexus, the deep petrosal nerve and the nerve of the pterygoid canal to reach the ganglion. The fibers pass through the ganglion without relay, and supply vasomotor nerves to the mucous membrane of the nose, the paranasal sinuses, the palate and the nasopharynx.

3. **The *sensory root*** comes from the maxillary nerve. Its fibers pass through the ganglion without relay. They emerge in the branches described below.

Branches of sphenopalatine ganglion

The branches of the ganglion are actually branches of the maxillary nerve. They also carry parasympathetic and sympathetic fibers which pass through the ganglion. The branches are as follows:

1. **Orbital branches** pass through the inferior orbital fissure and supply the periosteum of the orbit, and the orbitalis muscle.

2. **Palatine branches.** The greater (anterior) palatine nerve descends through the greater palatine canal, and supplies the hard palate and the lateral wall of the nose (inferior concha and adjoining meatuses). The *lesser (middle and posterior) palatine nerves* supply the soft palate and the tonsil.

3. **Nasal branches** enter the nasal cavity through the sphenopalatine foramen. The *lateral posterior superior nasal nerves* (about 6 in number) supply the posterior parts of the superior and middle conchae. The *medial posterior superior nasal nerves* (2 or 3 in number) supply the posterior part of the roof of the nose and of the nasal septum. The largest of these nerves is known as the *naso-palatine nerve* which descends up to the anterior part of the hard palate through the incisive foramen.

4. **The *pharyngeal branch*** passes through the palatovaginal canal and supplies the part of the nasopharynx behind the auditory tube.

LESIONS OF FACIAL NERVE

SUPRANUCLEAR LESIONS

Causes

At this level, cerebrovascular accidents and tumors are the most likely causes.

Clinical profile

In *supranuclear lesions* of the facial nerve (usually a part of the hemiplegia), only the lower part of the *contralateral face* is paralysed. The upper part (frontalis and part of orbicularis oculi) escapes due to its bilateral representation in the cerebral cortex.

INFRANUCLEAR LESIONS

- In *infranuclear lesions* of the facial nerve, the whole of the face of the ipsilateral side is paralysed, abolishing both voluntary and emotional movement. The face becomes asymmetrical and is drawn up to the normal side. The affected side is motionless. Wrinkles disappear from the forehead. The eye cannot be closed (lagophthalmos). Any attempt to smile draws the mouth to the normal side. During mastication, food accumulates between the teeth and the cheek. Articulation of labialis is impaired.

Causes of infranuclear lesions

The *common causes* of infranuclear facial nerve palsy are:

1. Bell's palsy which should be labelled when other pathology has been excluded since it is synonymous with the term idiopathic palsy

2. Diseases of the brainstem

3. Acoustic neuromas.

Clinical profile of infranuclear lesions

- *Lesions found distal to the chorda tympani* produce isolated facial palsy. In lesions proximal to the geniculate ganglion, the palsy is associated with loss of taste sensations on the anterior two-thirds of the tongue and diminished salivation.

- *Lesions proximal to the nerve to stapedius* are associated with an additional complaint of ipsilateral hyperacusis.

- *Ramsay-Hunt syndrome* occurs due to herpes zoster infection of the geniculate ganglion of the facial nerve. It is characterized by the lower motor neuron type of facial palsy associated with severe pain in the ear and vesicles near the ear.

- *Lesions at the level of pons* result in the involvement of both the abducent and the facial nerve.

- *Lesions at the cerebellopontine angle* result in the involvement of both the facial and auditory nerve.

BIBLIOGRAPHY

1. Ates O, Yoruk O. Unilateral anterior uveitis in Melkersson-Rosenthal syndrome: a case report. J Int Med Res 2006;34(4):428–32.
2. Coulson SE, O'Dwyer NJ, Adams RD, Croxson GR. Expression of emotion and quality of life after facial nerve paralysis. Otol Neurotol 2004;25(6):1014–9.
3. Duggan M, Ames W, Papsin B, et al. Facial nerve palsy: a complication following anaesthesia in a child with Treacher Collins syndrome. Paediatr Anaesth 2004;14:604–6.
4. Holland NJ, Weiner GM. Recent developments in Bell's palsy. BMJ 2004;329(7465):553–7.
5. Honda N, Hato N, Takahashi H, et al. Pathophysiology of facial nerve paralysis induced by herpes simplex virus type 1 infection. Ann Otol Rhinol Laryngol 2002;111(7 Pt 1):616–22.
6. Pitkäranta A, Lahdenne P, Piiparinen H. Facial nerve palsy after human herpes virus 6 infection. Pediatr Infect Dis J 2004;23(7):688–9.
7. Scriba H, Stoeckli SJ, Veraguth D, et al. Objective evaluation of normal facial function. Ann Otol Rhinol Laryngol 1999;108(7 Pt 1): 641–4.
8. Shafshak TS. The treatment of facial palsy from the point of view of physical and rehabilitation medicine. Eura Medicophys 2006; 42:41–7.
9. Teixeira LJ, Soares BDO, Vieira VP, et al. Physical therapy for Bell's palsy (idiopathic facial paralysis) Cochrane Database Syst Rev.; 2008 Jul 16(3):CD006283.
10. Yen TL, Driscoll CLW, Lalwani AK. Significance of House-Brackmann facial nerve grading global score in the setting of differential facial nerve function. Otol Neurotol 2003;24(1):118–22.

30 OCULAR MYASTHENIA GRAVIS

Neebha Passi, AK Khurana, Urmil Chawla

EPIDEMIOLOGY

PATHOPHYSIOLOGY
- Etiological profile
- Factors that worsen myasthenia gravis
- Associated conditions

CLINICAL FEATURES
- General considerations
- Lid dysfunctions
- Ocular motility dysfunctions
- Associated systemic symptoms

DIAGNOSIS
- Pharmacological and clinical tests for ocular myasthenia gravis

- Hematological tests
- Radiological investigations
- Electrodiagnostics

TREATMENT
- Medical treatment
- Surgical treatment
- Supportive therapy

PROGNOSIS
- Spontaneous remissions
- Course

EPIDEMIOLOGY

Myasthenia gravis (MG) is the paradigm of an auto-immune disorder, where anomalous antibodies are produced against the naturally occurring acetylcholine receptors in voluntary muscles causing fluctuating weakness. Generalized myasthenia gravis involves skeletal, respiratory or other striated muscles. Ocular myasthenia gravis is a subtype of MG where the muscles of the eye are involved, leading to abrupt onset of weakness/fatiguability of the eyelids or eye movement.

Presentation. Fifty percent patients present with ptosis or ocular motility abnormality only, and of this group, approximately half will remain ocular myasthenics, while the other half will progress to generalized MG, usually within 2 years of the onset of ocular symptoms.

Remission. There is approximately 22% spontaneous remission rate.

Prevalence of myasthenia gravis is approximately 3–30 cases for every 1 lac population

Age. Myasthenia gravis occurs at all ages with mean age of onset being 26 years for females and 31 years for males.

Sex. In ocular myasthenia, men are more frequently affected, especially after the age of 40 years.

Race. The disorder is seen in all races with a slight genetic predisposition: particular HLA types seem to predispose for myasthenia gravis (B8 and DR_3, with more specific for ocular myasthenia).

PATHOPHYSIOLOGY

Etiological profile

Reduction in number of available acetylcholine receptors of skeletal muscles results in a defect in neuromuscular transmission, resulting in muscle fatigue, and sometimes paralysis. In myasthenia gravis, the antibodies most commonly act against and block the nicotinic acetylcholine receptor (nAChR), the receptor in the motor endplate for the neurotransmitter acetylcholine that stimulates muscular contractions (Fig. 30.1). These antibodies prevent the molecule from binding to the receptor causing their blockade, accelerated degradation, and complement mediated damage, resulting in muscle fatigue and sometimes paralysis.

- Both production of high affinity IgG antibodies and sensitization of acetylcholine receptors antibody CD4 + T helper cells are observed.
- Randomness of neuromuscular blockade is the characteristic of ocular myasthenia gravis. It may be confined only to a small muscle of the eye or to one of the larger muscles.

Auto-antibodies against acetylcholine receptors are detectable in 70–90% of patients with generalized MG, but only 50% in ocular MG.

Idiopathic. Usually the cause of this autoimmune disorder is unknown.

Drug induced. However in some cases, it is drug induced in association with use of D-penicillamine, for instance. Other drugs like ainoglycosides, beta blockers, and quinidine may exacerbate myasthenia gravis by their direct effects on neuromuscular junction and neuromuscular blockade.

Thymus hyperplasia abnormality is found in up to 75% of patients of myasthenia gravis. Approximately 10–15% of adult patients have a thymoma (either benign or malignant).

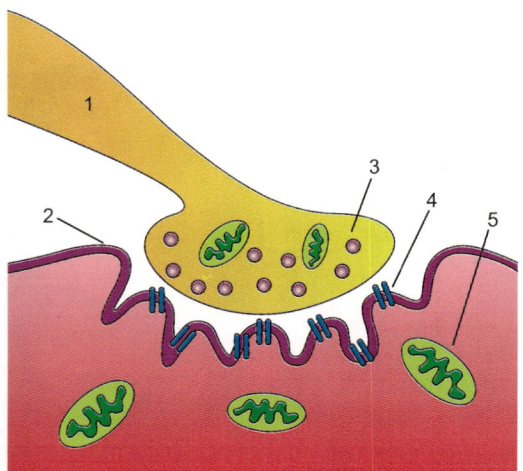

Fig. 30.1 *A neuromuscular junction: 1. Axon, 2. Muscle cell membrane sarcolemma, 3. Synaptic vesicle, 4. Nicotinic acetylcholine receptor and 5. Mitochondrion*

Factors that can worsen myasthenia gravis
- Fatigue
- Illness
- Stress
- Extreme heat
- Some medications such as beta blockers, calcium channel blockers, quinine and some antibiotics.

Associated conditions

MG is associated with various autoimmune diseases, like:
- Thyroid diseases, including Hashimoto's thyroiditis and Graves' disease.
- Diabetes mellitus type I
- Rheumatoid arthritis
- Systemic lupus erythematosus, and
- Demyelinating central nervous system diseases.

CLINICAL FEATURES

GENERAL CONSIDERATIONS

Onset. Ocular MG is characterized by an abrupt or insidious onset of weakness and fatiguability of one or both lids or eye muscles.

Hallmark features of ocular MG are variable and fatiguable ptosis, diplopia, chewing difficulties, dysarthria, dysphagia, dyspnea, and systemic weakness.

Diurnal variation is exhibited in most patients, as their weakness is better in the morning or after sleep than at the end of the day, when they are weakest.

Variations in clinical presentations are typical in patients with ocular MG, making the diagnosis elusive at times.

Common signs and symptoms of MG can be described under 2 main headings: Lid dysfunction and ocular motility dysfunction.

LID DYSFUNCTIONS

1. *Ptosis and fatiguability.* The most common manifestation of ocular MG is unilateral or bilateral ptosis, which can be symmetric or asymmetric. The degree of ptosis is variable and frequently will shift from one eye to the other. It typically becomes worse with fatigue, sustained upgaze and at the end of the day (Fig. 30.2). In

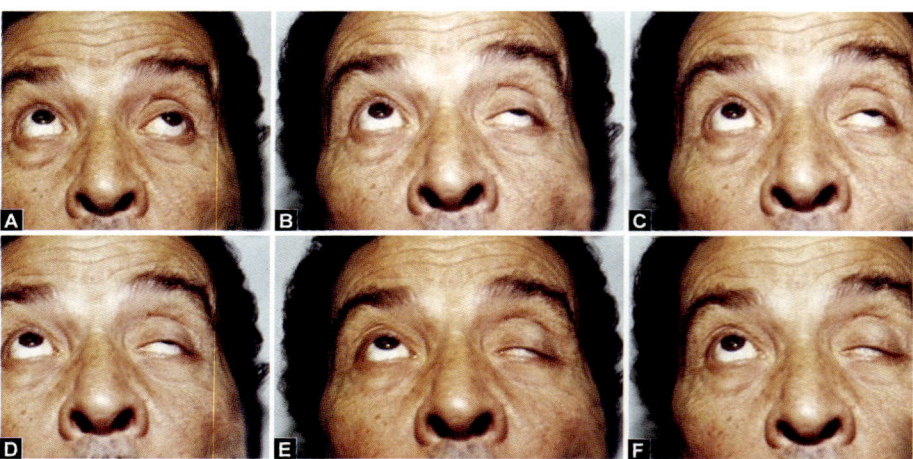

Fig. 30.2 *Fatiguability in a patient with myasthenia gravis (A through F). Note the limited elevation of the left eye denoting superior rectus palsy (A). (A, initially; C after around 20 seconds; F after 1 minute)*

cases where the ptosis is subtle, lid fatigue can be enhanced with repeated eyelid closure or sustained upward gaze. Levator function in myasthenia is related to the amount of ptosis; those with marked ptosis will have the most levator weakness. Normal levator function in the setting of marked ptosis argues against the diagnosis of myasthenia.

2. *Contralateral lid retraction.* May be present in some patients with unilateral ptosis which will assume its normal position when the ptotic eye is occluded or elevated, a result of Hering's law of equivalent innervations.

3. *Cogan's lid twitch* is characteristic of levator palpebrae superioris muscle involvement. This can be elicited by having the patient rapidly redirect gaze from downward to primary position. If a patient of myasthenic ptosis looks downward for 3–5 seconds, then looks up quickly into primary gaze, the eyelid appears to overshoot upward, then quickly falls (Fig. 30.3). This can be explained by a buildup of acetylcholine in neuromuscular junction of levator muscle fibers while the eyelid is resting in downgaze. Following upward fixation, the levator quickly fatigues and the eyelid droops.

4. *Lid hopping.* During the attempted lateral gaze, the fluttering of ptotic eyelid may be seen, known as lid hopping.

5. *Orbicularis oculi muscle weakness* is seen often in MG. Testing of orbicularis oculi muscle strength is helpful in the diagnosis of patients suspected of having MG. The characteristic "Peek" sign of orbicularis fatigue is seen in patients with MG. In such patients, upon gentle eyelid closure the orbicularis oculi muscle will initially contract to achieve eyelid closure. However orbicularis muscle rapidly fatigues resulting in widening of palpebral aperture.

6. *Curtaining and enhanced ptosis.* In asymmetric ptosis, when the more ptotic eyelid is

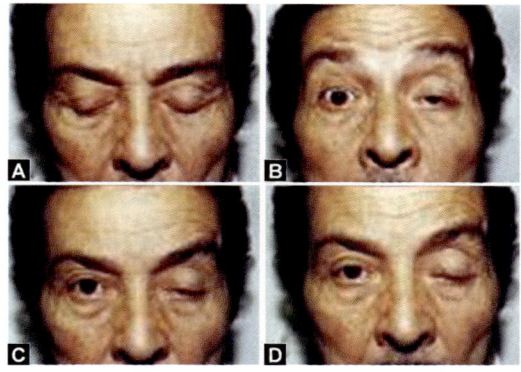

Fig. 30.3 *Cogan sign. The patient changes gaze from the downward position (A) to the primary position (B). Both lids are seen to overshoot in a twitch (C) before gaining their initial ptotic position (D). In this case, the Cogan sign is seen more obviously on the right, whereas the left lid is more ptotic.*

manually elevated, the fellow eye often droops (curtaining). This sign is nonspecific and can be seen in many other situations like, third nerve palsy. When the ptosis is symmetric, elevation of one eyelid will worsen the other eyelid (enhanced ptosis).

These eyelid signs are consequences of Herings law, as manual elevation of a ptotic eyelid reduces the patients required effort to elevate the eyelids and the other eyelid falls.

OCULAR MOTILITY DYSFUNCTIONS

1. *Diplopia.* Occurs due to weakness of one or more of the extraocular muscles. The medial rectus muscle is the most frequently involved isolated extraocular muscle. Involvement of the medial rectus may produce either a variable incomitant esotropia or a clinical picture simulating unilateral or bilateral internuclear ophthalmoplegia with weakness of adduction of one eye and an abducting nystagmus in the fellow eye.

EOM other than medial rectus also may be selectively involved.

Diplopia usually occurs with ptosis but may be the sole manifestation. It accounts for the initial complaint in 75% of patients with MG and eventually occurs in 90% of the patients with MG. About 80% of the patients will progress to involvement of other muscle groups within the Ist 2 years, thus only 20% of patients have pure ocular MG. If MG is confined to the ocular muscles for more than 3 years, there is a 94% likelihood that the symptoms will not worsen or generalize.

EOM involvement does not follow any set pattern, essentially any pattern of dysfunctional ocular movement may develop so that isolated muscle palsies or total immobility of eyes will accrue; sometimes mimicking other medical conditions such as strokes, tumors, thyroid, eye disease and multiple sclerosis, isolated or combined cranial nerve palsies.

2. *Other ocular motor abnormalities:* are also observed like saccadic eye movements which may be hypermetric or hypometric; quivering or small jerking eye movements and gaze evoked nystagmus. It is rare to have nystagmus as the sole manifestation of MG.

3. *Pupillary involvement* is a topic of controversy in MG. The possibility of iris sphincter involvement has been supported by several anecdotal reports. However, it is generally felt that if pupillary signs are present, other diagnoses like Horners syndrome and third nerve palsy, should be considered.

ASSOCIATED SYSTEMIC SYMPTOMS

- Difficulty in swallowing (dysphagia),
- Slurred speech (dysarthria), or nasal voice, due to involvement of oropharyngeal muscles
- Difficulty in chewing
- Difficulty in breathing
- Unstable or waddling gait
- Weakness in arms, hands, legs, neck, change in facial expression
- Myasthenic crisis is a life-threatening condition which occurs when the muscles controlling breathing are weakened or paralyzed leading to use of life support systems.
- Involvement of lower facial muscles will make the patient unable to smile, whistle, pucker, or hold air in the cheeks.

DIAGNOSIS

The variable course of MG may make the diagnosis difficult and it can mimic a variety of neuro-ophthalmic conditions. In brief, the diagnosis of MG relies mostly on the patients history and physical findings and various tests to elicit the condition.

A. PHARMACOLOGICAL AND CLINICAL TESTS FOR OCULAR MYASTHENIA GRAVIS

1. *Tensilon test.* It is a first line test for diagnosis of MG. It consists of injecting a small amount of tensilon (edrophonium chloride) intravenously. Edrophonium is a rapidly acting and quickly hydrolysed anticholinesterase which temporarily increases the level of acetylcholine at the neuromuscular junction. A 10 mg dose of tensilon is drawn up in a 1cc syringe. Initially, a 0.2 cc test dose is injected intravenously. If the lid or EOM function is not improved within 1 minute, the remaining 0.8cc is slowly injected over 30 seconds in 2 mg increments, and the lid positions and eye movements are reassessed for improvement (Fig. 30.4). The onset of action

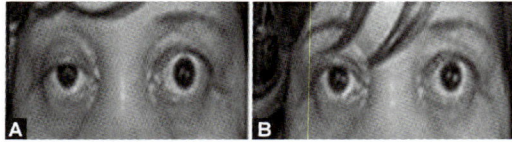

Fig. 30.4 *Ptosis in right eye (A), which disappears on Tensilon test (B).*

begins within 30–60 seconds of intravenous injection and the effect resolves within 5–10 minutes. The advantage of incremental method of administration is that the full 10 mg dose may not be required to produce a positive response. In infants, the dose of edrophonium chloride is 0.05 to 1.0 mg subcutaneously and 0.15 mg/kg in children.

Occasionally, patients develop salivation, lacrimation, increased sweating and mild gastrointestinal discomfort. Atropine 0.4 mg should be ready in a separate syringe and administered intravenously if symptomatic bradycardia occurs.

The Tensilon test is positive in 80–90% of patients with myasthenia gravis. The edrophonium test unfortunately has many false negative and false positive results. It can be false positive in other disorders of neuromuscular transmission, such as Lambert-Eaton myasthenic syndrome, botulism, and organophosphate toxicity, and also in some patients with skull base tumors. Therefore, a positive edrophonium test should not be the sole basis for making a diagnosis of myasthenia gravis.

2. *Neostigmine test.* Intramuscular Prostigmin (neostigmine bromide) may be used in children who are uncooperative or too agitated to monitor over a short period of time and also in adults whose signs are subtle and require longer period of observation. Usually 0.6 mg atropine sulphate and 1.5 mg Prostigmin are combined in a 3 cc syringe and injected intramuscularly. A change in ocular motility and ptosis is usually evident within 15–30 minutes following the injection.

3. *The 'Sleep test'.* It is based on the tendency for MG symptoms to improve following rest; may be used in small children and patients who have allergies or sensitivity to tensilon. The patient is placed in a quiet darkened room and

instructed to close their eyes for 30 minutes. The eye movement is measured before and after the rest. The test is considered positive if there is improvement in ptosis and/or eye movement following the 30 minutes rest period. The reappearance of the myasthenic signs over the next 30 seconds to 5 minutes adds further confirmation.

4. *The "Ice test".* It is a simple test for ocular MG in patients who have ptosis. A surgical glove filled with ice is held against the droopy eyelid for several minutes. After the ice pack is removed, improvement in ptosis is observed in patients with MG. The test is considered positive when the upper eyelid elevates by at least 2 mm following application of ice pack. The precise mechanism by which cooling improves myasthenic weakness is unclear. Reduced acetylcholinesterase activity and an increased receptor sensitization with lower temperature are the possible mechanisms. This test has a sensitivity and specificity of 76.9% and 98.3%, respectively.

5. *The morning/evening comparison test.* It is similar in concept to the sleep test. The patient is photographed and the ptosis and ocular motility are compared at different times during the day.

6. *The "Fatigue test".* The patient is asked to look at an object held up by the examiner in front of the patient. After a short period of time, the eyelid(s) will droop in person with ocular MG.

B. HEMATOLOGICAL TESTS

If the diagnosis is suspected, serological tests can be performed such as:

1. *Acetylcholine receptor antibody titre (AChR Ab):* Only about 70% of patients with ocular MG have detectable antibody level while 90% of patients with generalized MG have elevated titre. An elevated titre provides a baseline for future comparisons while monitoring the patients clinical course and the response to immunosuppressive treatment. Although the blood test when positive is highly specific but not particularly sensitive. The test has a reasonable sensitivity of 80–96%, but in ocular MG, the sensitivity falls to 50%, and they also suggest the presence of thymoma.

2. *Thyroid profile.* Thyroid dysfunction is found in approximate 5–10% of MG patients.

3. *Antibodies against MuSK protein.* A proportion of patients without antibodies against acetylcholinesterase receptors have antibodies against MuSK protein.

C. RADIOLOGICAL INVESTIGATIONS

Chest MRI or CT scan are done to rule out thyroid disorders as thymic tumors are present in 10–15% of MG patients, being more common in older individuals and rarely occurring before age of 30 years.

D. ELECTRODIAGNOSTICS

The fatiguability of the muscles in patients with MG can be measured by repetitive nerve stimulating test (RNS).

A decrement of the compound muscle action potential during electromyographic repetitive nerve stimulation (2 to 5 Hz) of limb or facial muscles is diagnostic in many cases of myasthenia gravis. However, this technique is relatively insensitive in ocular myasthenia. Additional single fiber electromyography (SFEMG) may be helpful in ocular myasthenia if the repetitive nerve stimulation, edrophonium test, and antibody studies are non diagnostic or cannot be performed. Normally, two muscle fibers innervated by the same motor axon will exhibit a variation, called jitter, in the time interval between their two action potentials during successive impulses. Jitter, can be increased in myasthenia gravis and other disorders of neuromuscular transmission. In patients with mild myasthenia, the combination of single fiber electromyography, antiacetylcholine receptor antibody studies, and the edrophonium test should provide the lab confirmation of myasthenia gravis in at least 95% of patients.

This is considered to be the most sensitive (but not the most specific) test for MG.

TREATMENT

The aims of treatment for ocular MG are improving the quality of life by returning the patient to a state of clear vision and to prevent the development or limit the severity of generalized MG while minimizing the side effects and possible risks. Treatment options may include medications/thymectomy/supportive therapy.

A. MEDICAL TREATMENT

1. Anticholinesterase agents

Patients with mild to moderate ocular MG are usually treated initially with oral anticholinesterase agents, pyridostigmine being the most commonly employed. It can be given orally at a starting dose of 30 mg every 4 hours while awake. The medication can be increased by 30 mg per dose, up to 120 to 150 mg every 4 hours. The onset of action is usually 30–45 minutes and lasts for up to six hours. A timespan preparation can be given at night to aid breathing, bulbar function, and weakness overnight. The response to pyridostigmine is variable. It seems most effective in alleviating most of the ocular and systemic symptoms, but relatively ineffective for diplopia.

The most common side effects are diarrhea and cramping, which resolve by lowering the dose or can be treated by anti-diarrheal medicines. The drug is contraindicated in patients with asthma, cardiac arrhythmias or urinary obstruction. It should also not be used in patients taking beta-blockers due to increased risk of hypotension and bradycardia.

2. Immunosuppressive drugs

Immunosuppressive therapy should be considered in all patients with MG whether or not serum AChR antibodies are detectable. Agent of choice is corticosteroids. Response to corticosteroids therapy is variable but some studies suggest that it decreases progression to generalized MG.

They are frequently used in patients with ocular myasthenia who fail to tolerate pyridostigmine or in patients who are not adequately controlled on pyridostigmine. Their use must be weighed against the possible short term and long term side effects. Common side-effects include obesity, diabetes, hypertension, threat of tuberculosis, esp. in underdeveloped/developing countries, opportunistic infections, osteoporosis, glaucoma, cataract and myopathy. Dosage usually starts at 20 mg/d of prednisolone. The dose can be titrated in patients individually by slowly increasing up to 1.0 mg/kg/d over several weeks. Maintenance dose is then continued for 6–12 weeks and then slowly tapered. Another suggested regimen starts patients of purely ocular myasthenia at low alternate day doses (prednisolone 10 mg qid) Once therapeutic efficacy is achieved, the dose can be tapered, after a few months. Most patients on steroids chronically require a small amount of alternate day dosing.

In patients with severe refractory symptoms, other **non-steroidal immunosuppressive agents** like azathioprine or cyclosporin are also used as supplementary agents or for steroid sparing effects.

- *Azathioprine* is given in doses of 2 to 3 mg/kg/day, with a time of onset of effect of 3 to 12 months and a time of maximal effect of 1 to 2 years. Common side-effects of azathioprine are hepatotoxicity, nausea and vomiting, infection and bone marrow suppression. Bone marrow and liver function should be monitored once every week for the first two months and then once every two months for the possible side-effects. The teratogenicity of azathioprine should also be kept in mind and not given in pregnant women.
- *Cyclosporin A* decreases the antigen stimulated IL-2 production in T cells. It is given in dose of 2.5 mg/kg BID, with a time of onset of effect of 2 to 12 weeks, and a time of maximal effect of 3 to 6 months. Side-effects of cyclosporin include myalgia, infection, hypertension and renal failure. For this, blood pressure, renal function and drug levels should be monitored. This drug is a third line drug, given in patients who are intolerant of steroids or azathioprine.

3. Mycophenolate mofetil

This is a new drug used in treatment of the MG It inhibits selectively T and B lymphocytes proliferation by blocking purine synthesis. It can be used as a steroid sparing drug or per se as a first line immunosuppressant. The dose for mycophenolate mofetil in MG is 1000–1500 mg twice a day. The effect is usually seen two months after initiation of treatment. The side-effects of this drug are usually mild. Studies have shown that this drug is safe and tolerable as a long-term immunosuppressant for ocular myasthenia gravis.

4. Plasmapheresis or intravenous immunoglobulins (IVIG) therapy

These are used for acute management of severe muscular weakness or mysthenic crisis. In plasmapheresis, plasma containing AChR antibodies is separated from whole blood and replaced with saline. Albumin or plasma protein fraction, leading to a decrease in serum AChR antibodies levels. Repeated exchanges are required to reduce AChR Ab titres and the total IgG levels.

IVIG involves injecting 0.4 g/kg/day of pooled human gamma globulins per kg of body weight for five days, followed by weekly or more frequent infusions to maintain effect.

These modalities are more appropriate for patients whose systemic symptoms are debilitating enough for hospitalization.

All these treatments offer only a temporary improvement and repeated treatments are necessary to sustain the effect. The ocular MG medications are used as treatment to improve muscle strength by suppressing the production of abnormal antibodies but these medications must be used with careful medical follow-up as they may cause major side-effects.

B. SURGICAL TREATMENT

Thymectomy is often recommended for patients with generalized MG who fail to respond to adequate medical therapy or in patients who show thymic enlargement on CT scans, but is rarely done in purely ocular MG unless a thymoma is suspected. The response to thymectomy is not immediate and may appear after several years.

C. SUPPORTIVE THERAPY

If the medications are ineffective or not tolerated, other modalities can be used to relieve the patients symptoms of ptosis, and diplopia like:

1. *Eyelid crutches*, which are devices that attach to glasses to keep eyelids open. Eyelid crutches are helpful for patients with significant eyelid droop that does not respond to medicine and for patients who want to avoid surgery.

2. *Eyelid tape,* which mechanically keeps eyelids open. Eyelid tape is helpful for patients with significant eyelid droop that does not respond to medicine and for patients who want to avoid surgery.

3. *Eyeglass prisms,* which are a simple, safe, solution for certain types of diplopia. Eyeglass prisms can be extremely helpful for individuals that require binocular vision for their livelihood.

4. *Eye patching,* to one eye, which eliminates troublesome diplopia.

PROGNOSIS

The prognosis tends to be good for patients with MG.

Spontaneous remissions can occur in any patient and sometimes persist for years. Most patients with MG show a fluctuating course.

Clinical course. MG is characteristically variable in course with the salient features of ocular MG, diplopia and ptosis, frequently being influenced by environmental, emotional and physical factors like bright sunlight, emotional stress, viral illness, surgery, pregnancy, etc. These may all precipitate a change in the expression of ocular MG.

BIBLIOGRAPHY

1. Chan W. Mycophenolate mofetil for ocular myasthenia. J Neurol 2008;255(4):510–3.
2. Gilbert ME, Savino PJ. Ocular myasthenia Gravis. Int Ophthalmol Clin 2007;47(4):93–103,ix.
3. Keesey JC. Clinical evaluation and management of myasthenia gravis. Muscle Nerve 2004; 29:484–505.
4. Oosterius HJGH. The natural course of myasthenia gravis: a long-term follow-up study. J Neurol Neurosurg Psychiatry 1989;52:1121–7.
5. Pascuzzi RM,Coslett HB, Johns TR. Long-term corticosteroid treatment of myasthenia gravis: Report of 116 patients. Ann Neurol 1984;15:291–8.
6. Seybld ME. Myasthenia gravis: A clinical and basic science review. JAMA 1983;250:2516–21.
7. Sommer N, Melms A, Weller M, et al. Ocular myasthenia gravis. A critical review of clinical and pathophysiological aspects. Doc Ophthalmol 1993;84(4):309–33.

31 | THYROID OPHTHALMOPATHY

Urmil Chawla, AK Khurana, Neebha Passi

INTRODUCTION
- Incidence

ETIOPATHOGENESIS
- Risk factors
- Pathophysiology

CLINICAL PROFILE
- Clinical features
  - Symptoms
  - Signs

- Classification of TAO
- Clinical course

MANAGEMENT
- Diagnostic considerations
- Investigations
- Histological features
- Treatment of TAO
- Consultations

INTRODUCTION

Graves' ophthalmopathy, also known as thyroid eye disease (TED), or dysthyroid/thyroid associated orbitopathy (TAO), or Graves' orbitopathy, is part of an autoimmune process that can affect the orbital and periorbital tissue, the thyroid gland, and rarely, the pretibial skin or digits (thyroid acropachy). Although the use of the term thyroid ophthalmopathy is pervasive, the disease process is actually an orbitopathy in which the orbital and periocular soft tissues are primarily affected with secondary effects on the eye.

Incidence. It is the most common cause of bilateral, symmetric proptosis in adults. Annual incidence of the disease is 16/1,00,000 in women and 3/10,000 in men. The ocular manifestations include eyelid retraction, proptosis, chemosis, periorbital edema, and altered ocular motility with significant functional, social and cosmetic consequences.

ETIOPATHOGENESIS

- Thyroid associated orbitopathy (TAO) is a multisystem disorder of unknown etiology.
- The thyroid gland itself does not cause thyroid associated orbitopathy and regulation of thyroid function does not abort this condition.
- Many patients are hyperthyroid (90%) but euthyroidism (6%), hypothyroidism (1%), Hashimoto's thyroiditis (3%), thyroid carcinoma and neck irradiation are also associated with thyroid orbitopathy.
- Severity of ophthalmopathy does not parallel with the levels of T3 or T4 in serum but is closely related to the level of thyroid stimulating hormone receptor antibodies (anti-TSHR).
- Graves' disease is basically caused by anti-TSHR and the ophthalmopathy related to an autoimmune reaction directed toward the orbital fibroblasts.

RISK FACTORS

- *Female sex.* There appears to be a female preponderance in which women are affected 2.5–6 times more frequently than men; however severe cases occur more often in men than women.
- *Middle age.* Most patients are in the age group of 30–50 years, with severity of disease increasing with age.
- *Smoking.* Cigarette smoking is a strong risk factor for TAO. The risk is directly related to the number of cigarettes smoked per day. Also patients treated with ^{131}I are at increased risk of developing the disease.
- *Autoimmune thyroid disease*
- *HLA-DR3 and HLA-B8*

PATHOPHYSIOLOGY

The underlying pathophysiology of TAO is thought to be an antibody-mediated reaction against the thyroid stimulating hormone (TSH) receptor with orbital fibroblast modulation of T cell lymphocytes. The inflammation results in a deposition of collagen and glycosaminoglycans in the muscles which leads to swelling of various tissues in the orbit and dysfunction of extraocular muscles in thyroid ophthalmopathy. This swelling of orbital tissue is the cause of eyelid edema, chemosis, proptosis, thickening of extraocular muscles and other signs of TAO. The following scheme for the pathophysiology has been proposed:

- T cell lymphocytes are believed to react against thyroid follicular cells with shared antigenic epitopes in the retro-orbital space. An active phase of inflammation is initially present.
- Lymphocytic infiltration of the orbital tissue causes a release of cytokines (e.g. tumor necrosis factor, interleukin I) from CD4 + T cells stimulating the orbital fibroblasts to produce mucopolysaccharides which by hyperosmotic shift, causes tissue edema in the extraocular muscles.
- Fibroblasts are believed to be the target and effector cells in TAO. They are extremely sensitive to stimulation by cytokines which activate previously quiescent fibroblasts to secrete hyaluronic acid, a glycosaminoglycan. Doubling the hyaluronic acid content in orbital

tissues causes a five-fold increase in tissue osmotic load. There is also induction of lipogenesis by fibroblasts and preadipocytes which causes orbital volume enlargement due to fat deposition.

- The increase in connective tissue volume and the fibrotic restriction of extraocular muscle movement leads to the clinical manifestation of TAO. The pretibial skin is also involved similarly resulting in expansion of dermal connective tissue which leads to the nodular or diffuse thickening characteristic of pretibial dermopathy.

Usually within 1–2 years of the onset of orbital involvement, the inflammation settles to a more quiescent phase predominated by scarring of the orbital tissues.

CLINICAL PROFILE

CLINICAL FEATURES

Thyroid associate orbitopathy usually has a self-limiting course lasting over one or more years. An acute or subacute stage of active inflammation occurs initially which later progresses to a more quiescent stage, which is characterized by fibrosis. Stable disease can occasionally reactivate, but this is uncommon. Signs and symptoms may vary and depend on the stage that the patient is experiencing.

SYMPTOMS

Ocular pain or discomfort is the most common ocular symptom which may be associated with dry eyes.

Other ocular symptoms include puffy eyelids, angry looking and bulging eyes, diplopia, blurred vision, dyschromatopsia, photopsia on upgaze and lacrimation.

Symptoms of hyperthyroidism, when associated include tachycardia, palpitation, nervousness, diaphoresis, heat intolerance, skeletal muscle weakness, tremors, weight loss, hair loss, irritability and goiter.

Symptoms of hypothyroidism, when associated include bradycardia, drowsiness, poor mentation, muscle cramps, weight gain, dry skin, husky voice, depression and cold intolerance.

SIGNS

1. Lid signs include (Fig. 31.1)

- *Retraction of the upper lids* which may be unilateral or bilateral. This produces the characteristic staring and frightened appearance (Dalrymple's sign) and is the most common sign of TAO seen in more than 90% of patients. The retraction of the lower eyelid results in inferior scleral show which is an early sign.

- Other eyelid signs are listed in Table 31.1

Table 31.1 *Eyelid signs in thyroid associated orbitopathy*

Characteristic features	Signs
Upper eyelid lags on down gaze	von Graefe's sign
Eversion of upper eyelid is difficult	Gifford's sign
Infrequent and incomplete blinking	Stellwag's sign
Eyelid-globe lag on supraduction	Kocher's sign
Tremors of eyelids on gentle closure	Rosenbach's sign
Fullness or edema of lower eyelid	Enroth's sign
Amplitude of blinking is reduced	Pochin's sign
Jerky movements of upper lid on down gaze	Boston's sign
Abnormal pigmentation of upper lid	Gellinek's sign
Bruit over eyelid	Riesman's sign

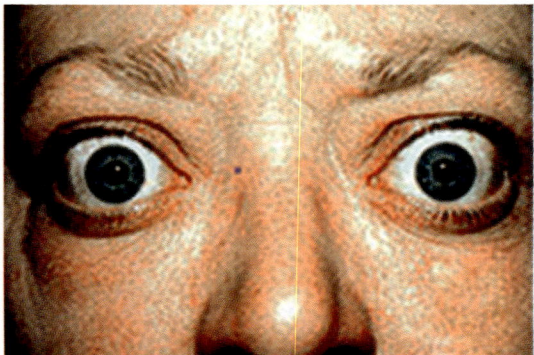

Fig. 31.1 *Patient with TAO showing proptosis and lid retraction.*

Note: When eyelid retraction is absent, then TAO may be diagnosed only if:

- Proptosis, optic nerve involvement, or restrictive extraocular myopathy is associated with thyroid dysfunction or abnormal regulation

- No other confounding ophthalmic features are apparent.

2. Conjunctival signs

Conjunctival signs include:

- Conjunctival injection usually over the rectus muscle insertions.

- Conjunctival chemosis.

3. Pupillary signs

These are of less importance and may be evident as inequality of dilatation of pupils.

4. Corneal signs

Corneal signs include:

- Corneal exposure with frank corneal ulceration may occur. Corneal exposure has been attributed to upper lid retraction, exophthalmos, lagophthalmos, inability to elevate the eyes and a decreased blink rate.

- Superior limbic keratoconjunctivitis is a chronic, often recurrent condition of ocular irritation. It has been considered to be because of mechanical trauma transmitted from the upper eyelid to the superior bulbar and tarsal conjunctiva. It is an indicator of severe thyroid associated orbitopathy.

5. Ocular motility defects

Ocular motility defects are common and include:

- Inferior rectus muscle followed by medial rectus muscle are the most commonly involved extraocular muscles leading to hypotropia or esotropia.

- Convergence insufficiency (Mobius's sign) is also an important finding.

- Restrictive myopathy sometimes can be confirmed with forced ductions or elevated intraocular pressure with eye movement. Inferior rectus muscle restriction may mimic double elevator palsy.

6. Exophthalmos

Exophthalmos (Fig. 31.1) is a common (60%) and classical sign of the disease. Although both eyes are symmetrically affected, often one eye may be more prominent than the other. Even unilateral proptosis is not uncommon. However, in majority of cases it is self-limiting. On exophthalmometry reading of >22 mm or asymmetry greater than 3 mm between two eyes is considered significant.

7. Pseudo nerve palsies and optic nerve compression

Pseudo-fourth nerve palsies have been described with TAO. In severe and active disease, with enlargement of the extraocular muscle at the orbital apex, the optic nerve is at risk of compression. The orbital fat or the stretching of the nerve due to increased orbital volume may also lead to optic nerve damage. It may manifest as papilledema or optic atrophy. The patient experiences a loss of visual acuity, visual field defect, afferent pupillary defect and loss of color vision. Optic nerve compression is an emergency and requires immediate surgery to prevent permanent blindness.

8. Cutaneous signs

Pretibial dermopathy (Fig. 31.2A) and thyroid acropachy (Fig. 31.2B) are less commonly encountered dramatic, cutaneous signs of dysthyroidism.

CLASSIFICATION OF TAO

Numerous classification systems exist for TAO, but all have shortcomings.

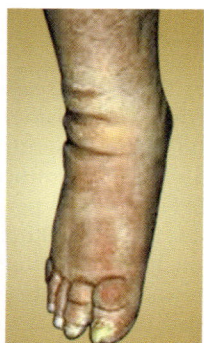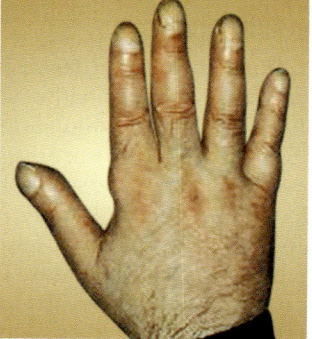

Fig 31.2 *Pretibial myxedema (A) and thyroid acropachy (B).*

I. NOSPECS

Werner's NOSPECS classification system given by American Thyroid Association (ATA) has classified TAO, irrespective of the hormonal status into the following classes, using a mnemonic NOSPECS.

NOSPECS is used to describe the presence or absence of signs or symptoms (NO) and grade and classify the severity and rank order of various clinical features as shown in Table 31.2.

Table 31.2 *American Thyroid Association Classification*	
Class 0	No signs and symptoms
Class 1	Only signs, no symptoms (signs are limited to upper lid retraction and stare, with or without lid lag and mild proptosis)
Class 2	Soft tissue involvement with signs (as described in class 1) and symptoms including lacrimation, photophobia, lid or conjunctival swelling and congestion
Class 3	Proptosis is well established
Class 4	Extraocular muscle involvement (limitation of movement and diplopia)
Class 5	Corneal involvement (exposure keratitis primarily due to lag ophthalmos)
Class 6	Sight loss due to optic nerve involvement with disc pallor or papilledema and visual field defects

For practical purposes it has been described as:
- *Early Graves' ophthalmopathy* (which include ATA class 1 and 2)
- *Late Graves' ophthalmopathy* (which includes ATA class 3 to 6)

Limitations of NOSPECS

Unfortunately, some weaknesses in NOSPECS classification may limit its prognostic value.
- Patients may not progress in an orderly fashion from Class 1 to Class 6 and may fall into more than 1 particular class.
- In addition, patients with visual loss from compressive optic neuropathy may not show marked proptosis or other signs of severe disease.

II. TAO: TYPE I AND II

The simplest classification for TAO is type I and type II; these 2 types are not mutually exclusive.

- **Type I TAO** is characterized by minimal inflammation and restrictive myopathy.
- **Type II TAO** is characterized by significant orbital inflammation and restrictive myopathy.

III. CLINICAL TYPES

1. **Thyrotoxic exophthalmos (exophthalmic goiter).** In this type mild exophthalmos and lid signs are associated with all signs of hyperthyroidism. Graves' disease is the commonest variety of hyperthyroid state. Women between the age group of 20 and 45 years of age are typically affected.

2. **Thyrotropic exophthalmos (Exophthalmic ophthalmoplegia).** This is a state of euthyroidism or hypothyroidism in which the patient clinically presents with an extreme exophthalmos and external ophthalmoplegia (due to infiltrative thyroid ophthalmopathy). The term ocular Graves' disease (OGD) is commonly used for this entity. Middle aged persons are usually affected with the disease running a self-limiting course characterized by remissions and relapses.

CLINICAL COURSE

Thyroid eye disease is a self-limiting disease that lasts from 1–5 years (longer in smokers as compared to non-smokers). Its clinical course is divided into three phases:

1. **Active phase** of increasing severity is characterized by active inflammation with marked lid edema, conjunctival chemosis and congestion and increasing exophthalmos.

2. **Regression phase** is of declining severity in which all of the above signs slowly settle down.

3. **Inactive plateau phase,** also known as quiescent burnt-out phase, ensues after regression phase.

Note. Reactivation of inflammation occurs in approximately 5–10% of patients over their lifetime.

4. **Rundle's curve** refers to the time course of the above phases and can be plotted graphically for each patient. Based on this the patients can be broadly categorized into mild, moderate, marked or severe disease (Rundle a–d).

MANAGEMENT

DIAGNOSTIC CONSIDERATIONS

Advanced cases of Graves' ophthalmopathy with bilateral proptosis are easily diagnosed. However, early cases having unilateral proptosis are difficult to diagnose and one should keep in mind the following differential diagnosis when evaluating a patient with suspected TAO.

a. **Orbital and preseptal cellulitis.** In this the onset of proptosis is much rapid, and patient has other evidence of infection (e.g. fever, leucocytosis). On radiography, the opacification of paranasal sinuses is often seen.

b. **Carotid-cavernous fistula.** In this the patient may have a cranial bruit, and the dilated episcleral vessels extend to the limbus.

c. **Orbital pseudotumor.** This orbital inflammatory syndrome is often more painful than TAO and has faster progress. It is associated more with ptosis than lid retraction. Isolated enlargement of the lateral rectus muscle more likely represents orbital inflammatory syndrome than TAO.

d. **Parinaud syndrome** (Dorsal midbrain syndrome). It is a condition in which patients present with lid retraction and upgaze problems. In this the globes elevate on the doll's head maneuver and the eye tends not to be injected or proptotic which is in contrast to TAO.

e. **Thickened muscles.** Other causes of thickened muscles are *sarcoidosis, metastases, lymphoma, amyloid* and *acromegaly*. However, a simple orbital ultrasound can quickly confirm if the patient has thickened muscles or an enlarged superior ophthalmic veins.

INVESTIGATIONS

1. **Thyroid function tests.** For thyroid disease screening, the combination of free T4 (thyroxine), and TSH (thyroid stimulating hormone) or serum TSH (thyrotropin) are highly sensitive and specific. Usually, the serum TSH is low in hyperthyroidism and high in hypothyroidism. Other blood tests that may be useful include calculated free T4 (thyroxine) index, thyroid stimulating immunoglobulin, antithyroid antibodies, and serum T3 (triiodothyronine). Estimation of radioactive iodine uptake is also an important marker.

2. *Positional tonometry.* The IOP may rise more than 8 mm Hg on upgaze because of restrictive myopathy. IOP may also increase due to decreased episcleral venous outflow. IOP recording helps in diagnosis of subclinical cases.

3. *Orbital imaging.* It is an interesting tool for diagnosing Graves' ophthalmopathy and also helps in monitoring the progression of disease. However, if the diagnosis can be established clinically, these tests are not warranted.

a. *Ultrasonography.* It helps to detect early Graves' orbitopathy in patients without clinical orbital findings, i.e. even in Class 0 and Class 1. It can demonstrate the increase in muscle thickness, erosion of temporal wall of orbit, accentuation of retrobulbar fat and perimural inflammation of optic nerve. However, the primary limitations of orbital USG are lack of visualization of the bony orbital architecture and inability to image the orbital apex.

b. *CT scan of orbit.* Excellent visualization of the extraocular muscles and intraconal fat as well as the orbital apex is possible. The thickening of the muscles is usually greater than 4 mm and it occurs uniformly within the muscle belly leaving the tendinous insertion (Fig. 31.3). Prominent intraconal fat can lead to anterior prolapse of orbital septum and show proptosis. The degree of globe proptosis relative to lateral orbital rim

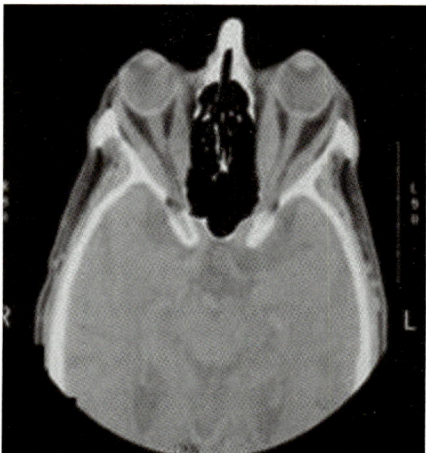

Fig 31.3: *Axial CT scan of orbit showing enlarged bellies of the extraocular muscle without involvement of tendinous insertion.*

can be measured with CT scan studies. Since CT scan shows better bony architecture it is must to be performed when an orbital decompression is required. However, cost and radiation exposure limit its use for serial examination.

c. *MRI of orbit.* This also provides excellent imaging of the extraocular muscles, their insertions and anatomy of the orbital apex. The amount of fat within the orbit and imaging of the optic nerve is better assessed and localized on MRI than CT scans. It is also better than CT in identifying other causes of proptosis, such as orbital tumors. Typically, however it is not an ideal imaging modality because of the associated increased cost.

4. *Orthoptic work-up.* Orthoptic work-up may include field of binocular single vision, field of uniocular fixation, and Hess/Lee charting.

HISTOLOGIC FEATURES

These include fibrosis with degenerative changes in the eye muscles, lymphocytic cell infiltration, enlargement of fibroblasts, accumulation of mucopolysaccharides, interstitial edema and increased collagen production.

TREATMENT OF TAO

The systemic management of patients with TAO lies in the domain of the endocrinologist. However, the therapy for the associated thyroid dysfunction usually does not alter the course of ophthalmic features. Hence, the ocular management is predominantly supportive and includes the following modalities:

A. Non-surgical management

1. *Smoking cessation* should be insisted with the patients as it may markedly influence the course of disease.

2. *Topical artificial tear drops* instilled frequently in the daytime and lubricating ointment at night and punctual plugs are useful for relief of foreign body sensation and other symptoms of dry eyes.

3. *Eyelid taping* at night prevents complication of exposure.

4. *Head elevation* while sleeping and cold compresses in the morning may help to decrease the morning lid edema.

5. *Guanethidine 5% eyedrops* may decrease the lid retraction caused by over action of Müller's muscle.

6. *Prisms* may be beneficial in patients with diplopia with small angle and relatively comitant deviations.

7. *Patient reassurance* about the self-limited but prolonged course of the disease with no immediate cure available.

8. *Systemic steroids* are usually reserved for patients with severe inflammation or compressive optic neuropathy in TAO. The European Group on Graves' orbitopathy (EUGOGO) suggests intravenous glucocorticoids for patient with advanced TAO. Steroids decrease the production of mucopolysaccharides by the fibroblasts. Pulse therapy may also be considered but if no response occurs after 48 hours, steroids probably will not work.

9. *Immunosuppressive therapy.* Antimetabolites like azathioprine and the role of plasmapheresis and intravenous immunoglobulin (IVIg) is not well delineated.

10. *Orbital radiation.* It is believed to damage orbital fibroblasts or perhaps lymphocytes. The radiation (1500–2000 cGy fractionated over 10 dose) is usually administered via lateral fields with posterior angulation. Since radiation may take several weeks to be effective and transiently causes increased inflammation it is advisable to maintain the patients on steroids during the first few weeks of treatment. Radiation is contraindicated in patients with diabetes mellitus because of the risk of worsening retinopathy. Cataract, radiation retinopathy and optic neuropathy are other possible risks of radiation.

11. *Combined therapy* with low dose steroids, azathioprine and irradiation is reported to be more effective than steroids or radiotherapy alone.

B. Surgical management

- *During active phase*, surgical orbital decompression may be required. If severe acute proptosis with corneal exposure and optic neuropathy does not respond to energetic steroid therapy or recurs after medical management, this may be performed.

- *During quiescent burnt-out phase* the surgical management is required to improve function and cosmesis. The disease is in quiescent stage for at least 6 months. Cosmetic improvement is the main indication for surgery which is done in a sequential manner in the following order:
  1. Orbital decompression
  2. Strabismus surgery
  3. Lid-lengthening surgery
  4. Blepharoplasty

1. Orbital decompression

Bony orbital decompression, may be carried out by an external or endoscopic approach and may involve 2, 3 or 4 walls.

- *Two-wall decompression.* To decompress the optic nerve, at least 2 orbital walls are usually decompressed (traditionally, the medial wall and floor of the orbit). This allows 3–6 mm of retroplacement of globe.

Medial wall removal should not extend above the frontoethmoidal suture to avert bleeding from the ethmoidal arteries and prevent CSF leaks. While removing the orbital floor, preservation of a strut of bone between the ethmoid and maxillary bones may reduce strabismus from inferomedial shift in the globe position.

- *Three-wall decompression.* It involves removal of parts of the floor, medial wall and lateral wall, and allows about 6–10 mm of retroplacement of the globe.

- *Four-wall decompression.* In addition to three-wall removal it involves removal of lateral half of roof and large portion of sphenoid at the apex. It requires a neurosurgical approach. This allows 10–16 mm of retroplacement of the globe and is indicated very rarely in patient with severe proptosis. The potential complications of orbital decompression are blindness, hemorrhage, diplopia, periorbital numbness, globe malposition, sinusitis and lid malposition.

Orbital fat decompression without bony removal is done for TAO without apical compression. These patients show predominant enlargement of the orbital fat compartment, rather than rectus muscles on orbital imaging.

In orbital fat decompression, fat is also removed posterior to equator of the globe unlike in cosmetic blepharoplasty. Reasonable and effective reduction in proptosis can be safely achieved by extensive orbital fat removal alone.

2. Strabismus surgery

Strabismus surgery in patients of TAO is generally delayed till the disease is inactive and the prism measurements have been stable for at least 6 months. It should always be carried out after the orbital decompression, since the latter may alter ocular motility. The goal of surgery is to minimize diplopia in primary and reading positions. Expecting binocular single vision in all positions of gaze may not be realistic.

Since TAO patients have restrictive myopathy, predominantly recessions are performed rather than resections. If possible, adjustable suture surgery is recommended. One should not operate simultaneously on more than 2 muscles per eye to prevent ocular ischemic syndrome.

3. Lid-lengthening surgery

Lid-lengthening surgery when required should be carried last, as the extraocular muscle surgery may affect eyelid retraction. It is considered if there is no improvement in lid retraction on restoration of the euthyroid state. It helps to decrease corneal exposure and can be used to deal with mild to moderate proptosis.

Botulinum toxin injection aimed at Müller's muscle and LPS muscle may be used as a temporary measure before definitive surgical correction, if desired by the patient. Eyelid surgery for definitive correction may include:

- *Müllerotomy,* i.e. disinsertion of Müller's muscle is the procedure of choice for mild lid retraction of 2–3 mm.
- *Levator recession/disinsertion* can be considered if further amounts of lid recession are required for moderate to severe upper eyelid retraction. Lateral levator tenotomy helps to decrease the temporal flare.
- *Scleral grafts* with LPS recession may be required in very severe cases.
- *Recession of lower eyelid retractors* may be required to correct more than 2 mm retraction of lower eyelid. Lower lid lengthening requires

a spacer material. Graft materials include human acellular dermis, tarsus and conjunctiva from the upper lid, hard palate. Horizontal tightening procedures (e.g. lateral tarsal strip) increase scleral show in patients with proptosis.

4. Blepharoplasty

This is the last phase of restorative surgery in TAO. Excess fatty tissue and redundant skin from around the eyelids is removed.

Upper lid blepharoplasty is performed transcutaneously with conservative skin excision. Brow fat resection may be considered.

Dacryopexy may be required if lacrimal gland prolapse occurs.

The transconjunctival approach to lower lid blepharoplasty can be used if no excess lower lid skin is present.

CONSULTATIONS

- Patients with TAO benefit from consultation and follow-up care with an endocrinologist.
- Orbital decompression can be performed in conjunction with an otorhinolaryngologist, especially when endoscopic procedures are contemplated.
- Neurosurgical consultation is required when decompression of the orbital roof is performed.

BIBLIOGRAPHY

1. Basic and clinical science course; section 5 Neuro-ophthalmology. American Academy of Ophthalmology 2009–10; chapter 14: 331–4.
2. Boulos PR, Hardy I. Thyroid associated orbitopathy: a clinicopathologic and therapeutic review. Current opinion in ophthalmology 2008;15(5): 389–400.
3. Luigi Bartelana, Claudi Marcocci, Aldo Pinchera. Graves' ophthalmology: a preventable disease? European Journal of Endocrinology 2006; 57–61.
4. Morax S, Ben Ayed H. Orbital decompression for dysthyroid orbitopathy: a review of techniques and indications. Journal francais ophthalmologie 2004;27(7):828–44.
5. Rose JG, Burkat CN, Boxrud CA. Diagnosis and management of thyroid orbitopathy. Otolaryngol Clin Nort Am 2005;38(5):1043–74.

32 | OCULAR MYOPATHIES

Ramesh Kekunnaya, Amit Gupta

INTRODUCTION AND CLASSIFICATION

INTRODUCTION

A variety of entities like fusional, neuronal, connective tissue (pulley) or optical disorder can cause strabismus. All these conditions can be either congenital or acquired. In addition, extraocular muscles can be directly, affected by various myopathies (inflammatory, infectious, benign or malignant conditions) and indirectly due to neuropathy. Below are the conditions that can be listed in this particular group. Congenital fibrosis of extraocular muscles (CFEOMs) has been studied extensively by many authors and now there is enough evidence to say that it is a primary neuropathy rather than, as formerly believed, a myopathy. CFEOMs is categorized under the group, congenital cranial nerve dysinnervation disorders (CCDDs). This chapter highlights in brief the clinical features and management aspects of all these disorders.

CLASSIFICATION

Extraocular muscle myopathies can be classified is as follows:

1. CFEOMs
2. Chronic progressive external ophthalmo-plegia (CPEO)
   a. Mitochondrial myopathy and encephalo-pathy, lactate acidosis, stroke-like episodes (MELAS)
   b. Kearns-Sayre syndrome/PEO plus
3. Oculopharyngeal muscular dystrophy
4. Myotonic dystrophy type 1
5. Ocular myocysticercosis
6. Ocular myositis
7. Thyroid associated ophthalmopathy
8. Tumors

CONGENITAL FIBROSIS OF EXTRAOCULAR MUSCLES

Congenital fibrosis of the extraocular muscles (CFEOMs) is a strabismus syndrome characterized by non-progressive, restrictive ophthalmoplegia of the extraocular muscles and congenital blepharoptosis. CFEOMs can be unilateral or bilateral. Three clinical phenotypes for familial CFEOMs (CFEOMs 1, 2, and 3) have been delineated, for which two genes have been identified to date: KIF21A for CFEOMs 1 and 3 and PHOX2A/ARIX for CFEOM2. The molecular genetics and MRI studies have strengthened the hypothesis that CFEOM results from the dysinnervation of the extraocular muscles supplied by the oculomotor (Fig. 32.1) and/or trochlear nerves (Demer et al. 2005).

CFEOM historically has been considered to be a primary myopathy in which there is fibrosis of the ocular musculature, fibrotic adhesions between Tenon's capsule and the extraocular muscles and in some cases, anomalous insertion of the muscles on the globe. More recent studies suggest that myopathic changes are secondary to aberrant innervation of the extraocular muscles. Evidence for a primary defect in innervation has emerged from neuropathologic and neuroimaging studies.

CFEOM1

CFEOM1 or "classic CFEOM" is characterized by bilateral blepharoptosis and ophthalmo-plegia with the eyes fixed in infraduction (hypotropia) approximately 20° to 30° below the horizontal midline (Fig. 32.2). Forced duction testing is positive for marked restriction of extraocular motility.

Patients typically assume a compensatory "chin up" head posture to fixate on objects.

Engle and colleagues used these findings to suggest that CFEOM1 may primarily be a neurogenic phenomenon with myopathy a secondary consequence of abnormal innervation. Inheritance of CFEOM1 is autosomal dominant with complete penetrance. The KIF21A gene encodes a kinesin microtubule associated motor protein that is associated with anterograde organelle transport in neuronal cells.

CFEOM2

CFEOM2 is characterized by bilateral blepharoptosis of varying severity and a partially or completely fixed large angle exotropia. Elevation, depression and adduction of the globes are essentially absent. Abduction is limited or absent. Forced duction testing is positive for marked restriction of extraocular motility. Patients undertake compensatory head posture such as a "chin up" posture or manual lid elevation to fixate on objects. There is phenotypic heterogeneity regarding the involvement of the vertical extraocular muscles and the degree of vertical misalignment of the eyes; Bosley and colleagues identified patients with varied

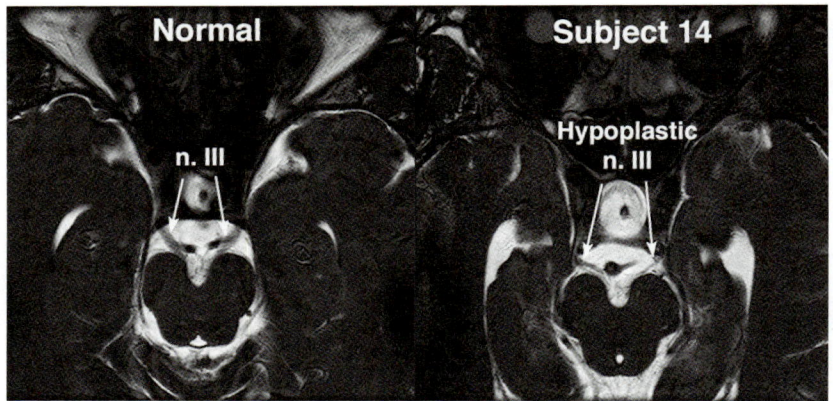

Fig. 32.1 *Case of CFEOMs where hypoplastic III nerve is noted (Courtesy: Demer et al.).*

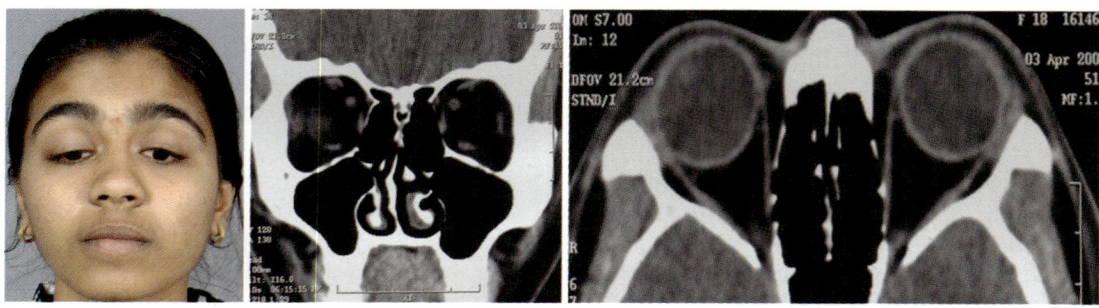

Fig. 32.2 *CFEOM1 with blepharoptosis and hypotropia. CT scan shows thinned out EOMs.*

presentations of vertical misalignment, including the absence of vertical strabismus, bilaterally infraducted eyes, bilaterally supraducted eyes, and a unilaterally misaligned eye, either supra- or infraducted. Synergistic convergent or divergent eye movements and Marcus Gunn jaw winking have not been identified as features of CFEOM2. Pupillary abnormalities in size as well as absent pupillary responses to light and near stimuli have been reported.

CFEOM3

CFEOM3 is characterized by a variable phenotypic presentation in which one of the affected family members does not fulfill the clinical criteria for classic CFEOM1. Affected individuals with CFEOM3 may have bilateral or unilateral (Fig. 32.3) disease. Blepharoptosis may be present. Motility varies from mild to complete ophthalmoplegia.

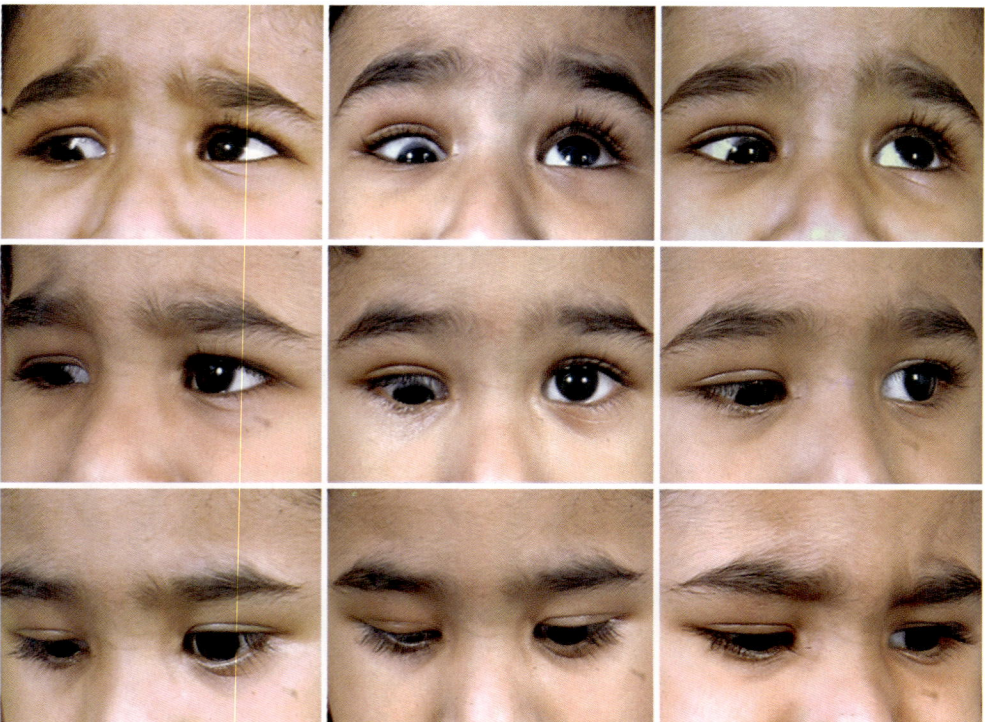

Fig. 32.3 *9-gaze picture showing CFEOM3 involving IR in the right eye.*

The patient may be orthotropic in primary position, and will adopt compensatory head postures depending upon the severity of the clinical phenotype. Aberrant synergistic and synkinetic eye movements are not consistently part of the CFEOM3 clinical spectrum. Pupillary abnormalities are not a feature of this subtype of CFEOM.

MANAGEMENT OF CFEOM

Treatment of CFEOM should incorporate both a surgical approach aimed at correction of strabismus (Fig. 32.4) and blepharoptosis and a non-surgical approach aimed at correction of refractive error with the ultimate goal of maximizing visual outcome, preventing the development of amblyopia, and improvement of head posture. Management should be individualized depending upon the severity of the clinical phenotype.

It is important to set expectations in patients and family members, as full eye movement cannot be restored and even alignment in primary position may not be attainable depending on the severity of involvement. Multiple procedures are likely to be required over time. Forced duction test should be performed after the rectus muscle has been detached in order to identify additional sources of globe restriction. It is best to avoid resection procedures. Botulinum toxin can serve as an adjunct to therapy in some cases with undercorrection if the residual tightness of the muscle is not profound. Surgical intervention can improve alignment but does not restore normal function.

PROGRESSIVE EXTERNAL OPHTHALMOPLEGIA

The diagnosis of mitochondrial myopathy depends upon a constellation of findings, family history, type of muscle involvement, specific laboratory abnormalities, and the results of histological, pathobiochemical and genetic analysis. The most common ocular manifestation of mitochondrial myopathy is progressive external ophthalmoplegia (PEO).

The most common form is late-onset bilateral progressive external ophthalmoplegia (PEO). PEO is characterized (Fig. 32.5) by ptosis and weakness of extraocular muscles leading to limitation of extraocular movements with relative sparing of downgaze and occasionally dysconjugate ocular movements.

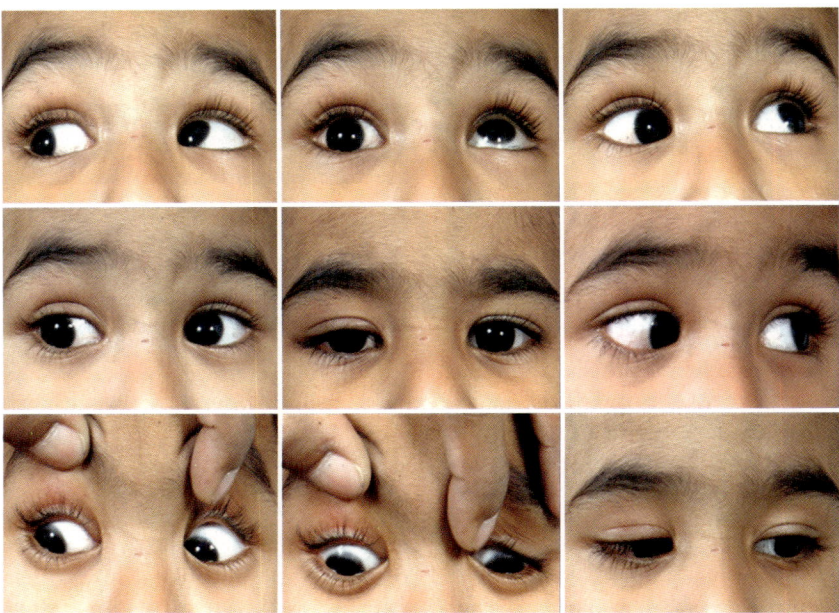

Fig. 32.4 *Postoperative 9-gaze showing the improvement in CFEOM involving right IR muscle.*

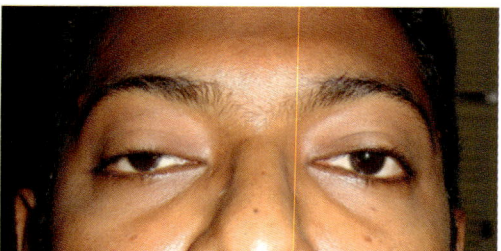

Fig. 32.5 *A patient with CPEO.*

Although, transient diplopia may occur, most patients seldom complain of it and are mostly unaware of their restrictions. The ptosis is often asymmetric. Up to 90% of PEO patients have additional weakness of the facial, bulbar or limb muscles. Thus, many patients may be classified as "PEO plus" because they present additional multisystem symptoms such as other neurological symptoms, hearing disturbances, or with diabetes.

Mitochondrial myopathy and encephalopathy, lactate acidosis, stroke-like episodes (MELAS)

The typical clinical manifestations of MELAS include stroke-like episodes (99–100%), seizures (85–96%), short stature (55–100%), muscle weakness (87–89%), headache/vomiting (77–92%), hearing loss (27–75%), encephalopathy (20–95%), optic atrophy (20%), pigmentary retinopathy (16%) and PEO (13%).

Kearns-Sayre syndrome/PEO plus

Kearns and Sayre first described PEO as a key feature of the Kearns-Sayre syndrome (KSS) in 1958. This syndrome is characterized by onset before age 20 years and encompasses PEO, atypical pigmentary retinopathy (salt- and pepper-like appearance), and frequently myopathic weakness, heart block, cerebellar ataxia and high cerebrospinal fluid (CSF) protein levels. KSS may include incomitant strabismus, mental deterioration, pyramidal signs, short stature, diabetes or delayed sexual maturation. An analogous syndrome-like entity of KSS is ptosis and ophthalmoplegia with additional organ involvement (PEO plus).

Both CPEO and Kearns-Sayre syndrome are associated with deficiencies in the respiratory chain complexes and mitochondrial DNA mutation or deletions. Muscle biopsy provides an important morphological clue for the diagnosis of mitochondrial disorders especially in patients presenting with predominant muscle involvement, as in CPEO. The characteristic morphological changes on muscle biopsy include ragged red fibers (RRF) on (Fig. 32.6) modified Gomori's trichrome (MGT) stain and lack of staining with a cytochrome C oxidase (COX) stain. However, muscle biopsy is normal in approximately 25% of patients with CPEO, thus necessitating molecular genetic analysis for more accurate diagnosis and to avoid the use of unnecessary drugs.

Muscle biopsy provides important clues to the diagnosis of patients presenting with CPEO. In muscle biopsy, combined COX-SDH is the most sensitive diagnostic histochemical stain. However, in about 40% of patients, histological studies may not be diagnostic of mitochondrial myopathy. Histological studies should be combined with genetic studies for the definitive diagnosis of CPEO syndrome.

Management is usually conservative. Some authors recommend Coenzyme Q, but the results are inconclusive. In some cases eye alignment surgery is helpful. Crutch glasses are generally used to correct blepharoptosis.

OCULOPHARYNGEAL MUSCULAR DYSTROPHY (OPMD)

Etiology

OPMD is caused by expansions in a 6-GCG trinucleotide repeat tract located in the first exon of the polyadenylate binding protein nuclear 1 gene on chromosome 14q. Genetic testing is available.

Clinical features

The combination of ptosis and pharyngeal weakness combined (Fig. 32.7) with ophthalmoparesis, dysphagia and weakness and wasting of face, neck, and distal limb muscles is quite characteristic for autosomal dominant, late onset OPMD.

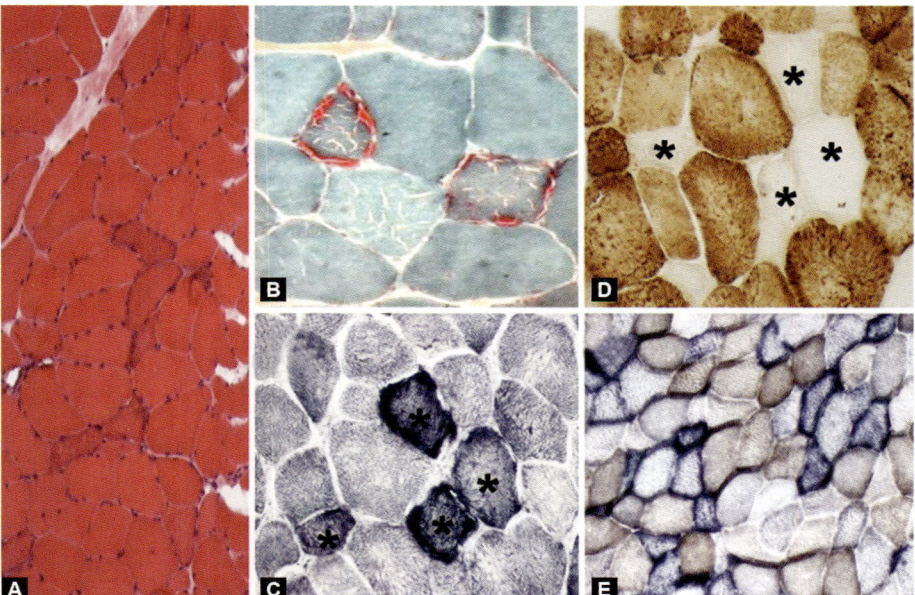

Fig. 32.6 *Various staining procedures showing: (A) Abnormal granular fibers (hematoxylin and eosin); (B) Characteristic red ragged fibers (modified Gomori's trichrome stain); (C) Blue ragged fibers (asterisks) (succinic dehydrogenase [SDH]); (D) Negative staining of blue ragged fibers with cytochrome C oxidase (asterisks) (COX); and (E) Combined staining showing more abnormal fibers (COX-SDH) (Sundaram C et al. 2011).*

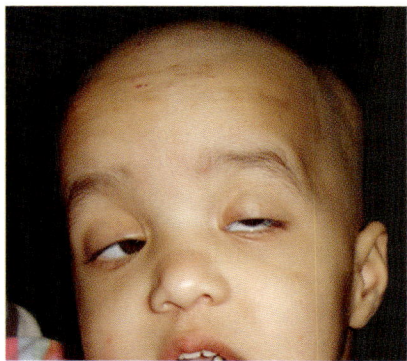

Fig. 32.7 *A patients with oculopharyngeal muscular dystrophy.*

MYOTONIC DYSTROPHY TYPE 1 (DM1)

Etiology

DM1 is caused by expansions in the CTG trinucleotide repeat tract located in the myotonic dystrophy protein kinase gene on chromosome 19q. Genetic testing is available.

Clinical features

Among the numerous well-known multisystemic features of the classic form of myotonic dystrophy (DM1), e.g. muscle weakness and myotonia, the eye is in any case affected. Not only myotonic cataracts but also retinal abnormalities, ptosis and blepharospasm are common features of the disease.

OCULAR MYASTHENIA GRAVIS

Clinical features

The term 'ocular myasthenia contrasting generalized myasthenia' is used to define the clinical subtype of myasthenia gravis with isolated eye muscle weakness and blepharoptosis or ophthalmoparesis, resulting in diplopia. Ocular dysfunction accounts for 50–80% of the initial manifestations of myasthenia gravis (Fig. 32.8). Asymmetric ptosis is most often associated with acquired and autoimmune myasthenia gravis. Furthermore, in young patients, inherited congenital myasthenic

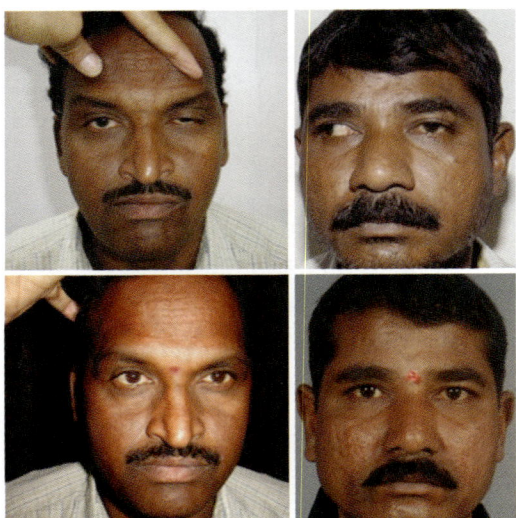

Fig. 32.8 *Pre- and post-treatment pictures of two patients with ocular myasthenia.*

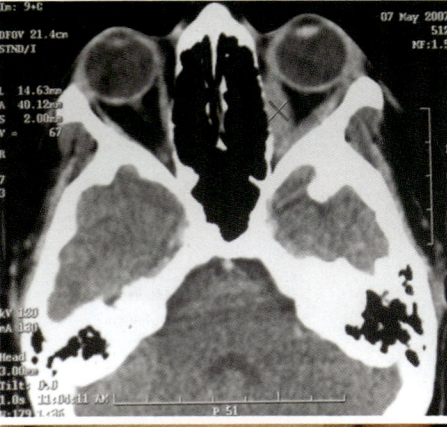

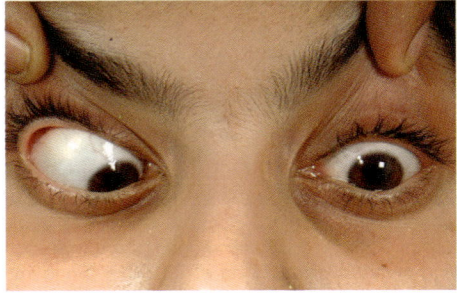

Fig. 32.9 *A case of myositis.*

syndromes are associated as an early feature with ptosis and ophthalmoplegia. The eyelid ice test, edrophonium test and nerve conduction studies with repetitive nerve stimulation of the facial nerves are helpful in making the diagnosis. Additionally, in 40–60% of the patients, acetylcholine receptor antibodies are present.

OCULAR MYOSITIS

Clinical features

In primary idiopathic orbital myositis, one or more extraocular muscles are affected. Acute onset, severe pain in and around the eye, pain on movement, occasional diplopia, chemosis and globe displacement are typical features. Beyond the acute form, a more chronic relapsing-remitting form is seen. Transorbital ultrasound and coronal MRI scans are helpful to further define the disease. Work up for the presence of any connective tissue disorder is essential. Imaging reveals enlargement of muscle belly as well as the tendinous portion (Fig. 32.9).

Treatment

Usually, there is a rapid response to systemic steroid therapy.

THYROID ASSOCIATED ORBITOPATHY

Thyroid orbitopathy is thought to be an organ specific autoimmune process and is associated with thyroid disease in 80–90% of cases. Bilateral muscle involvement (Figs 32.10 and 32.11) including inflammation, edema, and secondary fibrosis is very common. Imaging reveals fusiform posterior enlargement of extraocular muscles. For details, see Chapter 31.

MYOCYSTICERCOSIS

Etiology

Cysticercosis is a parasitic infestation by *Cysticercus cellulosae*, which is the larval form of *Taenia solium*. It is endemic in regions with poor sanitation. Human infection occurs by drinking contaminated water, eating uncooked vegetables infested with eggs of the worm, and auto-infection.

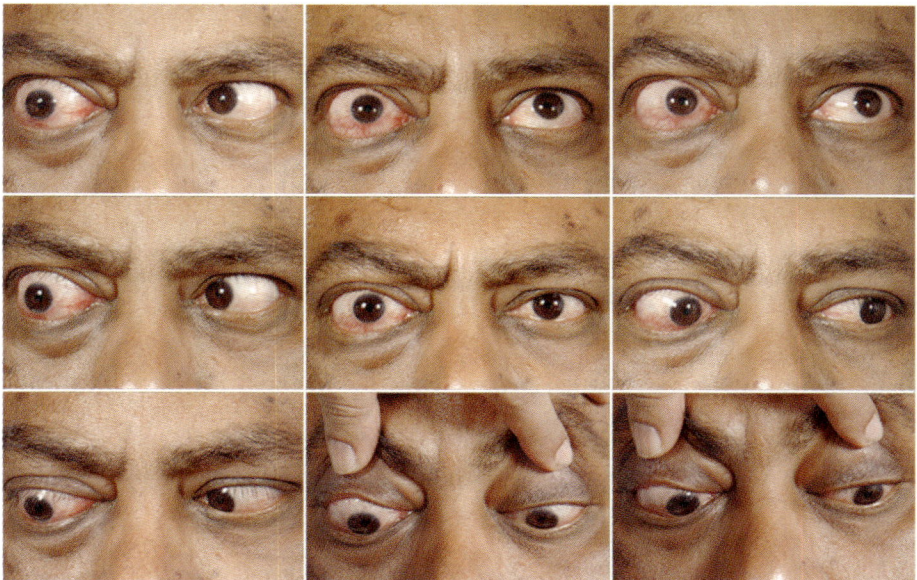

Fig. 32.10 *Thyroid associated orbitopathy.*

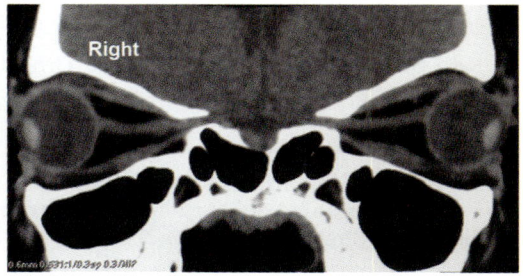

Fig. 32.11 *CT scan showing extraocular muscle involvement in thyroid associated orbitopathy.*

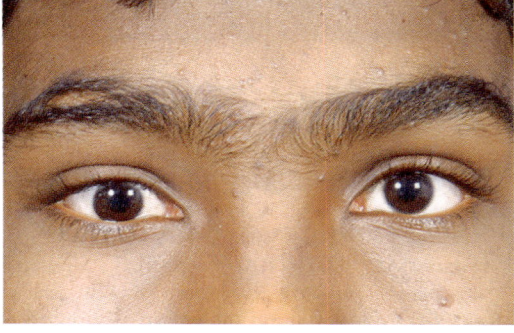

Fig. 32.12 *A case of right inferior rectus myocysticercosis.*

Clinical features

The most common form of systemic involvement is neurocysticercosis. Ocular and adnexal cysticercosis represents 13–46% of systemic disease. The three main symptoms at presentation were periocular swelling (38%), proptosis (24%), and ptosis (14%) with a median duration of 2 (range 0–24) months. The three main signs at presentation included ocular motility restriction (64.3%), proptosis (44.4%), and diplopia (36.8%). The cyst locations in the decreasing order of frequency were anterior orbit (69%), sub-conjunctival space (24.6%), posterior orbit (5.8%), and the eyelid (0.6%). In all, 80.7% of patients had cysts in relation to an extraocular muscle (Fig. 32.12). The superior rectus (33.3%) was the most commonly involved extraocular muscle.

USG B scan and/or CT scan of the orbit can confirm diagnosis.

Treatment

Myocysticercosis responds very well to a course of albendazole and oral prednisolone.

TUMORS OF EXTRAOCULAR MUSCLES

Primary tumors

The primary tumors which can involve the extraocular muscles are venous hemangioma, fibroangioma, neurilemoma, fibrous histiocytoma and paraganglioma.

Metastatic tumors

Malignancies that have been reported to metastasize to the orbit are adenocarcinomas of the breast and lung, melanomas of the skin, tumors of the genitourinary and gastrointestinal tracts as well as prostatic carcinoma. The commonest one is breast carcinoma, accounting for 10–61%. Metastatic carcinoma to the ocular muscles is extremely rare. There are few reports involving bilateral extraocular muscle metastasis following breast carcinoma.

Treatment

Treatment is mainly palliative.

BIBLIOGRAPHY

1. Bau V, Zierz S. Update on chronic progressive external ophthalmoplegia. Strabismus 2005; 13(3):133–42. Review.
2. Caballero PE, Candela MS, Alvarez CI, et al. Chronic progressive external ophthalmo-plegia: a report of 6 cases and a review of the literature. Neurologist 2007;13(1):33–6. Review.
3. Demer JL, Clark RA, Engle EC. Magnetic resonance imaging evidence for widespread orbital dysinnervation in congenital fibrosis of extraocular muscles due to mutations in KIF21A. Invest Ophthalmol Vis Sci 2005;46(2):530–9.
4. Engle EC, Goumnerov BC, McKeown CA, et al. Oculomotor nerve and muscle abnormalities in congenital fibrosis of the extraocular muscles. Ann Neurol. 1997;41(3):314–25.
5. He YJ, Lin TT, Song GX, et al. (Clinical analysis of primary extraocular muscles tumors.) Zhonghua Yan Ke Za Zhi Apr 2010;46(4):304–7.
6. Heidary G, Engle EC, Hunter DG. Congenital fibrosis of the extraocular muscles. Semin Ophthalmol 2008;23(1):3–8. Review.
7. Kekunnaya R, Bansal R, Vemuganti GK. Congenitally dysplastic inferior rectus muscle. J Pediatr Ophthalmol Strabismus 2010; 22;47:e1–4.
8. Kouvaris JR, Gkongkou PV, Papadimitriou CA, et al. Bilateral metastases to extraocular muscles from lobular breast carcinoma. Onkologie. 2008;31(7):387–9. Review.
9. Nakano M, Yamada K, Fain J, et al. Homozygous mutations in ARIX(PHOX2A) result in congenital fibrosis of the extraocular muscles type 2. Nat Genet 2001;29(3):315–20.
10. Oystreck DT, Engle EC, Bosley TM. Recent progress in understanding congenital cranial dysinnervation disorders. J Neuro-ophthalmol. 2011;31(1):69–77.
11. Rath S, Honavar SG, Naik M, et al. Orbital cysticercosis: clinical manifestations, diagnosis, management, and outcome. Ophthalmology 2010;117(3):600–5.
12. Schoser BG, Pongratz D. Extraocular mitochondrial myopathies and their differential diagnoses. Strabismus 2006;14(2):107–13.
13. Sundaram C, Meena AK, Uppin MS, et al. Contribution of muscle biopsy and genetics to the diagnosis of chronic progressive external opthalmoplegia of mitochondrial origin. J Clin Neurosci 2011;18(4):535–8.

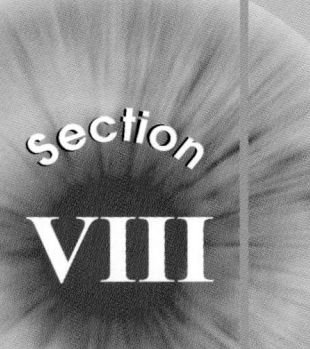

Neurological Disorders of Eyelids, Face, Orbital Syndromes, and Headache

NEUROLOGICAL DISORDERS OF EYELIDS AND FACIAL PAIN

Neebha Passi, AK Khurana, Urmil Chawla

NEUROLOGICAL DISORDERS OF EYELIDS

INTRODUCTION

Neurological disorders of eyelids can be enumerated as:

- Neurogenic Blepharoptosis
- Benign essential blepharospasm
- Marcus Gunn jaw winking syndrome
- Horner's syndrome
- Neurogenic eyelid retraction
- Plus minus lid syndrome
- Duane's retraction syndrome
- Blepharophimosis syndrome
- Parinaud's syndrome
- Chronic progressive external ophthalmoplegia
- Gluten ataxia

Majority of these have already been discussed in the previous chapters but there are some which need special mention.

BENIGN ESSENTIAL BLEPHAROSPASM

Benign essential blepharospasm (BEB) is a progressive neurological disorder characterized by involuntary muscle contractions and spasms of the eyelid muscles. It is a form of dystonia, a movement disorder in which muscle contractions cause sustained eyelid closure, twitching or repetitive movements.

BEB occurs in both men and women, although it is especially common in middle aged and elderly women.

Etiology

The anatomical origin and the biochemical basis of essential blepharospasm are unknown. It is believed that abnormalities in the basal ganglia or midbrain are responsible, but it is clear that the ultimate cause is multifactorial. Abnormal auditory brainstem response potentials have been noted in patients who have BEB and Meige's syndrome, which implicates involvement of the brainstem. Additionally, abnormal levels of neurotransmitters have been demonstrated in the midbrain and brainstem nuclei of patients with Meige's syndrome.

Clinical features

Benign essential blepharospasm begins gradually with increased frequency of eye blinking often associated with eye irritation. Salient features include:

- Bilateral involuntary spasmodic closure of the eyelids.
- Symptoms exacerbated by stress, fatigue, bright lights, interpersonal interactions.
- Fluctuation of symptoms marked by transient remissions and exacerbations.
- Generally, the spasms occur during the day, disappear in sleep, and reappear after waking.
- As the condition progresses, the spasms may intensify, forcing the eyelids to remain closed for long periods of time, and thereby causing substantial visual disturbance or functional blindness.
- Spasms improve with relaxation.
- Other symptoms may include increasing difficulty in keeping the eyes open and light sensitivity.

Associated features

- Decrease in tear production
- Dystonic activity of facial muscles (Meige's syndrome)
- Dystonic activity of the neck muscles (cranial cervical dystonia)
- Dystonic activity of the vocal cords (spastic dysphonia)
- Dysphagia, blepharoptosis, eyebrow ptosis, entropion, canthal tendon abnormalities.

Diagnosis

The diagnosis of essential blepharospasm is one of exclusion. The most common causes of secondary blepharospasm include blepharitis, trichiasis, dry eyes syndrome, corneal and external disease, glaucoma and uveitis.

Jankovic rating scale

0 : No spasms
1 : Minimal spasms with increased blinking only with external stimuli (e.g. bright light, wind, reading, driving)
2 : Mild, noticeable eyelid fluttering without functional disability
3 : Moderate, very noticeable spasm involving the eyelids causing some visual disability
4 : Severe, incapacitating spasms, often involving other facial muscles and causing functional blindness.

Treatment

The goal in the treatment of essential blepharospasm is to minimize or eliminate the disabling spasms. Pharmacological measures have variable success. Selective peripheral facial nerve avulsion, along with other surgical measures has been tried but complications such as facial paralysis, ectropion and high recurrences rates have decreased the success rate.

Pharmacological agents

Benzodiazepines, such as lorazepam 0.5–2.0 mg 2 to 3 times a day, or clonazepam 0.5–5 mg 3 times a day, or ozazepam 10–30 mg 3 to 4 times daily, have been sometimes effective.

Chemodenervation

The treatment of choice for the initial treatment of BEB is *botulinum toxin type A*. Botulinum neurotoxin blocks neuromuscular transmission by acting on peripheral cholinergic nerve endings to prevent acetylcholine release from the synaptic terminals. In most cases, there is a substantial relief of symptoms. Although some may experience side effects such as ptosis, diplopia, and eye dryness, these side effects are usually only temporary.

The onset of effect is within 24–72 hours with a plateau usually at 3–5 days but occasionally, onset may be delayed as long as 2–4 weeks. The duration of denervation averages 3 months for BEB and slightly longer for hemifacial spasm. Frequently, the procerus and corrugators muscles also are involved and so require injection. In the upper eyelid, the injections should be subcutaneous only in order to prevent migration of the toxin below the orbital septum, which otherwise results in paralysis of the levator muscle. Frequently, injections in the lower lid alone have a pronounced effect on spasms in the lower face, thus eliminating or decreasing the dosage required in the lower face for Meige's syndrome and hemifacial spasm. The recommended starting dosage for botulinum toxin type A is 1.25–5 units per injection site. If a suboptimal response occurs, the dosage should be doubled. Less toxin usually is required for dystonic activity following paresis.

Myectomy

Surgical myectomy is the major treatment for BEB in which the orbicularis, procerus and corrugators muscles are extirpated. A modified or limited myectomy has been introduced more recently, in which only the orbicularis muscle in the upper lid is removed. The limited myectomy offers a quicker recovery and most of the benefits of the radical myectomy with less morbidity.

Chemomyectomy is another type of myectomy under investigation. Local injections of doxorubicin produce permanent orbicularis oculi weakness. However, high concentrations of drug can result in skin ulceration, but a modified technique may be less deleterious. Although doxorubicin is known to be carried in a retrograde fashion to the brain and is a known neurotoxin, animal studies have been conducted to demonstrate a measurable loss of facial neurons.

NEUROGENIC EYELID RETRACTION

Causes

Mild retraction of the lower eyelid may occur as a variant of eyelid position in otherwise normal individuals. It may be associated with axial myopia, familial congenital shallow orbits, maxillary hypoplasia, or involutional lower lid laxity.

Neurogenic eyelid retraction encompasses a diverse group of diseases within which are several well known causes. Some of the common causes of lid retraction are listed as follows:

- Benign transient conjugate downward gaze in preterm infants
- "Eye-popping" reflex in infants
- Dorsal midbrain syndrome, Parinaud's syndrome, Sylvian aqueduct syndrome (Koerber-Salus-Elschnig syndrome)

- Pinealoma
- Hydrocephalus
- Basilar artery disease
- Disseminated sclerosis
- Bulbar poliomyelitis
- Closed head injury
- Impending tentorial herniation
- Guillain-Barré syndrome
- Oculogyric crisis
- Eyelid nystagmus
- Progressive supranuclear palsy
- "Levator spasticity" or failure of inhibition during coma ("coma vigil")
- Marcus Gunn (jaw winking) syndrome
- See-saw jaw winking
- Horizontal gaze palsy (congenital or acquired)
- Aberrant innervations or regeneration of the oculomotor nerve (congenital or acquired)
- Cyclic oculomotor paralysis
- Sympathetic irritation (Horner-Bernard syndrome)
- Weakness of orbicularis oculi (e.g. facial nerve paralysis)
- Orbital floor ("blowout") fracture
- Sympathomimetic eyedrops (phenylephrine, apraclonidine)

Evaluation and diagnosis

History

During initial patient evaluation, a careful history should be taken, especially the time of onset and progression. An extensive medical history helps to establish any further tests required to confirm a diagnosis. Particular attention should be directed to symptoms of thyroid disease.

Periocular examination

- *Position of eyelid margins.* A complete periocular examination should measure and document the position of the upper and lower eyelids with respect to the corneal limbus. Eyelid retraction is defined as a deviation from the normal position of the upper or lower eyelid margin with respect to the limbus of the eye. The normal upper eyelid margin rests 1–2 mm below the superior limbal border and the lower eyelid margin rests at the level of the inferior limbus. Elevation of the upper eyelid or depression of the lower eyelid results in a visible zone of white sclera above or below the limbal margin. Examination of the eyelid position should be completed in all fields of gaze and with movement of the mouth to uncover possible traumatic rectus muscle entrapment, Graves' disease, cranial nerve regeneration, jaw winking ptosis, and Duane's syndrome. Furthermore, retraction may be unilateral or bilateral.

- *Other helpful measurements* include the palpebral fissure height, degree of lagophthalmos or lid lag on downgaze, levator muscle function and the distances from eyelid margin to central corneal reflex.

- *Exophthalmometry* can also be used in suspected cases of exophthalmos.

- *Traction on the eyelids* may uncover fibrosis and scarring.

- *Forced duction testing* is helpful to diagnose the existence of fibrotic or incarcerated rectus muscles.

- *Palpation and observation of the orbital rims* may expose old bone trauma or maxillary hypoplasia.

- *Traction on the lower eyelid tissue* is helpful in diagnosing involutional laxity and cicatricial changes in the anterior and posterior eyelid lamellae.

- *Examination of ocular and orbital structures may detect several other causes* of the aberrant eyelid position.

- Buphthalmos, intraocular tumors, enlargement of the rectus muscles or orbital tumors may present with unilateral or bilateral proptosis and eyelid retraction.

- *Pseudoretraction* may be seen in cases of contralateral eyelid blepharoptosis with a Hering effect. In the presence of unilateral ptosis, equal central nuclear output to both levator muscles may result in elevation and retraction of the previously normal opposite eyelid. Pseudoretraction of the elevated eyelid is suggested when digital elevation of the more ptotic lid results in lowering of the retracted lid.

Management

Investigations

Proper diagnosis of the underlying disorder leading to eyelid retraction forms the basis for appropriate management of this condition.

- *Orbital imaging*: Orbital examination may be augmented by ultrasound or radiological studies. The latter are particularly helpful in the diagnosis of Graves' disease, orbital trauma, and orbital tumors.

- *Thyroid function tests* are commonly ordered in cases of upper eyelid retraction.

Conservative treatment

Mild forms of asymptomatic lid retraction can be simply managed with frequent instillation of topical lubricants

Medical treatment

Eyelid retraction related to systemic diseases, such as Guillain-Barré syndrome or myasthenia gravis should be treated using systemic medicines. Discontinuation of topical drops, such as apraclonidine, may also resolve drug induced retraction. Eyelid retraction associated with Graves' disease may show some improvement following high dose oral corticosteroids or radiotherapy.

Botulinum toxin. Till the time definitive surgery is performed, botulinum toxin can be used as a reliable adjunct to the treatment of lid retraction. An average drop in the upper lid of 2–3 mm can be achieved with a transconjunctival injection of 2.5–5 units for about 3 months. Patients must be explained that the procedure carries a 5–10 percent risk of overcorrection resulting in ptosis, and up to a 10 percent risk of transient diplopia.

Surgical treatment

Surgery is recommended to relieve or prevent persistent exposure of the cornea secondary to lid retraction and lagophthalmos or for cosmetic reasons. The choice of procedure depends upon whether the lid involved is upper or lower, severity of lid retraction and associated features like proptosis, status of extraocular muscles and corneal condition.

Surgical approaches which have been described for treatment of eyelid retraction include:

- Mullerectomy,
- Levator recession,
- Marginal myotomies, and
- Spacers

Injection of fillers like stabilized hyaluronic acid are useful in the treatment of mild lower lid retraction.

Orbital decompression. It may be necessary in cases with proptosis and indirectly relieves both upper and lower eyelid retraction to some extent.

PLUS MINUS LID SYNDROME

Plus minus lid syndrome is an ocular syndrome characterized by unilateral ptosis and contralateral lid retraction. Also when the ipsilateral lid is raised manually, the contralateral retracted lid does not revert.

Causes

Plus minus lid syndrome is an acquired neurological abnormality of eyelid position reported in the following conditions:

- *Ocular myasthenia,*
- *After lesions of ocular motor nerve,*
- *Ocular myositis,* and
- *Paramedian mesencephalic–diencephalic lesions.*
- Occasionally occur due to lesions involving the III nerve fascicles.

Neurological basis. Two muscles are involved in upper eyelid elevation, the tarsal smooth muscle of Müller that has a role limited to tonic control of eyelid position and the levator palpebrae, a skeletal muscle innervated by fascicles of the oculomotor nerve. These fascicles arise from a single medial nucleus called central caudal nucleus, a subdivision of the oculomotor nuclear complex. Nuclear lesions therefore, lead to bilateral ptosis; however fasicular lesions can cause unilateral ptosis. The nucleus of the posterior commissure provides inhibitory inputs to the central caudal nucleus. Each nucleus of the posterior commissure is connected with its contralateral counterpart through the posterior commissure but does not project directly on the central caudal nucleus. It projects on the levator palpebrae motor neurons in the supra-oculomotor area, located dorsolaterally to the oculomotor nucleus within the periaqueductal gray matter.

MARCUS GUNN'S JAW WINKING SYNDROME

The jaw winking syndrome was initially described by Marcus Gunn in 1883, also known as *trigemino oculomotor synkinesis*. This form of synkinetic ptosis is typically unilateral and not hereditary. There is intermittent elevation of the ptotic eyelid coinciding with contraction of the muscles of mastication, resulting in a "winking" movement during eating or chewing. The synkinesis commonly involves the ipsilateral external pterygoid muscle, which moves the jaw toward the opposite side. The severity of the ptosis and the amplitude of the wink are proportionately related. Measurable levator function is variable or decreased. The upper eyelid crease is usually intact. Hypotropia and other forms of strabismus may be seen in a jaw winking syndrome. The wink often becomes less noticeable with age, as patients learn to limit oral movements that stimulate the synkinesis.

Grading

Marcus Gunn phenomenon has been graded into:

- *Mild*: <2 mm
- *Moderate*: 2–5 mm
- *Severe*: >5 mm

Etiopathogenesis

The cause of this condition is unknown, although there appears to be misdirection of either the efferent motor innervations or afferent proprioceptive fibers of the third and fifth cranial nerves. A few authors have speculated that the jaw winking is due to disinhibition of pre-existing phylogenetically more primitive mechanisms.

Treatment

Mild cases can be treated with levator aponeurotic muscle resection.

Patients with *moderate to severe* Marcus Gunn jaw winking ptosis may require ablation of the levator, followed by frontalis suspension.

INVERSE MARCUS GUNN PHENOMENON

It is a condition that causes the eyelid to fall upon opening of the mouth. In this case, trigeminal innervation to the pterygoid muscles of the jaw is associated with an inhibition of the branch of the oculomotor nerve to the levator palpebrae superioris, as opposed to stimulation in Marcus Gunn jaw winking.

GLUTEN ATAXIA

Gluten ataxia is a rarely diagnosed and frequently overlooked condition responsible for a set of symptoms usually labelled *"sporadic idiopathic ataxia,"* meaning that symptoms arise spontaneously and sporadically, and cannot be traced to any definitive cause.

Etiopathogenesis

In the case of gluten ataxia, gluten cannot be properly digested in the body, and certain protein deposits develop in the brain, causing changes that affect the neurological system.

Clinical features

This condition usually occurs in adults and manifests in a variety of neurological symptoms:

• Drooping eyelids
• Severe headaches
• Lack of muscle coordination
• Gait and balance disturbances
• Numbness, tingling and weakness in the extremities
• Problems with speech and word finding

Diagnosis and treatment

• Usually the patient is worked up for multiple sclerosis, Parkinson's and other neurological disorders but is negative.
• *Repeated MRI scans* cannot pinpoint the exact cause of these symptoms, which can be severe and debilitating.
• Often the diagnosis of gluten ataxia is only made when the patient reveals a past positive test for gluten intolerance, family history of celiac disease, or a history of gastrointestinal problems like irritable bowel syndrome or colitis.

Supportive treatment

• *Supportive but not curative treatment* is given to patient, once the diagnosis "sporadic idiopathic ataxia" is made.
• *Complete avoidance of gluten* in addition to supportive physical and cognitive therapies can sometimes reverse many of the patient's symptoms but complete recovery is not always possible.

PARINAUD'S SYNDROME

Parinaud's syndrome, also known as *dorsal midbrain syndrome,* is a group of abnormalities of eye movement and pupil dysfunction. It is caused by lesions of the upper brainstem.

Clinical features

Parinaud's syndrome is a cluster of abnormalities of eye movement and pupil dysfunction, characterized by:

• *Eyelid retraction (Collier's sign)*
• *Paralysis of upgaze:* Downward gaze is usually preserved. This vertical palsy is supranuclear, so doll's head maneuver should elevate the eyes, but eventually all upward gaze mechanisms fail.
• *Pseudo-Argyll Robertson pupils*: Accommodative paresis ensues, and pupils become mid dilated and show light near dissociation.
• *Convergence retraction nystagmus*: Attempts at upward gaze often produce this phenomenon. On fast up gaze, the eyes pull in and the globes retract.
• *Conjugate downgaze in the primary position:* "setting sun sign".
• *Bilateral papilledema* is also commonly associated.

Etiology

Parinaud's syndrome results from injury, either direct or compressive to the dorsal midbrain, specifically, compression or ischemic damage of the mesencephalic tectum, including the superior colliculus adjacent oculomotor (origin of cranial nerve III) and Edinger-Westphal nuclei, causing dysfunction to the motor function of the eye.

Prognosis and treatment

- *Thorough workup*, including neuroimaging is essential to rule out anatomic lesions or other causes of this syndrome.
- *Treatment is primarily directed towards etiology* of the dorsal midbrain syndrome.
- *Bilateral inferior rectus recession* is useful to relieve visually significant upgaze palsy. Retraction nystagmus and convergence movements are usually improved with this procedure as well.

Prognosis

The eye findings of Parinaud's syndrome generally improve slowly over months, especially with resolution of the causative factor; continued resolution after the first 3–6 months of onset is uncommon.

FACIAL PAIN

GENERAL CONSIDERATIONS

Pain in the facial area may be due to neurological or vascular causes, but equally well may be dental in origin. All the neurological and vascular causes of facial pain (excluding headaches) are rare compared to the dental and temporomandibular causes. The risk factors for some of the conditions are known, but there is little information on natural history and prognosis.

Classification

A classification system is useful when attempting to make a diagnosis. The International Association for the Study of Pain (IASP) and the International Headache Society (IHS) have both classified these pains. The orofacial pain, as adapted from Hapak *et al.* (Table 33.1), can also be classified into:

- Musculoligamentous (Group 1),
- Dental (Group 2), and
- Neurological/vascular (Group 3).

Causes

Common causes of orofacial pain are summarized in Table 33.1.

Diagnosis

Diagnosis of the majority of these facial pains is based on a careful history and examination.

- *Brief pain inventory (BPI)* uses a visual analogue scale (0–10) to determine severity of pain and the impact on quality of life issues such as mood, relationships, and work.
- *Hospital anxiety and depression (HAD) scale* is used to determine if there is evidence for a diagnosis of depression or anxiety.

Management principles

In many respects treatment of a patient with chronic facial pain is no different from treating any patient with chronic pain, as the psychosocial and behavioral response patterns are the

Table 33.1 *Classification and causes of orofacial pain*

Musculoligamentous/soft tissue (Group 1)	Dentoalveolar (Group 2)	Neurological/vascular (Group 3)
Temporomandibular joint (TMJ) pain	Dentinal	Trigeminal neuralgia
Facial arthromyalgia, myofascial pain	Periodontal	Glossopharyngeal neuralgia
Atypical facial pain/idiopathic orofacial pain	Pulpal	Nerve compression
Salivary gland disease	Cracked tooth syndrome	Cluster headache
Optic neuritis	Maxillary sinusitis	Postherpetic neuralgia
Internal derangements TMJ		Cranial arteritis
Burning mouth	Thermal sensitivities	Pretrigeminal neuralgia
Candidiasis	Atypical odontalgia	SUNCT
Cancer, sinuses, nasopharynx, brain		Ramsay Hunt

same despite different medical and dental causes.

Referral for a patient with orofacial pain should be done as below:

- Group 1 patients are in general best referred to oral physicians or maxillofacial surgeons
- Group 2 to dentists, and
- Group 3 patients are referred to neurologists.

Aim of treatment can be summarized as below:

- Eliminate or minimize the facial pain
- Eliminate or minimize negative cognitive, behavioral, and emotional factors
- Increase efficacy of drug treatment by careful choice
- Encourage self management which increases control over pain.

Treatment modalities include: *medical, surgical,* and *alternative* (ranging from acupuncture to cognitive behavior therapy) and patients may need a variety of these.

SPECIFIC CONDITIONS

A few conditions which are important from an ophthalmological point of view are discussed here.

TRIGEMINAL NEURALGIA

Applied anatomy

The trigeminal nerve is the fifth (V) cranial nerve, which arises from the brainstem inside the skull. It divides into three branches and then exits the skull to supply feeling and movement to the face (Fig. 33.1).

- *Ophthalmic division* (V1) provides sensation to the forehead and eye.
- *Maxillary division* (V2) provides sensation to the cheek, upper lip, and roof of the mouth.
- *Mandibular division* (V3) provides sensation to the jaw and lower lip; it also provides movement of the muscles involved in biting, chewing, and swallowing.

Definition

Trigeminal neuralgia is defined by the Indian Association of Study of Pain (IASP) as "a sudden, usually unilateral, severe, brief, stabbing, recurrent pain in the distribution of one or more branches of the fifth cranial nerve".

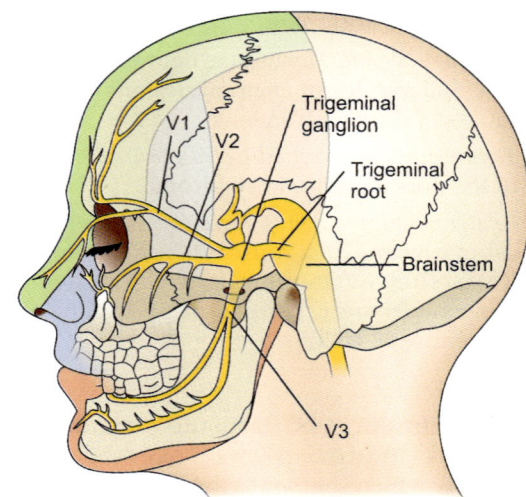

Fig. 33.1 *Three divisions of trigeminal nerve that branch from the trigeminal ganglion: ophthalmic division (V1) provides sensation to the forehead and eye, maxillary division (V2) provides sensation to the cheek, and mandibular division (V3) provides sensation to the jaw.*

Trigeminal neuralgia is characterized by extreme pain and muscle spasms in the face. Attacks of intense, electric shock-like facial pain can occur without warning or be triggered by touching specific areas of the face.

Etiology

It is believed that the protective sheath of the trigeminal nerve deteriorates, sending abnormal messages along the nerve, these abnormalities disrupt the normal signal of the nerve and cause pain. Several factors can cause the deterioration of this protective sheath: aging, multiple sclerosis, tumors, but most agree that it is caused by an abnormal vein or artery that compresses the nerve. Thus, etiology of this neuropathic pain remains unknown although it is postulated that the pathophysiological mechanism is that of compression of the trigeminal nerve by blood vessels such as the cerebral arteries in the root entry zone of the pons. In a minority of cases the trigeminal neuralgia is secondary to benign or malignant tumors.

Clinical features

- *An attack of intense pain,* which results when the trigeminal nerve becomes irritated, is also called *tic douloureux* because of the un-controllable facial twitching caused by the pain. Trigeminal neuralgia is serious because it interferes with many aspects of a person's life.

- *Typical trigeminal neuralgia* involves brief instances of intense pain, like an electrical shock in one side of the face. This pain comes in repeated waves that last an hour or more.
- Patient may initially experience short, mild attacks, with periods of remission. But trige-minal neuralgia can progress, causing longer, frequent attacks of searing pain.
- *Trigeminal neuralgia affects* 1 in every 25,000 people, and occurs slightly more in women than men.
- *Age.* Patients are usually middle age and older.
- *Patients describe an attack as* a "pins and needles" sensation that turns into a burning or jabbing pain, or as an electrical shock that may last a few seconds or minutes.
- *Triggering factors.* Everyday activities can trigger an episode. Other activities such as shaving or brushing teeth, can also trigger pain.
- *Trigger zones.* Some patients are sensitive in certain areas of the face, called *trigger zones*, which when touched cause an attack. These zones are usually near the nose, lips, eyes, ear, or inside the mouth.
- *Pain of typical trigeminal neuralgia* usually has the following features:
  – Affects one side of the face
  – Can last several days or weeks, followed by a remission for months or years
  – Frequency of painful attacks increases over time and may become disabling.
- *Atypical trigeminal neuralgia*, a less common form of the disorder, causes a less intense, constant, dull burning or aching pain. This pain sometimes occurs with occasional electric shock-like stabs that may last a day or more. Atypical facial pain is more difficult to treat.

Management

Diagnosis

When a person first experiences facial pain, a dentist is often consulted. If the pain requires further evaluation, a consultation with a neuro-logist or a neurosurgeon may be recommended.

The possibility of a tumor or multiple sclerosis must be ruled out. Therefore, a *magnetic resonance imaging* (MRI) scan may be performed. *Computed tomography* is useful to exclude tumors, whereas magnetic resonance imaging is used to assess whether compression of the trigeminal nerve has occurred. Although greater specificity and sensitivity is claimed for the latter, the evidence is not of high quality.

An MRI FIESTA scan can detect any blood vessels compressing the nerve. The diagnosis of trigeminal neuralgia is made after carefully assessing the patient's symptoms.

Treatment

A variety of treatments are available, including medication, surgery, needle procedures, and radiation. First line treatment is medication. When medications fail to control pain or cause intolerable side-effects, a neurosurgeon may be consulted to discuss other procedures.

Medication

Medications are the initial treatment for trigeminal neuralgia and are used as long as the pain is controlled and the side-effects do not interfere with a patient's activities. About 80% of patients experience at least short-term pain relief with medications. Anticonvulsants and muscle relaxants are prescribed to block the pain signals from the nerve.

- *Anticonvulsants,* such as carbamazepine (in the doses of 300–1000 mg/d), clonazepam (4–8 mg/d), oxcarbazepine (300–1200 mg/d), phenytoin (200–300 mg/d), and gabapentin (1800–3600 mg/d) are used to control trigeminal neuralgia pain. If the medication begins to lose effectiveness, the doctor may increase the dose or switch to another type. Side-effects may include drowsiness, unsteadiness, nausea, skin rash, and blood disorders. Therefore, patients are monitored routinely and undergo blood tests to ensure that the drug levels remain safe and that blood disorders do not develop. Multiple drug therapy may be necessary to control pain.
- *Muscle relaxants,* such as baclofen (in doses of 50–80 mg/d) are sometimes effective in treating trigeminal neuralgia. Side-effects may include confusion, nausea, and drowsiness.

Surgery

The goal of surgery is to stop the blood vessel from compressing the trigeminal nerve, or to cut the nerve to keep it from sending pain signals to the brain.

- *Microvascular decompression* (MVD) is a surgery to gently reroute the blood vessel from compressing the trigeminal nerve by padding the vessel with a sponge. MVD provides immediate pain relief in 95% of patients. About 20% of patients have pain recurrence within 10 years. The major benefit of MVD is that it causes little or no facial numbness. The major disadvantages are the risks of anesthesia and of undergoing an operation near the brain.
- *Sensory rhizotomy* is the irreversible cutting of the trigeminal nerve root at its connection to the brainstem. The motor root, which controls the chewing muscles, must be preserved. The sensory root fibers, which transmit the pain signals to the brain, are severed. Cutting the nerve causes permanent facial numbness and should only be considered for recurrent pain that has not responded to other treatments.

Outpatient needle procedures

Needle procedures are minimally invasive techniques of reaching the trigeminal nerve through the face without a skin incision or skull opening. They are performed with a hollow needle inserted through the skin (percutaneous) of the cheek into the trigeminal nerve at the base of the skull. The goal of rhizotomy or injection procedures is to damage an area of the trigeminal nerve to keep it from sending pain signals to the brain. Damaging the nerve causes mild to major facial numbness in that area.

- *Radiofrequency rhizotomy*, also called percutaneous stereotactic radiofrequency rhizotomy (PSR), uses a heating current to selectively destroy some of the trigeminal nerve fibers that produce pain. PSR provides immediate pain relief for 98% of patients. About 20% of patients experience pain recurrence within 15 years. Medication, repeat PSR, or another surgical procedure can be considered. Complications may include diplopia, jaw weakness, loss of corneal reflex, dysesthesia and very rarely anesthesia dolorosa. Partial facial numbness in the area where the pain existed is expected. Other complications, such as blurred vision or chewing problems, are usually temporary.
- *Glycerol injection* is similar to PSR in that a hollow needle is passed through the cheek to the nerve. The needle is positioned in the trigeminal cistern (a fluid-filled area in the ganglion). Glycerol is injected into the cistern to damage some of the trigeminal nerve fibers that produce pain. Because the location of the glycerol cannot be controlled precisely, the results are somewhat unpredictable. Glycerol injection provides immediate pain relief in 70% of patients. About 50% of patients experience pain recurrence within 3 to 4 years. As with PSR, partial facial numbness is expected and complications are similar.
- *Balloon compression* is similar to PSR in that a hollow needle is passed through the cheek to the nerve. However, it is performed under general anesthesia. A balloon is placed in the trigeminal nerve through a catheter. The balloon is inflated where fibers produce pain. The balloon compresses the nerve, injuring the pain-causing fibers. After several minutes the balloon and catheter are removed. Balloon compression provides immediate pain relief for 80% of patients. About 20% of patients experience pain recurrence within 3 years. Complications may include minor numbness, chewing problems, or double vision.
- *Peripheral neurectomy* can be performed to the nerve branches by exposing them on the face through a small skin incision. Cutting the supraorbital nerve (branch of V1 division) may be advised if pain is isolated to the area above the forehead. Cutting the infraorbital nerve (branch of V2 division) may be performed if pain is limited to the area below the eye along the upper cheekbone. Cutting the nerve causes complete facial numbness in the region the nerve supplies.

Radiation

The goal of radiation treatment is to deaden the trigeminal nerve root to interrupt the pain signals from reaching the brain. Stereotactic radiosurgery is a noninvasive outpatient procedure that uses radiation beams to destroy some of the trigeminal nerve. Highly focused beams of radiation are delivered to the trigeminal nerve root. Pain relief may not occur immediately but rather gradually over time. About 50% of patients have pain relief in 4 weeks; 75% of patients have pain relief in 8 weeks. Patients remain on medication for a period of time following treatment to control the pain while the radiation takes effect. Seventy percent of patients are relieved of pain for 2 years. In about 50% of patients, pain recurs 3 to 5 years after treatment. Complications include facial numbness and dry eye.

IDIOPATHIC OR ATYPICAL FACIAL PAIN

The definition for this condition is very unclear and remains a subject of controversy according to the International Association for the Study of Pain (IASP). Atypical Facial Pain (AFP, also termed *atypical facial neuralgia, chronic idiopathic facial pain, or psychogenic facial pain*), is a type of chronic facial pain which does not fulfill any other diagnosis. Both the International Headache Society (IHS) and the International Association for the Study of Pain (IASP) have adopted the term *persistent idiopathic facial pain (PIFP)* to replace AFP. In the 2nd Edition of the International Classification of Headache Disorders (ICHD-2), PIFP is defined as "persistent facial pain that does not have the characteristics of the cranial neuralgias and is not attributed to another disorder."

Clinical features

Main features of AFP are:

- No objective signs,
- Negative results with all investigations/tests,
- No obvious explanation for the cause of the pain, and
- A poor response to attempted treatments.

AFP has been described variably as a medically unexplained symptom, a diagnosis of exclusion, a psychogenic cause of pain (e.g. a manifestation of somatoform disorder), and as a neuropathy. It is usually burning and continuous in nature, and may last for many years.

Depression and anxiety are often associated.

Age. For unknown reasons, AFP is significantly more common in middle aged or elderly people, and in females.

Non-specific signs that may be associated with AFP include increased temperature and tenderness of the mucosa in the affected area, which is otherwise normal in every regard. Patient often reports symptoms of paresthesia, pain and throbbing.

Physical examination may be normal, but hypoesthesia, hyperesthesia, and allodynia may be found.

Diagnosis

AFP can be difficult to diagnose—and is often misdiagnosed.

- *Excluding an organic cause* for the pain is the most important part of the diagnosis.
- *Odontogenic pain* should especially be ruled out, since this accounts for over 95% of cases of orofacial pain.
- *Diagnosis of facial pain* generally is often multidisciplinary.

ICHD-2 diagnostic criteria

The International Classification of Headache Disorders (ICHD-2) lists diagnostic criteria for "persistent idiopathic facial pain" (the term that replaces AFP in this classification):

A. Pain in the face, present daily and persisting for all or most of the day, fulfilling criteria B and C,

B. Pain is confined at onset to a limited area on one side of the face, and is deep and poorly localized,

C. Pain is not associated with sensory loss or other physical signs,

D. Investigations including X-ray of face and jaws do not demonstrate any relevant abnormality.

Note. There are presently no accepted medical tests which consistently discriminate between facial pain syndromes or differentiate atypical facial pain from other syndromes. However, a normal radiograph, CT, and MRI may help to exclude other pathology such as arteriovenous malformation, tumor, temporomandibular joint disorder, or MS.

Management

Psychosocial interventions. Psychosocial interventions for AFP include:
- cognitive behavioral therapy, and
- biofeedback

Medical treatment. Medications such as analgesics, antidepressants, centrally acting muscle relaxants and anticonvulsants can be used to alleviate the pain.

Surgical treatment. Surgery is not an appropriate treatment for AFP, however, the frequent failure of medical treatment to relieve pain has occasionally led surgeons to attempt surgical treatments. Surgery may give a temporary remission from pain, but rarely there is a long term cure achieved via these measures. Sometimes the pain may be increased or simply migrate to an adjacent area following a surgical procedure.

GRADENIGO'S SYNDROME

As originally described, this is a syndrome triggered by mastoiditis which has extended to the petrous apex. At this site localized inflammation of the meninges is liable to affect the abducens nerve as it perforates the dura overlying the clivus. As a consequence the patient develops intense facial and ocular pain, associated with a sixth nerve palsy. There may be facial paresis in addition.

- Typically the pain antedates the appearance of the ophthalmoplegia.
- Occasionally, the meningeal infection becomes more widespread.
- The condition can be mimicked by other pathological processes, including aneurysm of the internal carotid artery and tumors.
- An alternative mechanism for abducens palsy in patients with mastoiditis is venous thrombosis of the inferior petrosal sinus. With modern imaging techniques it should be possible to distinguish these pathological entities.

POSTHERPETIC NEURALGIA

Herpes zoster (HZ) is a viral infection that usually presents as a childhood infection of varicella.

Epidemiology

Frequency. 1 month after onset of shingles is 9–14.3% and at 3 months is about 5%. At 1 year, 3% continue to have severe pain.

Family history as a risk factor for herpes zoster has been described. Older age appears to be the most significant risk factor for developing PHN.

Sex. No predilection for developing PHN is known. Although there is a usual predominance of women in the older age group.

Age. The association between greater age and PHN is strong. At age 60 years, approximately 60% of patients with shingles develop PHN, and at age 70 years, 75% develop PHN.

Etiology

The pathogen is human herpes virus-3 (HHV-3), also known as the varicella zoster virus (VZV). Following the acute phase, the virus enters the sensory nervous system, where it is harbored in the geniculate, trigeminal, or dorsal root ganglia and remains dormant for many years. With advancing age or immunocompromised states, the virus reactivates and an eruption occurs. Even after the acute rash subsides, pain can persist or recur in the affected areas. This condition is known as postherpetic neuralgia (PHN).

Risk factors

Normal risk factors for development of PHN include the following:
- Advancing age
- Site of HZ involvement
  - *Lower risk:* Jaw, neck, sacral, and lumbar
  - *Moderate risk:* Thoracic
  - *Highest risk:* Trigeminal (especially ophthalmic division), brachial plexus
- Severe prodromal pain (with HZ)
- Severe rash

Clinical features

- Area of previous HZ may show evidence of cutaneous scarring.
- Sensation may be altered over involved areas, in the form of either hypersensitivity or decreased sensation.

- Allodynia is pain produced by a non-noxious stimulus, such as a light touch, by a brush, and may be present over the involved area.
- Changes in autonomic function such as increased sweating over the involved area may be seen.
- Pain is intense and may be described as burning, stabbing, or gnawing.
- HZ can reactivate subclinically with pain in a dermatomal distribution without rash. This condition is known as zoster sine herpete and may be more complicated, affecting multiple levels of the nervous system and causing multiple cranial neuropathies, polyneuritis, myelitis, or aseptic meningitis.

Differential diagnosis

- Hemifacial spasm
- Cavernous sinus syndromes
- Chronic paroxysmal hemicrania
- Cluster headache
- Head injury
- Migraine headache
- Persistent idiopathic facial pain
- Tolosa-Hunt syndrome
- Traumatic peripheral nerve lesions

Laboratory studies

- *Viral culture* or immunofluorescent staining may be used to differentiate herpes simplex from herpes zoster in cases that are difficult to distinguish clinically.
- *Antibodies to herpes zoster* can be measured. A 4-fold increase has been used to support the diagnosis of subclinical herpes zoster (zoster sine herpete). However, a rising titer secondary to viral exposure rather than reactivation cannot be ruled out.

Treatment

Goal of therapy for postherpetic neuralgia (PHN) is to reduce morbidity through the use of tricyclic antidepressants (such as Amitryptyline and Nortryptyline), anticonvulsants, anesthetics, analgesics, corticosteroids, and antiviral agents.

Tricyclic antidepressants act by inhibiting reuptake of serotonin and/or norepinephrine by presynaptic neuronal membrane, may increase synaptic concentration in CNS. They are useful as analgesics for postherpetic neuralgia.

- *Amitryptyline* is given in the dose of 70 mg/d for at least 3 weeks.
- *Nortryptyline* is given in the dose of 10–25 mg at night (HS) or in two divided doses.
- *Gabapentin and nortriptyline* combination is more efficacious than either drug as monotherapy for neuropathic pain as per recent reports.
- **High-concentration capsaicin patch NGX-4010.** A single 60-minute treatment with this patch reduces PHN for up to 12 weeks regardless of concomitant systemic neuropathic pain medication use.

TOLOSA-HUNT SYNDROME

Tolosa-Hunt syndrome (THS) is a painful ophthalmoplegia caused by nonspecific inflammation of the cavernous sinus or superior orbital fissure. It is a rare disorder characterized by severe and unilateral headaches with extra-ocular palsies, usually involving the third, fourth, fifth, and sixth cranial nerves, and pain around the sides and back of the eye which is episodic and usually resolves spontaneously but can relapse and remit.

Etiology

Tolosa-Hunt syndrome was classified by International Headache Society (IHS) in 2004 and now is a part of classification ICHD-II. It is an idiopathic, sterile inflammation of the cavernous sinus. Its pathology is described as fibroblastic, lymphocytic, and plasmocytic infiltration of the cavernous sinus. Granulocytic and giant cell infiltrations have also been described. Pathology may extend to involve the superior orbital fissure (sphenocavernous or parasellar syndrome) or orbital apex and affect the optic nerve.

Clinical features

- Tolosa-Hunt syndrome is most often unilateral, although bilateral cases have been described.
- *Symptoms* are usually limited to one side of the head, and in most cases the individual affected will experience intense, sharp pain and paralysis of muscles around the eye. Symptoms may subside without medical intervention, yet recur without a noticeable pattern.

- In addition, affected individuals may experience paralysis of various facial nerves and drooping of the upper eyelid (ptosis).
- *Other signs* include diplopia, fever, chronic fatigue, vertigo or arthralgia. Headache, nausea, neck stiffness, photophobia, and a "boring" pain. Occasionally, the patient may present with exophthalmos.

Clinical work-up

In addition to the standard ophthalmic examination of the patient including vision, IOP, pupil check for APD and nystagmus, slit-lamp and dilated fundus exam, a complete sensorimotor examination should be done. This includes:

- *Oculomotor examination* (to check for esotropia, exotropia, hypertropia or hypotropia), ductions, vergence, saccades, pursuit, and head tilt/turn. A common finding is abduction deficit associated with esodeviation that increases with gaze to the affected side.
- *Lids should be checked* for ptosis or lid retraction or any change in lid aperture during eye movements (to check for aberrant regeneration). Lid strength, fatigue or variability should be noted.
- *Exophthalmometry* is a must examination.
- *Facial sensations* should be checked.
- *Stereopsis and color plates* should also be evaluated.

Differential diagnosis

Tolosa-Hunt syndrome is considered a diagnosis of exclusion. Thus, the following entities must be considered and ruled out before a diagnosis of Tolosa-Hunt syndrome is made:

- *Ischemic disease:* Hemorrhage, ischemic mononeuropathy
- *Infectious process:* post viral syndrome, chronic inflammation of petrous bone (recurrent ear infections), syphilis, basal meningitis
- *Anatomical malformation:* aneurysm, AVM, carotid-cavernous fistula, cavernous sinus thrombosis, pseudotumor cerebri, Duane syndrome/Moebius syndrome, Chiari malformation
- *Inflammatory disease:* Sarcoidosis, Wegeners, Behçet's disease
- *Autoimmune condition:* Myasthenia gravis, thyroid disease, lupus

- *Neoplastic disease:* Meningioma, neurogenic tumor, hemangioma, lymphoma/leukemia, schwannoma, pituitary adenoma, metastasis, CPA lesion, nasopharyngeal carcinoma, chordoma, chondrosarcoma, brainstem glioma in children
- *Demyelinating disease:* multiple sclerosis (MS)
- *Others:* Diabetes mellitus, head trauma, BBPV, Meniere's, ophthalmoplegic migraine.

Investigations

THS is usually diagnosed via exclusion, and as such a vast amount of laboratory tests are required to rule out other causes of the patient's symptoms.

- *Common tests* include a complete blood count, thyroid function tests and serum protein electrophoresis.
- *Imaging techniques:* The most appropriate imaging includes MRI/MRA (DWI series) which provides information about the cavernous sinus and orbital apex better than a CT. A CT with and without contrast can also be obtained (Fig. 33.2). Inflammatory change of the orbit on cross-sectional imaging in the absence of cranial nerve palsy is described by the more benign and general nomenclature of orbital pseudotumor.
- *Lumbar puncture* is recommended to check for opening pressure and CSF should be evaluated for infection/oligoclonal bands.
- *Biopsy* may need to be obtained sometimes to confirm the diagnosis, as it is useful in ruling out a neoplasm.

Treatment

- *Oral steroids* are the mainstay of treatment. Both symptoms and signs (headache, ptosis, ophthalmoplegia, etc.) can be expected to resolve rapidly with an oral steroid taper regimen over 3–4 months. Corticosteroids are the treatment of choice, usually providing significant pain relief within 24–72 hours of therapy initiation.
- Ophthalmoparesis usually requires weeks to months for resolution; indeed, ophthalmoparesis may not completely resolve in some cases depending on the degree of inflammation and the aggressiveness of therapy.

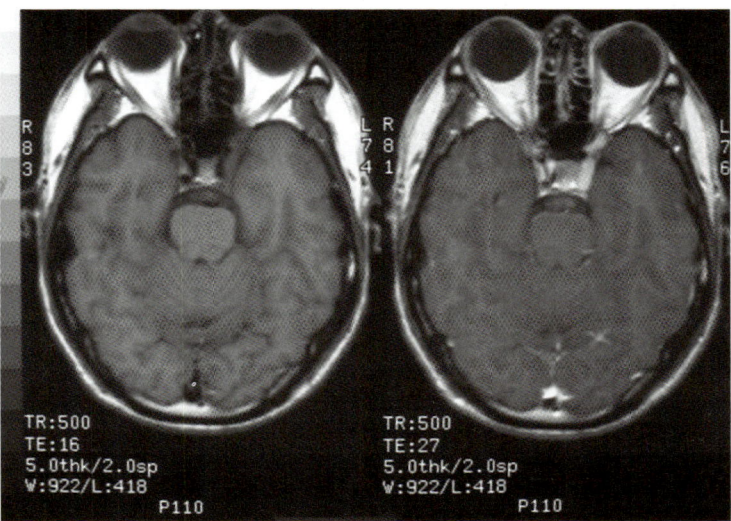

Fig. 33.2 *MRI of a 40-year-old man with severe periorbital pain OS, complete oculomotor nerve palsy OS, and partial abducens nerve palsy OS. Axial imaging without (left) and with (right) enhancement demonstrates nonspecific fullness involving the left cavernous sinus, consistent with Tolosa-Hunt syndrome within the context of the history.*

- *Immunosuppressants* like, azathioprine (Imuran) and methotrexate or *radiation therapy* are used for refractory cases.

Prognosis

Prognosis of Tolosa-Hunt syndrome is excellent. Full recovery is expected with steroid treatment. The disease may have a relapsing-remitting course.

BIBLIOGRAPHY

1. Anderson RL, Patel BC, Holds JB, et al. "Blepharospasm: past, present, and future". Ophthalmic Plastic and Reconstructive Surgery 1998;14(5):305–17.

2. Cates CA, Tyers AG. "Results of levator excision followed by fascia lata brow suspension in patients with congenital and jaw winking ptosis". Orbit 2008;27(2):83–9.

3. G Madland, C Fienmann. Chronic Facial pain. J Neurol Neurosurg Psychiatry 2001;71:716–9.

4. Hapak L, Gordon A, Locker D, et al. Differentiation between musculoligamentous, dentoalveolar, and neurologically based craniofacial pain with a diagnostic questionnaire. J Orofac Pain 1994;8:357–68.

5. International Association for the Study of Pain. Classification of chronic pain. Descriptors of chronic pain syndromes and definitions of pain terms. Seattle: International Association for the Study of Pain Press 1994:1–222.

6. International Headache Society. Classification and diagnostic criteria for headache disorders, cranial neuralgias and facial pain. Headache classification committee of the International Headache Society. Cephalalgia 1988;8 (suppl 7): 1–96.

7. Luke Bennetto, NK Patel, G Fuller. Trigeminal neuralgia and its management. BMJ 2007;334:201.

8. McQuay HJ, Tramer M, Nye BA, et al. A systematic review of antidepressants in europathic pain. Pain 1996;68:217–27.

9. Zakrzewska JM. Trigeminal neuralgia. Clinical Evidence 2001;5:916–23.

10. Zakrzewska JM. Trigeminal neuralgia. London: WB Saunders, 1995.

34 | ORBITAL APEX SYNDROME

Mahesh Kumar

INTRODUCTION

ETIOLOGY
- Inflammatory
- Infectious
- Neoplastic
- Iatrogenic
- Traumatic

- Vascular
- Others

CLINICAL FEATURES AND EVALUATION
- Clinical features
- Evaluation

TREATMENT
- Corticosteroids
- Immunosuppressant

INTRODUCTION

Orbital apex syndrome is a syndrome that involves the third, fourth, sixth, and ophthalmic division of the fifth cranial nerves in association with optic nerve dysfunction as they pass through the optic foramen and superior orbital fissure at the apex of the orbit.

Lesions causing this may be traumatic, inflammatory, infectious or neoplastic. The cavernous sinus syndrome (CSS) may include features of orbital apex syndrome along with features of involvement of the maxillary division of the trigeminal nerve and oculosympathetic fibers. Superior orbital fissure (SOF) syndrome denotes lesions immediately anterior to the orbital apex with involvement of 3rd, 4th and 6th cranial nerve without features of optic nerve involvement. The superior orbital fissure, orbital apex and the cavernous sinus are all contiguous structures and the etiologies of the syndromes involving these structures are similar.

Demographics. The disorder is rare during the first two decades of life. In people older than 20 years it has an even distribution between males and females.

ETIOLOGY

Nonspecific inflammation (non-caseating granulomatous or non-granulomatous) within the cavernous sinus or superior orbital fissure with extension into the orbital apex is the most common cause of this disorder. Infectious processes, neoplastic, iatrogenic/traumatic, or vascular processes are other causes of this disorder.

A. Inflammatory

- Sarcoidosis
- Systemic lupus erythematosus
- Wegener's granulomatosis
- Tolosa-Hunt syndrome
- Giant cell arteritis
- Inflammatory orbital pseudotumor
- Thyroid orbitopathy

B. Infectious

1. *Fungi.* Aspergillosis, mucormycosis

   Zygomycosis (also known as phycomycosis or mucormycosis) is the most common and virulent organism invading the orbit. It almost always extends into the orbit from the adjacent sinuses or nasal cavity and produces thrombosing vasculitis by invading the blood vessel wall. This leads to the characteristic clinical picture of a black, necrotic eschar in the nose or on the nasal turbinate. Unfortunately, the black eschar is often a rather late sign.

   The resultant tissue necrosis helps in further fungal invasion.

   Patients commonly present with proptosis and orbital apex syndrome. Elderly patients are more prone to this than younger individuals due to their relatively immuno-suppressed status and predisposing conditions include diabetes, metabolic acidosis, malignancies and treatment with antimetabolites and steroids.

   Therapy is aimed at control of underlying metabolic or immunological abnormality and local debridement. Antifungal therapy should be given as intravenous amphotericin-B or liposomal amphotericin-B.

2. *Bacteria: Streptococcus* sp. *Staphylococcus* sp., *Actinomyces* sp., gram-negative bacilli, anaerobes, *Mycobacterium tuberculosis.*

3. *Spirochetes: Treponema pallidum.*

4. *Viruses:* Herpes zoster.

C. Neoplastic

1. *Head and neck tumors:* Nasopharyngeal carcinoma, adenoid cystic carcinoma, squamous cell carcinoma, tumors of the sinuses, sphenoid wing and parasellar regions.

2. *Neural tumors:* Neurofibroma, meningioma, ciliary neurinoma, schwannoma.

3. *Metastatic lesions:* Lung, breast, renal cell, malignant melanoma.

4. *Hematologic:* Burkitt's lymphoma, non-Hodgkin's lymphoma, leukemia.

5. Perineural invasion of cutaneous malignancy.

D. Iatrogenic (post-sinonasal and orbital surgery)

Blindness following surgical procedures in the orbit and sinuses has been attributed to intra-operative or postoperative orbital haemorrhage, manipulation of the optic nerve, etc. Visual loss following intranasal endoscopic sinus surgery has been reported. Jaison et al. has reported a case of orbital apex syndrome as a complication of septorhinoplasty. In such situations, immediate and timely decompressive procedures might save the patient's vision.

E. Traumatic

1. *Penetrating injury*

2. *Nonpenetrating injury*

3. *Orbital apex fracture.* This occurs in association with other fractures of the face, orbit, or skull and may involve the optic canal, superior orbital fissure, and structures that pass through them. Associated complications may include damage to the optic nerves, with decreased visual acuity; cerebrospinal fluid leaks; and carotid cavernous sinus fistulas. Indirect traumatic optic neuropathy may result from stretching, tearing, twisting or bruising of the fixed intracanalicular portion of the optic nerve. Thin section CT of the section through the orbital apex and the anterior clinoid process demonstrates fractures at or adjacent to the optic canal.

4. *Retained foreign body.*

F. Vascular

1. *Carotid cavernous aneurysm*

2. *Carotid cavernous fistula.* CCF may cause pulsatile proptosis, severe conjunctival injection, and glaucoma from elevated episcleral venous pressure. A history of trauma is usually present but CCF can present spontaneously without trauma in patients with long-standing hypertension or connective tissue disorders such as Ehlers-Danlos syndrome.

3. *Cavernous sinus thrombosis*—septic cavernous sinus thrombosis usually spares vision and involves the contralateral cavernous sinus within 48 hours.

4. *Sickle cell anemia.*

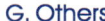

G. Others

Mucocele

The incidence of these different causes differed with the case series published. In one retrospective series of 151 patients, tumors were the cause in 45 patients (30%), iatrogenic (surgical)/ traumatic etiology was found in 53 patients (35%), self-limited inflammation was seen in 34 patients (23%), while vascular, infectious, and other causes constituted remaining 12%.

CLINICAL FEATURES AND EVALUATION

CLINICAL FEATURES

1. Visual loss from optic neuropathy and diplopia due to ophthalmoplegia involving multiple cranial nerves 3, 4 and 6 are the hall marks of this syndrome.
2. Most patients have retrobulbar pain. However, it may present without pain also, particularly those by tumors. Periorbital or facial pain may reflect involvement of the ophthalmic (V1) or the maxillary (V2) branch of the trigeminal nerve.
3. Pupillary dysfunction may be present and is related to injury to the sympathetic fibers or oculomotor nerve.
4. Trigeminal nerve involvement (particularly V1) may cause paresthesias of the forehead.
5. Infectious, inflammatory and neoplastic conditions may be associated with proptosis. Vascular conditions such as carotid-cavernous sinus fistula are associated with pulsatile proptosis.

EVALUATION

High-resolution MRI is the preferred modality of choice for lesions involving the orbital apex. MRI shows similar findings in both T1- and T2-weighted images with isointense tissue enhancing after gadolinium injection.

CT may show enlargement of the cavernous sinus, if involved, occupied by isodense soft tissue that may extend into the orbital apex and enhances following contrast injection. CT also is a useful tool in the setting of trauma, particularly to detect fractures in the orbital apex, and also in patients having magnetic foreign bodies, surgical clips, or who have other contraindications to MRI.

If a vascular lesion of the cavernous sinus is suspected, a magnetic resonance angiography (MRA) or CT angiography is helpful in the diagnosis.

Although laboratory studies may be useful adjuncts in the diagnostic evaluation of lesions involving the orbital apex, surgical biopsy may be required for definitive diagnosis. Lab testing should include base line investigations for inflammation and infection. (Erythrocyte sedimentation rate, complete blood count with differential count, treponema pallidum hemagglutination test, antinuclear antibody, Mantoux, chest radiograph, HIV) if the clinical findings suggest any of these processes.

Diagnosis is mainly clinical; the imaging differential diagnosis is with sarcoidosis, lymphoma, meningioma, metastatic tumor and dural AV fistula.

TREATMENT

Management of orbital apex syndrome is aimed at the underlying cause.

Corticosteroids are the treatment of choice, usually providing significant pain relief within 24–72 hours of therapy initiation. Ophthalmoparesis may require weeks to months for resolution. Judicious use of corticosteroids is recommended as it may aggravate any occult infectious disease, especially fungal disease.

Immunosuppressant like methotrexate and azathioprine have provided clinical benefit in a limited number of patients with THS.

BIBLIOGRAPHY

1. Ferry AP, Abedi S. Diagnosis and management of rhino-orbitocerebral mucormycosis (phycomycosis). A report of 16 personally observed cases. Ophthalmology 1983;90(9):1096–104.
2. Jaison SG, Bhatty SM, Chopra SK, Sajita V. Orbital apex syndrome. A rare complication of septorhinoplasty. Indian J ophthalmol 1994;42: 213–4.

3. Keane JR. cavernous sinus syndrome. Analysis of 151 cases. Arch Neurol 1996;53:967–71.

4. Kronish JW, Johnson TE, Gilberg SM, et al. Orbital infection in patients with human immuno-deficiency virus infection. Ophthalmology 1996;103(9):1483–92.

5. Lach B, Nair SG, Russel NA, et al. Spontaneous carotid-cavernous fistula and multiple arterial dissections in type IV Ehlers-Danlos syndrome. J Neurosurg 1987;66:462–7.

6. Long JC, Ellis PP. Total unilateral visual loss following orbital surgery. Am J Ophthalmol 1971;71:218.

7. Smith JR, Rosenbaum JT. A role for methotrexate in the management of non-infectious orbital inflammatory disease. Br J ophthalmol 2001; 85:1220–4.

8. Stankiewicz J. Blindness and intranasal ethmoidectomy-prevention and management. Otolaryngol Head and Neck Surg 1989;101:320–9.

9. Yeh S, Foroozan R. Orbital apex syndrome Curr opin Ophthalmol 2004;15:490–8.

35 VASCULAR DISORDERS OF THE ORBIT

Shikha Bassi, Mayav J, Movdawalla

INTRODUCTION AND CLASSIFICATION

INTRODUCTION

The vascular lesions of the orbit may include all the diseases affecting the orbit due to either a direct pathology in the orbital blood vessels, i.e. the capillaries, veins and the arteries or may be secondary to a pathology elsewhere and the signs being reflected in the orbit as is seen the carotid-cavernous fistula. Rootman has classified the vascular malformations of the orbit within the context of their hemodynamics. He has described three types of lesions. Type 1 (no flow) lesions have essentially little connection to the vascular system and include lymphangiomas or combined venous lymphatic malformations. Type 2 (venous flow) lesions appear as either distensible lesions with a direct and rich communication with the venous system or nondistensible anomalies that have minimal communication with the venous system. Types 1 and 2 can be combined with both features of distensible and nondistensible hemodynamics.

Arterial flow lesions, type 3, include arteriovenous malformations characterized by direct antegrade high flow through the lesion to the venous side. Cavernous hemangiomas are also malformations that demonstrate direct low flow through the lesion.

CLASSIFICATION

Orbital vascular lesions can be classified as:
A. **Primary vascular lesions**
  1. *Benign neoplasms of the orbital vessels* (without orbital hemodynamic implications)
      • Capillary hemangioma
      • Cavernous hemangiomas
      • Hemangiopericytoma
      • Hemangioblastoma

  2. *Orbital vascular malformations*
      • *No flow malformations*
        – Lymphangiomas
      • *Venous flow malformations*
        – Distensible
        – Nondistensible

- Mixed forms with venous and no flow components
- *Arterial flow malformations*
  - Arteriovenous malformations

B. **Secondary vascular lesions**
- Carotid cavernous fistula

PRIMARY ORBITAL VASCULAR PATHOLOGY

BENIGN NEOPLASMS OF ORBITAL VESSELS

CAPILLARY HEMANGIOMAS

These are the most common orbital tumors in infants. They arise early in life, grow rapidly during a proliferative phase and then slowly regress in an involutional phase. Though the hemangiomas usually regress spontaneously, they can lead to complications like astigmatism from corneal distortion and anisometropia and optic nerve compression. The incidence of amblyopia in periocular hemangiomas is documented to be 60% hence warranting an early intervention in selected cases. Mild cases are managed with periodic observation and amblyopia therapy.

Histopathology

Capillary hemangiomas are hamartomatous proliferations of vascular endothelial cells. They generally exhibit two phases of growth, a proliferative phase and an involutional phase. The proliferative phase of rapid growth typically occurs from 8 to 18 months. Pathologically, it is characterized by an increased number of endothelial and mast cells, the latter being a stimulus for vessel growth. Pathological findings include proliferation of a single layer of endothelial cells and pericytes. Endothelial cells of the basement membrane characteristically have large amounts of endoplasmic reticulum. The small vascular spaces lead to the formation of a high-flow lesion.

Natural history

The natural course of capillary hemangioma is that of progression during the first few months of life, followed by stabilization and then gradual regression of the lesion. One half of all lesions involute by age 5 years, and 75% will involute by age 7 years.

Clinical presentation

Patients usually present with a unilateral, superonasal eyelid or brow lesions. It typically blanches with pressure, unlike the lesions seen with port-wine stains. The mass lesion may be sufficient to cause a ptosis of the involved eyelid. Alternatively, if the lesion extends posteriorly in the orbit, proptosis and visual loss may be present. Amblyopia is seen in 43–60% of patients with eyelid hemangiomas. Anisometropia also can be found on examination as a result of the mass effect on the cornea. The axis of plus cylinder is usually toward the hemangioma.

Imaging

Ultrasonography shows a lesion with irregular contour and low-to-medium internal reflectivity. CT scan reveals a poorly circumscribed mass with no bony erosion. The lesion usually enhances with intravenous contrast. Magnetic resonance imaging (MRI) reveals a lesion that is hypointense to fat on T1-weighted scans and hyperintense to fat on T2-weighted scans. A well-circumscribed lobular pattern with prolonged parenchymal staining is seen with angiography. Involuting lesions tend to have less tissue staining.

Treatment

The first-line treatment of capillary hemangiomas is simple observation. Since most of these lesions regress on their own, there is no need to intervene unless there is occlusion of the visual axis, optic nerve compression, severe proptosis, and anisometropia.

Corticosteroids, in various formulations, also have been used in the treatment of capillary hemangiomas. Superficial periocular hemangiomas which threaten vision can be treated with topical steroids like clobetasol propionate. Injectable steroid formulations also are used in the treatment of these lesions. One study showed intralesional corticosteroid injections of 0.3 to 1.0 ml of a 50 : 50 mixture of triamcinolone (40 mg/ml) and dexamethasone phosphate

(4 mg/ml) given in infancy (between 2 and 10 months) resulted in a 63% reduction in the mean amount of astigmatism induced by periorbital capillary hemangioma. The study claims the astigmatism, not anisometropia or amblyopia, is the immediate indication for treatment of PCH with intralesional corticosteroids.

Although there may be a period of temporary enlargement, blanching usually is noted within 2–3 days and involution is seen by 2–4 weeks. Their effectiveness is most pronounced 2 weeks after injection but can be seen up to 2 months later. The overall success rate for this intervention is 75%. The most disconcerting adverse effect concerns reports of central retinal artery occlusion following the intralesional injection of corticosteroids. **To avoid this complication, it is recommended** to use 0.1 cc steroid aliquots injected slowly through a 30-gauge needle and avoid firm digital pressure on the lesion. Systemic corticosteroids are used for amblyogenic life-threatening lesions. An excellent response rate can be expected in 30% of patients, a questionable response in 40%, and no response in 30% when systemic corticosteroids are used under close observation. The response may be quite dramatic within the first 2 weeks, and the effect may last from 1–4 months. Doses of 2–3 mg/kg may be necessary for up to several months. Interferon alfa-2a has emerged as a new modality to combat the life-threatening and vision-threatening hemangiomas of infancy that are resistant to steroid treatment. While it has potent effects on these lesions, it is commonly associated with adverse effects of varying severity. Interferon alfa-2a exerts its effect by preventing endothelial cell migration in capillary hemangiomas. Patients with no cardiopulmonary contraindications can be treated with beta-blockers like topical timolol or oral propranolol also.

Laser surgery has been attempted to ameliorate capillary hemangiomas. The hemostatic effects of the carbon dioxide laser have been used with success to surgically remove these lesions. Other lasers used include the argon laser and the Nd:YAG laser. The pulsed dye laser is only effective for very superficial lesions; its mechanism of action is too slow for sight-threatening hemangiomas. Overall, variable results have been seen with various laser modalities, and the risks of scarring and ulceration often deter its use.

Surgery has generally been avoided because capillary hemangiomas are not encapsulated and piecemeal resection can produce significant bleeding. Surgical ligation of the heman-giomas produces equivocal results. Vascular embolization of the lesions should be used for large extraorbital hemangiomas only. Early surgical intervention can be considered as a primary treatment option in selected, isolated capillary hemangiomas without a significant cutaneous component. Surgery can provide definitive early treatment and prevent astigmatism and occlusion-related amblyopia.

CAVERNOUS HEMANGIOMA

Cavernous hemangioma is the most common vascular tumor of the orbit in adults and is the second most frequent cause of unilateral proptosis after thyroid-related orbitopathy.

Histopathology

Cavernous hemangiomas are presumed to be low-flow malformations or hamartomas. Histologically it consists of ectatic, largely thrombosed, and septate venous convulsions embedded by a compact capsule. The expression of progesterone receptors in epithelial cells of orbital cavernomas has been implicated for the high proportion of female patients.

Natural history

Cavernous hemangiomas are typically single, unilateral slow growing tumors and mostly do not recur after surgical excision. Patients with orbital cavernomas usually present in the fifth decade of life. Shields, et al. reported surgical removal of the lesion only in 52% of the cavernous hemangiomas referred to them. Many typical intraconal cavernous hemangiomas are recognized coincidentally during CT or MRI scanning for headache or other unrelated problems. In such cases, the patient can be followed up periodically and surgery can be withheld until vision is threatened or cosmetic appearance resulting from proptosis is unacceptable.

Clinical features

Painless exophthalmos with a slow onset is the leading clinical sign and often remains unnoticed by the patient. As cavernomas grow exceedingly slowly, and in some cases, not at all. The orbit and globe can accommodate to the mass without producing symptoms. Besides unilateral exophthalmos, blurred vision, visual field defects, restricted extraocular motility, choroidal folds, and papilledema are common ocular signs; optic atrophy is noted occasionally.

Imaging

Orbital ultrasound to confirm the diagnosis and localization of cavernomas in the anterior orbital compartment has been proven. Routine CT scanning or MRI sometimes reveals orbital tumors. With noncontrast CT, cavernous hemangiomas appear as lesions of about the same density as the cerebral parenchyma. A hard and compact capsule that can be proved by MRI is typical for orbital cavernomas.

Treatment

Indications for surgical treatment are visual impairment, diplopia due to ocular movement impairment, progressive and disfiguring unilateral proptosis, and severe retro-orbital pain clearly related to the orbital cavernoma. patients with orbital cavernomas may benefit more from a partial but uncomplicated excision compared with a complete removal associated with functional deficits. The majority of patients with orbital cavernomas can be managed primarily by ophthalmologists with experience in orbital surgery. Especially small orbital cavernomas located laterally or medially to the eyeball can be excised by a transconjunctival approach. Although this cosmetically and functionally very satisfying technique has occasionally been described for large cavernomas, it is generally recommended for small lesions that do not involve the orbital apex. The lateral orbitotomy is widely accepted as the technique of choice for lesions confined to the lateral aspect of the orbit. The transcranial approach is rarely indicated for lesions superior and medial to the optic nerve, especially if they involve the orbital apex.

HEMANGIOBLASTOMA

Hemangioblastoma is a benign vascular tumor associated with von Hippel-Lindau's (VHL) disease. VHL is a multisystem disease which includes cerebellar haemangioblastomas, endolymphatic sac tumors, renal cysts, renal cell carcinoma, pancreatic cysts and tumors, phaeochromocytomas. The characteristic ocular lesion of VHL is retinal capillary hemangioblastoma whereas retrobulbar or orbital hemangioblastomas are very rare. Almost always orbital hemangioblastomas are associated with retinal hemangioblastomas.

Histopathology

Histological examination demonstrated numerous small capillary like vascular channels intermixed with vacuolated stromal cells and positive neuron-specific enolase staining.

Natural history

The age of detection is in the 2nd or 3rd decade with an equal predilection for either sex.

Clinical features

Ocular features of hemangioblastoma are the earliest manifestations of von Hippel-Lindau's disease in about 50% of cases. Patients may be asymptomatic and a mass may be found on routine ophthalmoscopic examination. Hence, a routine ophthalmological examination in patients with a family history of hemangioblastoma is a must. Patients may sometimes present with deterioration in visual acuity, reduction in visual fields, reduction of colour vision and on examination may show afferent pupillary defect in the affected eye.

Imaging

Magnetic resonance scanning is the gold standard in diagnosis of hemangioblastomas. Hemangioblastomas have variable signal intensity on T1-weighted MRI, show high signal intensity on T2-weighted MRI, and typically enhance brightly with gadolinium contrast. Hemangioblastomas may show cystic spaces and curvilinear areas of flow void. Vascular flow voids on T2-weighted sequences in tumors in patients with VHL are highly suggestive of hemangioblastoma. As retrobulbar hemangioblastomas are often supplied by branches of the ophthalmic artery as demonstrated with angiography the high blood volume and permeability of these tumors result in a disproportionately large amount of edema for the size of the lesion.

Treatment

Treatment is mainly a wait and watch policy. If the tumor is impending on the optic nerve, affecting visual acuity and reducing visual fields, careful surgical excision of the tumor should be done as the tumor displaces rather than infiltrates the optic nerve. It has been seen that careful surgical excision of the hemangioblastoma has resulted in minimal or nil postoperative loss of vision. If there is early detection, cryotherapy or laser photocoagulation may be used to reduce the vascularity of the tumor.

HEMANGIOPERICYTOMA

Hemangiopericytoma is a rare mesenchymal neoplasm originating from the pericytes of blood vessels. This tumor is mesodermal in origin and it usually develops around a capillary network where maximum concentration of pericytes is present. It is a rare, slow growing neoplasm found mainly in the lower limbs and retroperitoneum with a frequency of about 5% in the orbit, paranasal sinuses and nasopharyngeal regions.

Histopathology

The histopathological appearance of the tumors is an irregular arrangement of spindleshaped tumor cells with oval nuclei interspersed in scanty cytoplasm around a complex network of capillaries and blood vessels and sometimes a few sinusoidal spaces. Additional features noted are myxoid, cystic and cellular changes along with areas of hemorrhages, necrosis and fibroblastic reactions. Three basic patterns have been documented—solid, sinusoidal and mixed.

Natural history

Hemangiopericytoma predominantly affects adults with a median age group of 42–45 years occurring equally in both males and females, however occurrence in orbit is more in males.

Clinical features

Orbital hemangiopericytomas present with slowly developing proptosis associated with or without pain and loss of visual acuity. Other manifestations are decreased extraocular movements, visual field loss, RAPD, disc edema and congested retinal and choroidal vessels. Depending on size and location of tumor, associated complaints of ptosis, impaired tear production and drainage leading to dry eyes has also been reported.

Imaging

Ultrasonography usually shows a well delineated lesion with low to medium internal reflectivity, internal structure of which shows features of solid, cystic, necrotic changes depending on the histological structure. Colour Doppler images indicate a highly vascular tumor which helps to differentiate from a capillary hemangioma. Computed tomography shows a well circumscribed mass with medium to high enhancement. The lesions may be well circumscribed and confined to the orbit, or they may have indistinct, irregular margins. When large, they may cause osseous erosion and re-modelling and may involve the central nervous system. Rarely, intralesional calcification is present. On magnetic resonance imaging, the intensity of signals from hemangiopericytomas is similar to T1- and T2-weighted images of the grey matter of the brain which helps to differentiate them from cavernous malformations. Digital subtraction angiography shows a prominent arterial supply, an early florid blush and late staining of the tumor.

Treatment

The standard treatment of choice is wide local excision of the tumor which may be technically demanding as osseous paranasal extensions of the tumor are seen. Post operative irradiation of 50–65 cGy provides better long-term survival. Long-term recurrence rates maybe almost up to 30%, 30 years after initial treatment. Large extensions of the tumor into paranasal sinuses, CNS, adjacent bones requires palliative chemotherapy and radiotherapy role of which is controversial.

ORBITAL VASCULAR MALFORMATIONS

NO FLOW MALFORMATIONS
LYMPHANGIOMA

Lymphangiomas are postulated to be congenital abnormal networks of lymphatic and venous tissue which invade the surrounding orbital tissues. Hence, the term orbital venous malformation is now synonymous with the term lymphangioma. They are hamartomatous malformations with a normal cell replication cycle. The pathophysiology is unclear but it is postulated that the venous lymphatic malformations isolate from their venous anlage having varying proportions of venous and lymphatic components. They are divided into superficial, orbital and combined lymphangiomas. Superficial affect the lids and conjunctiva, causing mainly a cosmetic blemish but no proptosis. Orbital lymphangiomas lie behind the orbital septum and invade the intraconal and extraconal space mainly presenting as proptosis. Combined include the above two forming an anterior and posterior compartment of the lymphangioma. Also lymphangiomas are classified according to the vascular flow within its substance into no flow, venous and arterial flow.

Histopathology

Pathologically it is a diffuse non-encapsulated mass that interdigitates with normal tissues. Histopathology reveals irregular vascular channels with thin walls, attenuated endothelial layer, interrupted basement membrane, absence of pericytes, loose fibrous stroma, few smooth muscle cells, and collections of lymphocytes. Studies using tritiated thymidine have shown that the endothelial lining has a turnover rate of normal mature cells, suggesting that lymphangiomas are areas of maldevelopment rather than true neoplasias.

Natural history

The natural history of lymph angiomas is usually variable and unpredictable. Though lymphangiomas are usually congenital their time of presentation is usually in childhood or adolescence in the 2nd decade. 60% are diagnosed before the age of 16 years.

Clinical features

The clinical features depend on the location of the tumor. The superficial variety apart from being cosmetically unacceptable may produce high astigmatism giving rise to anisometropic amblyopia. The orbital variety may be asymptomatic but may enlarge slowly giving rise to progressive proptosis, restriction of ocular motility and vertical globe displacement. A sudden increase in proptosis associated with pain usually indicates a spontaneous intralesional hemorrhage or a lymphoid proliferation within the tumor following a viral upper respiratory tract infection. This may lead to compressive optic neuropathy and secondary glaucoma as complications. Lid lesions include ptosis and ecchymosis.

Imaging

Ultrasound shows presence of hypoechoic cystic spaces in the tumor but blood filled spaces will be hyperechoic. On computed tomography, lymphangiomas are poorly circumscribed, multi-compartmental heterogeneous masses not confined by fascial planes which enhance minimally on administration of contrast material. Magnetic resonance scanning is the mainstay in diagnosing lymphatic malformations because it depicts the compartments accurately. Also T1-weighted images best depict lymphatic or proteinaceous fluid within the cysts while T1-weighted fat suppressed images depict blood and its components accurately. T2-weighted fat suppressed images provide enhanced visibility of components which contains non-hemorrhagic fluid. Multiple fluid-fluid levels present within the cysts are pathognomic of this condition.

Treatment

Observation and conservative management is the mainstay of treatment. Since the lesion arborises into surrounding tissue, complete surgical excision in difficult and recurrences common. However, in cases of severe proptosis, compressive optic neuropathy and impending amblyopia, surgical excision or debulking has to be undertaken. Newer techniques like injection of a sclerosing agent (sodium tetradecyl sulphate), OK432 intralesionally have been used but therapeutic side-effects, safety and efficacy is not yet known. Conjunctival lymphangioma is treated by CO_2 ablation, cryotherapy and surgical excision. Fractionated beta radiation has been used an adjunctive therapy for conjunctival lymphangioma.

VENOUS FLOW MALFORMATIONS

ORBITAL VARIX

Orbital varix is a rare orbital vascular lesion accounting for 0.3–1.3% of all orbital vascular tumors. They occur due to congenital weakness of the wall of the post-capillary vein (most commonly the superior ophthalmic vein). Venous stasis follows leading to proliferation of the venous system and dilatation of the proximal segment. This is further accentuated due to absence of valves in the orbital venous system and in conditions which increase intra-orbital pressures like the Valsalva maneuver. The sluggish venous flow and proximal dilatation of the segment lead to formation of a thrombus.

Natural history

Orbital varix usually presents in the 2nd and 3rd decades of life and affects males and females equally. Two types are seen. Primary orbital varix affects the orbital system primarily and is not associated with intracranial vascular mal-formations. Secondary orbital varix is associated with intracranial vascular AV malformations which shunt blood to the orbital venous system and lead to venous dilatation secondarily.

Clinical features

The most important clinical feature is positional or stress proptosis, i.e. the proptosis increases in prone position, while bending forward and during the Valsalva maneuver. Patient may present with an acute exacerbation and come with complaints of severe pain, subconjunctival hemorrhage and proptosis occurring after a spontaneous hemorrhage or thrombus forma-tion in the varix. Patient may also come with enophthalmos. Compressive optic neuropathy following hemorrhage may also result in profound visual loss and even blindness.

Histopathology

Histopathological examination of the lesion shows a markedly dilated and ecstatic vein with thickened walls and the presence of an orga-nized or recanalizing thrombus in the vessel wall. There is also deposition of hemosiderin pigments, fibroblastic proliferation, chronic inflammatory cells and intraluminal calcification (phleboliths).

Imaging

Modalities include B scan, color Doppler, CT and MRI. Ultrasonography of the orbit shows distensibility of the dilated segment on Valsalva which is indicative of a varix. The lesion appears as an intermittent anechoic retrobulbar lesion that exhibits intrinsic flow during the Valsalva maneuver. On color Doppler imaging there is reversal of flow towards the transducer during Valsalva. Axial CT on supine position shows an almost normal or mild dilatation of the vein which can be increased on applying a tourni-quet around the jugular venous system thereby increasing the intraorbital venous pressure. The varix now appears with a smooth contour, club like, segmentally dilated mass of tangled vessels. MR imaging shows a hypointense lesion on T1- and T2-weighted images when compared to the surrounding extraocular muscles in absence of hemorrhage and thrombus forma-tion. Presence of blood in the vessel lumen demonstrates increased signal intensity. CT, angiography demonstrates a homogeneously enhancing orbital apex lesion, providing excep-tional anatomic detail of inflow and outflow veins, confirming the diagnosis of an orbital varix.

Management

Surgical excision of the varix is the mainstay of treatment. However, exploration of the varices is technically demanding, hence, techniques which increase the intraorbital venous pressure have to be used to make visualization of the varix possible. Surgery involves excision of the anterior segment of the vessel wall, drainage of blood/thrombus and electrocauterization of the remain-der of the vessel. Embolization of the varix with cyanoacrylate glue prior to excision is beneficial in reducing intraoperative bleeding.

ARTERIAL FLOW MALFORMATIONS

ORBITAL ARTERIOVENOUS MALFORMATIONS

Intraorbital arteriovenous (AV) malformations are rare lesions of the orbit of congenital origin. They consist of multiple congenital micro-vascular connections between arteries and veins without an intervening capillary bed, but with cellular stromal tissue interspersed between the vessels. The feeder vessel is mainly the ophthalmic artery. Orbital arteriovenous malformations are mainly congenital hamartomas, with possibly trauma being the precipitating factor producing hemodynamic changes which gives rise to symptoms. They are classified on the basis of location into mainly three types: (i) Purely orbital, (ii) orbital, and (iii) periorbital. Orbital AV malformations with cerebral and retinal malformations also called *Wyburn-Mason syndrome*.

Histopathology

Histopathological features of orbital AV malformations include marked irregular muscularis thickness of the affected artery and vein with presence of partial thickness elastica and cellular stromal tissue around the vessels.

Natural history

There is no predilection for any sex and age of presentation is between 26 and 70 years. Lesions are usually unilateral. The lesions though congenital do not cause any symptoms in childhood. The precipitating causes postulated are menarche, pregnancy and trauma.

Clinical features

The most common clinical features are peri-orbital mass/swelling, proptosis, chemosis, and subconjunctival hemorrhage. In a high-flow type of AV malformation, pulsatile exophthalmos and bruit are important features. Associated features like pain, reduced visual acuity, reduced extraocular motility and corresponding diplopia have been noted. On straining and Valsalva maneuver, pain, chemosis and proptosis is increased. Also seen is an elevation of the episcleral venous pressure and a corresponding increase in IOP.

Imaging

Although angiography is the investigation of choice, computed tomography and magnetic resonance scanning have a role to play in the diagnosis of orbital AV malformations. CT scanning typically shows tubular or lobulated homogeneous and nonhomogeneous-enhancing mass lesions. Magnetic resonance imaging showed enhancing mass lesions with variable signal intensities depending on the flow, presence of hemorrhage, or thrombosis within the lesion. Doppler angiography shows an engorged and dilated proximal arterial segment, presence of malformation and the venous outflow. Feeder vessels may be from the internal carotid system 63% (ophthalmic artery and less commonly the ethmoidal artery) or external carotid system 38% (superficial temporal, maxillary and facial arteries).

Treatment

For asymptomatic cases, a wait and watch policy should be adopted. For symptomatic cases careful surgical excision is the treatment of choice. However, the major complication of surgery is intraoperative bleeding which has to be managed by preoperative ligation or embolization of the feeder vessel followed by careful tissue dissection and surgical excision of the AV malformation. Ligating the feeder vessel intraoperatively with clips, or by embolization with cyanoacrylate glue are newer methods to control intraoperative hemorrhage.

SECONDARY ORBITAL VASCULAR PATHOLOGY

CAROTID-CAVERNOUS FISTULA (CCF)

CCFs are abnormal communications between the cavernous sinus and the carotid arterial system. They can be classified as direct or indirect.

- *Direct CCFs* result from a direct connection between the cavernous segment of the intra-cavernous carotid artery and the cavernous sinus.
- *Indirect or dural CCFs* arise from abnormal shunts to the cavernous sinus from the meningeal branches of the carotid artery.

- Direct fistulas often demonstrate high-flow, whereas indirect fistulas are often low-flow lesions. Patients with CCF may initially present to an ophthalmologist with decreased vision, conjunctival chemosis, external ophthalmoplegia and proptosis.

Natural history

According to the Barrow classification on the basis of angiography there are four identifiable types of CCF: Type A, a direct shunt between the intracavernous internal carotid artery (ICA) and the cavernous sinus; type B, a dural arteriovenous (AV) fistula supplied by the ICA; type C, a dural AV fistula supplied by the external carotid artery (ECA); and type D, a dural AV fistula supplied by both the ICA and ECA. Type A fistulas usually are of the high-flow type and most often are post-traumatic. They can also arise from rupture of an intracavernous carotid artery aneurysm or from complications of surgery or percutaneous procedures. Because of the high blood flow rate, direct carotid-cavernous fistulas usually manifest with acute and severe symptoms, and they rarely resolve spontaneously. Dural fistulas are believed to be congenital arteriovenous connections that open spontaneously in older women or in the setting of hypertension, diabetes, atherosclerotic disease, childbirth, or collagen-vascular disease. Dural carotid-cavernous fistulas usually cause insidious and less severe symptoms. In contrast to direct fistulas, dural shunts are much more likely to be misdiagnosed initially and to resolve spontaneously.

Clinical presentation

The arterial blood can flow either anteriorly into the superior ophthalmic vein or posteriorly into the petrosal sinus. When arterial blood flow escapes posteriorly from the cavernous sinus through the petrosal sinuses, patients may not develop ocular symptoms or signs. When the arterial blood flows anteriorly into the superior or inferior ophthalmic veins, or both, ocular manifestations occur. High-flow, direct carotid-cavernous fistulas (type A) often present dramatically days or weeks after head injury with the classic triad of pulsating exophthalmos,

conjunctival chemosis, and bruit. Arterialization clinically appearing as corkscrew vessels is the hallmark of carotid-cavernous fistula. Dural fistulas present insidiously as a chronic red eye and the diagnosis usually is delayed and can be associated with vision loss due to glaucoma at the time of diagnosis. Common presenting symptoms of CCF are redness of eyes, decreased vision, pain, double vision and tinnitus. On examination the most common presenting sign is dilated episcleral vessels, proptosis, limitation of extraocular muscles, and thrill with bruit. Some patients may develop glaucoma secondary to raised episcleral pressure, fundus examination may show dilated vessels, and gonioscopy may reveal blood in Schlemm's canal. Vision loss may be due to glaucoma, traumatic optic neuropathy at the time of head injury, exposure keratopathy, vitreous hemorrhage, retinal venous stasis, central retinal vein occlusion, choroidal detachment, or anterior or posterior ischemic optic neuropathy.

Imaging

Ultrasound can show a dilated superior ophthalmic vein, thickened extraocular muscles and it may demonstrate a reversal of flow direction in the superior ophthalmic vein. With the A-scan method, dilated ophthalmic veins may be evident. The scans may also demonstrate evidence of arterialized blood coursing through the ophthalmic veins, which are seen as several low-amplitude spikes that are in constant motion.

CT scan findings in carotid-cavernous fistulas include enlargement of the ipsilateral cavernous sinus, prominent, dilated and tortuous superior ophthalmic vein and thickened extraocular muscles. MRI in CCF is characterized by abnormal flow voids in the affected cavernous sinus, lateral wall convexity of the cavernous sinus, dilated superior ophthalmic vein, and thickened extraocular muscles.

To accurately identify a carotid-cavernous fistula, selective catheterization of the right and left external and internal carotid arteries and the vertebral arteries is necessary. Including the entire skull in lateral projection imaging is important.

Treatment

The aim of treatment in CCF is to prevent vision loss. The ideal treatment would be a closure of the fistula while preserving internal carotid artery patency. High-flow CCF (type A) usually require urgent treatment. A variety of procedures can close the fistula, but unfortunately several involve occlusion of the internal carotid artery, occasionally, resulting in ipsilateral cerebral infarction and even the ocular ischemic syndrome. Therefore, selective closure of the fistula without occlusion of the internal carotid artery is the treatment of choice. Direct surgical obliteration of the fistula is technically difficult. Selective embolization and detachable balloon occlusion is the treatment of choice in direct carotid-cavernous fistulas. The balloon is usually placed into the cavernous sinus either by an arterial route, through the tear in the internal carotid artery, or by a venous route, through the inferior petrosal sinus or the superior ophthalmic vein. Balloon occlusion of a carotid-cavernous fistula may be followed by transient worsening of ocular signs, particularly proptosis, ophthalmoplegia, and pain, with subsequent resolution within a few weeks. In addition to occlusion of the fistula, secondary glaucoma and ischemic retinopathy may require medical treatment and photocoagulation therapy, respectively. For non-traumatic dural carotid-cavernous fistulas (types B, C, and D), initial conservative management is usually recommended because spontaneous resolution can occur in 20–50% of cases. This is thought to result from partial or complete thrombosis of the cavernous sinus or its tributaries. When indirect carotid-cavernous fistulas produce progressive visual loss, persistent diplopia, or intolerable proptosis, bruit, or headache, selective embolization is usually performed.

BIBLIOGRAPHY

1. Alexander Friedreich Scheuerle, Hans H. Steiner, Gerold Kolling, et al. Treatment and Long-term Outcome of Patients With Orbital Cavernomas. Am J Ophthalmol 2004;138: 237–44.

2. Assaf A, Nasr A, Johnson T. Corticosteroids in the management of adnexal hemangiomas in infancy and childhood. Ann Ophthalmol 1992; 24(1):12–8.

3. Aydin A, Velioglu M, et al. Orbital varix presenting with enophthalmos-A case report-J. Fr. Ophthalmology 2010;33(5):344. Epub 2010 May 7.

4. Barlow CF, Priebe CJ, Mulliken JB, et al. Spastic diplegia as a complication of interferon alfa-2a treatment of hemangiomas of infancy. J Pediatr. 1998;132(3 Pt 1):527–30.

5. Barrow DL, Spector RH, Braun IF, et al. Classification and treatment of spontaneous carotid-cavernous sinus fistulas. J Neurosurg 1985; 62:248-56.

6. Bastin KT, Mehta MP. Meningeal hemangiopericytoma defining the role for radiation therapy. J neuro-oncol 1992;14:277–87.

7. Blindness for orbital varices-Phan IT, Hoyt WFG, McCulley TJ Orbit 2009;28(5):303–5.

8. Bomiuk M, et al. Hemangiopericytoma of meninges of Optic Nerve-a clinicopathologic report and electron microscopic observations Ophthalmol 1985;92:178–1787.

9. Boon LM, MacDonald DM, Mulliken JB. Complications of systemic corticosteroid therapy for problematic hemangioma. Plast Reconstr Surg. 1999;104(6):1616–23.

10. Bose B, et al. Hemangiopericytoma, a clinicopathologic and ultrastructural study World J Surg 1981;863–71.

11. Brown Dn, MacCarty CS, et al. Orbital Hemangiopericytoma—review of literature and case report of 4 cases. J Neurosurg 1965;22:354–61.

12. Bytne, et al. Ultrasound of the Eye and Orbit-St. Louis Mosby 1992;339–42.

13. Capillary Hemangioma Author: Stuart Seiff, MD, FACS; Chief Editor: Hampton Roy Sr, MD medscape,emedicine.

14. Chaudhry Imtiaz A, Elkhamry Sahar M, Al-Rashed Waleed, et al. Carotid cavernous fistula: Ophthalmological implications. Middle East African Journal of Ophthalmology 2009; 16:(2):57–63.

15. Chew EY. Ocular manifestations of von Hippel Lindau disease: Clinical and genetic investigations. Trans Am Ophthalmol Soc. 2005;103: 495–511.

16. Choyke PL, Glenn GM, Walther MM, et al. von Hippel-Lindau disease: genetic, clinical, and imaging features. Radiology 1995;194:629–42.

17. Clinical course of Retinal Hemangioblastomas in von Hippel-Lindau disease. Catherine B, Sam S, et al. Ophthalmology 2008;115:1382–89.

18. Couch SM, Garrity JA, et al. Embolisation of orbital varices with n-butyl cyanoacrylate as an aid in surgical excision. American Journal of Ophthalmology 2009;148(4):614–8.

19. Craven JP, Quigley TM, et al. Current Management and clinical outcome of hemangiopericytoma. Ann J Surg 1992:162;490–3.

20. Croxatto JO. Hemangiopericytoma of the orbit- a clinicopathologic study of 30 cases. Hum Pathol 1982;13:210–8.

21. Cruz OA, Zarnegar SR, Myers SE. Treatment of periocular capillary hemangioma with topical clobetasol propionate. Ophthalmology 1995; 102(12):2012–5.

22. Deans RM, Harris GJ, Kivlin JD. Surgical dissection of capillary hemangiomas. An alternative to intralesional corticosteroids. Arch Ophthalmol Dec 1992;110(12):1743–7.

23. Demonstration of orbital varix with computed tomography and Valsalva manoeuvre-Shields JA, Dolinkas BC, et al. American Journal of ophthalmology 1984;(97):108–10.

24. Di Tommaso L, Scarpellini F, Salvi F, et al. Progesterone receptor expression in orbital cavernous hemangiomas. Virchows Archiv 2000;436:284–8.

25. Elsas FJ, Lewis AR. Topical treatment of periocular capillary hemangioma. J Pediatr Ophthalmol Strabismus 1994;31(3):153–6.

26. Elster AD, Chen MY, Richardson DN, Yeatts PR. Dilated intercavernous sinuses: an MR sign of carotid-cavernous and carotid-dural fistulas. AJNR Am J Neuroradiol 1991;12(4):641–5.

27. Enzinger FM, Smith BH, et al. Hemangiopericytoma an analysis of 106 cases. Hum Pathol 1976;61–82.

28. Friling R, Axer-Siegel R, Ben-Amitai D, et al. Intralesional and sub-Tenon's infusion of corticosteroids for treatment of refractory periorbital and orbital capillary haemangioma. Eye. 2008;117:110–113.

29. Gerald J. Harris, for the Orbital Society. Orbital Vascular Malformations: A Consensus Statement on Terminology and its Clinical Implications. American Journal of Ophthalmology 2001;127(4):453–55.

30. Goldberg RA, Garcia GH, Duckwiler GR. Combined embolization and surgical treatment of arteriovenous malformation of the orbit. Am J Ophthalmol 1993;116(1):17–25.

31. Goldberg RA, Goldey SH, Duckwiler G, et al. Management of cavernous sinus-dural fistulas: Indications and techniques for primary embolization via the superior ophthalmic vein. Arch Ophthalmol 1996;i 14:707–14.

32. Graeb DA, Rootman J, et al. Orbital lymphangiomas: Clinical, radiologic and pathologic characteristics. Radiology 1990;175:417–21.

33. Grove AS. The dural shunt syndrome: Pathophysiology and clinical course. Ophthalmology 1984;91(3):l–44.

34. Gunalp Gunduz et al. Vascular Tumors of the orbit. Doc Ophthalmol 1995;89(4):337–45.

35. Harris G, Sakol P, Bonavolonta G, et al. An analysis of thirty cases of orbital lymphangioma. Pathophysiologic considerations and management recommendations. Ophthalmology 1990;97:1583–92.

36. Harris GJ, Frederick AJ. Cavernous hemangioma of the orbit. J Neurosurg 1979;51:219–28.

37. Harris GJ, Sakol PJ, Bonavolonta G, et al. An analysis of thirty cases of orbital lymphangioma. Pathophysiologic considerations and management recommendations. Ophthalmology 1990;97:1583–92.

38. Harris GJ. Orbital vascular malformation: A consensus statement on terminology and its clinical implications. Orbital society. Am. J. Ophthalmol 1999;127:453–5.

39. Hasenfratz G. Orbital tumors—the importance of standardized echography. Acta Ophthalmol Suppl 1994;204:82–6.

40. Hassler W, Schaller C, Farghaly F, et al. Transconjunctival approach to a large cavernoma of the orbit. Neurosurgery 1994;34:859–61.

41. Hayes BH, Shore JW, Westfall CT, et al. Management of orbital and periorbital arteriovenous malformations. Ophthalmic Surg 1995; 26(2):145–52.

42. Hejazi N, Classen R, Hassler W. Orbital and cerebral cavernomas: Comparison of clinical, neuroimaging, and neuropathological features. Neurosurgical Review 1999;22:28–33.

43. Henderson JW, Farrow GM, Garrity JA. Clinical course of an incompletely removed cavernous hemangioma of the orbit. Ophthalmology 1990;97:625–8.

44. Iliff WJ, Green WR. Orbital lymphangiomas. Ophthalmology 1979;86:914–29.

45. Jalil A, Maino A, Bhojwani R, et al. Clinical review of periorbital capillary hemangiomas of infancy. J Pediatr Ophthalmol Strabismus 2010;1–8.

46. Jeremy H, Allan J, et al. Diagnosis and anatomic mapping of an orbital varix by computed tomographic analysis. American Journal of Ophthalmology. 2005;140(5):945–7.

47. Jerry A. Shields, Carol L. Shields, Richard Scartozzi Survey of 1264 Patients with Orbital Tumors and Simulating Lesions. The 2002 Montgomery Lecture, Ophthalmology 2004; 111(5Pt1):997–1008.

48. Karcioglu ZA, Nasr AM, Haik BG. Orbital hemangiopericytoma: Clinical and morphologic features. Am J Ophthalmol 1997;124:661–72.

49. Katz SE, Rootman J, Vangveeravong S, et al. Combined venous lymphatic malformations of the orbit (so-called lymphangiomas): Association with noncontiguous intracranial vascular anomalies. Ophthalmology 1998;105:176–84.

50. Kavanagh EC, Heran MK, Peleg A, et al. Imaging of the natural history of an orbital capillary hemangioma. Orbit 2006;25(1):69–72.

51. Keltner JL, Satterheld D, Dublin AB, et al. Dural and carotid-cavernous sinus fistulas: Diagnosis, management, and complications. Ophthalmology 1987;94:1585–600.

52. Kennerdell JS, Maroon JC, Garrity JA, Abla AA. Surgical management of orbital lymphangioma with the carbon dioxide laser. Am J Ophthalmol 1986;102:308–14.

53. Kersten RC, Kulwin DR. Surgical management of orbital cavernous angiomas: prognosis for visual function after removal (letter, comment). Neurosurgery 1995;36:1058.

54. Kim AW, Kosmorsky GS. Arteriovenous communication in the orbit. J. Neuro-ophthalmol 2000; 20(1):17–9.

55. Kouri JG, Chen MY, Watson JC, et al. Resection of suprasellar tumors by using a modified trans-sphenoidal approach: Report of four cases. J Neurosurg 2000;92:1028–35.

56. Kupersmith MJ, Vargas EM, Warren F, et al. Venous obstruction as the cause of retinal/choroidal dysfunction associated with arteriovenous shunts in the cavernous. J Neuro-ophthalmol 1996;16:1–6.

57. Kushner BJ. Intralesional corticosteroid injection for infantile adnexal hemangioma. Am J Ophthalmol 1982;93(4):496–506.

58. Lacey B, Rootman J, Marotta TR. Distensible venous malformations of the orbit: Clinical and hemodynamic features and a new technique of management. Ophthalmology 1999;106:1197–209. Kupersmith MJ, Satterfield D, Dublin AB, et al. Dural and carotid cavernous sinus fistulas: Diagnosis, management and complications. Ophthalmology 1987;94:1585–1600.

59. Lonser RR, Glenn GM, Walther M, et al. von Hippel-Lindau disease. Lancet 2003;361: 2059–67.

60. Lymphangiomas: Clinical, radiologic and pathologic characteristics. Radiology 1990;175: 417–21.

61. McMaster Mj, et al. Hemangiopericytoma-a clinicopathologic study and long-term follow-up of 60 patients. Cancer 1975;2232–44.

62. McNab AA, Wright JE. Cavernous hemangioma of the orbit. Aust N Z J Ophthalmol 1989; 17:337–45.

63. Mena H, Ribus JL, et al. Hemangiopericytoma of the central nervous system. A review of 94 cases. Hum Pathol 1991;22:84–91.

64. Miller NR. Carotid-cavernous fistula. In: Miller NR, Newman NJ (Eds). Walsh and Hoyt's clinical neuro-ophthalmology. 5th ed. Baltimore: Williams & Wilkins, 1998.

65. Mulliken JB, Glowaski J. Hemangiomas and vascular malformations in infants and children: A classification based on endothelial characteristics. Plast Reconstr Surg 1982;69:412–22.

66. Nina Ni, Suqin Guo, Paul Langer. Current concepts in the management of periocular infantile (capillary) hemangioma. Current opinion in ophthalmology 2011;22:102–106.

67. O'Keefe M, Lanigan B, Byrne SA. Capillary haemangioma of the eyelids and orbit: a clinical review of the safety and efficacy of intralesional steroid. Acta Ophthalmol Scand 2003;81(3): 294–8.

68. Orbital arteriovenous malformations. Sunil Warrier, C Prabhakran, et al. Archives of Ophthalmology 2008;126(12):1669–76.

69. Orbital lymphangioma: Clinical features and management. Kalisa P, Van Zieleghem B, Roux P, Meire F. Bull. Soc. Belge Ophthalmol 2001; 282: 59–68.

70. Orbital varix thrombosis—Bullock JF, Goldberg SH, et al. Ophthalmology 1990;(97):251–6.

71. Orbital Venous malformations—Current Multi-Disciplinary Treatment Approach; Yonca Ozkan, M Mawad, et al. Archives of Ophthalmology 2004;122:1151–8.

72. Orcutt JC, Wulc AE, Mills RP, et al. Asymptomatic orbital cavernous hemangiomas. Ophthalmology 1991;98:1257–60.

73. Ossoinig KC. Echographic differentiation of vascular tumors in orbit. The Netherlands Junk 1981;283.

74. Peralta R, Glavas I. Review of capillary hemangioma. Eyenet 2009;35–7.

75. Phelps CD, Thompson HS, Ossoinig KC. The diagnosis and prognosis of atypical carotid-cavernous fistula (red-eyed shunt syndrome). Am J Ophthalmol 1982;93:423–36.

76. Preliminary observations of embolisation treatment of orbital varices with Glubran 2 acrylic glue Xiao LH, Lu XZ, et al. Zhongua yank e za zhi May 2009;45(5):436–40.

77. Raila FA, Zimmerman J, Azordegan P, et al. Successful surgical removal of an asymptomatic optic nerve hemangioblastoma in von Hippel-Lindau disease. J Neuroimaging 1997;748–50.

78. Rootman J. Vascular malformations of the orbit: hemodynamic concepts. Orbit 2003;22(2):103–20.

79. Rosca TI, Pop MI, Curca M, et al. Vascular tumors in the orbit—capillary and cavernous hemangiomas. Ann Diagn Pathol 2006;10(1): 13–9.

80. Schwartz SR, Blei F, Ceisler E, et al. Risk factors for amblyopia in children with capillary hemangioma of the eyelids and orbit. J AA PO S 2006;10:262–8.

81. Searl, et al. Hemangiopericytoma Int ophthalmol Clinic 1982:22:141–62.

82. Seregard and Sahlin Panaroma of Orbital space occupying lesions Acta Ophthalmol Scand 1999; 77(1):91–8.

83. Shields JA, Bakewell B, Augsburger JJ, et al. Classification and incidence of space-occupying lesions of the orbit: A survey of 645 biopsies. Arch Ophthalmol 1974;102:1606–11.

84. Shields JA, Bakewell B, et al. Space occupying orbital masses in children. A review of 250 consecutive biopsies-Ophthalmology 1986; 93(3):379–84.

85. Shields JA, Shields CL. Atlas of Orbital Tumors. Philadelphia:Lippincott Williams and Wilkins 1999;2–231.

86. Shields JA. Diagnosis and Management of Orbital Tumors. Philadelphia: Saunders 1989; 89–388.

87. Shorr N, Seiff SR. Central retinal artery occlusion associated with periocular corticosteroid injection for juvenile hemangioma. Ophthalmic Surg 1986;17(4):229–31.

88. Sklar EL, Quencer RM, Byrne SF, et al. Correlative study of the computed tomographic, ultrasonographic and pathological characteristics of cavernous versus capillary hemangiomas of the orbit. J Clin Neuro-ophthalmol 1986; 6:14–21.

89. Slaughter K, Sullivan T, Boulton J, et al. Early surgical intervention as definitive treatment for ocular adnexal capillary haemangioma. Clin Experiment Ophthalmol 2003;31(5):418–23.

90. Spector RH. Echographic diagnosis of dural carotid-cavernous sinus fistulas. Am J Ophthalmol 1991;111(1):77–83.

91. Stenhouse D, Mason DK. Oral Hemangio-pericytoma, a case report. Br J Oral Surg 1968; 114–7.

92. Stout Ap, Murray MR, et al. Hemangiopericytoma: vascular tumor featuringv Zimmermann's pericytes. Ann Surgery 1942;116:26–33.

93. Suzuki Y, Obana A, Management of orbital lymphangioma using intralesional injection of OK432. Br J Ophthalmol 2000;84:614–7.

94. Tunc M, Sadri E, Char DH. Orbital lymphan-gioma: An analysis of 26 patients. Br J Ophthalmol 1999;83:76–80.

95. Tunc M, Sadri E. Orbital lymphangioma: An analysis of 26 patients. Br J Ophthalmol 1999; 83:76–80.

96. Uchino A, Hasuo K, Matsumoto S, et al. MRI of dural carotid-cavernous fistulas. Comparisons with postcontrast CT. Clin Imaging 1992; 16(4):263–8.

97. Uehara T, Tabuchi M, Kawaguchi T, et al. Spontaneous dural carotid-cavernous sinus fistula presenting isolated ophthalmoplegia: Evaluation with MR angiography. Neurology 1998;50(3):814–6.

98. Valérie Biousse, Maria E Mendicino, Deborah J Simon, et al. The ophthalmology of intracranial vascular abnormalities. American journal of ophthalmology 1998;125(4):527–44.

99. Vinuela F, Fox AJ, Debrun GM, et al, Drake CG. Spontaneous carotid-cavernous fistulas: clinical, radiological, and therapeutic considerations: experience with 20 cases. J Neurosurg 1984;60:976–84.

100. Vu BL, Harris GJ. Orbital vascular lesions. Ophthalmol Clin North Am 2000;13:609–31.

101. Wanebo JE, Lonser RR, Glenn GM, Oldfield EH. The natural history of hemangioblastomas of the central nervous system in patients with von Hippel-Lindau disease. J Neurosurg 2003; 98:82–94.

102. Weiss AH, Kelly JP. Reappraisal of astigmatism induced by periocular capillary hemangioma and treatment with intralesional corticosteroid injection. Ophthalmology 2008;115(2):390–7.

103. Wendy R, Lindell R, et al. Vascular lesions of the orbit-more than what meets the eye. 2008; 28:185–204.

104. Wendy R, Lindell R, et al. Vascular lesions of the orbit—more than what meets the eye. 2008; 28:185–204.

105. Wendy R, Lindell R, et al. Vascular lesions of the orbit-more than what meets the eye. Radiographics 2008;28:185–204.

106. Wesley RE, Bond JB. Carbon dioxide laser in ophthalmic plastic and orbital surgery. Ophthalmic Surg 1985;16:631–3.

107. Wetzel SG, Bilecen D, Lyrer P, et al. Cerebral dural arteriovenous fistulas: Detection by dynamic MR projection angiography. AJR Am. J Roentgenol 2000;174(5):1293–5.

108. Wright JE, Sullivan TJ, Garner A, et al. Orbital venous anomalies. Ophthalmology 1997;104: 905–13.

109. Yamasaki T, Handa H, Yamashita J, et al. Intracranial and orbital cavernous angiomas. J Neurosurg 1986;64:197–208.

110. Zeynel A, Karcioglu, et al. Orbital Hemangiopericytoma—Clinical and Morphologic features. Am J Ophthal. 1997 vol 124, no 5 Nov 1997.

MIGRAINE AND OTHER HEADACHE SYNDROMES

AK Khurana, Ankita Phogat, Aruj K Khurana,
Bhawna Khurana

GENERAL AND ANATOMICAL CONSIDERATIONS

GENERAL CONSIDERATIONS

Every ophthalmologist attends to a number of patients presenting with headache and facial pain. At one end of spectrum, are the benign causes such as tension type headache and refractive errors, and on the other end are the headaches due to conditions resulting in raised intracranial tension. Hence, the role of an ophthalmologist lies in:

- Recognizing benign causes for pain like migraine, tension type headache.
- Diagnosing correctly and treating ocular causes.
- Identifying and promptly referring cases with serious intracranial or systemic pathologies.

APPLIED ANATOMICAL CONSIDERATIONS

Before evaluating a case of headache, it will be worth while to be familiar with the applied anatomical aspects to be considered with headache:

Pain sensitive structures within the cranium
- Great venous sinuses and their tributaries
- Dura at the base of skull, and
- Dural and cerebral arteries at the base of brain

Anatomical basis of intracranial headache

Traction due to any pathology on:
- Tributary vein or displacement of great venous sinuses
- Middle meningeal arteries, and
- Large cerebral arteries or branches at the base

Distension and dilatation of intracranial arteries

Inflammation of pain sensitive intracranial structures

Direct pressure on cranial or cervical nerves:
- 5th cranial nerve above tentorium
- 9th, 10th, 11th and 12th cranial nerves and upper cervical nerves below the tentorium.

Extracranial structures producing headache
- Fasciae and muscles of scalp and face
- Galea
- Arteries and veins of scalp, face and neck
- Mucous membranes and tympanic membrane

EVALUATION OF A CASE OF HEADACHE

History

A thorough, meticulous and intelligent history is the key for diagnosing the cause for headache, since 95% cases of headache have a normal examination.

Important points to be covered in the history are as follows:
- *Site of pain* (unilateral or bilateral, diffuse or localized).
- *Type of pain, daily pattern and duration* (sharp/dull, throbbing, constant, squeezing, worse in morning or evening, waking the patient from sleep).
- *Age at onset*, frequency of attacks and if any recent change in pattern.
- *Associated symptoms* such as nausea, vomiting, vertigo, scintillating scotoma, flashing lights, tearing, weakness.
- *Precipitating or relieving factors* (supine, bending over, food, sleep)
- *Preceding symptoms* especially in vascular headaches where autonomic disturbance may precede headache by 24 hrs (drowsiness, irritability, insomnia, depression).

Important clues in history are as below:
- *Patients presenting with headache for the first time after 50 yrs of age* should be suspected of having giant cell arteritis or some intracranial pathology. These can be identified after proper history and examination of patient as the former is associated with jaw claudication, fever, weight loss, scalp tenderness, raised ESR, the latter is usually worse in morning, increases on bending or moving the head and also with Valsalva, projectile vomiting may occur, associated focal neurologic signs and papilledema may be present.
- Any *headache which awakens the patient* from sleep is pathological.
- *Headache due to intracranial hemorrhage* is severe, with neck stiffness and changes in mentation or focal neurological signs.
- *Meningitis headache* is usually chronic without focal deficits but neck stiffness and pain on flexion are present associated with photophobia and pain on eye movements.

Systemic examination

A patient with headache should undergo a detailed systemic examination which includes:
- *Blood pressure* and pulse.
- *Neurological examination* for meningeal signs, point tenderness and symmetry of cranial nerve and motor functions.
- *Visual fields* should be tested if any associated visual phenomenon is present.

Investigations and neuroimaging

Investigations and neuroimaging required will depend on the suspected causes and are mentioned with each syndrome.

HEADACHE SYNDROMES

Commonly encountered headache syndromes include:
Migraine and other headache syndromes
- Cluster headache
- SUNCT syndrome
- Stress-tension headache
- Temporal arteritis
- Headache due to raised intracranial tension
- Sinus disease headache
- Reader's headache
- Other causes of headache

MIGRAINE

Migraine is characterized by repetitive bouts of headache, with a strong familial tendency and is more frequent in females. Typically, the headache starts at puberty or early adulthood and may decrease after menopause. *Diagnosis is* supported by unilateral location, pulsating/throbbing character, associated nausea/vomiting, photophobia and aggravation with physical activity. *Precipitating factors* may include menstruation, hunger, pregnancy, stress, certain food (chocolate, wine) and sleep deprivation.

PATHOPHYSIOLOGY

Vascular theory of migraine is now secondary to primary brain dysfunction.

Brain dysfunction theory of migraine consists of an ion channelopathy in brainstem nuclei modulating sensory input.

A phenomenon called *cortical spreading depression*, in which neurological activity is depressed over an area of cortex, causes release of inflammatory mediators irritating the cranial nerve roots. The dysfunction mainly involves the afferent sensory neurons of trigeminal nerve.

Three important factors in pathogenesis include:
- Cranial blood vessels.
- Trigeminal innervation of these vessels, and
- Reflex connection of trigeminal system with cranial parasympathetic outflow (C2 nerve roots).
- *The spreading depression in occipital region* may be responsible for aura and changes in blood vessels result in pain.
- *Genetic factors* with significant familial incidence may be present (e.g. familial hemiplegic migraine, rare autosomal dominant inherited form of migraine, has been mapped to chromosome 19).

TYPES OF MIGRAINE
- Migraine without aura (common migraine or hemicranias simplex)
- Migraine with aura (classic migraine)
- Ophthalmoplegic migraine
- Retinal migraine
- Chronic migraine
- Migraine equivalent or variant

Migraine without aura (common migraine)
Diagnostic criteria

Common migraine is diagnosed when at least 5 attacks of headache fulfilling the following criteria are reported:

Headache attack of 4 to 72 hrs (untreated or unsuccessfully treated)

Pain with at least two of the following characteristics:
- Unilateral location
- Pulsating
- Moderate to severe in intensity
- Aggravated by routine physical activity

At least one of the following associated phenomenon:
- Nausea and/or vomiting
- Photophobia or phonophobia.

Characteristic features of common migraine
- It usually starts in second or third decade.
- When migraine persists for longer than 3 days, it is called "status migrainosis".
- *Common sites* for migraine can be temporal, supraorbital, parietal, post auricular, occipital.
- *Prodrome* in common migraine is usually similar to that seen in classic migraine, starting hours to days before headache, consisting of psychological, neurological, constitutional and autonomic features like depression, euphoria, irritability, restlessness, drowsiness, diarrhea, anorexia, food cravings, etc. It is directly followed by headache without any intervening aura stage.
- *Ocular symptoms* in addition to photophobia include conjunctival injection and tearing. Visual aura is typically absent.
- *Differential diagnosis:* Distinguishing this from tension type headache is difficult.

Migraine with aura (classic migraine)
Diagnostic criteria

Classic migraine is diagnosed when at least 2 attacks fulfilling following criteria are reported:

Aura, fully reversible, without any motor weakness and consisting of at least one of the following:
- *Visual phenomenon* which may be positive (flickering lights, spots or lines) and/or negative (loss of vision).
- *Sensory dysfunction* which may be positive (pins and needles) and/or negative (numbness).
- *Speech disturbances*.

At least two of the following features:
- Homonymous visual phenomenon and/or unilateral sensory disturbances.
- At least one aur symptom develops gradually over ≥ 5 mins and/or different aura symptoms occur in succession over ≥ 5 mins.
- Each symptom last ≥ 5 mins and ≤ 60 mins.

Headache fulfilling of above criteria for migraine without aura within 60 mins.

Characteristic features

Classic migraine usually starts in teens followed by simple periodic headache or isolated auras in later life.

Classic migraine may present in following forms:
- Typical syndrome
- Basilar artery syndrome (Bickerstaff's migraine)
- Acephalic migraine (migraine aura without headache)

Typical syndrome of classic migraine

The classic attack of migraine can be divided into five stages:

1. *Prodrome.* It occurs hours to days before headache and consist of irritability, restlessness, depression, euphoria, anorexia, diarrhea, food craving, etc.

2. *Aura* refers to reversible focal neurological symptoms preceding or accompanying a migraine attack. It develops over 5–20 mins and lasts <60 minutes. Headache occurs within 60 mins after the aura ends. Most commonly, patients complain of homonymous scintillating scotoma seen as multicolored shimmering lights, beginning in paracentral area and expanding in a crescent shaped fashion over a large portion of the homonymous hemifields of both eyes. Leading edge of the scintillating scotoma may be positive and trailing edge usually negative (dark). Less frequently, there may occur hemisensory disturbances in the form of paresthesia or numbness.

3. *Headache* builds over 1–2 hrs on the side opposite to aura and lasts for few hours to a day, is exaggerated by physical activity and is usually associated with photophobia, phonophobia, nausea and drowsiness. So, patient prefers to sleep in the dark quiet room.

4. and 5. *Termination* and *Postdrome.* These stages last for 24 hrs or so. Patient feels tired and washed out or less commonly elated and refreshed.

Important notes

- Structural lesions like arteriovenous malformations (AVMs) of occipital region may present with transient homonymous visual loss with scintillating scotoma and headache. The differentiating features are:
  - *Headache* consistently is localized to the same site (unlike migraine where site may change with episode)

- *Visual phenomenon* persists intermittently throughout the period of headache (unlike migraine where aura completes before the onset of headache).
- In any case, where aura is prolonged or persists even during or after headache, neuroimaging is mandatory.
- Migraine with aura is sometimes called "ophthalmic migraine" (different from typical ophthalmoplegic migraine).
- Aura persisting beyond headache used to be referred to as "complicated migraine".

Treatment

- *Aspirin, ibuprofen or caffeine* at first sign of attack may abort the headache in some patients.
- *Sumatriptan (5HT agonist)* given by oral, nasal or subcutaneous route can terminate acute attack.
- *Prophylactic treatment* with β-blockers, calcium channel blockers, anticonvulsants, methylsergide (causes retroperitoneal fibrosis) or vasodilators (nitroglycerine/nifedipine), is indicated for those with frequent attacks and not responding even to sumatriptan.

Basilar artery migraine (Bickerstaff's migraine)

Characteristic features include:
- *Young women* with strong family history of migraine are usually affected.
- *Neurological finding* include bilateral visual loss, vertigo, tinnitus, hearing loss, dysesthesia, ataxia, and altered consciousness. These symptoms usually clear, but permanent deficit can occur sometime.

Differential diagnosis. Basilar artery migraine mimicks vertebrobasilar insufficiency seen in elderly patients. Distinguishing features include severe headache and vomiting following the onset in migraine.

Acephalic migraine (migraine aura without headache)

Acephalic migraine, as the name indicates, refers to occurrence of migraine aura without a headache phase. This is one of the most common forms of migraine seen by the ophthalmologists.

Features of migraine aura include:
- *Visual symptoms* such as scintillating scotoma, transient hemianopia, amaurosis fugax, altitudinal field defects, tunnel vision and diplopia.
- *Neurological symptoms* noted include hemiparesthesia, hemiparesis, dysphasia, cloudy thinking.

Diagnosis of acephalic migraine is made from the history of typical scintillating scotoma. In the absence of typical scotoma, diagnosis is one of exclusion.

Ophthalmoplegic migraine

Characteristic features

- *Onset* is in early childhood (usually before the age of 10 years), rare in adults.
- *Nerve most commonly involved* is 3rd cranial, with ptosis, loss of accommodation and mydriasis occuring during the attack. Rarely 6th or 4th cranial nerve may also be involved.
- *Ophthalmoplegia occurs* during (rarely, just before) a typical migrainous attack, i.e. during height of headache and persists after the headache resolves.
- *Resolves* completely in few days to weeks.
- *Residual ptosis and ophthalmoplegia* may remain after repeated attacks.
- *Headache* usually unilateral but may become bilateral and lasts for several hours to days.

Differential diagnosis

Differential diagnosis includes intracranial aneurysms/tumor (neuroimaging), diabetes mellitus (GTT), sphenoid sinus mucocele (radiological study), myasthenia gravis (painless, edrophonium/neostigmine test), Tolosa-Hunt syndrome (persisting pain).

Diagnostic criteria

- Onset in first decade of life,
- History of typical migraine,
- Ophthalmoplegia ipsilateral to headache,
- MRI normal or may show thickening and contrast enhancement of nerve root as it exits midbrain.

Retinal migraine (ocular migraine, anterior visual pathway migraine)

Characteristic features

- More frequent than ophthalmoplegic migraine.

- Transient (rarely permanent) monocular visual disturbance (scotoma/blindness) accompanying a migraine attack or in an individual with strong history of migrainous episodes.
- Visual loss shorter than occipital variety (around 5–15 mins).
- Amaurosis, in some, may occur during rather than before headache.
- Retinal vasospasm, seen ophthalmoscopically, in some.
- Headache is frequently absent during the spell.
- Diagnosis is of exclusion.

Chronic migraine

Migraine headache, for 15 or more days per month, for more than 3 months in the absence of medication over use.

OTHER HEADACHE SYNDROMES

CLUSTER HEADACHE

Clinical features. Cluster headache, also known as, Horton's headache or histamine cephalgia has following features:
- *Age.* Occurs in third and fourth decade.
- *Sex.* More common in males.
- *Pain.* Strictly unilateral and pain very severe in intensity, lasting for 15–180 mins (around 45 mins). Pain occurs in the distribution of the external carotid (frontal or frontotemporal pain)
- *Patient hyperactive*, pacing around room until the pain subsides.
- *Ipsilateral sympathetic dysfunction* during attack may occur in the form of Horner's syndrome, conjunctival injection, nasal congestion, rhinorrhea, eyelid swelling.
- *Time.* Attack may occur at night waking the patient from sleep. Typically awakens patient early in the morning.
- *Attacks cluster in time*, at least once a day (same time each day), with progression frequency increases. Cluster period lasts 4–12 weeks followed by asymptomatic period till next cluster (usually same time of year).

Treatment includes:
- Sumatriptan may be used for acute attack.

- Prednisolone may halt bouts of headache.
- Lithium is required for more resistant cases.

SUNCT SYNDROME

Short lasting **U**nilateral **N**euralgiform headache with **C**onjunctival injection and **T**earing (SUNCT) can be:
- Idiopathic, or
- Secondary to prolactin secreting tumors, or secondary to brainstem infarction.

STRESS TENSION HEADACHE

Etiology. Stress tension headache, also known as, anxiety headache or acute contraction headache occurs due to sustained contraction of neck and scalp muscles.

Characteristic features of stress tension headache are as below:
- *Frequency.* Most common (accounts for 90% of all headaches).
- *Features of pain.* Mild to moderate, pressing/squeezing type, non-pulsatile like a band encircling the head.
- *Site of pain.* Bifrontal/biooccipital.
- *Radiation.* Pain may radiate to posterior neck or jaw.
- *No specific factors* aggravating or relieving pain.
- *Non-specific pattern,* may last 30 mins to a day, may occur once a year or several times a week or month with symptom free interval.
- *Emotional trigger* is usually present and patient may be suffering from depression.

TEMPORAL ARTERITIS

Temporal arteritis is systemic disorder with inflammatory obliterative arteritis especially involving external carotid and ophthalmic arteries.

Characteristic features are:
- Dull pain/ache around temporal arteries throughout day.
- Scalp tenderness.
- Jaw claudication, diplopia, transient visual loss, AION.
- Polymyalgia rheumatic, elevated ESR

Histopathological diagnosis is made after temporal artery biopsy.

HEADACHE DUE TO RAISED INTRACRANIAL TENSION (ICT)

- New onset or new pattern headache.
- Worst headache patient ever had.
- *Associated signs* of meningeal irritation include neck stiffness, projectile vomiting, nausea and fever.
- Exaggerated by coughing, sneezing or bending over.
- Associated with focal or non-focal neurological signs like weakness/numbness, aphasia, personality change.

SINUS DISEASE HEADACHE

Etiology. Chronic sinusitis may be associated with sinus disease headache.

Clinical features are as below:
- *Character.* Low to moderate, dull aching pain, present almost daily.
- *Site.* Mostly located over frontal and maxillary area with associated sinus tenderness.
- *Nasal congestion with mucopurulent discharge* are important presenting features.
- *Exaggerated with* bending, sneezing or blowing nose.
- *Associated respiratory allergy* usually present.

Diagnosis is made from typical clinical features
- *Plain X-ray* film helps in diagnosis.
- *CT scan of sinuses* helps in planning management. *Tumors, abscess and mucoceles* arising in sinuses and nasopharynx can give rise to facial or periorbital pain, associated with proptosis and are diagnosed on radioimaging.

RAEDER'S SYNDROME

Raeder's syndrome, also known as paratrigeminal neuralgia, refers to painful Horner's syndrome characterized by pain in the distribution of first division of 5th cranial nerve.

Etiology. Raeder's syndrome is caused by migrainous dilatation of internal carotid artery with compression of ophthalmic division of trigeminal nerve and sympathetic plexus in the middle cranial fossa.

Clinical features
- *Age.* Middle aged or elderly males are more frequently involved.

- *Clinical types.* Two presentations are known:
  - *Type one Raeder's syndrome* is typically characterize by pain in ophthalmic division with post-ganglionic Horner's syndrome only. Pain may last for days to weeks or even months. Rarely, in this type there may occur fibrovascular dysplasia or spontaneous internal carotid artery dissection.
  - *Type two Raeder's syndrome* is characterized by involvement of other cranial nerves and thus requires complete neuroradiographic investigations to rule out a parasellar mass.

TRIGEMINAL NEURALGIA (TIC DOULOUREUX)

Clinical features
- *Pain* is usually sudden, severe and stabbing lasting for a few seconds, recurring in episodes over several minutes.
- *Unilateral* and localized to one of the divisions of trigeminal nerve (most commonly 2nd and 3rd divisions).
- *Age.* Middle age or latter.
- *Triggered by* chewing, swallowing, tooth brushing or light touch to face (cold wind).

Etiology. Most commonly due to vascular compression of trigeminal nerve (demyelinating lesion or posterior fossa mass should be ruled out).

Treatment includes:
- *Medical therapy* with gabapentine, carbamazepine, phenytoin, baclofen, clonazepam and valproic acid.
- *Selective destruction* of trigeminal fibres (rhizotomy) of surgical decompression of trigeminal in recalcitrant cases.

ICEPICK HEADACHES (JABS AND JOLTS SYNDROME)

Characteristic features include:
- *Pain* which is usually severe stabbing and lasts for a few seconds.
- *Site.* In periorbital, forehead and frontal regions.
- *Etiology.* May be associated with migraine or occur independently.
- *Treatment* includes indomethacin.

MISCELLANEOUS CAUSES OF HEADACHE SYNDROME

Other causes of headache known are:
- *Hypertension,* is a common cause of headache and needs to be excluded.
- *Temporomandibular joint dysfunction* may also be associated with headache.
- *Ocular inflammation,* fever, eye strain (asthenopia), Conversion reaction, herpetic disease and greater occipital neuralgia are other causes of headache.

BIBLIOGRAPHY

1. Barrett Katz and Colin R. Bamford. Migrainous ischemic optic neuropathy, Neurology January 1985;35(1):112.

2. Brian M. Grosberg, Seymour Solomon, Richard B. Lipton. Retinal migraine, Current Pain and Headache Reports 2005;9(4):268–71.

3. David O. Harrington, Milton Flocks. Ophthalmoplegic migraine, AMA Arch Ophthalmol 1953; 49(6):643–55.

4. E. Wayne Massey. Pupillary Dysautonomia and Migraine: Is Adie's Pupil Caused by Migraine, Headache: The Journal of Head and Face Pain, July 1981;21(4):143–6.

5. Gerald P Durkan, B Todd Troost, Thomas L Slamovits, et al. Recurrent Painless Oculomotor Palsy in Children. A Variant of Ophthalmopegic Migraine, Headache: The Journal of Head and Face Pain, March 1981;21(2):58–62.

6. Hugh C. Donahue. Migraine and its ocular manifestations, Arch Ophthalmol 1950; 43(1):96.

7. J. Pearce. The ophthalmological complications of migraine, Journal of the Neurological Sciences, 1968;6(1):73–81.

8. Lanning B. Kline, Christopher L. Kell. Ocular Migraine in a Patient with Cluster Headaches, Headache: The Journal of Head and Face Pain, September 1980;20(5):253–7.

9. Morris Levin, Thomas N. Ward: Ophthalmoplegic migraine, Current Pain and Headache Reports 2004;8(4):306–9.

10. Vinod Kumar Gupta. Migrainous scintillating scotoma and headache is ocular in origin: A new hypothesis, Medical Hypothesis 2006; 66(3)454–60.

Index

Reader's Note

Reader's Note

Reader's Note